Handbook of Clinical Automation, Robotics, and Optimization

Edited by
Gerald J. Kost, M.D., Ph.D.
Professor of Medical Pathology and Biomedical Engineering
University of California, Davis
Davis, CA

With the collaboration of

Judith Welsh, R.N., M.L.S.
Associate Librarian
University of California, Davis
Davis, CA

A Wiley-Interscience Publication
JOHN WILEY & SONS, INC.
New York · Chichester · Brisbane · Toronto · Singapore

This text is printed on acid-free paper.

Copyright © 1996 by John Wiley & Sons, Inc.

All rights reserved. Published simultaneously in Canada.

Reproduction or translation of any part of this work beyond
that permitted by Section 107 or 108 of the 1976 United
States Copyright Act without the permission of the copyright
owner is unlawful. Requests for permission or further
information should be addressed to the Permissions Department,
John Wiley & Sons, Inc., 605 Third Avenue, New York, NY
10158-0012.

Library of Congress Cataloging in Publication Data:
Handbook of clinical automation, robotics, and optimization / edited
    by Gerald J. Kost.
        p.   cm. — (Wiley interscience series on laboratory
    automation)
    Includes bibliographical references and index.
    ISBN 0-471-03179-8 (cloth : alk. paper)
    1. Diagnosis—Data processing.   2. Computers in medicine.
  3. Robotics in medicine.   4. Expert systems (Computer science)
  I. Kost, Gerald J.   II. Series.
  RC78.7.D35H36   1996
  610'.285—dc20   95-38368

Printed in the United States of America

10 9 8 7 6 5 4 3 2

To the authors
for their creative contributions
and hard work
and
To my mother, Ora Imogene Kost,
and my father, Edward William Kost,
for their love and support

Contributors

JOHN E. AGAPAKIS, PH.D., *Acuity Imaging, Inc., 9 Townsend West, Nashua, NH 03063-1217*

MARK A. ARNOLD, PH.D., *Professor, Department of Chemistry, 230 IATL, University of Iowa, Iowa City, Iowa 52242*

GEOFFREY F. AUCHINLEK, B.A.SC., P. ENG., *Vice President, Product Development, AutoMed Corporation, Suite 140, 13120 Vanier Place, Richmond, British Columbia, Canada V6V 2J2*

JEFFREY K. BELKORA, M.SC., *Department of Engineering–Economic Systems, Stanford University, Stanford, CA 94305-4025*

DANIEL W. CHAN, PH.D., DABCC, *Associate Professor, Departments of Pathology and Oncology, Johns Hopkins University; Director of Clinical Chemistry, Johns Hopkins Hospital, Meyer B-125, 600 N. Wolfe Street, Baltimore, MD 21287-7065*

ROBERT P. DE CRESCE, M.D., M.B.A., *Director of Clinical Laboratories, Rush-Presbyterian-St. Luke's Medical Center; Assistant Professor of Pathology, Rush Medical College, Department of Pathology, Rawson 409, 1653 West Congress Parkway, Chicago, IL 60612*

LAURA J. ESSERMAN, M.D., M.B.A., *Assistant Professor of Surgery, Department of Surgery, University of California, San Francisco; Mount Zion Medical Center, San Francisco, CA 94115*

RALPH E. FARNSWORTH, *Program Manager, Belcan Business Consulting, 10200 Anderson Way, Cincinnati, OH 45242*

MICHAEL R. FEHLING, PH.D., *Associate Professor, Research, Department of Engineering–Economic Systems, Stanford University, Stanford, CA 94305-4025*

ROBIN A. FELDER, PH.D., *Associate Professor and Associate Director of Clinical Chemistry, Toxicology and Robotics Laboratories; Department of Pathology, Box 168, University of Virginia Health Sciences Center, Charlottesville, VA 22908*

WILLIAM J. GODOLPHIN, PH.D., *Professor, Department of Pathology and Laboratory Medicine, University of British Columbia; Director of Research and Development, Division of Clinical Chemistry, Vancouver Hospital and Health Sciences Centre, 855 West 12th Avenue, Vancouver, B.C., Canada V5Z 1M9*

CLIFFORD HAGUE, *Vice President, Marketing and Business Development, MiniMed Technologies, Inc., 12744 San Fernando Road, Sylmar, CA 91324*

JUN IMAMURA, M.D., *Department of Blood Transfusion, Kochi Medical School, Kohasu, Okoh-cho, Nankoku-city, Kochi-pref. 783, Japan*

ELLIS JACOBS, PH.D., DABCC, *Assistant Professor of Patholgoy, Mount Sinai School of Medicine; Director of Stat Laboratories, Box 1519, Mount Sinai Medical Center, One Gustave L. Levy Place, New York, NY 10029-6574*

HIROMI KATAOKA, *Clinical Laboratory, Kochi Medical School, Kohasu, Okoh-cho, Nankoku-city, Kochi-pref. 783, Japan*

JOSEPH H. KEFFER, M.D., *Professor and Director, Clinical Pathology, Southwestern Medical Center, University of Texas, CS 3.114, 5323 Harry Hines Boulevard, Dallas, TX 75235-9072*

GERALD J. KOST, (VOLUME EDITOR), M.D., PH.D., *Professor of Medical Pathology and Biomedical Engineering, Medical Pathology, School of Medicine, University of California, Davis, CA 95616*

LARRY J. KRICKA, D. PHIL., F.R.C. PATH., *Professor, Department of Pathology and Laboratory Medicine; Director, General Chemistry Laboratory, Hospital of the University of Pennsylvania, 3400 Spruce Street, Philadelphia, PA 19104-4283*

SARATH KRISHNASWAMY, M.S., *Acuity Imaging, Inc., 9 Townsend West, Nashua, NH 03063-1217*

MARTIN H. KROLL, M.D., *Associate Professor, Department of Pathology; Associate Director of Clinical Chemistry, Johns Hopkins Hospital, Meyer B-125, 600 N. Wolfe Street, Baltimore, MD 21287-7065*

MICHAEL LAPOSATA, M.D., PH.D., *Associate Professor, Harvard Medical School; Director of Clinical Laboratories, Gray Building 2, Massachusetts General Hospital, 55 Fruit Street, Boston, MA 02114*

KENT B. LEWANDROWSKI, M.D., *Assistant Professor of Patholgoy, Harvard Medical School; Assistant Director of Clinical Laboratories, Gray Building 2, Massachusetts General Hospital, 55 Fruit Street, Boston, MA 02114*

MARK S. LIFSHITZ, M.D., *Director of Clinical Laboratories, New York University Medical Center; Clinical Professor, Department of Pathology, New York University School of Medicine, 560 First Avenue, Room TH-351, New York, NY 10016*

ROGER B. LINES, B.A.SC., P. ENG., *Manager of Research and Development, Auto-Med Corporation, Suite 140, 13120 Vanier Place, Richmond, B.C., Canada V6V 2J2*

KATHLEEN LUCZYK, M.T. (ASCP), M.A., M.B.A., *Administration Manager, Clinical Chemistry Laboratory, Hartford Hospital, 80 Seymour Street, Hartford, CT 06102*

LAWRENCE C. MAGUIRE, M.D., *President, Medical Robotics, Inc., 366 Waller Avenue, Suite 119, Lexington, KY 40504; Lexington Clinic, 1221 South Broadway, Lexington, KY 40504*

RODNEY S. MARKIN, M.D., PH.D., *Professor, Department of Pathology and Microbiology; Director of Laboratory Information System, University of Nebraska Medical Center, Box 983135, 600 South 42nd Street, Omaha, NE 68198-3135*

JACK MARTIN, PH.D., *Senior Technical Staff Specialist, IBM Corporation, 2108 Bridgeport Avenue, Lexington, KY 40502*

VINCENT A. MEMOLI, M.D., *Professor, Department of Pathology, Dartmouth-Hitchcock Medical Center, One Medical Center Drive, Lebanon, NH 03756*

MR. STEPHEN MIDDLETON, *Director, Technology Design and Development, Auto-Lab Systems, 100 International Boulevard, Etobicoke, Ontario, Canada M9W 6J6*

ROBERT MOORE, PH.D., DABCC, *Associate Director, Clinical Chemistry Laboratory, Hartford Hospital, 80 Seymour Street, Hartford, CT 06102*

PAUL MOUNTAIN, B.SC., M.SC., M.T. (ASCP), *Vice President, Science and Technology, AutoLab Systems, 100 International Bouldvard, Etobicoke, Ontario, Canada M9W 6J6*

KATSUMI OGURA, *Clinical Laboratory, Kochi Medical School, Kohasu, Okoh-cho, Nankoku-city, Kochi-pref. 783, Japan*

MASAHIDE SASAKI, M.D., *Director of Clinical Laboratories, Kochi Medical School, Kohasu, Okoh-cho, Nankoku-city, Kochi-pref. 783, Japan*

SERDAR UCKUN, M.D., PH.D., *Rockwell International Science Center, 444 High Street, Suite 400, Palo Alto, CA 94301*

FRANK T. VERTOSICK, JR., M.D., F.A.C.S., *Associate Chief, Division of Neurosurgery; Associate Director, The Center for Neuro-oncology, West Pennsylvania Center for Neuro-oncology, Western Pennsylvania Hospital, Suite 1614, 4800 Friendship Avenue, Pittsburgh, PA 15224-1722*

DONNA WEBER, M.T. (ASCP), M.B.A., *Marketing Director, TransLogic Corporation, 10825 East 47th Avenue, Denver, CO 80239*

WENDY A. WELLS, M.D., M.SC., *Assistant Professor, Department of Pathology, Dartmouth-Hitchcock Medical Center, One Medical Center Drive, Lebanon, NH 03756*

PETER WILDING, PH.D., *Professor, Department of Pathology and Laboratory Medicine, Hospital of the University of Pennsylvania, 3400 Spruce Street, Philadelphia, PA 19104-4283*

EMILY S. WINN-DEEN, PH.D., *Group Leader, Human Genetic Analysis, Applied Biosystems, Perkin Elmer, 850 Lincoln Center Drive, Foster City, CA 94404*

ALAN H. B. WU, PH.D., DABCC, *Director, Clinical Chemistry Laboratory, Hartford Hospital, 80 Seymour Street, Hartford, CT 06102*

JANE M. YANG, M.D., *Clinical Fellow in Pathology, Gray Building 2, Massachusetts General Hospital, 55 Fruit Street, Boston, MA 02114*

Preface

The objective of this book is to provide essential information needed to redesign diagnostic testing in order to conserve resources and improve patient outcomes. Our philosophy was to assemble a comprehensive resource that would meet the future needs of medical diagnosis, from basic science to bedside. A major challenge facing healthcare systems today is containing costs and increasing productivity while still maintaining or improving the quality of patient care. This is stimulating highly competitive reorganization. Societal needs and professional objectives intensify demands for rethinking the ways things are done. The imperative is to accomplish more with less, and do it quickly. The strategies in this book will be invaluable to those actively restructuring diagnostic testing services to meet these demands. The shared visions, professional expertise, and clinical judgment will help the reader to make high quality decisions, focus on the welfare of patients, and meet current challenges successfully during this period of tumultuous change in the delivery of medical care.

As the first critical appraisal of an exploding field, this book will increase awareness of valuable opportunities and cost-effective alternatives for the future. Diagnostic testing is a vital component of clinical medicine and acute care. To be financially competitive, we must not only plan and implement an automated and robotic clinical laboratory, but also assure its operational and economic efficiency. Total laboratory automation is one part of the anticipated solution. However, integrated healthcare systems also require, for example, real-time process optimization, robotic diagnostic workstations, and a continuum of data communications that extends to the point of care, wherever the medical care is needed. The book explores these timely and practical topics in depth. In addition, it includes several user-friendly features, such as easily-understood graphics, well-organized tables, extensive literature summaries, and explanations of new diagnostic methods (e.g., molecular diagnostics and patient monitoring).

The reader can use this book to customize an educational or instructional program. We start with a perspective of the field and its future (Part I). Then, major sections focus on theory and fundamental principles (Part II), areas such as robotics, visual processing, or integrated systems (Part III), and how to implement these new technologies efficiently and cost-effectively, as well as carefully reengineer the organization where they are used (Part IV). In response to critical medical needs for rapid diagnosis and dramatic changes in healthcare delivery, rapid response testing is shifting out of the traditional clinical laboratory. A

comprehensive section provides explanation and advice for this new discipline—
point-of-care testing (Part V). Technical advances in diagnostic testing lead to discoveries that expand medical knowledge exponentially. One must, therefore, consider
the extraordinary value of diagnostic information and how to create and manage
the knowledge. Thus, we conclude with a section (Part VI) that addresses how to
optimize medical knowledge and clinical decision making.

Davis, California   Gerald J. Kost, M.D., Ph.D.

Contents

Handbook of Clinical Automation, Robotics, and Optimization

I

THE FUTURE

CHAPTER

1

Overview and Challenges

ROBIN A. FELDER

CONTENTS

Handbook of Clinical Automation, Robotics, and Optimization, Edited by Gerald J. Kost with the collaboration of Judith Welsh.
ISBN 0-471-03179-8 © 1996 John Wiley & Sons, Inc.

1.1. INTRODUCTION

Revolutionary changes occurring in the healthcare delivery system are forcing clinical laboratories to provide analytical services under increasing cost containment pressures. Reducing the cost of laboratory tests while maintaining the high quality and rapid turnaround required by physicians and patients will present many challenges for clinical laboratories. Considerable attention is being directed toward reengineering the laboratory by the use of new automation techniques. Novel approaches for managing the laboratory will have to be applied to best utilize modern robotic and automation technology. This paradigm shift toward automation will provide exciting new professional opportunities to every technologist, supervisor, manager, and administrator involved in providing clinical laboratory services.

Laboratory automation, until recently, focused on the simplification of the analytical process. Analytical instruments have become smaller and easier to use, and have been increasing the number of available analytical tests. However, analytical instruments have operated as islands of automation with little knowledge of the laboratory world around them. Analytical instruments need to be linked through automatic transportation of specimens, electronic transmission of data, and a minute-to-minute knowledge of the flow of specimens and operation of the laboratory system.

Such enhancement in laboratory automation will provide dramatic reductions in operating costs for the laboratory as well as the medical institution. Lower costs to the laboratory will come from reducing labor at the levels of both medical technologist and laboratory administration. Lower costs to the hospital will result from improved patient care brought about by a laboratory more quickly able to provide test results to physicians. Redundant instrumentation and underutilized instrumentation will be eliminated. Additional benefits will undoubtedly result from automation of the laboratory: improvement in speed, superior minute-to-minute control of quality, reductions of laboratory errors, improvement in safety, reduction in waste, less iatrogenic blood loss (smaller samples are required), improved communication between the physician and laboratory, and savings in space needed for laboratory services. The laboratory will become a more exciting place to work since many mundane tasks will be reduced and replaced with an emphasis on production management, development of new laboratory tests, and the provision of skilled laboratory test interpretation.

Laboratory automation will benefit from application of the same approaches that have streamlined the manufacturing industry. Robots will naturally play an important role in laboratory automation; however, many other technologies and disciplines can be equally useful in improving the analytical process. Many of these technological areas described briefly below will form the basis for chapters to appear later in this book.

1.2. SELECTED DISCIPLINES ASSOCIATED WITH LABORATORY AUTOMATION AND ROBOTICS

Laboratory automation has borrowed heavily from manufacturing practices used in industry. Much of the technology associated with laboratory automation was created to support and improve manufacturing of durable goods for automotive, electronic, and military industries. The subdisciplines of laboratory automation are listed in Table 1.1. Several of the more developed fields are described in detail as follows.

TABLE 1.1. Laboratory Automation Subdisciplines

Systems engineering
  Simulation modeling
  Artificial intelligence
    Expert systems
    Neural networks
    Fuzzy logic
    Genetic algorithms
  Process control
  Process optimization
Accessioning (specimen processing)
  Labeling and reading
    Bar codes
    Machine vision
  Sorting
  Separation (centrifugation)
  Interfacing
    Mechanical
    Electronic
  Conveyance
    Conveyor belts
    Automated guided vehicles (mobile robots)
Point-of-care automation
Storage retrieval
Waste disposal
Laboratory–hospital integration

1.2.1. Laboratory Robotics

The definition of laboratory robotics is becoming increasingly blurred with the introduction of advanced automated devices for the clinical laboratory. By definition, a robot is "an automatically controlled, reprogrammable, multipurpose, manipulative machine with several degrees of freedom, which may be either fixed in place or mobile for use in automation applications."[1,2] Many "robotic" clinical analyzers do not come under the definition of a laboratory robot because they have limited reprogrammability. The ability to change a dilution volume or the number of repeat samplings from a primary tube is not sufficient reprogrammability to be defined as robotic. On the other hand, a pipetting station that can be programmed to pipette any volume of liquid anywhere in a cartesian space of a half a cubic meter (0.5 m³) is clearly a robot. Some devices will fall on the border with limited reprogrammability yet more versatility than a clinical analyzer. For the purposes of this book, clinical laboratory robotics constitute the next generation of reprogrammable automated devices for the clinical laboratory, which will be described here in detail and have an obviously greater versatility than the clinical analyzers of the past.

Robotics is becoming an increasingly popular solution to the analytical needs of the medical laboratory due to the low cost and improving versatility of robots. A wide variety of laboratory robots are available to suit almost any automation need.[3] Briefly, three basic robot types are commercially available.

The most widely accepted laboratory robot has been the cartesian robot capable of pipetting liquids. The pipetting robot began as a device whose primary purpose was only the transfer of liquids. Today, the pipetting robot is a multifunctional device capable of performing complex analytical procedures. Multifunctional pipetting laboratory robots should probably be redefined as a cartesian laboratory workstation. Pipetting robots have seen wide applications in clinical laboratories and have paved the way for the acceptance of more complex robotic automation. Five major companies have created successful cartesian workstations. Beckman Instruments (Brea, Orange County, CA, USA) has been the market leader with the Biomek workstation (Fig. 1.1). The Biomek was the first workstation to incorporate novel designs such as interchangeable tools to allow single or multiple simultaneous pipetting, disposable tips, and an integral spectrophotometer. Hamilton Co. (Reno, NV, USA) has created the Fully Automated Microplate Elisas (F.A.M.E.) system, which is a workstation based on their successful high-throughput, 12-channel cartesian workstation, the microlab AT (Fig. 1.2). The FAME system allows interchangeability of workstation components to perform complete analysis such as enzyme-linked immunosorbent assays (ELISAs). Rosys Inc. (Hombrechtikon, Switzerland) has created a state-of-the-art cartesian workstation that allows multiple pipetting with three sizes of disposable tips, capacity for 16 microplates, and an integral incubator and spectrophotometer (Fig. 1.3). This station is unique in its ability to move microplates around the surface of the workstation. Tecan Inc. (Hillsborough, NC, USA) has the largest market share of cartesian workstations in clinical laboratories. Tecan

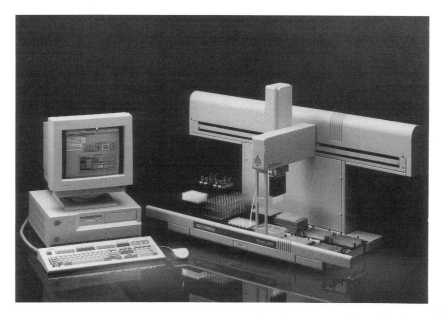

Figure 1.1. The Beckman Biomek 2000 pipetting station features interchangeable pipet-ting tools, removal deck to facilitate placement of instruments within reach of the robotic arm, and a microsoft-proprietary windows-based programming environment.

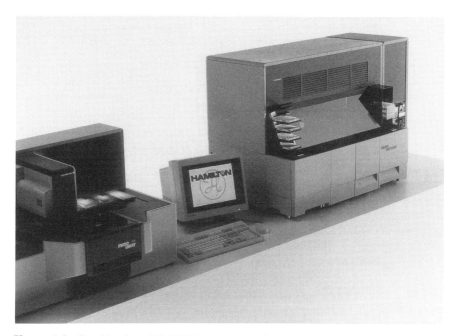

Figure 1.2. The Hamilton F.A.M.E. has been engineered to automatically manipulate microplates. Plates may have reagents added in any order or number, incubated, washed, and quantitated in a spectrophotometer without the need for technologist interaction.

7

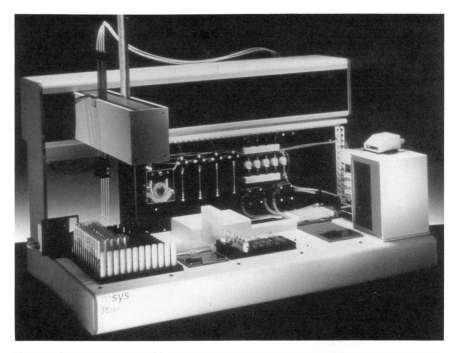

Figure 1.3. The Rosys Plato 3300 is a versatile pipetting station that allows the pipetting arm to also move microplates. A built-in incubator and spectrophotometer can perform all the functions required to complete microplate elisa assays. This system can also be used for nonstandard containers.

cartesian workstations are currently used in blood grouping, immunoassays, and solid-phase extraction in many laboratories (Fig. 1.4). The major feature offered by Tecan cartesian workstations is the option of dual robotic arms capable of simultaneously performing independent tasks. A relatively recent arrival on the market is the MultiProbe (Packard Instruments, Meriden, CN, USA), a versatile cartesian workstation featuring a simple design that fits into any area of the laboratory (Fig. 1.5). Many laboratories do not need the complexity offered by the more multifunctional cartesian workstations. Additional cartesian worksta-tions are offered by other companies such as Matrix Technologies (Lowell, MA), Denley (Durham, NC), and Dynatec (Chantilly, VA).

Cylindrical robots have been popularized by Zymark Inc. (Hopkinton, MA) (Fig. 1.6). The performance envelope of a cylindrical robot is, as the name implies, a cylinder defined by the height of the central column and the limit of extension for the robotic arm. Zymark has patented many features of their cylindrical robot. For example, the ability to change hands to perform different laboratory unit operations. The Zymate robot has also been successfully applied to microplate handling.[4] Articulating arms are also becoming increasingly popu-

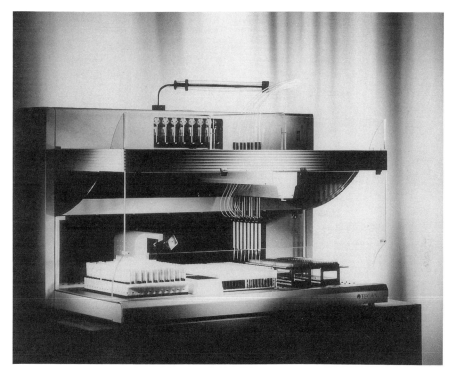

Figure 1.4. The Tecan RSP 5052 has been equipped with independently operated pipetting devices that also incorporate liquid-level sense. A similar version with dual arms provides a multitasking robot capable of high throughput.

lar for laboratory work. Commercial vendors include Mitubishi, CRS (Burlington, Ontario, Canada) (Fig. 1.7), and Sagian (Concord, CA).

Hybrid systems have been created that borrow the better features of robots and dedicated instruments and combine them to create a device specifically designed for laboratory tasks. The Scitec (Lausanne, Switzerland) system is a multifunctional microplate handling environment that relies on the Sagian Orka arm to move microplates to various laboratory stations (Fig. 1.8). Although this system has found initial popularity in the pharmaceutical industry, it would be suitable for commercial clinical laboratories that perform high-volume immunoassays. The K-Tech (Demaurex, Romanel s/Lausanne, Switzerland) system was designed to provide clinical laboratory immunoassay automation to laboratories with either low- or high-throughput needs. The K-Tech system combines conveyance and robotic manipulation to perform its tasks.

Selection of a robot will be most highly dependent on the cycle time for pick–place operations. Currently, industrial robots are capable of extremely rapid movements. In loading food or candy boxes, for example, a pick–place

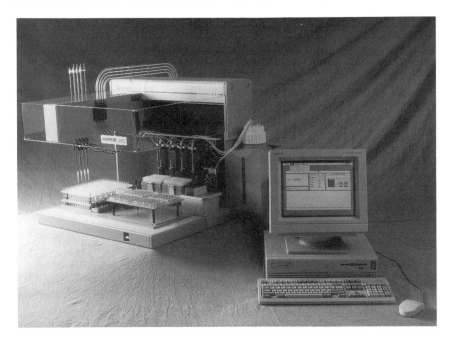

Figure 1.5. The Packard MultiProbe has four independently operated pipetting devices that incorporate liquid-level sense and can pick up either 200- or 20-μL tips. This device has been successfully used for the automation of the PCR (polymerase chain reaction) reaction.

movement covering 50 cm (19.7 in.) is possible in less than one second (<1 s). In designing these systems, however, clinical chemists will have to be cautious about the possible deleterious effects of extremely rapid accelerations and decelerations on sample integrity. The most cost-efficient robots for pipetting tasks and specimen sortation have been the cartesian robot because of their low cost and the limited specimen manipulation required in a clinical laboratory. The greatest savings can be realized with task-specific automation that has the flexibility to adapt to changes in testing methodology.

It is not immediately obvious to laboratorians who are used to purchasing instruments for specific tasks how one might use a laboratory robot. At the University of Virginia we have created three robotic applications that demonstrate the feasibility of using a variety of robotics in the clinical laboratory. For example, we have created a novel device on a cartesian robotic workstation to perform a complex column chromatographic extraction of glycated hemoglobin for monitoring averaged blood glucose concentrations in diabetic patients. We have also used a cylindrical robotic workstation for the solid-phase extraction of cyclosporin prior to high-performance liquid chromatography (HPLC) (see Fig. 1.9). These two applications will be described to highlight the versatility of robotics for solving complex laboratory tasks. We have also designed, built, and implemented a workstation based on an articulating arm for the performance of whole-blood analysis in an unmanned critical care laboratory. This application is described in detail in Chapter 24.

The Benchmate (Zymark Inc, Hopkinton, MA, USA) cylindrical robotic workstation was used to automate the solid phase extraction of cyclosporin from whole blood.[5] Cyclosporin in a cyclic peptide that has unique immunosuppressive properties that render it useful in organ transplantation. Whole-blood specimens, which had been previously dosed with internal standard and whose red blood cells had been lysed, were placed on the Benchmate for unattended extraction of cyclosporin. Automation of this procedure reduced analytical imprecision of the assay over the manual procedure by 5.1% for between-run coefficient of variation. Throughput was calculated at over 100 specimens per day with a substantial reduction of labor costs to perform this procedure. This study demonstrated that significant cost savings could be realized using commercially available automation and could be rapidly implemented in the clinical laboratory with a minimal amount of operator training.

Glycohemoglobin measurement by boronate affinity chromatography is becoming the method of choice for the monitoring of long-term glucose control in diabetic subjects. The boronate chromatography method, however, is a tedious

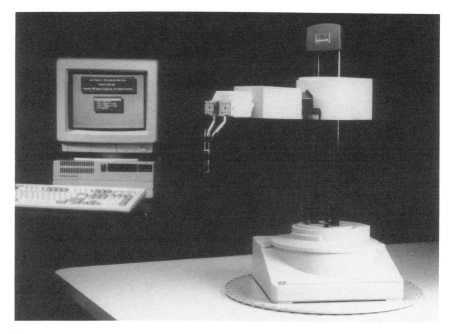

Figure 1.6. The Zymate cylindrical robot is proven technology that has been used in thousands of laboratories. A wide variety of peripheral devices complement this arm to provide any laboratory with a complete turnkey solution to any automation task.

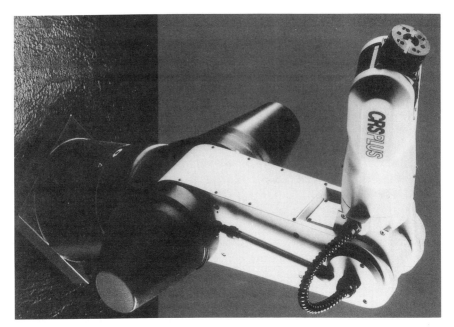

Figure 1.7. The CRS PLUS articulating arm operates with a high degree of precision to perform many laboratory tasks. This robust arm is easily programmed to lift payloads of ≤1 kg and has a repeatability of <1 mm.

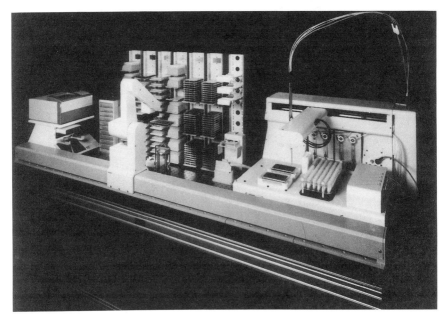

Figure 1.8. Scitec S.A. has engineered a system that combines the use of a Sagian ORCA arm and peripheral devices from Tecan and SLT to manipulate many microplates. This system is ideally suited for large-scale screening assays in pharmaceutical laboratories and for clinical assays in commercial clinical laboratories.

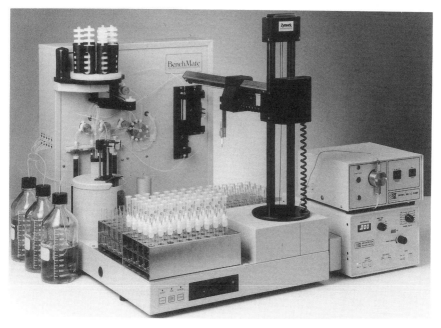

Figure 1.9. The Bechmate is a hybrid between a cylindrical robot arm and a chromatography processor. The system will do solid-phase extraction and filtration on specimens while keeping an electronic database of each step (including specimen weights) in the procedure. This easily programmed device can also serve as an autoinjector for any HPLC.

procedure requiring manual manipulation of individual disposable columns. Furthermore, there are many steps necessary to both prepare the columns and elute the products of interest that require a significant amount of operator time. We created a novel trolley system when placed on the bed of a Hamilton 2200 (Hamilton Co., Reno, NV) cartesian workstation allowed complete automation of specimen preparation, transfer to prepared columns, and elution of hemoglobin fractions prior to spectrophotometric analysis in a microplate[6] (Fig. 1.10). The automated method allowed 96 specimens to be analyzed simultaneously including controls. Within-run and between-run precision of the method were equal to that obtained by the manual procedure. Automation of this procedure reduced operator time from approximately 5 h to less than 45 min (hands-on time reduced by 80% and analysis time reduced by 40%). This study resulted in a robust method that has significantly reduced laboratory costs for this analysis.

After evaluation of the economic benefits of robotic automation, careful planning of the system development, assigning capable engineers to the task, and a thorough validation of the completed system, considerable cost savings can be realized over a relatively short period of time. With today's commercially available tools, modular, task-specific automation is generally more profitable than laboratorywide automation.

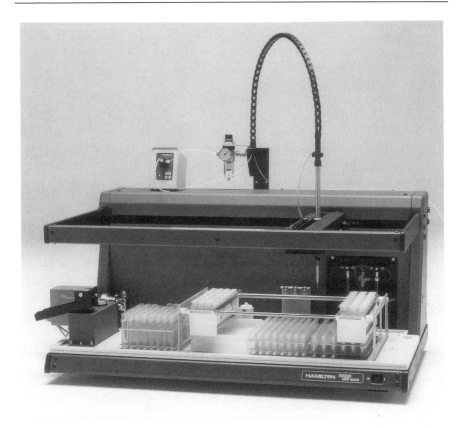

Figure 1.10. The Hamilton Company configured the 2200 pipetting device to perform automated glycated hemoglobin analysis on 48 samples. The boronate affinity chromatography eluates are then placed in a microplate for insertion into a microplate spectrophotometer.

1.2.2. Simulation Modeling and Process Control

Simulation is to the clinical laboratory what a budget forecast is to a hospital administrator. Simulation modeling is performed most often today on computers using algorithms that allow forecast of events based on input parameters. Ideally, simulation modeling will allow laboratory directors to predict the impact of new technology, alternative operating procedures, and increasing and decreasing demand on laboratory services. Simulation is the subject of Chapter 5, which describes this seldom used technique to predict the effects of new technology on laboratory efficiency. Commercially available simulation products that may be used on laboratory problems are listed in Table 1.2.

An extension of simulation modeling is process control, which uses real-time data as an input. Some process controllers can be run off line and thus become simulation models. A process controller provides computer integration of the

TABLE 1.2. Simulation Modeling Software: Simulation Modeling Companies

Company	Telephone #	Contact Person	Name of Product
AutoSimulations	(215) 245-2228	Scott Freedman	3-D
CACI Products Company	(619) 457-9681	Scott Swegles	SIMSCRIPT II.5 NETWORK II.5 COMNET II.5 L●NET II.5 MODSIM II SIMFACTORY II.5
Wolverine Software Corporation	(703) 750-3910	Douglas S. Smith	GPSS/H
ProModel Corporation	(801) 756-9893	Robert E. Bateman	ProModel PC 5.01
Pritsker Corporation	(317) 463-5557	Jenny Mishler	SLAMSYSTEM
Micro Analysis & Design Incorporated	(303) 442-6947	Lori Hood	Micro Saint

many decision-making tasks that occur in the daily activity of a laboratory, such as specimen tracking, monitoring specimen queues at analytical instruments, monitoring instrument functions and failures, scheduling technologists as well as analytical processes and robots, and monitoring quality control efforts. Since very few laboratories count the numbers of specimens they process at each analytical stations of the laboratory on a minute-to-minute basis, automated methods must be installed that can gather the volumes of input data necessary to feed a process controller. Process controllers will someday include user-definable algorithms for automatic reflex testing. Only a few process controllers include optimization algorithms that will determine the most efficient processes to use. Paul Mountain and Stephen Middleton discuss process controllers in detail in Chapter 20.

1.2.3. Artificial Intelligence

The field of applying computer processing to perform human reasoning is known as *artificial intelligence* (AI). Artificial intelligence encompasses a variety of disciplines including, knowledge-based reasoning, speech recognition and synthesis, and machine vision and processing. Knowledge-based reasoning has a number of evolving subfields including expert systems, fuzzy logic, genetic algorithms, and neural networks. Laboratory medicine could benefit enormously from fully evolved products based on these disciplines. Therefore, research is being done in many institutions focusing in these areas. Since the application of artificial intelligence has progressed further in applying these techniques to manufacturing, many products are being borrowed from industry and used in the laboratory environment.

Knowledge-based reasoning—including expert systems, fuzzy logic, neural networks, and genetic algorithms—is being used effectively to interpret laboratory data.[7,8] An entire section of this book (Part VI) is dedicated to knowledge optimization by computer. We are beginning to see the use of neural networks and fuzzy logic for process management and data interpretation. These machine interpretive methods attempt to deal with the uncertainty in data interpretation that results from medical decision making. Using these methods, decisions can be made in a much more rapid timeframe than by other more precise methods that require developing the mathematical relationships between many variables that are encountered in the dynamic process of human disease. Neural networks do not require encoding into the computer a precise set of quantifiable rules. They automate the task of acquiring knowledge by allowing the user to provide the computer a set of input examples. The computer than outputs a set of interpretations. Correct interpretive pathways are then strengthened by the user by indicating the correct output data. Following this iterative training exercise, the computer can then make probability predictions based on additional input data.

Fuzzy logic, on the other hand, automates the process of decision making in a similar, but simpler, way as an expert system. The important distinction between fuzzy logic and expert systems is the presence of tools that allow interpretation and interpolation at boundaries. For example, if a process is either slow or fast, fuzzy logic allows the use of additional modifiers such as fairly slow or fairly fast. Overlap is allowed between adjacent discrete regions. Therefore, fuzzy logic is simply a way of automating the programming of a process.

1.2.4. Machine Vision

Chapter 14 discusses image analysis in detail, focusing on many of the fundamentals of image processing. Basically, image processing begins with digitizing the output of a videocamera in a microcomputer. The digitized information is a numerical representation of the shade of gray "seen" by each pixel in a charge-coupled device (CCD). The digitized image is then mathematically interpreted by software that determines features from each region of interest (ROI). For example, the user may wish to find the edge of a black test-tube rack on the top of a white table. Image analysis software would then look for a line of pixels in which one group has primarily white values (the tabletop) and the other group would have black values (the edge of the rack). Circular groups of pixels may then be interpreted to have "seen" the top rim of a vacutainer tube. The coordinates of these numerical values can then be used to drive a robot to a desired location within the field of view of the videocamera.

The primary application of image processing and analysis has been on the interpretation of radiology and anatomic pathology images. However, there are indications that application of image processing to the clinical laboratory is beginning (see the proceedings of the ICAR 1995 conference). The cost of imaging hardware and processing software has begun to fall to affordable levels. The advent of the Apple Power PC (Trademark, Apple Computers) and Pentium

(Trademark, Intel Corp.) computers equipped with 32-bit bus architecture has made image processing fast enough to be useful in the laboratory environment.

1.2.5. Specimen Identification

Bar coding is gaining wider acceptance in the clinical laboratory. Estimates calculate that 35% of clinical laboratories are currently using bar codes. Bar codes allow rapid data reading and writing, which is essential for automated processors that have $\leq$500-tube/h throughput. Data transcription errors using bar codes have been estimated to be 1 billion times more reliable than manually keyed-in data.[9] The series of bars and spaces that characterize all bar codes are used in laboratories in three popular formats, Code 3 of 9, Code 49, and Code 128. Bar coding is a visual representation of a digital code in which bars and intervening spaces represent ASCII (American Standard Code for Information Interchange) characters and symbols. For example, Code 3 of 9 has a format in which three of the 9 characters are wide bars and the remainder are narrow bars. Laser readers have two elements: a laser light that is scanned across the code and a light-sensitive diode that detects the reflected light. The voltage coming from the light-sensitive diode is measured and a threshold is established that determines the reflections from spaces. Lasers scan the bar code rapidly and gather repeated digital codes, which are then compared so that a consensus is reached. Bar code scanners can read code at rates between 6 and 40 characters per second.

Newer codes are being invented each year. A poplar code that has been adopted by the Japanese Medical Association is the Matrix code. Matrix code appears more like a collection of squares and spaces. Advantages of Matrix code include higher data densities, readability in any orientation and on curved surfaces, internal redundancy that allows reading with 20% obliteration of the code, and low-contrast requirements. Matrix code is particularly good for machine vision applications since it does not require a high-contrast environment in which to be read. Olympus-Symbol Inc. has commercialized a two-dimensional (2D) code (PDF417), which has been in use for many years. The 2D code is read by a scanning laser reader. High data densities are achievable, and even machine executable code can be encoded into the technology. PDF417 and Matrix code are the only codes that contain error-correcting capabilities. In Europe, the dot code has been proposed by Impeco (Milano, Italy) as a possible method to label medical specimens. This code is described in Chapter 12.

1.3. CHALLENGES

1.3.1. Automation and Healthcare Reform in the United States

Healthcare reform in the United States is an attempt to put limits on growth of healthcare costs, making healthcare affordable to all Americans.[10,11] Healthcare reform in the United States is being closely scrutinized by European countries who are looking for successful systems to apply to their own rapidly spiraling healthcare costs. Two major elements form the basis of medical reform: managed competition and global budgeting. The former provides regulations that require both the private and public sectors to pay for healthcare. Costs containment under managed competition would rely on the proliferation of several large health maintenance organizations (HMOs). Global budgeting, on the other hand, would require a commission of healthcare providers to set a national limit on healthcare costs.

How will these two methods for cost containment affect the market for advanced automation? The increased emphasis on early diagnosis and prevention of disease will result in an increase in large-volume laboratory screening tests. In particular, be an increased demand for tests aimed at early detection, such as bone panels for osteoporosis and tumor markers for cancer, is expected. Another example is the screening for spina bifida and other related diseases by measuring alphafetoprotein, human chorionic gonadotropin, and unconjugated estriol. The need for large numbers of screening tests will require the use of automated systems to perform these tests at low cost. The most likely target of cost containment in laboratories is capital expenditures for large equipment. Clinical chemists, may not be able to buy the latest clinical analyzer every 3–5 years as has been customary in the past. There will be an increased emphasis on flexible automation which will have a longer lifespan and can adapt to the changing needs of the laboratory environment. Advanced laboratory automation is being designed to meet this goal.

Healthcare reform will also try to reduce overutilization of laboratory tests. There will be an increased need for "intelligent" software that can guide the laboratory director and physician to the most efficient testing strategies. Reflex testing and the extensive use of chemometrics will become an important cost-saving measures. Intelligent software coupled with automated analysis will result in the most efficient use of laboratory resources.

Another area targeted by regulatory agencies is the analytical tests produced in house. Clinical Laboratory Improvement Act (CLIA) regulations specifically dictate what steps must be taken to validate the performance of in-house tests. The FDA also wishes to regulate these tests. Robotics will be able to provide fixed protocols that would automatically perform the necessary validation protocols and provide the necessary documentation to satisfy any number of regulatory agencies that wish to regulate clinical laboratories. Undoubtedly, the robots themselves will also be subject to FDA and CLIA regulations and so will have to be designed with self-validation and documentation steps built in.

Healthcare reform has difficulty dealing with the apparently high costs of near-patient testing. Hidden-cost reduction will result from patient-focused care initiatives. For example, improving turnaround time will often result in cost savings to the patient and institution. Rapid pathogen identification during an office visit eliminates the need for a return visit, allows more rapid patient recovery since antibiotics are started sooner, and increases patient satisfaction. A happy customer is a return customer. Rapid turnaround near-patient testing may come at a higher cost to the laboratory but result in a net saving to the hospital.

1.3.2. Workforce

The greatest challenge to implementing laboratory automation will be the downsizing of the laboratory workforce. Laboratory automation has, as its fundamental goal, to reduce the labor associated with providing laboratory services. While automation can reduce the labor shortages associated with the current 15% vacancy rate in medical technologists in the United States, it provides a degree of efficiency that could reduce the labor needs of a laboratory by up to 50%.[12]

The attrition rate of technologists is not fast enough in many laboratories, particularly in rural areas, to accommodate the need to reduce personnel. Layoffs will undoubtedly be necessary. The remaining workforce must be trained to provide the support services to maintain advanced automation since these skills are not present in today's medical technologist. For example, federal regulations (CLIA regulations, Subpart M, Section 493.1421) allow high-school graduates with on-the-job training to perform many clinical laboratory tests. Recall, that most high-school graduates have no exposure to basic electronics, mechanical design, only a cursory knowledge of human physiology, and virtually no understanding of the basis of many of the tests they will be trained to perform. Up to 75% of the 9 billion tests performed annually will fall under a category of tests that can be performed by this group. Virtually no effort has been made to change the curriculum in medical technology programs to prepare graduates for the automated laboratory.

1.3.3. Service Patterns

Service patterns will also have to be examined and modified as a result of laboratory automation. We will have to modify the tendency to separate the subdisciplines of clinical pathology in distinct building locations as a result of the need of laboratory directors to have their own identity and space. For example, in the past the director of endocrinology was provided with laboratory and technologists to perform endocrine tests despite the fact that the main high-throughput analyzer in the central laboratory could have done many of these tests at a fraction of the cost. Many of the disciplines of clinical pathology will be provided in the same room, attached to the same delivery system, and managed by a central process controller. The laboratory director will have to evolve to manage many more medical disciplines, or the laboratory directors will have to work more closely together as a coordinated team.

Consolidation will affect not only intralaboratory service patters but also interlaboratory relationships. Regional laboratories will also have to consolidate to provide cost containment. Smaller laboratories coexisting in the same community are being forced to combine their services to reduce overhead costs.

These networking arrangements reduce many redundancies in equipment, personnel, and management. At the same time that cost containment is being practiced, there is also a need to increase revenue from outreach programs and novel methods to provide laboratory services. The home market and physician laboratory are seen as two potential growth areas for laboratories.

1.3.4. Research and Development

Research and development are often the first target of administrator's budget cuts. The next generation of laboratory tests and instrumentation come from the creative efforts of clinical laboratory scientists. Consolidation and downsizing will reduce the number of laboratory scientists actively doing applied research as well as the money available for research supplies. Cooperative agreements between industry and laboratories will probably replace a small percentage of hospital laboratory-funded research. The remainder of the research effort will probably take place within the diagnostic companies themselves. However, research performed in the laboratories of diagnostic companies is rarely as innovative as the research that takes place in academic hospitals. The daily exposure to patients and human disease serves as the catalyst for the inventive process. Therefore, countries that are willing to invest in research and development will become the next market leaders in the diagnostic field.

1.3.5. Error Rates

The clinical laboratory has error rates that are considered high when compared to the manufacturing industry. The error rate of clinical laboratories is quoted to be approximately 0.01% or 100 parts per million (ppm). Although 0.01% seems like an acceptable figure, it is relatively large when compared to Motorola's manufacturing error rates (0.003% or 3 ppm) and the number of airline crashes per flight (0.00003% or 0.3 ppm).[13] Furthermore, the error rate per proficiency test (our best objective way of determining laboratory quality) is misleading since it is considerably lower than the true laboratory error rate (0.22% or 2200 ppm). Even with automation, there is a calculable error rate below which no system can go.[14]

Increasing interest in reducing errors is coming at a time when cost containment is imperative. On one hand, legislation has been passed (CLIA '88) ensuring that "safe and accurate testing occurs throughout the laboratory testing system while still enabling health care providers to offer convenient, low cost laboratory services in a broad range of environments." The implementation of the Clinical Laboratory Improvement Act of 1988 is estimated to increase the cost of each laboratory test by 25 cents (9 billion tests per annum). On the other hand, many laboratories are trying to reduce costs by over 30% in order to survive. Automation, hopefully, will provide a solution to this dilemma.

1.3.6. Instrument Maintenance

Automated laboratory systems that have been manufactured in Japan have been quoted to need only minor service. In fact, manufacturers of these systems are quoting mean time between failures (MTBFs) of 3 months. On the other hand, many clinical analyzers require minute-to-minute supervision to monitor errors that occur in routine pipetting and analysis. Recently, instrument manufacturers have made great strides in designing instruments to be more reliable. For example, the Ciba Corning 850 blood-gas analyzer requires only minimal weekly maintenance. Many expendable parts need be replaced only once a year. The calculated efficiencies of automated laboratory systems should be include the realities of instrument failure and the labor required to maintain functional systems. Therefore, industry will have to design more reliability into instrumentation because frequent breakdowns will become more evident in automated systems.

1.3.7. Market Acceptance

The acceptance of advanced laboratory automation depends on the ease of integration with existing laboratory facilities, hardware, and disposables. Many laboratories will be unable or unwilling to obtain capital dollars to purchase a labwide automation system. Furthermore, few laboratories can afford the downtime necessary to install and debug a labwide system. Laboratory automation systems will be more successful if they use the computer and analytical systems already in place in the laboratory. Furthermore, modular systems will be easier to integrate and will appeal to a broader market. Laboratories will be more comfortable purchasing one automated unit with which to gain experience and confidence and then expand to more complete systems as time and capital allows. For example, an automatic aliquoter systems would immediately provide cost savings most laboratories as well as increase safety. As needs increase in the laboratory, automation should be expandable to meet the increased demand. Small laboratories such as the physician's office or group practice, initially will require only modest automation. However, as many laboratories consolidate services into regional laboratories, they will need to increase their ability to handle large workloads.

1.3.8. Data Management

Information management becomes a priority in an automated laboratory. The use of a laboratory information management system (LIMS) will improve the efficiency of automated systems. Interface design will allow real-time querying of the database to compare the test requisitions with specimen volume, identification, and attributes (cap color, serum quality etc.). Therefore, a necessary component of a LIMS system is bar-coded specimen containers. Bar codes will provide positive specimen ID, allow the automation to route the specimen, provide information for specimen processing, determine the number and volume of aliquots to be created, and direct the proper storage and disposal of the specimen. Analytical data as well as interpretive information provided by the technologist or computer must be sent into the medical records, printed, and archived for later retrieval.

1.3.9. Standardization

The need for standardization in laboratory automation was made alarmingly clear by a recent survey of users of personal computers. The survey attempted to measure the time wasted by users of personal computers in nonproductive activities, such as learning how to use software or waiting for technical support and system configuration.[15] Nonstandard human interfaces and nonstandard computer hardware are major contributors to nonproductive activities. American businesses loose in excess of $100 billion annually to nonproductive computer time or almost 2% of the GNP (gross national product). Robotics and automation are more complex than personal computers; therefore the percentage of nonproductive activities related to installing and operating robotic hardware are expected to be substantial.

To address these needs, several groups have formed in the last several years whose primary focus is the creation of standards that will apply to virtually all aspects of laboratory automation. The Consortium on Automated Analytical Laboratory Systems (CAALS) has been formed at the National Institutes of Standards and Technology (NIST) and is currently headed by Gary Kramer, Ph.D. [NIST, Center for Analytical Chemistry, Gaithersburg, MD, USA, Tel (301)-975-4142]. CAALS is a consortium between NIST and members of U.S. industry interested in promoting the development of standards for the automation of chemical laboratories. They have embarked on the creation of a "standard laboratory module" (SLM), which is a set of hardware and software specifications for devices to be sold commercially that will work together in a seamless fashion to perform inorganic and organic chemical analyses. Therefore, the automation platform becomes vendor-independent; that is, hardware purchased from one vendor will work and interact with another without the usual need to develop proprietary interfaces. SLMs can be combined into larger systems that will easily interact and share data with each other. Groups of SLMs may be combined to form even larger standard analytical methods that will create data that does not differ from site to site.

While CAALS focuses their activities on analytical laboratories, the National Committee for Clinical Laboratory Standards (NCCLS) is where the clinical laboratory standards are defined.[16] The priorities of this organization for creating automation standards were recently defined by the chairman of the NCCLS, Charles F. Galanaugh. It was suggested that approximately 20% of the standardization problems that affect 80% of the laboratory process should be identified. Three major areas of concern were suggested as areas that should be addressed first: standardization of the blood collection tube, creation of a "plug and play" electronics standard for interfaces, and defining mechanical standards for sample input and output from analytical instruments. Emery Stephens (Enterprise Analysis, Stanford, Conn), chair of the NCCLS subcommittee on data management, has organized his group to complete two proposals for standards: user interface and software validation standards. They are currently under review at the NCCLS. His next initiative will be to focus the subcommittee on mechanical and electronic interfaces to laboratory instruments.

It is not clear why the NCCLS should choose to create their own standards when other organizations have also addressed many of the interconnectivity concerns facing clinical laboratories. The American Society for Testing and Materials (ASTM) have already published recommendations for many laboratory standards as well as medical standards that can be applied to many aspects of laboratory testing. The ASTM standard E1384 is already widely used by most clinical laboratory instrument manufacturers.[17] Table 1.3 lists the standards that have already been published by this group. Specific standards that apply to robotic automation and systems integration are missing from this list. Perhaps it is the desire of the NCCLS to fill in this gap.

Standards developed in the United States will not necessarily be adopted in foreign countries. One European initiative to standardize clinical laboratory automation was centered with the European Committee for Clinical Laboratory Standards (ECCLS). However, this group was recently disbanded. A new group administered from the International Federation for Clinical Chemistry is currently becoming organized. Guidelines for patient and specimen identification have been published.[18] In this document, the committee provides suggestions for assessing the effectiveness of systems for specimen identification and track-

TABLE 1.3. Published Standards Related to Medical Computing

E 792	Standard guide for computer automation in the clinical laboratory
E 1029	Standard guide for documentation of clinical laboratory systems
E 1238	Standard specifications for transmitting clinical observations between independent systems
E 1239	Standard guide for description of reservation/registration-admission, discharge, transfer (R-ADT) systems for automated patient care information systems
E 1384	Standard specifications for the low-level protocol in transferring messages between clinical laboratory instruments and computer systems
E 1384	Standard guide for description for content and structure on an automated patient health record
E 1394	Standard specifications for transferring information between clinical instruments and computer system
E 1466	Standard specification for the use of bar codes on specimen tubes in the clinical laboratory

Source: ASTM standards, ASTM Committee E-31.

ing through the analytical process. Standardized terminology is suggested followed by a general description of optimal flow for laboratory diagnostic activities, whether performed manually or with automated equipment. An assessment checklist is provided so that users may determine whether their system is providing optimal identification and tracking of specimens. Although this document has been written in broad general terms (i.e., it suggests that automated systems be fault-tolerant without discussing the many options in this area), it is helpful for laboratories who wish to look at the options available for optimal specimen flow from patient to laboratory.

Another European standard that is gaining in popularity is OPENLABS,[19] which is a knowledge-based system that will provide a common architecture that will integrate the various functions of the laboratory. Estimates suggest that only 10% of laboratory tests actually influence medical decision making while 60% are considered unnecessary. The remainder of analytical tests are necessary for medical and/or legal documentation. OPENLABS contains a knowledge-based system to facilitate appropriate test ordering, automatic scheduling of additional tests (dynamic test rescheduling), and result interpretation. The OPENLABS architecture has been built to accommodate classification schemes (nomenclature) from existing classifications such as those developed by IUPAC, IFCC, WCC, and ASTM/CPT.

OPENLABS takes the creation of standards one step further. It not only suggests standard communication protocols but also has links to various administrative functions of the laboratory. It incorporates data interpretation tools that follow established medical reasoning and uses historical data from the same patient. Neural networks are used to assist with interpretation hematology cell counting and sizing images. A simulation tool is included in the management software module. Automated patient results validation, remote instrument fault diagnosis and instrument maintenance, and results validation will also appear in this software communication tool. Any syntax format will be accommodated, including HL7, ASTM, EDIFACT, and ASN1.

The Consortium de Reims is yet another European standardization initiative that is coordinated by Alain Donzel at Scitec (Lausanne, Switzerland). This organization seeks to create a forum where instrument manufacturers and organizations representing users, such as the International Conference on Automation and Robotics, can influence the direction of standards development. Although this effort seems to duplicate other initiatives.

Currently, there is no dearth of standards or groups who are creating them. However, what is missing is a consensus as to what standard or group of standard will be adopted for clinical laboratories. For example, there are a plethora of electronic interface standards already in use, such as IEEE 488, HPIB, GPIB, or RS-232C.[20,21] An electronic interface standard for clinical robotic applications was published first by Margrey and coworkers at The University of Virginia.[22,23] A mechanical docking interface standard has also been proposed by Markin at The University of Nebraska.[24] A steering committee was formed in 1994 at the American Association for Clinical Chemistry. This initial meeting was funded by Beckton Dickenson who is the market leader for specimen containers that are used in the United States. Further efforts of this committee will be funded by other agencies and take place at popular gatherings such as the AACC, CLMA, and ICAR. Initial meetings by this group have agreed to develop standards on

1. Interfaces: electronic, mechanical, user–instrument
2. Specimen identification, containers, and their carriers
3. Error and exception management
4. Information about the entire system performance

1.3.10. Modular and Flexible Automation

Standards will facilitate the lengthy process of installing automated systems in clinical laboratories because less time will have to be devoted to writing interfaces, designing novel tube carriers, or creating dedicated hardware to load and unload analytical instruments. Instrument manufacturers will be able to more effectively compete in the upcoming marketplace by providing several of these standards on their instruments. Laboratories will be less dependant on one manufacturer for the entire laboratory automation system since they will be able to mix and match any analyzer to the automation scheme. Laboratories will hopefully eliminate the compatibility dilemma with standardized, self-configuring instruments similar to the "plug and play" approach to computer peripherals. Currently instrument interfacing is a "plug and pray," or "plug and pay," nightmare.

1.4. RESOURCES

1.4.1. Books

A number of books have been written on laboratory automation. A well-known and useful series is the *Proceedings of the ISLAR Symposium,* which has been published since 1984 (Zymark Corporation, Hopkinton, MA, ISBN 0-931565-01-4). The *Laboratory Robotics Handbook* is also useful for beginners (ISBN 0-931565-08-1). In the field of laboratory medicine, however, there is very little introductory material.

1.4.2. Journals

Journals whose contents are dedicated to the discipline of laboratory automation are listed in Table 1.4. Several journals were started exclusively to act as a vehicle for this expanding field. However, they have had difficulty filling their pages because of the lack of research in this area. Future prospects for these journals appear to be better.

TABLE 1.4. Journals Dedicated to the Field of Laboratory Automation and Robotics

Primary Journals

Clinical Laboratory Automation
Journal of Automatic Chemistry—Taylor & Francis publishers
Journal of Laboratoy Automation and Robotics—VCH Publishers, Inc., 220 East 23rd
Street, Suite 909, New York, NY 10010, tel (212) 683-8333
Laboratory Automation and Information Management (formerly Laboratory Information
Management)—Elsevier Science B.V., P.O. Box 330, 1000AH, Amsterdam, The
Netherlands; fax 31-20-589-2845

Related Journals

Ameican Biotechnology Laboratory (Lowell, MA)
American Clinical Laboratory (Shelton, CT) (fax 203-926-9310)
American Laboratory
Journal of Clinical Chemistry (Charlottesville, VA)
LC-GC (Eugene, OR)

1.4.3. Conferences

Conferences are another ideal place to become familiar with what is taking place in laboratory automation. Established and new conferences in this area are listed in Table 1.5. Recently, established clinical meetings have been devoting more time to the presentation of robotics-related information.

TABLE 1.5. Conferences, Meetings, and Symposia on Laboratory Automation and Robotics

Primary Meetings and Symposia

The International Conference on Automation, Robotics, And Artificial Intelligence
Applied to Analytical Chemistry and Laboratory Medicine (ICAR)—chairpersons:
Robin Felder, Ph.D., Charlottesville, VA, fax 804-924-5718; Jan Van Der Greef, Ph.D.,
Zeist, Netherlands, fax 31-3404-5-7224
International Symposium on Laboratory Automation and Robotics (ISLAR), Organized
by Zymark Inc. Hopkinton, MA, USA, fax (508)-435-3439

Related Meetings

Scientific Computing and Automation
The Pittsburgh Conference
Clinical Laboratory Management Association
The Annual Meeting of the American Association for Clinical Chemistry (contact the
American Association for Clinical Chemistry, Washington, DC, USA)
The Oak Ridge Conference (contact the American Association for Clinical Chemistry,
Washington, DC, USA)

1.5. PREDICTIONS FOR THE FUTURE

The clinical laboratory of the future will be closer to the patient bedside and distributed throughout the hospitals and in community health clinics. In the near term, up to 80% of the laboratory work will be performed on instruments within a few steps of each patient. In the long term, most analytes will be quantitated by noninvasive biosensors. Central facilities will exist to process and analyze the esoteric specimens that have not yet evolved to the bedside instrument.

All laboratory related events will be monitored in real time (i.e., each second). A process controller will guide the flow of materials, activities, and information using sophisticated optimization algorithms. The laboratory will automatically adjust to changing workflow and prioritized turnaround time based on patient outcomes. Specimens will be obtained in standardized prelabeled containers that are electronically matched with the patient at the moment they are collected. Only the amount of specimen will be obtained that is required for the tests requested.

The data that is produced from the laboratory will be available locally. Like client/server architecture used in distributed corporate databases, laboratory information will reside where it is used the most and only be transmitted to the host when it is most efficient to do so. Wire transmission of data will be replaced with wireless transmission of packets of information [e.g., cellular digital packet data (CDPD)] using the same commercial carriers for wrist pagers and cellular phones (e.g. Motorola).

The era of prepackaged reagents will end when the highly versatile laboratory robot will be able to manufacture reagents on an as-needed basis. Raw materials have a longer shelf life than commercially available reagents. Therefore, robots will be able to mix the proper reagents, quality-control and validate each lot, and put the new material into service without the need for human intervention.

The clinical laboratory will be largely devoid of medical technologists since it will operate by robot and process controllers. Laboratory medicine professionals will add value to laboratory data by providing interpretation beyond the capabilities of the computer system. Laboratory directors and technologists will be concentrated in the R&D area looking for new clinically relevant analytes and preparing new assays for automation.

ACKNOWLEDGMENTS

Contributions for this chapter were made by the Laboratory Robotics Engineering Group at The University of Virginia Health Sciences Center; Keith Margrey, William Holman, John Savory, and Jim Boyd. Editorial and organizational assistance was provided by Silvia Dowell.

REFERENCES

1. Kingston HM, Kingston ML: Nomenclature in laboratory robotics and automation. *Pure Appl Chem* 66:609–630, 1994.

2. *Manipulating Industrial Robots: Vocabulary,* International Organization for Standardization, ISO/TR, 8373, 1988.

3. Felder RA, Boyd JC, Margrey KS, Holman W, Roberts J, Savory J: Robots in health care. *Anal Chem* 63:741A–747A, 1991.

4. Little JN, Proulx A, Connelly J: Recent advances in robotic automation of microplate assays. *Lab Info Management* 26:89–99, 1994.

5. Holman JW, Felder RA: Robotic automation of cyclosporin analysis in whole blood. *Clin Chem* 38:1440–1443, 1992.

6. Herold CD, Andree K, Herold DA, Felder RA: Robotic chromatography: development and evaluation of automated instrumentation for assay of glycohemoglobin. *Clin Chem* 39:143–147, 1993.

7. Pribor H: Expert systems and laboratory medicine. *Lab Management* 36–41, Nov 1988.

8. Pribor H: Expert systems in laboratory medicine: a practical consultative application. *J Med Sys* 13:103–109, 1989.

9. Maffertone MA, Watt SW, Whisler KE: Automated specimen handling: bar codes and robotics. *Lab Med* 21:436–443, 1990.

10. Bucher WF, Brown JW: The impact of health care reform on the clinical laboratory. *MLO,* March 30–35, 1994.

11. Bissell MG: Health care reform and the clinical laboratory. *MLO,* June, 24–29, 1993.

12. Middleton S, Mountain P, Kemp A: Laboratory automation: a model. *Leader Health Serv* 2:20–24, 1993.

13. Laboratory error rates should be reported in parts per million (PPM) rather than percent—moreover, proficiency tests do not measure true blunders. *Lab Report* 16:22–23, March 1994.

14. Lincoln TL, Korpman RA: *Science* 210:257–263, 1980.

15. Metcalf B: Are you still futzing around with your PC? *Info World* 25, Jan 11, 1993.

16. National Committee on Clinical Laboratory Standards (NCCLS), 771 E Lancaster Ave, Villanova, PA, 19085, tel (610) 525-4383, fax 610-526-9603.

17. American Society for Testing and Materials (ASTM), 1916 Race St, Philadelphia, PA 19103-1187, tel (215) 299-5400, fax (215) 299-2630.

18. Bonini PA, Alpert N, Luzzana M, Rubin R: Guidelines for the identification and distribution of patient samples in the medical laboratory. Recommendation of the European Committee for Clinical Laboratory Standards (ECCLS) and approved document of the International Federation of Clinical Chemistry (IFCC). *J Auto Chem* 16:25–32, 1994.

19. McAllister B: OPENLABS: Application of advanced informatics and telematics for optimization of clinical laboratory services. Project code A2028. Irish Medical Systems, Clara House, Glenageary Park, Glenageary Co, Dublin, Ireland. Tel 353.1.284.05.55, fax 353.1.284.08.29.

20. Selmyer J: Clinical laboratory instrument interfacing: basic considerations and functional types of interface applications, Part 1. *Am Clin Lab* Nov 28–30, 1994.

21. Selmyer J: Clinical laboratory instrument interfacing: interface architecture and communication standards, Part 2. *Am Clin Lab* Jan 16–18, 1994.

22. Margrey K, Martinez A, Vaughn DP, Felder RA: A standard clinical instrument interface for robotic applications. *Clin Chem* 36:1572–1575, 1990.

23. Margrey KS, Felder RA, Boyd JC, Holman WJ, Roberts JH, Savory J, Martinez A: Robotically operated laboratory system. US Patent 5,366,896.

24. Markin RS: Challenging the future of clinical laboratory automation: a paradigm shift. *Clin Lab Management Rev* 243–251, May/June 1993.

2

Historical Perspectives and Critical Issues

RODNEY S. MARKIN

CONTENTS

2.1. INTRODUCTION

The application of automation strategies in the healthcare industry has been slow to develop. In part, this delay may be attributed to a lack of ingenuity and a laboratory perspective; however, the primary determinate is related to the historical financial aspects of healthcare financing. In the past, hospitals and other healthcare providers have been reimbursed on a cost-plus scheme. Over the last several years, the reimbursement mechanism has changed from a fee-for-service to a global reimbursement structure, such as diagnosis-related groups (DRGs) or other contractual mechanisms.

As the technology and testing volume in healthcare advances, costs continue to rise. The work of the clinical laboratory continues to accelerate along with advances in technology and therapy. New methodologies for operating the clini-

Handbook of Clinical Automation, Robotics, and Optimization, Edited by Gerald J. Kost with the collaboration of Judith Welsh.
ISBN 0-471-03179-8 © 1996 John Wiley & Sons, Inc.

cal laboratory are needed to maintain a necessary level of service and to support the technologically advanced treatments.

During the past 50–70 years, the clinical laboratory has evolved, driven primarily by technological advances. Tests or assays were performed manually in the early years of clinical laboratory science; the 1920s through the 1940s. These first tests included chemistry assays, such as sodium and potassium, and examination of peripheral blood films for cell morphology, microorganisms, and parasites. With advances in medical therapy, basic science, and technology, the development of clinical laboratory instrumentation began (Fig. 2.1; see also Tables 2.1 and 2.2).

2.1.1. Analytical Instruments

The evolution of clinical laboratory automation began in the 1950s with the application of flame photometry for clinical measurements and the introduction of peripheral blood cell analysis using the aperture method.[1] The Coulter counter was introduced in 1957, revolutionizing the counting of a variety of peripheral blood cells, including red blood cells and leukocytes.[2,3] In the 1960s single and multichannel analyzers were developed for performing chemistry analyzers such as the sequential multiple analyzer (SMA).[4,5] By 1970, the automatic clinical analyzer (ACA) from DuPont and the automatic blood analyzer (ABA) has been unveiled.[6] A large variety of centrifugal analyzers, including the Centrichem from Baker Instruments, was introduced at this time. By the late 1970s, methods for mass production of monoclonal antibodies were perfected. Technologies such as enzyme-linked immunosorbent assays (ELISAs), enzyme-multiplied immunoassay techniques (EMITs), and other similar techniques measured particular protein epitopes to find clinical applications. In the 1980s, ion-selective electrodes changed the equation for laboratory testing in a radical way; electrolyte analysis could be performed on whole blood, removing the need for centrif-

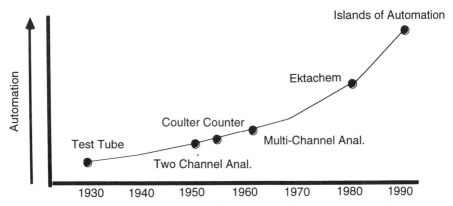

Figure 2.1. Graphic representation of the history of laboratory automation.

TABLE 2.1. Major Technological Advances in Laboratory Automation

Sequential multiple analyzer (SMA)
Automated clinical analyzer (ACA)
Automated blood analyzer
Fast centrifugal analyzer (e.g., centrifichem)
Development of monoclonal antiobodies
Enzyme-linked immunosorbent assay (ELISA technology)
Enzyme multiplied immunoassay techniques (EMIT)
Fluorescence polarization immunoassay (FPIA)
Ion-specific electrodes
Substrate-specific electrodes
Therapeutic drug monitoring using antibody-based reagents (TDM)
Automated hemogram, CBC with automated differential
Automated microbiology identification system (e.g., Bactek)
Flow cytometry
Chromogenic coagulation assays
Immobilized enzymes and reagent strip technology
DNA probes
Fluorescence *in situ* hybridization (FISH)
Image analysis–vision systems

ugation and precise volume measurements. By 1985, ion-specific electrode techniques replaced most, if not all, flame photometry units.[7]

At the same time, immunoassay techniques began to impact the drug testing arena. Concepts such as therapeutic drug monitoring (TDM), once considered very sophisticated chromatographic techniques, were replaced by antibody-based reagent methodologies. The need for automation was driven by two factors: (1) the increasing demands from clinicians and other users of laboratory services for more rapid turnaround of results and (2) a move to decrease the

TABLE 2.2. Issues That Have Shaped the History and Will Continue to Impact the Future of Laboratory Automation

Emphasis on decreasing the overutilization of testing
Wellness testing
Expansion of managed care
Point-of-care testing; near-patient testing
Staff shortages in specialized areas
Cost containment pressures
Medical and legal issues regarding test performance in managed care
Federal government laboratory regulations
Consolidation of laboratories and opportunity streamline operations
New breakthroughs in testing (e.g., methods, analytes)
Laboratory managers and supervisors managing testing operations
Optimizing laboratory costs and performing cost/benefit ratios

costs of producing laboratory results and consolidate laboratory testing into more concise workstations. Larger multitest or multichannel analyzers became available providing one unit the functionality that previously existed at multiple workstations. Over time the laboratory divided into two conceptual sections: automated areas and specialized manual areas. The automated sections consist of large multichannel chemistry analyzers, large multiparameter hematology analyzers, and a variety of immunoassay analyzers that perform drug, hormone, and other analyte assays.[8] The more manual procedures require a significant amount of interpretative evaluation, including blood banking, microbiology, coagulation testing, electrophoresis, and chromatography.

Historically, the automation arena centered around chemistry and hematology. Coagulation and some areas of microbiology testing (e.g., blood culture) were eventually brought into the fold. Blood banking, the most difficult arena to automate, remains the question on the horizon.

Applying automation to blood banking has been approached by different vendors with a variety of results. The most striking application of automation to blood banking is currently operating in Japan. Japan for the most part is a racially pure nation. The majority of the population possess blood type O and a limited number of antibodies. Applying automation to this population is simplified because the statistical chance of discovering a noncompatible donor is very low. In the United States and Europe, however, the population is divided among four specific blood types split into multiple subcategories. A significant number of circulating antibodies is present in the population, further complicating the application of automation to blood banking.

2.1.2. New Technologies

In the late 1980s and early 1990s, the development of "impregnated tape technologies," containing either ion-specific electrodes[9] or immobilized enzymes (substrate-specific technologies), provided the basis for developing near-patient testing (known as *point-of-care testing* or *bedside testing*). This development in technology permitted new testing possibilities for physician office laboratories, nursing homes, at-home testing, and to a certain extent, hospital testing. Analytes such as glucose, electrolytes, and even blood gases are now easily monitored in a single disposable monitoring methodology.

An extremely significant technological breakthrough in the last 50 years, is the application of DNA (deoxyribonucleic acid) probes. DNA probes enable us to measure extremely small quantities of the genetic material important to detecting organisms that cause disease (i.e, bacteria and viruses) and enable genetic testing. These applications were thrust to the forefront primarily by the legal system with respect to determining innocence or guilt through forensic evidence collected at the crime scene. Current DNA testing appears to be experiencing another quantum leap in laboratory testing with the application of fluorescence *in situ* hybridization (FISH) for specific identification of genetic-based diseases.[10,11]

A variety of different issues fueled the historical progression of automation in the clinical laboratory. First and most important is the continuation of discovery at the basic science level. Techniques such as ion-specific electrodes, immobilized enzymes, and DNA probes were not developed for specific medical applications but for research applications that span the gamut of analytical testing. Coupling of these technologies with the government and third-party payers cost containment pressures has driven opportunities in laboratory automation.[12] Staff shortages will continue, particularly in the areas of cytology, cytogenetics, and toxicology. The need for laboratory testing will not decline and will, in fact, increase as new technologies are developed for discovering and treating diseases. Historically, both solid organ and bone marrow transplantation drive the increase in laboratory test volume in transplant test centers around the world.[13] This is a result of the application of a new technology monitored by both existing technologies and new technologies developed to support the field. The future of laboratory automation remains bright despite significant changes in government regulation. Over the last 25 years, government regulations increased significantly, including Food & Drug Administration (FDA) rules and regulations enacted via CLIA 67 and CLIA 88 and the Occupational Safety & Health Administration (OSHA) entering the clinical laboratory in the late 1980s. The use of automation will help laboratories conform to all of the regulations conceived or constructed during this evolutionary period.[14]

2.2. MANAGED CARE AND UTILIZATION

Two of the most critical issues in healthcare are (1) *the cost of each service or procedure* and (2) *the utilization of medical services and procedures.*

The cost of each service or procedure is composed of several subcomponents, such as labor, materials, disposables, overhead, depreciation, and other allocated expenses. The clinical laboratory is one of the hospital operation leaders in developing cost accounting of procedures and services.[15]

In the clinical laboratory the cost of performing each test follows a similar formula. In a typical clinical laboratory operation, the costs of labor, supplies, and reagents are approximately equal halves of the total budget. These operational costs continue to rise every year. The cost of labor is increasing at approximately 4% per year. The cost of reagents and supplies is increasing at a rate of approximately 8–12% per year. The cost of performing a specific test may be heavily dependent on the method used and the number of tests performed (an economy of scale). In general, as the number of a specific test increases, the cost per test will decline.

The cost of labor in the clinical laboratory may be the cost containment most amenable to change. During the last 10 years, the period of time when the most significant changes in clinical laboratory technology have occurred, we have substituted reagent and equipment dollars for labor dollars. All clinical laboratory operations have experienced the use of a cost justification model to move from a manual procedure such as radioimmunoassay (RIA) to a semiautomated immunoassay or automated immunoassay method. This methodology served us well in an era when the entire industry experienced significant growth in testing volume. The same cost justification models may be used to justify the acquisition of clinical laboratory automation solutions.[16–19]

Utilization of procedures and services is the most significant issue in the long-term operation of the clinical laboratory. The "managed" component of managed care refers to the management of utilization of procedures and services (utilization management). Historically, the management of utilization has been the purview of the attending or consulting physician. In the new managed care model, the control of utilization is transferred from the physician to the third-party payer [insurance company or health maintenance organization (HMO)], the hospital, or a physician hospital organization (PHO) in which the physician, the hospital, and possibly a third-party payer, share the financial risk of the healthcare operation. In the future, the responsibility for the management of laboratory test utilization will be at the level of the clinical laboratory as mandated by one of the utilization management organizations. Physician hospital organizations or groups of hospitals will be organized into health alliances or health enterprises. These enterprises will determine the evaluation and treatment of patient populations. Physicians treating the patients may be associated with more than one health alliance or hospital and be bound to follow a different set of rules for patient evaluation and treatment depending on where the patient is hospitalized or treated (Fig. 2.2).

When teaching differential diagnosis skills to medical students, emphasis is placed on the use of testing algorithms as a method for deriving a diagnosis and subsequent therapy. This method is based on the use of "screening" tests or procedures when the patient evaluation begins. Throughout the process, more advanced and potentially diagnostic tests and procedures are used. The method used requires working through the diagnostic possibilities in sequential order to arrive at the diagnosis or diagnoses for a particular patient. This method is

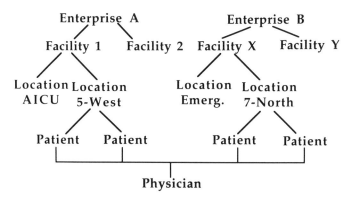

Figure 2.2. Organizational structure of a healthcare alliance representing two alliances with multiple facilities within the same geographic area.

sound and has been used successfully since the time of Sir William Osler, the father of diagnostic medicine.

In the current paradigm, the speed of the diagnosis and treatment, the avoidance of litigation, and the satisfaction of the patient are paramount. With the transition to managed care, new scenarios may arise that result in conflict. The balance between the financial outcome (dollars spent) and the patient's medical outcome (including patient satisfaction) may not be maintained. The result may be a patient outcome that is less than optimal since we are measuring the costs and charges incurred by the third-party payer with better-defined metrics than the patient's medical outcome.

The optimal solution is a system that allows for the most cost-efficient testing mechanism to occur in the least amount of time using the same algorithmic approach as taught in medical school. Figure 2.3 shows a schematic representation of a testing algorithm that represents either a series of clinical laboratory tests performed in sequential order based on the previous result or a combination of clinical laboratory testing and nonlaboratory testing. Several mechanisms are used to accomplish this goal. The first requires that a tight communications link be established with each physician or healthcare provider. Through this link, the results of screening tests and other tests ordered by the provider are transmitted and the next order in the sequence is executed. The difficulty with this mechanism is the need for intermittent communication with the provider and the possibility that the provider is not aware of all of the rules or management conditions that have been set up by the PHO, hospital, or third-party payer.

The second mechanism is to have the physician interact with the hospital information system or clinic information system software on a frequent basis (four or more times per day) to evaluate clinical information and the results of clinical laboratory tests and nonlaboratory tests and procedures. The difficulty with this mechanism is that the healthcare industry is shifting the provision of the majority of patient care from the inpatient arena to the outpatient arena. In this situation, the physician may not have access to an information system, either a patient or a clinic system, for a variety of reasons. As healthcare alliances are created, independent physicians and small physician groups tend to sign up with every available health plan. This behavior is understandable given the climate. However, each health plan creates its own set of guidelines to follow on the basis of their patient population, their experience with a population, and their medical direction. In these situations, the physician is required to know and understand several different sets of rules for the treatment of patients. These rules vary from hospital to hospital and from patient to patient according to the patient's choice of enrollment plans. This translates to a formidable task that most, if not all, information systems are able to contend with at their current level of functionality.

The most likely scenario for the future is that the clinical laboratory will bear the responsibility for providing the service that will invoke the rules for testing. Some clinical laboratory operations have the ability to provide the option for rules-based testing for their clients. Conventional wisdom suggests that clinical

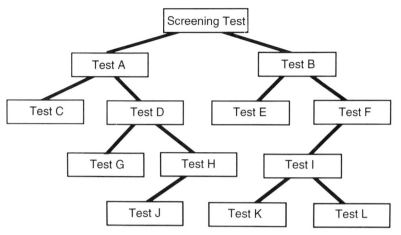

Figure 2.3. Hierarchical testing algorithm for both clinical laboratory and nonlaboratory testing and procedures.

laboratories should not invoke reflex testing since the laboratory may profit from the "self-referral" process. Indeed, the federal and state governments, patients, and the patients' physicians are opposed to the practice. *In the near future, utilization management and risk sharing will mandate that the clinical laboratory take the lead in the implementation of algorithmic testing.*

2.3. LABORATORY ORGANIZATION AND PHYSICAL LAYOUT

The current paradigm for the clinical laboratory operation is best described by Figure 2.4, which is a schematic representation of the individual component

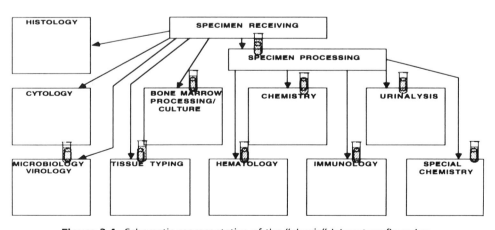

Figure 2.4. Schematic representative of the "classic" laboratory floorplan.

sections of the clinical laboratory and the flow of specimens from a central specimen receiving area and specimen processing area to the individual sections. In this paradigm most of the laboratory sections have names that would be found either as the title of a textbook (e.g., *Chemistry, Microbiology, Hematology,* or *Immunology*) or as a chapter in a major textbook (e.g., Urinalysis, Bone marrow processing and culture). As medicine has advanced, so has the clinical laboratory. The current boxlike structures in the laboratory organization represent specific and sometimes highly specialized services provided by a hospital or clinic. There is usually one pathologist and a laboratory section administrator who manage each section. The pathologist responsible for the section provides continuity and a direct information transfer mechanism to the clinical service in addition to serving as a consultant.[20]

In this paradigm, there are well-defined walls and spaces that are easily understood and fairly easily managed. Specimens and technologies are usually confined to the purview with minimal overlap. Some clinical laboratories are arranged in a more technology-based or methods-based operation where certain methods are utilized in certain sections of the laboratory. This type of operation is difficult to manage from a global administrative perspective and occasionally causes conflict. Understanding this operation depends entirely on the direction of your approach. From a medical perspective, antibodies measured in serum should be in the purview of the immunology section. If you are measuring an analyte using an antibody, you will most likely perform that assay in a section or subsection of chemistry or, possibly, hematology. In the global aspect, however, the entire clinical laboratory operation is based on the fundamentals of chemistry, whether this is identifying bacteria using chemical analysis, simple chemistry such as sodium and potassium, staining peripheral blood cells, or using antibodies as reagents.

2.3.1. The Paradigm Shift

The new paradigm arises from the current manufacturing industry technology. This paradigm is modeled around the assumption that the assay of clinical laboratory specimens be based on the specimen matrix, such as, plasma, serum, and whole blood.[21] Compared to the current operation (Fig. 2.4), different components of each clinical laboratory section are attached to a product line such as serum/plasma or whole blood. The ideal organization for such a product line is presented in Figure 2.5. Figure 2.5 describes a mode of operation where specimens are placed into the clinical laboratory flow and routed through different product lines based on the matrix type. Specimens enter through a specimen receiving area and are immediately analyzed for glucose and ionized calcium, or blood-gas determinations, or both, if ordered by the physician. Specimens may also pass through the line without undergoing analysis, moving to a specimen processing station where, if necessary, specimen centrifugation and serum or plasma separation will occur. Specimens are further gated to individual analyzers down the product line based on current automated technol-

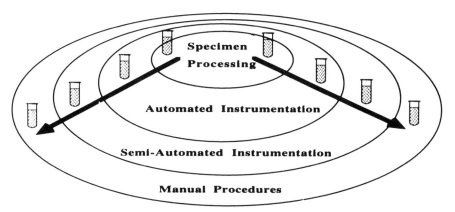

Figure 2.5. Schematic representation of optimal specimen flow–specimen processing scheme for laboratory automation platform: based on assaying specimens, based (in turn) on their matrix.

ogy (e.g., automated chemistry or hematology analyzers), turnaround time, and cost-effectiveness. At the end of the product line, a specimen archiving station stops specimens for quality-assurance purposes or to retain a serum bank for research studies. An alternative to the "product line" floorplan organization is shown in Figure 2.6. This type of organization allows laboratory sections to maintain some cohesion.

The results from these assays return to the laboratory information system (LIS) through the electronic interface of each instrument or through the entry of results via a terminal session. If appropriate to a specific institution, results could be released according to their relationship to predetermined limits. Accumula-

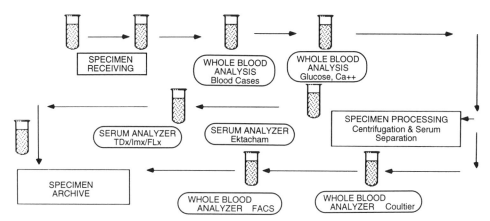

Figure 2.6. Schematic representation of a laboratory floor plan based on automation levels.

tion of and collating results for production of the cumulative report would continue to be the primary function of the LIS. From the database of results and other transactions, quality control and other statistical information that discusses the laboratory operation can be described. LIS functionality will evolve over time to include the information necessary to manage the operation of the clinical laboratory of the future.[22–24]

2.4. CONCLUSIONS AND SUMMARY

The evolution of the clinical laboratory[25] parallels the advances in clinical medicine. The technical advances of the clinical laboratory surpass the precision requirements of medical practice and possibly human physiology.

Changes in healthcare financing are driving significant changes in the practice of medicine. As the clinical laboratory product (the test result) transforms from a specialized or custom product to a commodity available from a variety of sources, the competition between laboratories will increase substantially. To compete, clinical laboratories are required to produce the same level of quality and service for a lower price. The mechanism to obtain this constantly moving target requires a greater level of automation in the clinical laboratory. The implementation of a clinical laboratory automation system in a laboratory operation enhances the financial performance of the operation as well as addresses issues of quality and turnaround time. In addition, the use of the enabling technology of specimen transportation allows the laboratory to meet the demands of the newly forming healthcare alliances.

The overriding issue in the managed healthcare scenario is managing procedure and service utilization. The rules for utilization or the algorithms for the evaluation of the patient will be determined by the third-party payer, hospital, or physician hospital organization. In an environment where most physicians are either independent operators or members of independent groups, many providers are working across healthcare alliances. The same physician, or possibly the same hospital, working across alliances will result in different rules or algorithms being used for evaluating the same symptoms in different patients. The responsibility to implement algorithmic testing will be delegated to the clinical laboratory. A clinical laboratory automation system with functional hardware and highly "intelligent" software will be invaluable in controlling the process.

The evolution of laboratory automation will continue. As described in the chapters dealing with robotics, docking devices, and transportation systems, the implementation of computer integrated manufacturing applications in the laboratory arena sets the stage for making the laboratory a cost-effective, integral piece in operating a managed care enterprise. Developing a standard to connect a docking device to disparate instruments and automation technology will continue along the trajectory set by this historical path.

REFERENCES

1. Saunders AM, Scott F: Hematologic automation by continuous flow systems. *J Histochem Cytochem* 22:707, 1974.

2. Mansfield HP: Optical techniques of particle counting. Technicon International Congress 1969, *Adv Auto Anal* 1:213, 1970.

3. Bull BS, Schneiderman MA, Brecher G: Platelet counts with the Coulter Counter. *Am J Clin Pathol* 44:678, 1965.

4. Gambino SR, Schreiber H: The measurement of CO_2 content with the AutoAnalyzer. *Am J Clin Pathol* 45:406, 1966.

5. Mabry CC, Gevedon RE, Roeckel IE, Gochman N: Automated submicrochemistries. A system of rapid sodium, potassium, chloride, carbon dioxide, sugar, urea nitrogen, total and direct-reacting bilirubin, and total protein. *Am J Clin Pathol* 46:265, 1966.

6. Gilbert HS: The clinical application of automated cytochemical techniques in patient management. In *Advances in Automated Analysis,* Technicon International Congress, Madiad, Inc, Tarrytown, NY, 1973, p 51.

7. Burtis CA: Recent technological developments and their impact on laboratory automation. In Okuda K, ed: *Automation and New Technology in the Clinical Laboratory,* Oxford: Blackwell Scientific Publications, 1988, pp 1–6.

8. Chan DW: *Immunoassay Automation: A Practical Guide.* San Diego: Academic Press, 1993.

9. Pelleg A, Levy GB: Determination of Na^+ and K^+ in urine with ion-selective electrodes in an automated analyzer. *Clin Chem* 21:1572, 1975.

10. Lifshitz MS, DeCresce RP, eds: *Perspectives on Clinical Laboratory Automation: Clinics in Laboratory Medicine.* Philadelphia: Saunders, 1988.

11. Lifshitz MS, DeCresce RP: New technologies in chemistry instrumentation: The basis for clinical chemistry automation. In Lifshitz MS, DeCresce RP, eds: *Perspectives on Clinical Laboratory Automation. Clinics in Laboratory Medicine.* Philadelphia: Saunders, 8:623–632, 1988.

12. Maclin E, Young DS: Automation in the clinical laboratory. In Burtis CA, Ashwood ER: *Tietz Textbook of Clinical Chemistry.* Philadelphia: Saunders, 1994, Chap 11, pp 313–382.

13. Markin RS: The impact of transplantation on the clinical laboratory: experience at the University of Nebraska with bone marrow and liver transplantation. *Arch Pathol Lab Med* 116:1004–1011, Oct 1992.

14. Ward KM, Lehmann CA, Leiden AM: *Clinical Laboratory Instrumentation and Automation: Principles, Applications and Selection.* Philadelphia: Saunders, 1994.

15. Cerda V, Ramis G: *An Introduction to Laboratory Automation.* New York: Wiley, 1990.

16. Asper R, Vonderschmitt DJ: Laboratory mechanization and automation. In Vonderschmitt DJ, ed: *Laboratory Organization and Automation.* New York: Walter de Gruyter, 1991, Chap 12, pp 271–325.

17. Brunner LA: The laboratory of the nineties. Planning for total automation. *Lab Robot Auto* 4:227–231, 1992.

18. DeCresce RP, Lifshitz MS: Integrating automation into the clinical laboratory. In Lif-

shitz MS, DeCresce RP, eds: *Perspectives on Clinical Laboratory Automation. Clinics in Laboratory Medicine.* Philadelphia: Saunders, 8:759–774, 1988.

19. Leiken AM, Lehmann CA: The impact of instrumentation on laboratory costs. In Ward KM, Lehmann CA, Leiken AM, eds: *Clinical Laboratory Instrumentation and Automation: Principles, Applications and Selection.* Philadelphia: Saunders, 1994, Chap 18, pp 469–487.

20. Vonderschmitt DJ, ed: *Laboratory Organization and Automation.* New York: Walter de Gruyter, 1991.

21. Markin RS: Clinical laboratory automation: a paradigm shift. *Clin Lab Management Rev* 7:243–251, 1993.

22. Liscouski J: *Laboratory and Scientific Computing: A Strategic Approach.* New York: Wiley, 1995.

23. Griffiths J: Automation and other recent developments in clinical Chemistry. *Am J Clin Pathol (Path Patterns).* 98 (Suppl 1):S31–S34, 1992.

24. Markin RS: Laboratory automation systems. An introduction to concepts and terminology. *Am J Clin Pathol (Path Patterns).* 98 (Suppl 1):S3–S10, 1992.

25. Markin RS: Clinical laboratory automation systems: Concepts designs, and future directions. *Clin Lab Automat* In Press, 1995.

II

THEORY AND FUNDAMENTAL PRINCIPLES

CHAPTER

3

Micromechanics and Nanotechnology

LARRY J KRICKA AND PETER WILDING

CONTENTS

Handbook of Clinical Automation, Robotics, and Optimization, Edited by Gerald J. Kost with the collaboration of Judith Welsh.
ISBN 0-471-03179-8 © 1996 John Wiley & Sons, Inc.

3.1. INTRODUCTION

Academic and commercial interest in the miniaturization of instrumentation using silicon micromachining techniques is growing. Small micromachined devices ranging in complexity from a cantilever beam to an electric motor have been constructed from micrometer-sized (10^{-6} m) silicon components (Table 3.1).[1-5] Ultimately, still smaller, nanometer-sized [1 nanometer (nm) = 1×10^{-9} m), devices constructed from individual atoms and molecules using the emerging nanotechnological techniques are envisaged.[5-13] In the analytical laboratory micromachined devices are currently in transition from a laboratory curiosity to key components of routine biomedical analyzers and test devices. This is in contrast to other applications, where micromachined components such as sensors for measuring blood pressure, fuel flow in automobile engines, and triggering airbags in automobiles, have already become established, and have superseded their macroscale counterparts (Fig. 3.1).[14] This existing and successful application for micromachined components provides a firm basis for the continuing development of other devices for use in the analytical sciences.

Miniaturization of analytical devices down to the micrometer (μm) scale has a number of advantages:

Ease of Manufacture and Design. For devices fabricated from silicon, the existing microelectronics industry manufacturing processes are already geared to high-volume production (millions of wafers per year). Device density per wafer is high (e.g., 24 different designs of a 17 × 14-mm device can be fitted onto a 4-in.-diameter wafer) (Fig. 3.2), and thus many different designs can be simultaneously fabricated on the same wafer and then tested. This permits rapid design cycles and the potential for more design iterations than would be normally possible for a macroscale device.

Reduced Cost of Manufacture and Operation of the Analyzer. In devices with total volumes of <1 μL, the per test reagent consumption is greatly reduced, thus decreasing the reagent component of the overall cost per test.

Portability. Microminiaturization facilitates the fabrication of compact, lightweight, handheld analyzers that have low power consumption and are suitable for use in nonlaboratory settings, such as point-of-care testing (e.g., bedside, physician's office), remote/on-line process monitoring, and environmental testing (e.g., stream-side).

Speed of Operation. Faster response times are possible using microscale devices.

Complex High Volume Analysis. Miniaturized arrays of different reagents on planar surfaces (e.g., plastic, glass, or silicon) permits simultaneous testing of a sample for specific components.

Sample Size. The volume of sample required for analysis is greatly reduced, with nL to pL (nanoliter to picoliter) volumes as compared to the μL

TABLE 3.1. Micromachined Devices

Device	Reference
Accelerometer	74–76
Acoustic filter	5
Actuator	77
Air turbine	4
Beam	78
Bearing	9
Blood flow meter	79
Cantilever	80–82
Comb actuator	83,84
Diaphram valve	85
Elastic force motor	86
Electroporation system	87
Fabry–Perot interferometer	88
Fluidic amplifier	4
Gas chromatograph	64,89
Gears	9
Glass electrode	90
Gripper	91
Heat exchanger	92
Incandescent light	93
Infrared imaging array	94
Ink-jet printhead	95
Interferometer	96
Lever	97
Magnetic field sensor	98,99
Microphone	100–102
Mirror array	103
Motion detector	104
Motor	105–107
Neural connector	108
Particle filter	109
Pirani vacuum gauge	110
Plate-wave sensor	111
Positioning system	112
Pressure switch	113
Pressure sensor	114
Pump	115–120
Read/write head	121
Refrigerator	122
Relay	4
Robot	123
SFM and STM tips	80–82
Sieve electrode	124
Solenoid	98

(continued)

TABLE 3.1. (*Continued*)

Device	Reference
Strain gauge	4
Switch	125
Thermal detector	126
Tuning fork	127
Turbine	4
Tweezers	4
Vacuum tube	4
Valve	119,128–133
Voltage sensor	134

volumes used in current analyzers. In a clinical setting this is beneficial to the patient and more convenient for the phlebotomist (fingerstick versus venepuncture). It is also a specific advantage for neonatal and pediatric patients where total blood volume is relatively small and removal of large samples medically contraindicated.

Disposal and Safety. The small sample size reduces the exposure of health workers to potentially hazardous samples. The low capacity of devices minimizes the volume of waste fluids. It is also possible to entomb the contents of a device (unreacted sample and reagents and reaction mixtures) for safe disposal.

Reliability. Multiple test sites for simultaneous multiplicate assays can be designed on one device. This built-in redundancy provides an analytical safeguard not easily achieved in a conventional macroscale system, where duplicate assays represent the normal extent of repetitive assay of a specimen. Also, encapsulated microscale devices may provide extended operation over a wider range of environmental conditions of humidity and temperature.

System Integration. Microscale fabrication makes possible system integration. The various steps of sample addition, processing, analysis and readout can be integrated in a single device.

In practice, miniaturization also has some disadvantages and difficulties. Connecting different microcomponents can be complex. Access to interior surfaces for selective surface modification, such as coating microcapillaries, is not facile. Measurement of minute quantities of components present in nano- or picoliter volumes contained within devices challenges the limits of detection of some of the current analytical methods. Optimal packaging of some types of chips into final products has not been adequately addressed. Despite such difficulties, the range of microanalytical devices is growing rapidly, and there is an extensive applications literature and a burgeoning industrial manufacturing infrastructure.

This chapter surveys the range and current state of development of micro-

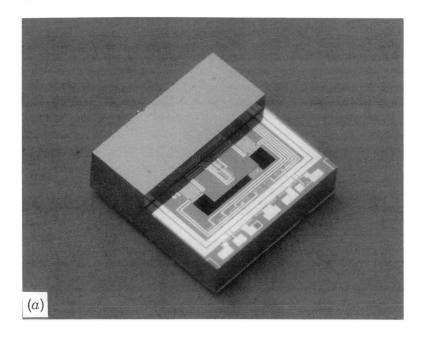

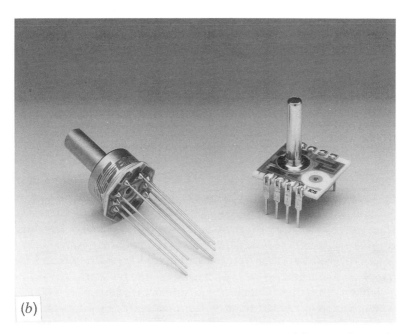

Figure 3.1. Examples of micromachined devices and sensors: (a) automotive accelerometer chip; (b) pressure sensor (photographs courtesy of ICSensors, Milpitas, CA).

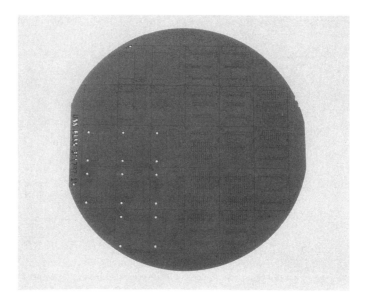

Figure 3.2. Etched silicon wafer illustrating a series of microchannel devices laid out on the mask in a repeating serpentine pattern.

machined devices and structures and discusses the future role of this technology in analysis. It also examines various glass and silicon devices that are chemically modified to form two-dimensional (2D) surface arrays of reactions zones and test areas that have micrometer dimensions. In an analytical context the new devices are variously referred to as *chips, microchips,* or *planar chips.*

3.2. MICROMACHINING TECHNIQUES AND MATERIALS

A range of techniques and materials are available for the fabrication of micro-devices (Table 3.2). Although photolithography of silicon is the most common combination, other materials and processes are in use or under investigation, including embossing, laser ablation, molding, and atomic force microscopic etching.

The size of features that can be fabricated in or on a surface is determined by the choice of fabrication process. Conventional photolithography (405 or 436 nm) is limited to features of approximately 1 μm. Deep-ultraviolet (UV) (230–260-nm) lithography has a minimum feature size of 0.3 μm, and x-ray and electron-beams (e-beams) can be used to generate features as small as 0.1 μm. The advent of the new high-power microscopes capable of imaging individual atoms and molecules has provided a means to produce even smaller features sizes. For example, a scanning tunneling microscope was used to etch a 150-nm-long, 8-nm-wide, <1-nm-deep groove on the surface of a rubidium molyb-

TABLE 3.2. Materials and Techniques for Micromachining

Materials Suitable for Micromachining

Alumina[135]
Aluminium[136]
Ceramics[137]
Copper[92]
Diamond[138]
Fluorocarbon polymers[139]
Gallium arsenide[140]
Glass (Pyrex, Corning 7059, 7740, Tempax, Schott B270, soda)[141,142]
Gold[143]
Indium phosphide[140]
Quartz[144]
Rubidium molybdenum oxide[15]
Silicon (110, 111)[3]
Silicon carbide[145]

Microfabrication Techniques

Atomic force microscopy[136,146]
Anisotropic etching[3]
Electron-beam (e-beam)[147]
Embossing[148]
Focused ion-beam (FIB)[149]
Isotropic etching[3]
Laser[150]
   Copper vapor[151]
   Excimer[137,152]
   Stereo[153]
   X-ray[154]
Reactive-ion etching (RIE)[155,156]
Scanning probe microscope[157,158]
Scanning tunneling microscope (STM)[73,159,160]
Solvent softening[148]

denum oxide crystal.[15] This type of techniques is still at an experimental stage but provides a means of fabricating nanometer sized structures.

Table 3.2 lists some of the different materials that are suitable for fabrication purposes. Silicon and glass are the most popular and are discussed in detail below.

3.2.1. Silicon

The micromachining of silicon to produce mechanical devices, using photolithographic etching procedures established by the microelectronics industry, is a relatively recent development. Multilayer etching using sacrificial layer techniques has permitted the fabrication of complex three-dimensional (3D) multi-component micrometer-sized devices such as electric motors. Silicon photo-lithography involves a series of steps:[1,3,16]

1. A photomask defining the shapes of the structures to be etched on the silicon wafer is generated (Fig. 3.3).
2. The silicon wafer is oxidized to produce a thin surface layer of chemically resistant silicon dioxide.
3. The wafer is evenly coated with a polymeric photoresist using a spin-coating procedure, and patterned using a photomask and a UV light source. The photoresist can be a positive resist (photoresist in areas of the wafer exposed to light is rendered soluble) or a negative resist (photoresist in areas of the wafer unexposed to light is rendered soluble). The insoluble polymerized resist remaining on the wafer forms a image of the photomask on the silicon dioxide surface of the water.
4. The wafer is dipped in hydrofluoric acid, and any exposed oxide layer is etched away (areas of oxide coated by the photoresist are protected from the etchant)

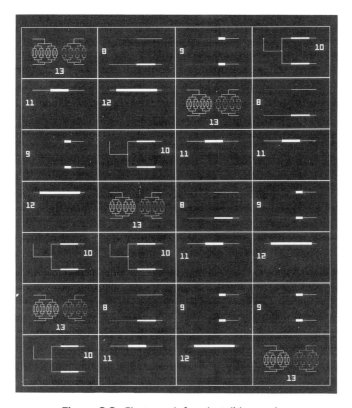

Figure 3.3. Photomask for photolithography.

5. The photoresist is removed from the surface of the wafer to give a silicon dioxide duplicate of the original photoresist pattern.

6. The exposed silicon is etched using either an isotropic etchant (e.g., hydrofluoric acid–nitric acid–acetic acid mixture) or an orientation-dependent anisotropic etchant [e.g., KOH (potassium hydroxide), hydrazine–water, ethylenediamine–pyrocatechol–water].

7. In the final step, the silicon dioxide layer is removed to give the final etched silicon wafer.

By using multiple masks and sacrificial layers, that permit undercutting to produce movable components,[17] it is possible to fabricate complex multicomponent structures on the surface of a silicon wafer. All of these fabrication steps must be performed in a cleanroom environment, thus permitting the production of sterile devices suitable for *in vivo* or clinical application.

3.2.2. Glass

Etching of glass is usually achieved using hydrofluoric acid. The etch is anisotropic, but this has not proved problematic in applications such as fabrication of capillary-zone electrophoresis chips. Microstructures in glass can also be formed by laser ablation techniques.

3.2.3. Molding

The LIGA process (Lithographie, Galvanoformung, Abformung) provides a way to manufacture a mold for a microstructure. It consists of the following steps. A resist-coated substrate is patterned using a mask and a source of synchrotron radiation (oriented x-rays). After development the resist structure is electroplated. This electroforming produces a metal microstructure (a negative replica of the structure) and this is then used as the mold for the final structure. Advantages of the LIGA process are that high aspect ratios can be attained (e.g., lateral dimensions of a few micrometers and vertical dimensions of ≤ 1000 μm), and the molds can be used to prepare multiple replicas of the structure in a variety of materials (e.g., polyimide, polymethylmethacrylate).[14]

Direct molding using a silicon master and a thermoplastic fluoropolymer (e.g., Hostaflon) at 150°C and at a pressure of 50 kg/cm^2 has been employed to fabricate channels for performing electrophoresis.[18] The plastic molded part was then clamped between two plates in order to complete the sealing of the channel.

3.2.4. Bonding and Sealing

Sealing structures to produce liquidtight enclosures (chambers, channels) is a key step in the fabrication of an analytical test device. Several different processes are available depending on the materials employed:[19]

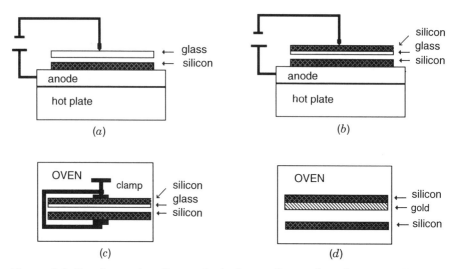

Figure 3.4. Bonding and sealing methods: (a, anodic bonding of glass to silicon; b, anodic bonding of silicon to silicon using a sputteref glass layer; c, low-melting glass bonding of silicon to silicon; d, eutectic bonding of silicon to silicon using a gold layer.

Anodic Bonding. Pyrex glass can be bonded to silicon using an anodic bonding (electrostatic, field-assisted) technique[20] (Fig. 3.4A). The thermal expansion coefficients of the two materials are similar; thus residual stress after bonding is minimized. A mirror-polished clean flat piece of glass is placed on top of a clean piece of polished silicon and heated to near the annealing point of the glass (180–500°C). A negative voltage of 200–1000 V is applied by attaching electrodes to the silicon (anode) and glass (cathode) The DC (direct-current) voltage creates an electric field between the two surfaces and pulls them into contact. This electrostatic attraction arises as follows: glass behaves as an electrolyte at high temperature, and there is a migration of ions (mostly Na^+ from the dissociation of Na_2O) toward the cathode that leaves a residual negative charge on the glass surface adjacent to the silicon surface. The actual bond is believed to be chemical, possibly a thin layer of silicon dioxide. Other materials can also be bonded using this process, including gallium arsenide–glass, and silicon–silicon. The latter is achieved by first sputtering a thin layer of Pyrex glass (4 μm thick) onto one of the silicon' surfaces (Fig. 3.4B).

Thermal Bonding. Glass can be bonded to glass using a simple thermal cycle process. An example of the sequence of steps in the bonding of Pyrex to Pyrex is shown in Table 3.3.[21]

Low-Temperature Glass Bonding. This process does not require an electric field (Fig. 3.4C). A thin layer of a low-melting glass, such as phoshosilicate glass, is coated onto one surface of a silicon wafer by a thermal growth or a

TABLE 3.3. Conditions for Glass–Glass Bonding

Step	Conditions
1	Clean surfaces place in furnace (optionally use weights to ensure close contact of two surfaces to be bonded)
2.	40°C/min to 550°C (total time 30 min)
3	20°C/min to 610°C (total time 30 min)
4	20°C/min to 635°C (total time 30 min)
5	10°C/min to 650°C (total time 6 h)
6	Natural cooling

Source: Reference 21.

sputtering process. The two wafers are then clamped together, forced into intimate contact using a vacuum pump, and then heated in a furnace at 1100°C for 30 min.[19]

Eutectic Bonding. This can be used for bonding two silicon surfaces.[19] A thin layer of gold is coated onto the surface of one of the wafers, or a thin sheet of gold–silicon or gold–tin mixture is placed between the two surfaces (a preform) (Fig. 3.4D). The assembled device is then clamped together and heated in a vacuum chamber above the eutectic temperature for the particular materials (e.g., eutectic temperature for Si/Au is 363°C). The preform melts and a diffusion process (gold into the silicon surface) leads to the formation of a silicon alloy between the contacted surfaces. As this cools, a bond is formed between the two surfaces.

Direct Bonding. Two mirror-polished flat silicon wafers can be bonded together as follows. The wafers are first washed (H_2O_2/H_2SO_4, followed by HF) and then dipped in dilute H_2SO_4 to form a hydrophillic surface layer. After washing and drying, the two surfaces are contacted whereupon a strong bond is formed (stable to 200°C).[22] In some cases a final heating step is included (1100°C for 2 h), which forms a permanent seal between the surfaces.[23]

Clamping. Structures may be sealed by simply forcing a cover into intimate contact with the molded part using a clamp.[18]

3.2.5. Drilling

It is important to be able to provide direct access into structures formed, for example, by bonding a glass top to a micromachined silicon part. Holes can be formed in both silicon and glass by deep etching. This is a relatively simple process, but does have the disadvantage of being slow and can damage existing surface structures. Mechanical, ultrasonic, and laser drilling are alternative procedures. Laser drilling is particularly well suited for drilling very small size holes (e.g., μ2 um using a deep-UV excimer laser). Holes can also be drilled through glass by means of an electrodischarge process in which the glass is submerged in an alkaline solution (e.g., NaOH) and a needle (30-μm-diameter tip) contacted with the glass and a negative potential applied (40 V).[24]

3.3. MICROMACHINED ANALYTICAL DEVICES

This section reviews some of the emerging clinical applications of micromachined devices. In many instances the opportunity for system integration to produce total chemical analysis systems (TAS) on a microminiature scale (μ-TAS) has been a key motivating factor in the development of these devices.[25]

3.3.1. Micromachined Silicon–Glass Structures for Semen Analysis

Silicon microchannels capped with Pyrex glass have proved to be an effective environment for the qualitative and quantitative assessment of sperm motility.[26–28] Figure 3.5A shows an example of one of the "SpermChip" devices. A semen sample (typically, 2 μL) is applied through a hole in the Pyrex glass cover into an open chamber at one end of a 100-μm-wide, 40-μm-deep fluid-filled microchannel. Progress of individual sperm along the tortuous channel constructed with a series of right-angle turns is monitored visually using a microscope (600× magnification), and a numerical scale next to the channel permits exact location of the sperm. The distribution of sperm along the length of the channel provides a measure of the motility and forward progression of sperm in the semen sample. Poorly motile sperm will migrate only a short distance along the channel, whereas in a sample containing large numbers of highly motile sperm, the number of sperm at the far end of the channel will be higher. Microchannels and microchambers can also be used for other tests of sperm function including immunoassays for sperm antibodies and sperm–cervical mucus penetration tests. Microchannel devices have also been adapted for the simultaneous testing of the effect of different spermicides and spermicide concentrations on motile sperm.

3.3.2. IVF Devices

A range of glass-capped microchips forming two chambers connected by tortuous 100-μm-wide × 40-μm-deep microchannel are under investigation for use in *in vitro* fertilization procedures. Eggs are placed in one of the chambers and semen added into the other chamber at the far end of the channel (Fig. 3.5B). Sperm must reach the eggs via the channel, and this has the advantageous effect of selecting the fastest, most motile sperm for the fertilization step.

3.3.3. Nucleic Acid Amplification

A range of nucleic acid amplification procedures are now available that require repetitive analytical steps and cycles of temperature changes. The polymerase

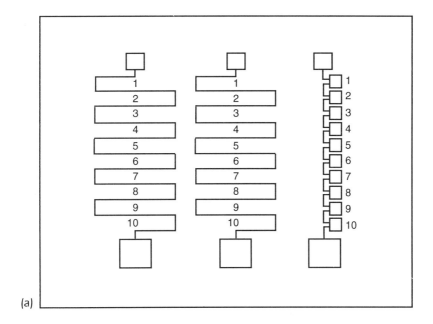

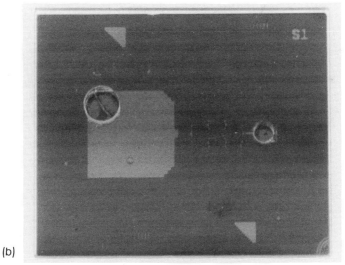

Figure 3.5. Schematic of a silicon glass sperm testing chip (*a*) and an *in vitro* fertilization chip (*b*).

chain reaction (PCR), because of its importance in research and routine applications, has been targeted by several groups for miniaturization using silicon microchambers. The thermal properties of silicon (e.g., high thermal conductivity, 1.57 W/cm °C; low thermal expansion coefficient, $2.33 \times 10^{-6}/°C$) make it an ideal fabrication material for reaction chambers designed for performing the rapid cycles of repeated heating and cooling required by the polymerase chain reaction. Several different designs of Pyrex-capped silicon micro-PCR chambers are in use with volumes ranging from 5 to 50 μL (Fig. 3.6).[29,30] Thermal cycling is achieved either by heaters built onto the chip, or by an external Peltier device. Very rapid cycle times can be achieved, thus shortening the overall time needed to complete a PCR reaction. The PCR reaction product is expelled from the chamber at the end of the reaction and analyzed electrophoretically. Figure 3.7 compares the amplification of a 500-bp sequence of lambda phage DNA in a micro-PCR chamber (9 μL; 14 × 8 mm, 80 μm deep) cycled using a Peltier device and the same mixture in a microtube in a conventional thermocycler. Comparable results are obtained indicating that there are no adverse effects in scaling down and performing the PCR reaction in a silicon–glass device. Miniaturization of the PCR reaction will make possible small handheld PCR machines. Proposed uses for such devices include on-site testing of human remains as an aid to identification of military personnel, and testing for biological weapons.[31]

3.3.4. DNA Analysis

Micromachined devices and microdimensioned arrays of oligonucleotides are being exploited in quantitative analysis of DNA and in DNA sequencing.

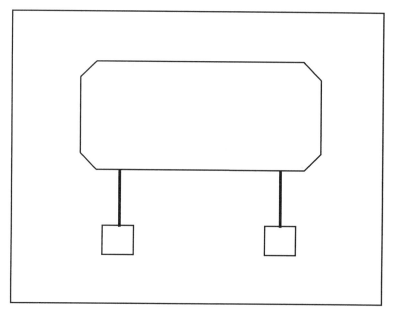

Figure 3.6. Schematic of a PCR chip (square inlet and outlet ports are connected by channels to a central microchamber, 9 μL).

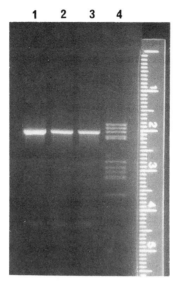

Figure 3.7. Gel electrophoresis of PCR reaction mixture (500-bp lambda phage target) stained with ethidium bromide (Lanes 1, conventional PCR in a microtube in a Perkin Elmer 9600 thermocycler; 2, 3, PCR performed in a silicon microchamber; 4, DNA-size markers).

3.3.4.1. TOTAL DNA. A silicon-based light-addressable potentiometric sensor (LAPS) detects total DNA according to the scheme shown in Figure 3.8. Denatured DNA in the sample reacts with biotinylated-DNA binding protein, anti-single-stranded DNA–urease, and avidin assay reagents. The resulting complexes are captured onto a biotinylated membrane. After washing the membrane is placed into contact with a LAPS to form a microchamber containing approximately 0.5 μL of a urea substrate solution. The conversion of urea to ammonia by the urease label produces a significant change in the pH of the solution and this is detected by the LAPS. As little as 2 pg (picograms) of DNA can be detected using this microanalytical device.[32,33]

3.3.4.2. SPECIFIC DNA SEQUENCES. LAPS devices are also used to detect specific DNA sequences. Sample DNA is reacted with biotinylated and fluorescein-labeled DNA probes specific for the target sequences. The reaction product is then reacted with an antifluorescein–urease conjugate, and complexes are captured onto a biotinylated membrane. Bound urease label is quantitated via change in pH using a LAPS. This 2-h assay detected 20×10^6 target molecules.[34] Vast arrays of nucleic acid probes immobilized on the surface of a small piece of glass or silicon ("DNA chip") are being developed by several groups for numerous purposes, including secondary structure analysis, analysis of basepairing properties, sequence comparison, optimization of PCR primers and antisense oligonucleotides, and sequencing.[35–37]

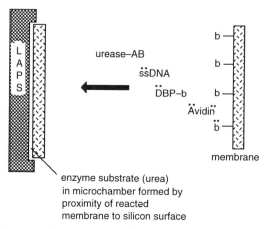

Figure 3.8. DNA assay using a urease label and a LAPS detector. (AB, antibody to DNA; b, biotin; DBP, DNA binding protein; ssDNA, single stranded DNA).

Two different preparative procedures are in development for the production of the arrays. One utilizes a simple microscope slide. The surface is activated chemically, and then clamped onto a glass plate that has a parallel array of 1-mm-diameter silicon rubber tubing spaced at 3-mm intervals (synthesis mask).[38] The channels formed by the spaces between the tubing define oligonucleotide synthesis sites on the activated glass surface. Rotation of the plate through 90° with respect to the mask permits reaction to be performed across the first line of reactions, thus producing a 2D array.[37,39,40]

The second procedure (light-directed parallel chemical synthesis) produces arrays with much smaller reaction zones, typically 50×50 μm or 100×100 μm in size. Oligonucleotide probes are immobilized at discrete locations on the surface of a glass chip by first activating the surface with a silanizing reagent that has reactive amino or hydroxyl groups. Photolabile protecting groups are then attached to the amino (or hydroxyl) groups and then different locations selectively addressed using a photolithographic mask and a light source.[36] Clear areas of the photomask expose the surface to light, and the protecting group is photolysed to unmask the reactive group. This group then becomes the site of attachment of an particular oligonucleotide. Repetition of this process with different masks exposes different surface locations, and hence it is possible to prepare a 2D oligonucleotide array. Studies with fluorescein labeled DNA probes and a scanning confocal microscope indicate that less than 100 fluorescein labels can be detected on a 1-μm^2 area, and that detection limits of 5–10 fluorescein labels/μm^2 may be achievable.[36] Using the current system it is possible to produce 10^5 synthesis sites per square centimeter, and an increase to 10^6 sites/cm^2 is anticipated.[41] Arrays of 256 eight-mer probes have been synthesized and recently all 65,536 eight-mers prepared as an array on a 1.28-cm^2 chip using a 32-step reaction.[42,43]

The reagent-array approach to analysis has several benefits. Very little reagent is required, and hence overall reagent costs are low. The eventual mass production of the devices will lead to a further economic benefit. Much of the surface is covered with reagent, hence minimizing nonspecific binding problems. Analysis using reagent arrays is particularly well suited to the testing for genetic diseases with many disease-causing mutations, for example, cystic fibrosis, which can be caused by >200 different mutations. Simultaneous testing for all of these mutations could be accomplished in a single assay on an array device.

Arrays of immobilized DNA probes in miniature test wells (100 μm^2) containing embedded microelectrodes form the basis of a novel test device for DNA analysis and sequencing. Hybridization of target DNA to a specific probe immobilized in a well changes the local electrical properties (dielectric dispersion) inside the well, and this is detected by measuring the dielectric relaxation frequency.[35]

Recently, the use of a CCD (charge-coupled device) to detect reactions of DNA with arrays of oligonucleotide arrays has been described.[44] The oligonucleotides were either immobilized directly onto the 420 × 420-pixel array of the CCD, or onto a silicon chip that was then pressed into contact with the CCD for measurement purposes. This format was adapted for detection of ^{32}P, fluorophore, and chemiluminogenic labels.

3.3.5. Immunoassay

Fluorescent bead latex–agglutination immunoassays for alphafetoprotein (AFP) have been performed in parallel in a series of four microchannels (0.4 μL; 10 mm long, 80 μm deep, 500 μm wide) etched in Pyrex glass.[45] The rate of agglutination of the 1.66-μm-diameter beads was enhanced using an alternating electric field and agglutination assessed by means of a fluorescent microscope and an image analyzer. The assay was rapid (1 min) and had a detection limit for AFP of 10 pg/mL.

A biotinylated capture membrane–LAPS combination used for DNA analysis (see Section 3.3.3) is also applicable to immunologic assays.[33,34] A model two-site immunoassay for mouse IgG, using a biotinylated antimouse antibody, a fluorescein-labeled antimouse antibody, an antifluorescein–urease conjugate, and avidin was linear over the range 25–5000 pg. This assay format was also been used to test for potential contaminants of recombinant protein products (e.g., *E. coli* protein, protein A), hormones (e.g., hCG), and infectious agents (e.g., *Yersinia pestis*). Antigen:antibody binding constants (e.g., antiricin antibody) have also been measured using a LAPS-based technique.[46]

A polished silicon wafer is highly reflective, and this property can be exploited in an optical biosensor immunoassay for hCG.[47] Aminopropyltriethoxysilane is used to activate the wafer surface, and then the activated surface reacted with an anti-hCG antibody. The wafer surface is then illuminated (short-wavelength UV radiation) through a quartz photomask having a periodic pattern of opaque and clear lines. This creates a surface grating pattern representing immunologically active and inactive antibody. Next, the wafer is diced into chips (4 × 5 mm), which are then mounted onto dipsticks. Reaction of active antibody on the surface of the chip with hCG (human chorionic gonadotropin) in a sample produces a biological diffraction grating. Illumination of the reacted chip with a diode laser (670 nm) produces a diffraction signal that is proportional to the hCG concentration in the sample [detection limit 5 international units per liter (IU/L)].

Microspot assays based on an array of 100-μm^2 zones of Texas Red labeled capture antibody deposited on a substrate (e.g., polystyrene) and a fluorescein labeled conjugate are being developed for immunoassays.[48] Also, fluorescence capillary-fill devices (FCFDs) constructed of two pieces of glass (30 mm long) spaced 100 um apart are under development for a range of immunoassays (e.g., prostate specific antigen, chorionic gonadotropin). A capture antibody is immobilized onto the inside surface of the glass, and a fluorescently labeled conjugate is microdosed into the device. Analyte present in the sample reacts with the antibodies to form sandwiches on the surface of the glass, and these are detected by an evanescent-wave technique.[49]

3.3.6. Cell Analysis

The microphysiometer (Cytosensor) measures the minute changes in pH that occur as a consequence of alterations in cellular metabolism.[50,51] It consists of a flow chamber (e.g., 50 μm deep × 6 mm diameter) which is in contact with the pH-sensitive silicon surface of a LAPS chip. A 1-mm^2 array of wells (50 × 50 × 50 μm: nominal volume 125 pL) is etched on the wafer surface and these trap the test cells.[52] A test substance is introduced into the flow chamber and its effect on cells trapped in the silicon wells assessed by monitoring changes in pH. The silicon microphysiometer is effective in a variety of applications, including studies of cellular-receptors[53,54] [e.g., granulocyte-macrophage colony-stimulating factor (GM-CSF) receptors],[55] muscarinic receptors,[52] cholinergic receptors,[54] viral infection (e.g., HIV-1), response to therapeutic agents (e.g., azidothymidine), cellular response to energy sources (e.g., glucose), and second-messenger pathways (e.g., protein kinase C).[34]

Physical properties of cells can be determined using micromachined silicon devices. For example a silicon microhemorheometer can be used to measure red cell deformability.[56] This silicon–silicon bonded structure comprises an array of 8 channels (5 × 5 × 100 μm) that are viewed through a SiO_2 window. An imaging system monitors the flow and deformation of red cells in the microchannels.

It is also possible to separate cells using micromachined silicon devices. Micromachined filters of different geometries, fabricated across the width of a 500-μm-wide × 5–40-μm-deep flow channel, effectively separate red and white blood cells, and also filter suspensions of latex microbeads from mixtures flowing along the channel (Fig. 3.9).[30] The filters are relatively easy to manufacture in a range of sizes and can thus be designed for a particular size separation. The

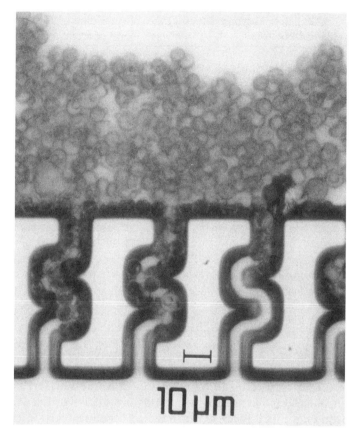

Figure 3.9. Silicon filter (5-μm spacings) in a 500-μm-wide channel

ability to perform size-based separations in a microfabricated device has numerous benefits in terms of sample handling and processing.

3.3.7. Chemical Analyzers

Integration of all of the components of an analyzer onto a single chip is an attractive proposition. A selection of miniature analyzers produced using microfabrication techniques are collected in Table 3.4. A blood pH analyzer (internal volume 50 nL) has been fabricated from a pH ion-selective electrode field-effect transistor (ISFET) in a silicon–glass structure. The device required a 10-μL sample of blood and the pH measurement was performed in a 5-nL measuring cell.[57] Similarly, a potassium sensitive ISFET was incorporated into a miniature analyzer.[58] Integration of sample and reagent addition in these miniature analyzers is due largely to the successful development of micropumps and microvalves[57] and microdetectors.[59,60] The flow rates in the microvalves can be as low as 1 μL/min and the valves have dead volumes <20 nL. Detector cells with

TABLE 3.4. Micromachined Chemical Analyzers and Detectors

Analyzers
Chlorine[161]
Flow injection[24]
Glucose[162]
pH[163]
pH, K, Ca[164]
Lactate[59]
p_{O_2}, p_{CO_2}, pH[165,166]
O_2[167]
K[58]
Titrator[168]
Na, K, Cl, urea nitrogen, glucose, hematocrit[72]

Detectors
Chemiluminescence[59]
Electrochemical[169]
Optical[170,171]
Thermal conductivity[64]

volumes in the range 1–100 nL have been constructed.[61] The degree of complexity that can be achieved with micromachining is illustrated by the chemiluminescent glucose and lactate analyzer.[59] This analyzer is fabricated on a 15 × 20-mm silicon chip capped with Pyrex glass (total internal volume of the analyzer is 15 μL). A microchamber filled with enzyme immobilized beads (100-μm diameter) reacts specifically with the analyte to generate hydrogen peroxide. This is transported to a mixing chamber, where it is mixed with the chemiluminescent reagent added via an inlet port. The reaction mixture is then pumped into a spiral flow cell and light emission detected using a photodiode. In a separate study, chemiluminescent light emission from alkaline phosphatase and horseradish peroxidase catalyzed reactions, and from the peroxyoxalate reaction in nanoliter reaction chambers was successfully detected using either a photomultiplier tube or a CCD camera.[62]

3.3.8. Chromatography

Miniaturization of separation techniques (Table 3.5) is a natural extension of the miniaturization of chromatographic media and the column dimensions of macroanalyzers.

3.3.8.1. GAS CHROMATOGRAPHY. In 1975 Terry described the fabrication of a gas chromatograph on a 5 cm diameter silicon wafer.[63] The chromatograph consisted of a 1.5-m-long spiral column (20 μm wide × 40 μm deep coated with OV-101 silicone oil) capped with a Pyrex glass cover plate. A thermal conduc-

TABLE 3.5. Micromachined Separation Devices

Electrophoresis
    Capillary[21,61,68,172–179]
    DNA[67]
    Polyacrylamide gel electrophoresis (PAGE)[179]
Chromatography
    Gas–liquid[64,89,180]
    Liquid[65,181,182]
Field-flow fractionation[183]
Filtration[109,184,185]

tivity detector was clamped onto the wafer, and a diaphragm valve (4-nL internal volume) was used for sample injection.[64] Separation times were short, and in a demonstration analysis a mixture of nitrogen, pentane, and hexane was resolved in <5 s. This early development provided a solid demonstration of the feasibility and capabilities of microfabrication techniques as applied to analytical instrumentation. Unfortunately, the scientific and commercial communities were not enthusiastic and this pioneering device did not gain acceptance for routine applications.

3.3.8.2. LIQUID CHROMATOGRAPHY. Hitachi have described a miniature liquid chromatograph that consists of a 5 × 5 × 0.4-mm chip capped with Pyrex glass. A 15-cm-long spiral column (6 μm wide, 2 μm deep, total volume 1.8 nL) is etched into the silicon surface. Separations on the column are monitored with a 1.2-pL detection cell.[65,66]

3.3.9. Electrophoresis

Electrophoretic separation of DNA based on length is simply accomplished using an obstacle course constituting an array of 2 million silicon posts (0.15 μm high, 1 μm diameter, 2.0 μm center-to-center) on a 2.7 × 2.7-mm piece of silicon wafer capped with Pyrex glass. Individual DNA molecules were stained with ethidium bromide and visualized by means of a fluorescence microscope and a CCD camera.[67]

There is widespread interest in the design and fabrication of capillary electrophoresis (CE) chips. Practical benefits of miniaturization of CE are valveless injections, zero dead volumes, and the small column dimensions, high thermal conductivity, and large mass of the glass substrate enable efficient dissipation of Joule heat. The latter feature permits the devices to be operated at higher electric field strengths and this leads to faster separations. Theoretical studies predict that reduction in size of capillaries leads to improved analytical performance. Separation efficiency is proportional to voltage applied across the separation capillary; thus it is possible to use very short length capillaries. Figure 3.10 illustrates the design and layout of a typical CE chip. Some examples of the dimensions of the separation and sample channels are collected in Table 3.6. CE

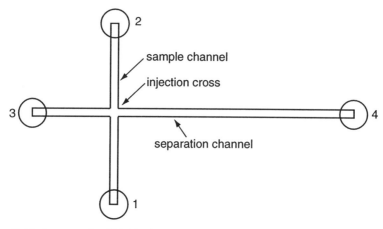

Figure 3.10. Layout of a CE chip (reservoirs; 1, waste; 2, analyte; 3, buffer; 4, waste).

chips have been fabricated from glass, silicon, and plastics. Glass is preferred because of its good dielectric properties. Silicon can be used but the surface of the capillary must be coated with an insulating layer of silicon dioxide or a double layer of silicon dioxide–silicon nitride because silicon is conductive. The use of plastics to fabricate CE chips has been described in the patent literature. A 5–8-cm serpentine channel (250 μm wide, 50 μm deep) was made using an etched silicon mold. The plastic replica was clamped between two glass plates to cap the channel and to provide mechanical rigidity.[18]

In CE chips sample injection is achieved by means of electroosmosis/ electrophoresis. The intersection of the separation and sample channel defines the injection volume and this can be pumped into the separation channel by

TABLE 3.6. Capillary Electrophoresis (CE) Chips

Channels Separation l(mm)/ w(μm)/ d(μm)	Sample l(mm)/ w(μm)/ d(μm)	Substrate	Reference
21.6/94/15	16.8/94/15	Glass	173
177.4[b]/90/10	18.8/90/10	Glass	172
16/10/5	8/10/5	Silicon	175
16/10/9	8/50/9	Silicon	
16/50/15	8/50/15	Silicon	
16/1000/10	8/30/10	Glass	68
16/30/10	8/30/10	Glass	
16/30/10	8/30/10	Glass	21
16/30/10	8/70/10	Glass	
16/70/10	8/70/10	Glass	

[a]*Key:* l = length; w = width; d = diameter.
[b]Serpentine channel.

switching voltages between the reservoirs at the ends of the channels (sample applied to reservoir 2 and voltages applied between reservoirs 2 and 3). Picoliter volumes are easily and reproducibly injected and separations achieved in the milliseconds to seconds time period. Detection of resolved components is usually by means of laser-induced fluorescence. CE separation can also be imaged using a charge coupled device (CCD) camera in conjunction with a laser. Resolution of mixtures of fluorescent dyes and FITC-labeled amino acids has demonstrated the analytical utility of CE chips.[68]

3.4. NANOTECHNOLOGY

Nanotechnology can be defined as "a technology giving nearly complete control of the structure of matter on a nanometer scale."[13] The proposed nanomachines will be two to three orders of magnitude smaller than the current silicon micromachines. A nanomachine represents the ultimate goal in microengineering. Individual atoms and molecules will be used to fabricate devices.[69] Biological structures and biomolecules have reexamined by engineers from a nanotechnological perspective. A ribosome is viewed as a production line, a binding site on a molecule is seen as a clamp, an enzyme is considered a tool for accomplishing a specific modifications, and the flagella of bacteria are seen as drive shafts to power the new nanomachines. Nanomachines are not practical realities, but nevertheless they represent an important direction in miniaturization research.

Nanotechnology is also being investigated from the viewpoint of the chemist. The new area of nanochemistry is concerned with the synthesis and properties of molecules that will spontaneously associate (molecular self-assembly) to produce nanostructures.[70] For example, nanotubules can be formed from certain cyclic polypeptides. On protonation these molecules crystallize to form tubules >100 nm long and 0.7–0.8 nm in diameter.[71]

3.5. CONCLUSIONS

Silicon and glass micromachined devices are emerging as viable alternatives to conventional macroscale analytical systems, and in some applications providing analytical capabilities not possible using macroscale systems. An increasingly diverse range of analytical devices are being fabricated and tested, but as yet few of these devices have been commercialized for use in routine clinical laboratories. In many cases there is only preliminary information on assay performance and reliability, and economic issues.

The i-STAT (i-STAT Corporation, Princeton, NJ), Cytosensor, and Threshold (Molecular Devices, Menlo Park, CA) are among the first commercial analyzers to exploit silicon technology. The i-STAT is a whole-blood analyzer that is based on a silicon chip biosensor array.[72] The Cytosensor and Threshold exploit measurements of minute pH changes due to cellular metabolism or the activity of a urease label to study cells or measure macromolecules, respectively. Success of these devices should promote interest in the analytical applications of silicon-based microanalyzers.

In the distant future nanotechnological analytical devices may gain widespread popularity. Progress in this area has been slow, but the results obtained with scanning tunneling microscopes (STMs) already indicate that nanometer and sub-nanometer-sized features can be created on surfaces.[15,73] Armed with routine nanometer-scale micromaching, the next step will be to assemble complete analyzers or at least analytically useful structures in order to demonstrate proof of principle.

REFERENCES

1. Angell JB, Terry SC, Barth PW: Silicon micromechanical devices. *Sci Am* 248:44–55, 1983.

2. Amoto I: Small things considered: Scientists craft machines that seem impossibly tiny. *Sci News* 136:8–10, 1989.

3. Petersen KE: Silicon as a mechanical material. *Proc IEEE* 70:420–456, 1982.

4. Mallon J: Nanotechnology from a micromachinist's point of view. In Crandall BC, Lewis J, eds.: *Nanotechnology—Research and Perspectives.* Cambridge: MIT Press, 1992, pp. 215–240.

5. Stix G: Micron machinations. *Sci Am* 267:106–117, 1992.

6. Crandall BC, Lewis J: *Nanotechnology—Research and Perspectives.* Cambridge, MA: MIT Press, 1992.

7. Drexler KE: Molecular engineering: an approach to the development of general capabilities for molecular manipulation. *Proc Natl Acad Sci* (USA) 78:5275–5278, 1981.

8. Drexler KE: *Engines of Creation.* Garden City, NY: Anchor Press, 1986.

9. Drexler KE: Nanomachinery: atomically precise gears and bearings. *Proceedings of IEEE Micro Robots and Teleoperators Workshop.* New York: IEEE, 1987, pp 1–6.

10. Drexler KE: Molecular machinery and molecular electronic devices. In Carter F, ed: *Molecular Electronic Devices II.* New York: Marcel Dekker, 1987, pp 549–571.

11. Drexler E, Peterson C, Pergamit G: *Unbounding the Future. The Nanotechnology Revolution.* New York: William Morrow, 1991.

12. Drexler KE: Molecular directions in nanotechnology. *Nanotechnology* 2:113–118, 1991.

13. Drexler KE: Machines of inner space. In Crandall BC, Lewis J, eds: *Nanotechnology—Research and Perspectives.* Cambridge: MIT Press, 1992, pp 325–346.

14. Bryzek J, Petersen K, McCulley W: Micromachines on the march. IEEE *Spectrum* 31:20–31, 1994.

15. Garfunkel E, Rudd G, Novak D, et al: Scanning tunneling microscopy and nanolithography on a conducting oxide, $RB_{0.3}$ MoO_3. *Science* 246:99–100, 1989.

16. Sze SM: *VLSI Technology,* 2nd ed. New York: McGraw-Hill, 1988.

17. Fan L-S, Tai Y-C, Muller RS: Integrated movable micromechanical structures for sensors and actuators. *IEEE Trans Electron Devices* 35:724–730, 1988.

18. Ekström B, Jacobson G, Öhman O, Sjödin H: Microfluidic structure and process for its manufacture. WO Patent 16966, 1991.

19. Ko WH, Suminto JT, Yeh GJ: Bonding techniques for microsensors. In Fung CD, Cheung PW, Ko WH, Fleming DG, eds: *Micromachining and Micropackaging of Transducers.* New York: Elsevier Science, 1985, pp 41–61.

20. Wallis G, Pomerantz DI: Field-assisted glass-metal sealing. *J Appl Phys* 40:3946–3949, 1969.

21. Fan ZH, Harrison DJ: Micromachining of capillary electrophoresis injectors and separators on glass chips and evaluation of flow at capillary intersections. *Anal Chem* 66:177–184, 1994.

22. Stengl R, Ahn K, Gosele U: Bubble-free silicon wafer bonding in a non-cleanroom environment. *Jpn J Appl Phys* 27:2364–2366, 1988.

23. Shimbo M, Furukawa K, Fukuda K, Tanzawa K: Silicon-to-silicon direct bonding method. *J Appl Phys* 60:2987–2989, 1986.

24. Shoji S, Esashi M: Microfabrication and microsensors. *Appl Biochem Biotechnol* 41:21–34, 1993.

25. Manz A, Graber N, Widmer HM: Miniaturized total analysis systems: a novel concept for chemical sensors. *Sens Actuators* B1:244–248, 1990.

26. Kricka LJ, Wilding P: Mesoscale sperm handling devices. US Patent 5296375, 1994.

27. Kricka LJ, Nozaki O, Heyner S, Garside WT, Wilding P: Applications of a microfabricated device for evaluating sperm function. *Clin Chem* 39:1944–1947, 1993.

28. Kricka LJ, Ji X, Nozaki O, Heyner S, Garside WT, Wilding P: Sperm testing with microfabricated glass-capped silicon microchannels. *Clin Chem* 40:1823–1824, 1994.

29. Northrup MA, Ching MT, White RM, Watson RT: DNA amplification with a microfabricated reaction chamber. *IEEE International Conference on Solid-State Sensors and Actuators* (Transducers '93). New York: IEEE, 1993.

30. Wilding P, Shoffner M, Kricka LJ: PCR in a silicon microstructure. *Clin Chem* 40:1815–1818, 1994.

31. Stix G: Gene readers. *Sci Am* 271:149–150, 1994.

32. Kung VT, Panfili PR, Sheldon EL, et al: Picogram quantities of total DNA using DNA-binding proteins in a silicon sensor-based system. *Anal Biochem* 187:220–227, 1990.

33. Briggs J, Fanfili PR: Quantitation of DNA and protein impurities in biopharmaceuticals. *Anal Chem* 63:850–859, 1991.

34. Owicki JC, Bousse LJ, Hafeman DG, et al: The light-addressable poteniometric sensor. *Annu Rev Biophys Biomol Struct* 23:87–113, 1994.

35. Beattie K, Eggers M, Shumaker J, et al: Genosensor technology. *Clin Chem* 39:719–722, 1993.

36. Sheldon EL, Briggs J, Bryan R, et al: Matrix DNA hybridization. *Clin Chem* 39:718–719, 1993.

37. Southern EM, Maskos U, Elder JK: Analyzing and comparing nucleic acid sequences by hybridization to arrays of oligonucleotides: evaluation using experimental models. *Genomics* 13:1008–1017, 1992.

38. Southern EM, Maskos U: Parallel synthesis and analysis of large numbers of related chemical compounds: applications to oligonucleotides. *J Biotechnol* 35:217–227, 1994.

39. Maskos U, Southern EM: A novel method for the parallel analysis of multiple mutations. *Nucl Acids Res* 21:2269–2270, 1993.

40. Maskos U, Southern EM: A novel method for the analysis of multiple sequence variants by hybridization to oligonucleotides. *Nucl Acids Res* 21:2267–2268, 1993.

41. Fodor SPA, Rava RP, Huang XC, Pease AC, Holmes CP, Adams CL: Multiplexed biochemical assays with biological chips. *Nature* 364:555–556, 1993.

42. Jacobs JW, Fodor SPA: Combinatorial chemistry—applications of light-directed chemical synthesis. *Tibtech* 12:19–26, 1994.

43. Lipschutz RJ, Fodor SPA: Advanced DNA sequencing technologies. *Curr Opin Struct Biol* 4:376–380, 1994.

44. Eggers M, Hogan M, Reich RK, et al: A microchip for quantitative detection of molecules utilizing luminescent and radioisotope reporter groups. *BioTechniques* 17:516–524, 1994.

45. Song MI, Iwata K, Yamada M, et al: Multisample analysis using an array of microreactors for an alternating-current field-enhanced latex immunoassay. *Anal Chem* 66:778–781, 1994.

46. Dill K, Lin M, Poteras C, et al: Antibody-antigen binding constants determined in solution-phase with the threshhold membrane-capture system: binding constants for anti-fluorescein, anti-saxitoxin, and anti-ricin antibodies. *Anal Biochem* 217:128–138, 1994.

47. Tsay YG, Lin CI, Lee J, et al: Optical biosensor assay (OBA). *Clin Chem* 37:1502–1505, 1991.

48. Ekins R, Chu FW: Multianalyte microspot immunoassay—microanalytical "compact disk" of the future. *Clin Chem* 37:1955–1967, 1991.

49. Fletcher JE, O'Neil PM, Stafford CG, Daniels PB, Bacarese-Hamilton T: Rapid, biosensor-based, assay for PSA in whole blood. *Tumor Marker Update* 5:99–101, 1993.

50. Parce JW, Owicki JC, Kercso KM, et al: Detection of cell-affecting agents with a silicon bioisensor. *Science* 246:243–247, 1989.

51. McConnell HM, Owicki JC, Parce JW, et al: The cytosensor microphysiometer: biological applications of silicon technology. *Science* 257:1906–1912, 1992.

52. Baxter GT, Young M-L, Miller DL, Owicki JC: Using microphysiometry to study the pharmacology of exogenously expressed m1 and m3 muscarinic receptors. *Life Sci* 55:573–583, 1994.

53. Miller DL, Olson JC, Parce JW, Owicki JC: Cholinergoic stimulation of the Na^+/K^+ adenosine triphosphatase as revealed by microphysiometry. *Biophys J* 64:813–823, 1993.

54. Bousse LJ, Miller DL, Owicki JC, Parce JW: Rapid determination of cellular metabolic rates with a silicon microphysiometer. *IEEE International Conference on Solid-State Sensors and Actuators* (Transducers '91). New York: IEEE, 1991, pp 74–77.

55. Baxter GT, Miller DL, Kuo RC, Wada HG, Owicki JC: PKce is involved in granulocyte-macrophage colony-stimulating factor signal transduction: evidence from microphysiometry and antisense oligonucleotide experiments. *Biochemistry* 31:10950–10954, 1992.

56. Tracy MC, Kaye PH, Shepherd JN: Microfabricated microhaemorheometer. *IEEE International Conference on Solid-State Sensors and Actuators* (Transducers '91). New York: IEEE, 82–84, 1991.

57. Shoji S, Esashi M, Matsuo T: Prototype miniature blood gas analyser fabricated on a silicon wafer. *Sens Actuators* 14:101–107, 1988.

58. Van der Schoot B, van den Berg A, Jeanneret S, de Rooij N: A miniaturized chemical analysis system using two silicon micro pumps. *IEEE International Conference on Solid-State Sensors and Actuators* (Transducers '91). New York: IEEE, 1991, pp 789–791.

59. Suda M, Sakuhara T, Karube I: Miniaturized detectors for a chemical-analysis system. *Appl Biochem Biotechnol* 41:3–10, 1993.

60. Liu CC: Applications of microfabrication techniques in electrochemical sensor development. *Appl Biochem Biotechnol* 41:99–107, 1993.

61. Manz A, Harrison DJ, Verpoorte EMJ, et al: Planar chips technology for miniaturization and integration of separation techniques into monitoring systems. Capillary electrophoresis on a chip. *J Chromatogr* 593:253–258, 1992.

62. Kricka LJ, Ji X, Nozaki O, Wilding P: Imaging of chemiluminescent reactions in mesoscale silicon-glass microstructures. *J Biolumin Chemilumin* 9:135–138, 1994.

63. Terry SC: A gas chromatograph system fabricated on a silicon wafer using integrated circuit technology. PhD thesis, Stanford University, 1975.

64. Terry SC, Jerman JH, Angell JB: A gas chromatograph air analyzer fabricated on a silicon wafer. *IEEE Trans Electron Devices* ED-26:1880–1886, 1979.

65. Manz A, Miyahara Y, Miura J, Watanabe Y, Miyagi H, Sato K: Design of an open-tubular column liquid chromatograph using silicon chip technology. *Sens Actuators* B1:249–255, 1990.

66. Prohaska O, Prohaska OJ: Thin-film capillary chromatography device. Eur Patent Appl 307530, 1989.

67. Volkmuth WD, Austin RH: DNA electrophoresis in microlithographic arrays. *Nature* 358:600–602, 1992.

68. Harrison DJ, Fan Z, Seler K, Manz A, Widmer HM: Rapid separation of fluorescein derivatives using a micromachined capillary electrophoresis system. *Anal Chim Acta* 283:361–366, 1993.

69. Kaehler T: Nanotechnology: Basic concepts and definitions. *Clin Chem* 40:1797–1799, 1994.

70. Whitesides GM, Mathias JP, Seto CT: Molecular self-assembly and nanochemistry: a chemical strategy for the synthesis of nanostructures. *Science* 254:1312–1319, 1991.

71. Ghadiri MR, Granja JR, Milligan RA, McRee DE, Khazanovich N: Self-assembling organic nanotubes based on cyclic peptide architecture. *Nature* 366:324–327, 1993.

72. Erickson KA, Wilding P: Evaluation of a novel point-of-care system, the i-STAT portable clinical analyzer. *Clin Chem* 39:283–287, 1993.

73. Kobayashi A, Grey F, Williams RS, Aono M: Formation of nanometer-scale grooves in silicon with a scanning tunneling microscope. *Science* 259:1724–1726, 1993.

74. Allen HV, Terry SC, de Bruin DW: Accelerometer systems with built-in testing. Sensors and Actuators A-Physical vol 21, no 1–3, p 381–386, 1990.

75. Tschan T, de Rooij NF, Bezinge A: Damping of piezoresistive silicon accelerometers. *Sens Actuators* A32:375–379, 1992.

76. Weinberg MS, Greiff P: Permanent magnet force rebalance micro accelerometer. US Patent 5,060,039, 1991.

77. Minami K, Kawamura S, Esashi M: Fabrication of distributed electrostatic micro actuator (DEMA). *J MEMS* (Microelectromechanical Systems) 2:121–127, 1993.

78. Linder C, de Rooij NF: Investigations on free-standing polysilicon beams in view of their applications as transducers. *Sensors and Actuators A-Physical* vol 23, no 1–3 p 1053–1059, 1990.

79. Rapoport SD, Reed ML, Weiss LE: Fabrication and testing of a microdynamic rotor for blood flow measurement. *J Micromech Microeng* 1:60–65, 1991.

80. Brugger J, Buser RA, de Rooij NF: Silicon cantilevers and tips for scanning force microscopy. *Sens Actuators* A34:193–200, 1992.

81. Buser RA, Brugger J, de Rooij NF: Micromachined silicon cantilevers and tips for scanning probe microscopy. *Microelectronic Eng* 15:407–410, 1991.

82. Buser RA, Brugger J, de Rooij NF: Micromachined silicon cantilevers and tips for bidirectional force microscopy. *Ultramicroscopy* 42:1476–1480, 1992.

83. Jaecklin VP, Linder C, de Rooij NF, Moret JM: Micromechanical comb actuators with low driving voltage. *J Micromech Microeng* 2:250–255, 1992.

84. Jaecklin VP, Linder C, de Rooij NF, Moret J-M: Comb acuators for *xy*-microstages. *Sensors and Actuators A-Physical* vol 39, no 1, p 83–89, 1993.

85. Jerman JH: The fabrication and use of micromachined corrugated silicon diaphragms. *Sensors and Actuators A-Physical* vol 23, no 1–3, p 988–992, 1990.

86. Racine GA, Luthier R, de Rooij NF: Piezoelectric position sensor for ultrasonic EFM motors. *Sensors and Actuators A-Physical* vol 42, no 1–3, p 661–665, 1994.

87. Murakami Y , Motohashi K, Yano K, et al: Micromachined electroporation system for transgenic fish. *J Biotechnol* 34:35–42, 1994.

88. Jerman JH, Clift DJ, Mallinson SR: A miniature Fabry-Perot interferometer with a corrugated silicon diaphragm support. *Sens Actuators* A29:151–158, 1991.

89. Bruns MW: High-speed portable gas-chromatograph—silicon micromachining. *Erdol Kohle Erdgas Petrochem* 47:80–84, 1994.

90. Suzuki H, Sugama A: Micromachined glass electrode. *Sens Actuators* B20:27–32, 1994.

91. Suzuki Y: Fabrication and evaluation of flexible microgripper. *Jpn J Appl Phys* 33:2107–2112, 1994.

92. Friedrich CR, Kang SD: Micro-heat exchangers fabricated by diamond machining. *Prec Eng J Am Soc Prec Eng* 16:56–59, 1994.

93. Muller RS, Mastrangelo CH: Vacuum-sealed silicon incandescent light. US Patent 5,285,131, 1994.

94. Pham L, Tjhen W, Ye C, Polla DL: Surface-micromachined pyroelectric infrared imaging array with vertically integrated signal-processing circuitary. *IEEE Trans Ultrasonics Ferroelectrics Freq Control* 41:552–555, 1994.

95. Smith L, Soderbarg A, Bjorkengren U: Continuous ink-jet print head utilizing silicon micromachined nozzles. *Sens Actuators* A43:311–316, 1994.

96. Aratani K, French PJ, Sarro PM, Poenar D, Wolffenbuttel RF, Middelhoek S: Surface micromachining tunable interferometer array. *Sens Actuators* A43:17–23, 1994.

97. Brugger J, Blanc N, Renaud P, de Rooij NF: Microlever with combined integrated

sensor actuator functions for scanning force microscopy. *Sens Actuators* A43:339–345, 1994.

98. Kawahito S, Sasaki Y, Sato H, Nakamura T, Tadokoro Y: A fluxgate magnetic sensor with micro-solenoids and electroplated permalloy cores. *Sens Actuators* A43:128–134, 1994.

99. Kadar Z, Bossche A, Mollinger J: Integrated resonant magnetic-field sensor. *Sens Actuators* A41:66–69, 1994.

100. Murphy P, Hubschi K, de Rooij NF, Racine C: Subminiature silicon integrated electret capacitor microphone. *IEEE Trans Elec Insul* 24:2495–2498, 1989.

101. Schneider U, Schellin R: A phase-modulating microphone utilizing integrated-optics and micromachining in silicon. *Sens Actuators* A42:695–698, 1994.

102. Muller RS, Kim S: IC processed piezoelectric microphone. US Patent 4,783,821, 1988.

103. Mognardi MA: Digital mirror array for projection TV. *Solid State Technol* 37:63ff, 1994.

104. Kenny TW, Waltman SB, Reynolds JK, Kaiser WJ: Micromachined silicon tunnel sensor for motion detection. *Appl Phys Lett* 58:100–102, 1991.

105. Paratte L, Racine G-A, de Rooij NF, Bornand E: A rigid ring electrostatic harmonic wobble motor with axial field. *IEEE International Conference on Solid-State Sensors and Actuators* (Transducers '91). New York: IEEE, 1991, pp 890–893.

106. Paratte L, Racine G, de Rooij NF, Bornand E: Design of an integrated stepper motor with axial field. *Sens Actuators* A25–A27:597–603, 1991.

107. White RM: Method and apparatus for using ultrasonic energy for moving microminiature elements. US Patent 5,006,749, 1991.

108. Cocco M, Dario P, Toro M, Pastacaldi P, Sacchett R: An implantable neural connector incorporating microfabricated components. *J Micromech Microeng* 3:219–221, 1993.

109. Kittilsland G, Stemme G: A sub-micron particle filter. *Sens Actuators* A21–A23:904–907, 1990.

110. Weng PK, Shie JS: Micro-Pirani vacuum gauge. *Rev Sci Instrum* 65:492–499, 1994.

111. Wang AW, Costello BJ, White RM: An ultrasonic flexural plate-wave sensor for measurement of diffusion in gels. *Anal Chem* 65:1639–1642, 1993.

112. Tomita Y, Koyanagawa Y, Satoh F: A surface motor-driven positioning system. *Prec Eng J Am Soc Prec Eng* 16:184–191, 1994.

113. de Bruin DW, Allen HV, Terry SC, Jerman JH: Electrically trimmable silicon micromachined pressure switch. *Sens Actuators* A21–A23:54–57, 1990.

114. Buser R, de Rooij NF: Silicon pressure sensor based on a resonating element. *Sens Actuators* A25–A27:717–722, 1991.

115. Fuhr G, Hagedorn R, Müller T, Benecke W, Wagner B: Pumping of water solutions in microfabricated electrohydrodynamic systems. *Proceedings of the Microelectromechanical Systems Conference* (MEMS '92). New York: IEEE, 1992, pp 25–30.

116. Gass V, van der Schoot BH, Jeanneret S, de Rooij NF: Micro liquid handling using a flow-regulated silicon micropump. *J Micromech Microeng* 3:214–215, 1993.

117. Rapp R, Schomburg WK, Maas D, Schulz J, Stark W: LIGA micropump for gases and liquids. *Sens Actuators* A40:57–61, 1994.

118. Richter A, Plettner A, Hofmann KA, Sandmaier H: A micromachined electrohydrodynamic (EHD) pump. *Sens Actuators* A29:159–168, 1991.

119. Schomburg WK, Fahrenberg J, Maas D, Rapp R: Active valves and pumps for microfluidics. *J Micromech Microeng* 3:216–218, 1993.

120. Stemme E, Stemme G: A valveless diffuser/nozzle-based fluid pump. *Sens Actuators* A39:159–167, 1993.

121. O'Connor L: Micromachining read-and-write heads. *Mech Eng* 116:126, 1994.

122. Little W: Microminiature refrigeration. *Rev Sci Instrum* 55:661–680, 1984.

123. Yasuda T, Shimoyama I, Miura H: Microrobot actuated by a vibration energy-field. *Sens Actuators* A43:366–370, 1994.

124. Akin T, Najafi K, Smoke RH, Bradley RM: A micromachined silicon sieve electrode for nerve regeneration applications. *IEEE Trans Biomed Eng* 41:305–313, 1994.

125. Müller A, Göttert J, Mohr J: LIGA microstructures on top of micromachined silicon wafers used to fabricate a micro-optical switch. *J Micromech Microeng* 3:158–160, 1993.

126. Quataishat S, Davidsson P, Desling P, et al: Design of microelectronic thermal detectors for high-resolution radiation spectroscopy. *Nucl Instr Meth Phys Res A* 342:504–508, 1994.

127. Buser R, de Rooij NF: Tuning forks in silicon. *Proceedings of IEEE Micro-Electro Mechanical Systems* (Workshop). Salt Lake City, UT: IEEE; New York, 1989, pp 94–95.

128. Gordon GB: Thermally-actuated microminiature valve. US Patent 5,058,856, 1991.

129. Jensen OS, Gravesen P: Flow characteristics of a micromachined diaphragm valve designed for liquid flows above 1 ml min^{-1}. *J Micromech Microeng* 3:236–238, 1993.

130. Perers GEL: Valve devices. US Patent 5,197,517, 1993.

131. Shoji S, Van der Schoot B, de Rooij N, Esashi M: Smallest dead volume microvalves for integrated chemical analysing system. *IEEE International Conference on Solid-State Sensors and Actuators* (Transducer '91). New York: IEEE, 1991, pp 1052–1055.

132. Trah H-P, Baumann H, Döring C, Goebel H, Grauer T, Mettner M: Micromachined valve with hydraulically actuated membrane subsequent to a thermoelectrically controlled bimorph cantilever. *Sens Actuators* A39:169–176, 1993.

133. Zdeblick M: Integrated, microminiature electric to fluidic valve and pressure/flow regulator. US Patent 4,943,032, 1990.

134. Xiao Z, Norrman S, Engstrom O: A fiber optical voltage sensor prepared by micromachining and wafer bonding. *Sens Actuators* A41:334–337, 1994.

135. Knapp J, Andreae G, Petersohn D: Ceramic sensor technology for the measurement of mechanical quantities at high temperature. *Sens Actuators* A21–A23:1080–1083, 1990.

136. Chen LL, Guay D: Selected dissolution of aluminium initiated by atomic-force microscope tip-surface interaction. *J Electrochem Soc* 141:L43–L45, 1994.

137. Goller M, Lutz N, Geiger M: Micromachining of ceramics with excimer-laser radiation. *J Eur Ceram Soc* 121:315–321, 1993.

138. Herb JA, Peters MG, Terry SC, Jerman JH: PECVD diamond films for use in silicon microstructures. *Sens Actuators* A21–A23:982–987, 1990.

139. Jansen HV, Gardeniers JGE, Elders J, Tilmans HAC, Elwenspoek M: Applications of

fluorocarbon polymers in micromechanics and micromachining. *Sensors and Actuators A-Physical,* vol 41, no 1–3, p 136–140, 1994.

140. Khare R, Hu EL, Brown JJ, Melendes MA: Micromachining in III-V semiconductors using wet photoelectrochemical etching. *J Vac Sci Technol B* 11:2497–2501, 1993.

141. Lom B, Healy KE, Hockberger PE: A versatile technique for patterning biomolecules onto glass coverslips. *J Neurosci Meth* 50:385–397, 1993.

142. Dietrich TR, Abraham M, Diebel J, Lacher M, Ruf A: Photoetchable glass for microsystems: tips for atomic force microscopy. *J Micromech Microeng* 3:187–189, 1993.

143. Abbott NL, Kumar A, Whitesides GM: Using micromachining, molecular self-assembly, and wet etching to fabricate 0.1–1 um scale structures of gold and silicon. *Chem Mater* 6:596–602, 1994.

144. Danel JS, Delapierre G: Quartz: a material for microdevices. *J Micromech Microeng* 1:187–198, 1991.

145. Muller G, Krotz G: SiC for sensors and high-temperature electronics. *Sens Actuators* A43:259–268, 1994.

146. Kim Y, Lieber C: Machining oxide thin films with an atomic force microscope: pattern and object formation on the nanometer scale. *Science* 257:371–377, 1992.

147. Brünger WH, Kohlmann KT: E-Beam-induced fabrication of microstructures. *J MEMS* 2:30–32, 1993.

148. Columbus RL: Liquid transport device. US Patent 4,233,029, 1980.

149. Khamsehpour B, Davies ST: Angle lapping of multilayer structures for thickness measurement using focused ion-beam micromachining. *Semicond Sci Technol* 9:249–255, 1994.

150. Osvay K, Bor Z, Racz B, Hertz J: Direct writing and in-situ material processing by a laser-micromachining projection microscope. *Appl Phys A Sol Surf* 58:211–214, 1994.

151. Editorial. Notes on micromachining with copper-vapor lasers. *Opt Laser Technol* 26:200–201, 1994.

152. Seddon BJ, Shao Y, Fost J, Girault HH: The application of excimer-laser micromachining for the fabrication of disc microelectrodes. *Electrochim Acta* 39:783–791, 1994.

153. Bloomstein TM, Ehrlich DJ: Laser-chemical three-dimensional writing for micro-electromechanics and application to standard-cell microfluidics. *J Vac Sci Tech B* 10:2671–2674, 1992.

154. Hawryluk AM, Ciarlo DR, Rambach GD: X-ray laser fabrication by aniosotropic etching of silicon. *J Vac Sci Technol B* 3:276–281, 1985.

155. Shaw KA, Zhang ZL, MacDonald NC: SCREAM I: A single mask, single-crystal silicon, reactive ion etching process for microelectromechanical structures. *Sens Actuators* A40:63–70, 1994.

156. Li YX, Wolffenbuttel MR, French PJ, Laros M, Sarro PM, Wolffenbuttel RF: Reactive ion etching (RIE) techniques for micromachining applications. *Sens Actuators* A41:317–323, 1994.

157. Sumomogi T, Endo T, Kuwahara K, Kaneko R, Miyamoto T: Micromachining of metal surfaces by scanning probe microscope. *J Vac Sci Technol B* 12:1876–1880, 1994.

158. Stroscio JA, Eigler D: Atomic and molecular manipulation with the scanning tunneling microscope. *Science* 254:1319–1326, 1991.

159. Eigler D, Schweizer E: Positioning single atoms with a scanning tunnelling microscope. *Nature* 344:524–526, 1990.

160. Foster J, Frommer J, Arnett P: Molecular manipulation using a tunnelling microscope. *Nature* 331:324–326, 1988.

161. van den Berg A, Grisel A, Verney-Norberg E, van der Schoot BH, Koudelka-Hep M, de Rooij NF: On-wafer fabricated free-chlorine sensor with ppb detection limit for drinking-water monitoring. *Sens Actuators* B13:396–369, 1993.

162. Murakami Y, Takeuchi T, Yokoyama K, Tamiya E, Karube I: Integration of enzyme-immobilized column with electrochemical flow cell using micromachined techniques for a glucose detection system. *Anal Chem* 65:2731–2735, 1993.

163. Shoji S, Esashi M, Masuo T: Prototype miniature blood gas analyzere fabricated on a silicon wafer. *Sens Actuators* 14:101–107, 1988.

164. van der Schoot BH, van den Vlekkert HH, van den Berg A, Grisel A, de Rooij NF: A flow injection analysis system with a glass-bonded ISFETs for the simultaneous detection of calcium and potassium and pH. *Sens Actuators* B4:239–241, 1991.

165. Shoji S, Esashi M: Micro flow cell for blood gas analysis realizing very small sample volume. *Sens Actuators* B8:205–208, 1992.

166. Arquint P, Kouldelka-Hep M, van der Schoot BH, van der Wal P, de Rooij NF: Micromachined analyzers on a silicon chip. *Clin Chem* 40:1805–1809, 1994.

167. Suzuki H, Tamiya E, Karube I: Fabrication of an oxygen electrode using semiconductor technology. *Anal Chem* 60:1078–1080, 1988.

168. van der Schoot B, Bergveld P: An ISFET-based microlitre titrator: Integration of a chemical sensor-activator system. *Sens Actuators* 8:11–22, 1985.

169. Aoki A, Matsue T, Uchida I: Electromechanical response at microarray electrodes in flowing streams and determination of catecholamines. *Anal Chem* 62:2206–2210, 1990.

170. Verpoorte E, Manz A, Ludi H, Widmer HM, van der Schoot BH, de Rooij NF: A novel optical detector cell for use in miniaturized total chemical analysis system. *IEEE International Conference on Solid-State Sensors and Actuators* (Transducers '91). New York: IEEE, 1991, pp 796–799.

171. Verpoorte E, Manz A, Ludi H, et al: A silicon flow cell for optical detection in miniaturized total chemical analysis systems. *Sens Actuators* B6:66–70, 1992.

172. Jacobson SC, Hergenröder R, Koutny LB, Warmack RJ, Ramsey JM: Effects of injection schemes and column geometry on the performance of microchip electrophoresis devices. *Anal Chem* 66:1107–1113, 1994.

173. Jacobson SC, Hergenröder R, Koutny LB, Ramsey JM: High-speed separations on a microchip. *Anal Chem* 66:1114–1118, 1994.

174. Harrison DJ, Manz A, Fan Z, Lüdi H, Widmer HM: Capillary electrophoresis and sample injection systems integrated on a planar glass chip. *Anal Chem* 64:1926–1932, 1992.

175. Harrison DJ, Glavina PG, Manz A: Towards miniaturized electrophoresis and chemical analysis systems on silicon: an alternative to chemical sensors. *Sens Actuators* B10:107–116, 1993.

176. Harrison DJ, Fluri K, Seiler K, Fan Z, Effenhauser CS, Manz A: Micromachining a miniaturized capillary electrophoresis-based chemical analysis system on a chip. *Science* 261:895–897, 1993.

177. Effenhauser CS, Manz A, Widmer HM: Glass chips for high-speed capillary electrophoresis separations with submicrometer plate heights. *Anal Chem* 65:2637–2642, 1993.

178. Seiler K, Harrison DJ, Manz A: Planar glass chips for capillary electrophoresis: repetitive sample injection, quantitation, and separation efficiency. *Anal Chem* 65:1481–1488, 1993.

179. Pace SJ: Silicon semiconductor wafer for analyzing micronic biological samples. US Patent 4,908,112, 1990.

180. Saadat S, Terry SC: A high-speed chromatographic gas analyzer. *Am Lab* 16:90, 1984.

181. Manz A, Verpoorte E, Effenhauser CS, et al: Miniaturization of separation techniques using planar chip technology. *J High Res Chromatogr* 16:433–436, 1993.

182. Miura J, Manz A, Watanabe Y, Miyahara Y, Miyagi H, Tsukada K: Liquid chromatograph. US Patent 5,132,012, 1992.

183. Yue V, Kowal R, Neargarder L, Bond L, Muetterties A, Parsons R: Miniature field-flow fractionation system for analysis of blood cells. *Clin Chem* 40:1810–1814, 1994.

184. Wilding P, Kricka LJ, Zemel JN: Fluid handling in mesoscale analytical devices. US Patent 5,304,487, 1994.

185. Wilding P, Pfahler J, Bau HH, Zemel JN, Kricka LJ: Manipulation of biological fluids in straight channels micromachined in silicon. *Clin Chem* 40:1–5, 1994.

CHAPTER

4

Neural Networks

FRANK VERTOSICK, JR.

CONTENTS

Handbook of Clinical Automation, Robotics, and Optimization, Edited by Gerald J. Kost with the collaboration of Judith Welsh.
ISBN 0-471-03179-8 © 1996 John Wiley & Sons, Inc.

4.1. INTRODUCTION

4.1.1. What Is a Neural Network?

Neural networks are computational devices consisting of simple nodes, called units or *processing elements* (PEs), which are linked by weighted connections. A neural network maps input to output data in terms of its own internal connectivity. The term *neural network* derives from the obvious nervous system analogy, with the PE serving as neurons and the connection weights equivalent to variable synaptic strengths.

A variety of neural network models have been devised. However, only a single example will be considered here in detail: the feedforward, backpropagation (FFBP) network. Presently, the FFBP network is the one of the most popular architectures for practical applications.

Like other artificial intelligence (AI) constructs, FFBP networks are input/output algorithms customized to solve specific problems. Unlike expert systems, neural networks function without the need for human experts or ad hoc rules. FFBP networks are trained using a *training set* of known input/output data points. During training, the network alters the connection weights among its component PE to provide some stable, quantitative mapping of inputs to outputs in the training set. Once this is accomplished, the trained network can then be deployed to find solutions to novel problems.

The expert system, by way of contrast, is built from a priori rules that relate the various input parameters to the output. For example, suppose we wish to construct a model to predict left ventricular output (LVO) as a function of a panel of several different serum enzymes obtained 24 h after myocardial infarction. Each enzyme value would constitute an input *field,* while LVO would be the single output field.

To build an expert system for this problem, cardiologists would be asked to construct rules correlating enzyme levels with LVO. The rules are then programmed into a predictive algorithm. In this case, the training set consists of the patients treated by the expert cardiologists during their careers and the feature extraction process occurs within the brains of the experts, not in the software per se.

To build a network model, on the other hand, a large set of known enzyme–LVO relationships is obtained and used to train the network connections. The network derives its own rules relating the enzyme levels to cardiac performance using the data in the training set. Given a large enough training set, a person with no cardiology experience could set up a usable FFBP for the enzyme–LVO problem.

Each approach has unique advantages and disadvantages. For example, expert systems require experts in the problem to be solved in addition to significant programming expertise. Furthermore, setting up quantitative rules is not straightforward. A cardiologist may know that LVO negatively correlates with age, but is that correlation linear? If so, what is the slope of the age–LVO plot?

Neural networks, on the other hand, can be applied to problems for which no experts may yet exist. With the help of commercial software packages, furthermore, they can be quickly implemented with little programming experience. Unfortunately, large training sets are necessary and the network's behavior can be idiosyncratic, leading to poor performance.

4.2. DEFINING THE PROBLEM

Before building a specific network, the nature of the problem to be solved should be considered. Does it involve classifying old data or predicting new data? Are the available training data clean or noisy? Are the data numerical and continuous, or are they discrete and nonnumerical, for example, male versus female, days of the week?

The nature of the problem will determine what analytical method to use. For example, if the problem involves only a few continuous input fields that are linearly separable (i.e., each input has an independent quasilinear effect on output), then techniques based on linear regression may be more effective than a neural network approach.

Few problems are neatly separable into independent, quasilinear relationships, however. More typically, nonlinear interactions among input fields complicate the problem. Consider a network designed to predict the product of an enzyme-catalyzed reaction in which the enzyme's activity is pH dependent. Three input fields are used: concentration of substrate, concentration of enzyme and pH of the buffer, with the concentration of product as the output field. In this problem, there will be a nonlinear effect introduced by the interaction of the enzyme and the pH input fields. This problem is ideal for neural network analysis but may prove difficult or impossible to approach using other methods.

4.2.1. Classification versus Prediction

Neural networks can be used to categorize existing data (classification) or to forecast new data (prediction). FFBP networks can be applied to both problems.

Classification problems seek meaningful subsets within a larger set of known data. *Example:* Suppose that some industrious molecular biologist has sequenced the genes encoding key serum proteins in a hundred different species of birds. The biologist wishes to create a taxonomy of the species using the molecular data and compare it to an accepted taxonomy based on gross morphologic features. Thus, the biologist does not seek to predict new data but to extract a coherent pattern from data already at hand.

The enzyme–LVO example described previously is a prediction problem. Based on enzyme–LVO relationships extracted from the training set of prior patients, a network is fashioned to predict the LVO of new patients.

The two types of problems are not mutually exclusive. For instance, the enzyme–LVO problem could be reformulated as a classification problem. A network could be used to classify patterns of serum enzyme levels in the training set into high- or low-LVO subgroups. If this cannot be done reliably, then there is no point in trying to predict LVO in patients outside the training set.

4.2.2. Clean versus Noisy Data

The "cleanliness" of data is the degree to which random noise and not the input fields affect outcome. Consider a published FFBP model predicting the behavior of a simple enzyme-linked immunosorbent assay (ELISA). There are four input fields (coating antigen, primary antibody titer, secondary antibody titer, and chromagen development time) and one output field [optical density (OD)]. In this problem, although there are the usual small random errors in pipetting reagents, the relative contribution of this noise to OD is minimal compared to the contribution of the input fields, making this problem quite clean.

As an example of a noisy problem, consider a prediction network designed to estimate the survival of patients after the diagnosis of a malignant brain tumor. The input fields are the clinical parameters at the time of surgical biopsy, such as age, clinical performance scores, tumor type, and so on. In this problem, even though input fields such as age and tumor type are known to affect survival significantly, the impact of unpredictable events is also large. A patient with a benign tumor may be killed in an auto accident and perish years before a patient with a more malignant lesion. The effect of this noise is equal to or greater than the effect of any one of the input variables.

Networks can address noisy problems, but the size of the training set must increase with the degree of noise. The ultraclean ELISA network works well even if trained with only 20 or 30 input/output examples.[1] However, the brain tumor network performs miserably despite a training set containing many hundreds of patients (data unpublished). Taken to the extreme limit, totally random problems have no network solution at all. The best network can never predict tomorrow's lottery numbers no matter what input fields are chosen or how many training examples are provided.

Clean problems can be solved nicely with networks, but, as statisticians will point out, they can be solved by other methods as well, particularly when there are few nonlinearities. Somewhere between the perfectly linear problems that can be approached without neural networks and the totally random problems that can't be solved by any approach are those problems best suited for network analysis.

The take-home message: Don't expect magic from a neural network. The literature contains many examples of FFBP networks applied to noisy clinical problems in which only a hundred or less training examples are used, even though thousands may be needed to create a trustworthy predictive network. Unlike statistical methods in which the number of examples needed for a "significant" result can usually be calculated, network analysis currently provides few methods, beyond trial and error, for determining the reliability of network outcome.

4.3. ANATOMY OF A FFBP NETWORK

4.3.1. The Processing Elements

The PEs are simple I/O devices that receive multiple inputs but produce only a single output. Information flows in one direction only through the PE. The multiple inputs are summed linearly and then converted to a PE output, also called the PE's *activation,* using a *transfer function.* Figure 4.1 illustrates typical transfer functions. The most commonly used transfer function is the sigmoidal function:

$$\text{Output} = (1.0 + e^{-\text{input}})^{-1} \qquad\qquad (4.1)$$

or some variation thereof. Networks composed totally of linear PE are of little practical value, although some networks function well if a few PE are allowed to have a linear transfer function.

EXAMPLES OF TRANSFER FUNCTIONS

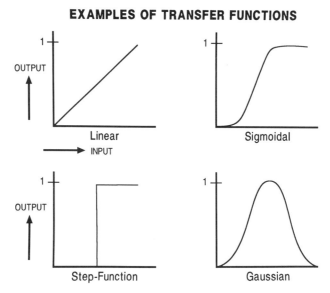

Figure 4.1. The processing elements (PEs) of a neural network utilize a transfer function to convert their summated inputs into a single output. The *x* axis is input; the *y* axis, output. The most commonly used transfer function is the sigmoidal function.

4.3.2. Connection Weights

The output of PE A is transferred as input to another PE B in the network according to the equation

$$\text{Input}_B = (W_{AB})(\text{output}_A) \tag{4.2}$$

where W_{AB} is the *connection weight* between A and B. If W_{AB} is zero, the activation of A has no effect on B at that point in time; a large connection weight allows A to have a major impact on B. The weights form an $N \times N$ matrix, where N is the total number of PE in the network. The weights can be modified over time to alter the behavior of the network.

4.3.3. The FFBP Architecture

Figure 4.2 shows a typical FFBP architecture. The network has at least three layers of PE: an input layer, a hidden layer, and an output layer. Information flows forward only (feedforward), that is, from input layer to hidden layer and from hidden layer to output layer. Any two adjacent layers are maximally interconnected, while there are typically no connections directly from input to output. A bias PE is used to translate the sigmoidal activation curves along the input axis. Note that this network is not *recursive,* in that no connections from output to hidden or hidden to input are included. Any of these rules can be modified, however, to fit a specific problem. For example, two or more hidden PE layers can be used.

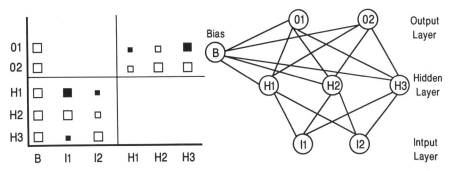

Figure 4.2. The architecture of a neural network is shown on the right. Note that there are three layers of PE not counting the bias PE, which serves to translate the transfer functions of the PE along the input axis. Note also that adjacent layers are maximally interconnected, and that there are no direct connections between the input and output layers. This is the classic feedforward backpropagation (FFBP) network. On the left is a Hinton diagram of the pictured network, which shows the magnitude and sign of the various connection weights in a schematic way (see text).

To the left of the network on Figure 4.2 is a Hinton diagram, named after the network pioneer Geoffrey Hinton. The Hinton diagram is shorthand for the connection weight matrix. Open squares are positive connection weights while black squares are negative weights. The size of the square correlates with the magnitude of the weight. The designated square states the scaling of the activation of the PE on the horizontal axis to the input side of PE in the vertical axis. Since the outputs of the output PE are not scaled, they are not listed in the horizontal axis. Likewise, since the inputs to the input PE are not scaled, they are not included in the vertical axis. In other words, the connection weights linking the network to its external environment are all unity and do not vary with time, so they are not shown.

The Hinton diagram provides a quick overview of the connectivity after a network has been trained. Note that in this trained network hidden PE-1 is weakly connected to both output PE-1 and output PE-2, while hidden unit PE-3 is strongly connected to both output PEs. Thus, hidden PE-1 might be deleted without affecting network behavior.

Some software packages display the Hinton diagram to allow a quick visual assessment of which PE make no contribution to the problem. During the solution of the brain tumor problem above, for example, the input PE corresponding to patient sex could be found to have no significant connection to the hidden layer, signifying that the patient's sex has no impact on the problem of survival prediction. This input field could then be deleted. The computer must grind through the calculations of all PE, contributory or otherwise, and so the deletion of meaningless PE speeds up the solution to the problem.

4.3.4. The Learning Rule

The learning rule is an algorithm that modifies the connection weights during the period of network training. The FFBP network uses the backpropagation of errors, also known as *backpropagation* or simply *backprop*. A rigorous exposition of backpropagation theory is beyond the scope of the present discussion, but the basic concepts can be outlined here. Interested readers are referred to excellent discussions of backpropagation and neural networks in general that are available elsewhere.[2-5]

The connection weights of an untrained network are initialized at random. Thus, when the inputs are put through for the first time, they will generate only random outputs. These random outputs can then be compared to the desired outputs contained in the training set. The difference between the actual and desired outputs constitutes the error, e_i, for output PE_i. For example, consider a data "vector" from the training set of the ELISA model:

$$1.0 \quad 1:1000 \quad 1:1000 \quad 15 \quad 0.124$$

where the first four numbers are input fields (antigen coating concentration, 1.0 picomolar; primary antibody titer, 1:1000; secondary antibody titer, 1:1000; chromagen development time, 15 min) and the last number is the output (optical density). When the inputs fields are put through an untrained network, let's say the output PE yields a value of 0.258, versus the real output of 0.124. For this training set vector, the error of the output PE on the first pass of the input fields through this random network is $0.258 - 0.124 = +0.134$. This error in the output PE can then be backpropagated to determine the output error of the other PE in the network. Once all the output errors are known, corrections to the connection weights are made according to the equation

$$\Delta W_{ij} = (R)(e_i^l)(A_j^{l-1}) \tag{4.3}$$

where ΔW_{ij} is the correction to weight W_{ij}, R is the learning rate, e_i^l the error of the ith PE in layer l, and A_j^{l-1} the activation of the jth unit in layer $l - 1$.

Thus, each pass, or iteration, of the training set data consists of two steps: (1) the input data are fed forward to yield outputs, the output errors computed and then backpropagated to determine the output errors of all the PE; and (2) the output errors are converted to connection weight corrections and the weights updated.

These iterations are repeated over and over again, the weights adjusted after each iteration, until each training set input generates the desired output within a predetermined level of uncertainty (e.g., ±5%). Once this is accomplished, the network is trained and the process stops. The final connection weight matrix now carries one "solution" to the I/O mapping. For typical FFBP network problems, hundreds or even many thousands of iterations may be needed to achieve a trained network.

The goal of the backpropagation method is to minimize the sum of the squared output errors for the training set by adjusting the connection weights. This technique is also known as *gradient descent,* in that it pushes the network into a minimum on the network's error surface.

Although this technique is quite successful, it has two drawbacks: (1) since the weight corrections during each iteration of the data set are proportional to the size of the errors, the training process becomes slower and slower as the errors decrease and a minimum is approached; and (2) there is nothing to guarantee that the error minimum that the network falls into is indeed the lowest, or best, of the available minima. Mimima that represent one solution, but not the best solution, to the training set mapping are known as *local minima.* Networks in local minima are solved on the training set; that is, they predict the outputs in the training set, but they may fail when deployed to predict new outcomes.

A set of known inputs and outputs independent of the training set is referred as the *cross-validation* set (or CV set). In the enzyme–LVO network, for example, a series of enzyme/LVO relationships can be measured after a network has been trained. The performance of the network in the cross-validation set can be used as a test of whether the network can generalize adequately or whether it is in a local minimum. If the correlation between predicted and desired outputs is high in the training set, but low in the CV set, then the network is in a local minimum.

Many schemes have been developed to compensate for these drawbacks. For example, the learning rate, *R,* can be increased as the network approaches an error minimum, increasing the magnitude of the weight corrections [see Eq. (4.3)] and driving the network to a solution more quickly. Moreover, algorithms such as *simulated annealing* and the introduction of "noise" into the training set have been devised to jolt the network out of local minima during the training process.

4.3.5. What a Neural Network Does

Many people use neural networks without an intuitive feel for what they do. Consequently, networks are often applied in a "cookbook" fashion.

Despite its elaborate architecture, a trained FFBP network is simply an equation that relates input variables to output variables. The network diagram in Figure 4.2 can be considered as a graphical representation of that equation, much as Feynmann diagrams are representations of complicated scattering equations in high-energy physics. If we were to plug in the final values for the trained connection weights and the activation functions for the various PEs, a very long equation with the inputs on the left side of the equal sign and the outputs on the other could be displayed.

During training the network uses the hidden PE to provide a "best fit" of the input data to the output data in the training set. In a sense, the network is doing a multidimensional *curve-fitting* routine using an expansion series of the PE transfer functions. This makes neural network analysis a cousin of other series expansions, such as polynomial series and Fourier transforms. The connection weights then become analogous to the coefficients of the series—adaptable to different sets of problems.

Like any curve-fitting routine, a neural network seeks not just seek to fit the data but to allow interpolation of the data as well, that is, to fill in the gaps between known data points. In the network case, the known data is in the training set and the interpolation occurs when the network is used to predict a CV set. As anyone who has used a curve-fitting routine on a standard graphics software package can verify, it is possible to create a curve which goes precisely through all the known data points yet behaves so bizarrely between points that it is useless for data interpolation. This is a equivalent to a local minimum of a network, wherein the training set is completely and accurately predicted by the training network's "equation" while the CV sets are not.

4.4. OPTIMIZING AN FFBP NETWORK

Optimizing a neural network remains a largely trial-and-error affair. A typical neural network software package will allow the user to vary a number of parameters including the number of PE in each layer, the transfer functions of the different PE, the learning rate and the exact form of the backpropagation algorithm (there are many variations on the backprop theme), among others. From a practical standpoint, two of the biggest factors that impact the performance of a network are (1) the number of PEs, particularly the number of hidden PE, and (2) the quality of the input data.

4.4.1. The Number of PEs

There are no limits to the number of PEs in a network. Each PE, however, adds a computational burden to the problem. The work environment plays a role here: a supercomputer or workstation will handle larger networks than a desktop PC (personal computer).

There has been much written about the optimal number of hidden PE, and about whether two or more layers of hidden PE are better than one. For most common laboratory applications a single layer of hidden PE should suffice. A number of rules of thumb have been devised for setting the optimal number of hidden PE. For example, one commonly cited rule is

$$H = \frac{I + O}{2} \tag{4.4}$$

where H is the number of hidden PEs, I is the number of input PE, and o is the number of output PEs.

In truth, however, the optimal number of hidden PEs must be customized to a given problem. Too few hidden PEs and the network may not be able to learn the training set; too many hidden PEs, and the network will overlearn the training set and will be rendered unusable for interpolation. Again, consider the curve-fitting analogy: too simple a function (e.g., polynomial series, Fourier transforms) and the fit will be poor and too complex, and the fit will behave erratically between data points.

4.4.2. Transforming the Data

For most problems, the use of raw, untransformed data will yield suboptimal results. For theoretical reasons, networks train best when the PEs are active over their full range. For example, in Eq. (4.3) the corrections to the connection weights during backpropagation are a function of the activation values of the PE. If a PE's activation is always zero, then that PE will not participate.

How can this occur? Neural network software programs scale the range of input values to between zero and one. Suppose a network is being constructed in which one of the input fields is serum sodium concentration. The values for this field in the training set may look like this:

139, 140, 135, 136, 137, 140, 141, 140, 136, 138, 193

In this case, most patients fall in the range of 135–141, with the single exception being a severely abnormal serum sodium of 193. However, this lone outlier point is sufficient to define the range of this field as 135–193 and, when the software scales this range, most of the input values lie near the lower end of the range (zero). In effect, the lone high value clamps this unit at an activation of zero and eliminates the contribution of serum sodium to the problem. The solution? If only a few aberrant points are responsible for extending the data range, try tossing them out.

In some cases, however, there are too many points to toss out. Figure 4.3 shows a histogram of data points. Most are clustered near the upper end of the range such that the corresponding input PE effectively acts as if it had a constant activation of 1.0; in other words, it acts like a bias PE and not an input PE. If the square root of the data are used, however, the distribution over the range becomes more even, permitting this input field to have a greater impact during training.

4.4.3. Discontinuous Data

How best to input discontinuous data? Suppose an investigator wants to compare the performance of an assay at three different laboratories: A, B, and C. Remember that the FFBP network represents an equation and so must have numerical inputs.

The simplest way would be to assign a single PE to represent the "laboratory" input field and encode the laboratories numerically—A = 0, B = 0.5, C = 1.0, but this will nearly always produce poor results. Why? Because the network will rank the networks according to number. As a numerically driven device, the network cannot consider the labs as equivalent since they carry different quantitative values.

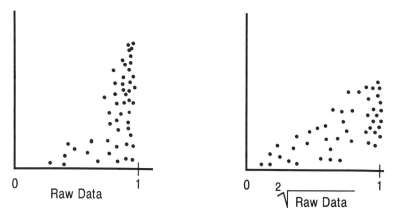

Figure 4.3. An illustration of data transformation. The raw-data histogram on the left is too clustered and can be spread out more evenly by taking the square root of the data. This type of transformation allows the input PE corresponding to the data field to be active over the complete range of its transfer function, allowing it to participate in network learning (see text).

A better way is to use three input PE and encode the laboratories in a binary fashion:

	PE-1	PE-2	PE-3
Laboratory A	1	0	0
Laboratory B	0	1	0
Laboratory C	0	0	1

In this way, the laboratories are different, yet equivalent, states of a 3D "lab vector."

4.5. SOME EXAMPLES OF NEURAL NETWORKS IN THE LABORATORY

With this brief overview of FFBP networks as a background, several published applications of this method to clinical laboratory problems will be discussed and critiqued.

4.5.1. The ELISA Prediction Network

This application was mentioned above. Vertosick and Rehn used an FFBP network to predict the behavior of an ELISA for measuring the concentration of human albumin. The training set consisted of approximately one 96-well microtiter plate treated with random combinations of the four input fields described above, together the corresponding OD as measured in the laboratory. After being trained on these random values, the network was used to predict a variety of curves, such as the dependence of OD on antigen concentrations. The actual curves were then run in the laboratory and found to be in remarkable agreement with the network simulations.[1]

Thus, with only a tray's worth of reagents, a network capable of predicting the entire range of ELISA behavior could be trained. Optimization of the assay for various antigen concentrations could then be done on a PC, without the consumption of valuable antibodies and technician time.

Although there was nothing wrong with the application of a neural network to this problem, it was overkill. The problem could have been solved as easily using conventional numerical methods. However, the basic principle was sound and networks should prove useful for the optimization of lab assays in which the input fields are more numerous, such as flow cytometry or DNA sequencing.

4.5.2. Predicting Pancreatitis

Kazmierczak et al. compared the performance of an FFBP network to that of a rule-based program for predicting the diagnosis of pancreatitis using as inputs the serum levels of serum amylase and lipase measured at five points in time. There were nine input PEs corresponding to the five enzyme levels and the four time intervals between them, 10 hidden PEs, and two output PE corresponding to the two possible outcomes (pancreatitis versus no pancreatitis).[6]

Note that these authors correctly used two output PEs for their discontinuous outputs. As discussed above, using a single PE for output and postulating pancreatitis = 1 and no pancreatitis = 0 would have been incorrect since it would mislead that network into thinking pancreatitis is a more meaningful outcome than no pancreatitis.

A total of 508 patient data points were available; 254 were used for the training set and the remainder, as the CV set. The diagnostic accuracy of the trained network in the CV set was 76% when amylase was used, 82% when lipase was used, and 84% when a combination of the two was used. The rule-based protocol had a 92% accuracy.

The paper is flawed, however, in that the authors made no attempt to optimize network performance. There is no mention of the use of data transformation or manipulations of the hidden layer to improve network performance, and the authors admit that they used only the software's default values for the various network parameters. Ten hidden PEs may have been too many for this problem, causing the network to fall into a local minimum. The authors may have also "overtrained" their data (see Astion et al.[7] for a discussion of overtraining).

This does not invalidate their conclusion that neural networks can be applied to this problem; it just makes their comparisons of one method to another suspect. To truly compare two methods, both must be optimized by experts.

4.5.3. Other Diagnostic Networks

Schweiger et al. used an FFBP network to predict the presence or absence of lung carcinoma when presented with seven tumor markers. The total number of patients was relatively small (63 with cancer, 43 without), yet the network compared favorably with multivariate stepwise discriminant analysis in that the network could "learn" all the training points. There is no mention of CV set testing. The authors note that using large numbers of hidden PE (>25) or more than one layer of hidden PE caused a degradation of network performance.[8]

Astion and Wilding employed an FFBP network to predict the presence or absence of breast cancer nine input fields, including patient age and a series of serum lipid values and tumor markers. Again, the network could "learn" all of the training points (57 patients) and was 80% accurate in predicting outcome in a CV set of only 20 patients.[9]

It should be noted here that excessive significance should not be attached to the ability of a network to solve the entire training set (or even a large part of it) to the designated output error tolerance. Remember, a linear regression line through a scatterplot can be very useful even if it does not actually pass through a single data point. Likewise, a network may be trainable on only two-thirds of the training set elements and yet still be a very usuable network. Conversely, as has been mentioned repeatedly, a network that learns 100% of the training set may prove to be 100% worthless in CV testing.

4.5.4. Other Examples

Space does not permit a discussion of all of the uses of FFBP networks in biomedical settings. Just to mention a few others, the neural network technique has been applied to: classifying mammograms,[10] classifying electrophoretic patterns,[11,12] analyzing electroencephalograms,[13] and interpreting SPECT images.[14]

4.6. CONCLUSION

This chapter has been intended as an introduction to the use of a particular type of neural network, the FFBP network. Other types of networks are gaining favor, such as the self-organizing maps.

There is no substitute for experience. The reader is urged to try available software packages. Several companies produce inexpensive introductory programs with excellent documentation that permit the beginner to learn how to use this method. The introductory programs can then be upgraded to more expensive, "expert" versions. Even better, a number of courses are offered throughout the country which provide both theoretical and practical teaching of network applications.

The surface of neural network applications in the clinical laboratory has yet to be scratched. When combined with improving hardware and other methods, such as fuzzy logic, this AI paradigm will almost certainly have a major impact in laboratory science in the years ahead.

REFERENCES

1. Vertosick FT, Rehn T: Predicting behavior of an enzyme-linked immunoassay model by using commercially available neural network software. *Clin Chem* 39:2478–2482, 1993.

2. Rumelhart DE, Hinton GE, Williams RJ: Learning representations by back-propagating errors. *Nature* 323:533–535, 1986.

3. Lippmann RP: An introduction to computing with neural nets. *IEEE ASSP Mag* 4:4–22, 1987.

4. Wasserman P: *Neural Computing: Theory and Practice.* New York: Chapman & Hall, 1989.

5. Hecht-Nielsen R: *Neurocomputing.* New York: Addison-Wesley, 1990.

6. Kazmierczak SC, Catrou PG, Van Lente F: Diagnostic accuracy of pancreatic enzymes evaluated by use of multivariate data analysis. *Clin Chem* 39:1960–1965, 1993.

7. Astion ML, Wener MH, Thomas RG, Hunder GG, Bloch DA: Overtraining in neural networks that interpret clinical data. *Clin Chem* 39:1998–2004, 1993.

8. Schweiger CR, Soergi G, Spitzauer S, Maenner G, Pohl AL: Evaluation of laboratory data by conventional statistics and by three types of neural networks. *Clin Chem* 39:1966–1971, 1993.

9. Astion ML, Wilding P: Application of neural networks to the interpretation of laboratory data in cancer diagnosis. *Clin Chem* 38:34–38, 1992.

10. Wu Y, Doi K, Giger ML, Nishikawa RM: Computerized detection of clustered microcalcifications in digitial mammograms: applications of artificial neural networks. *Med Phys* 19:555–560, 1992.

11. Sondergaard I, Krath BN, Hagerup M: Classification of crossed immunoelectrophoretic patterns using digital image processing and artificial neural networks. *Electrophoresis* 13:411–415, 1992.

12. Manner GA, Scweiger CR, Soregi G, Pohl AL: Detection of monoclonal gammopathies in serum electrophoresis by neural networks. *Clin Chem* 39:1984–1985, 1993.

13. Bankman IN, Sigillito VG, Wise RA, Smith PL: Feature-based detection of the K-complex wave in the human electroencephalogram using neural networks. *IEEE Trans Biomed Eng* 12:1305–1310, 1992.

14. Fujita H, Katafuchi T, Uehara T, Nishimura T: Application of artificial neural networks to computer-aided diagnosis of coronary artery disease in myocardial SPECT bull's eye images. *J Nucl Med* 33:272–276, 1992.

5

Simulation Modeling

WILLIAM GODOLPHIN

CONTENTS

5.1. INTRODUCTION

The leading edge in large clinical laboratories is rapidly approaching a mature industry. Economic, social and regulatory factors are both driving and pulling them toward factory-ization. They are being thought of and operated more like systems. There is demand for greater productivity, better response to the customer needs and increasing substitution of technology and systems for people. One of the major problems with this development is that capital costs can be very high for experimentation and mistakes.

The typical large hospital or private-sector clinical laboratory is a very complex system with many semiautonomous parts. It has many different machine

Handbook of Clinical Automation, Robotics, and Optimization, Edited by Gerald J. Kost with the collaboration of Judith Welsh.
ISBN 0-471-03179-8 © 1996 John Wiley & Sons, Inc.

modules (analytical instruments) and operators (technologists, technicians, and clinical scientists) but processes a relatively small variety of specimens. The challenge is to provide, as in modern manufacturing, a consistent service and uniform product reliably and flexibly over a wide range of customer demand levels.[1–3]

Management must design the workflow and select the automation to achieve this and the usual tools are experience, intuition, and vendors' claims. Major changes and purchases are seldom made unless there is a high degree of certainty that the result will be much better. Small gains are too risky. Computer simulation modelling is a tool widely used in the manufacturing and service industries to assist such system design and hardware selection. It is a valuable technique routinely used in apparently very different settings such as military strategic planning, meteorologic services, communications networks as well as manufacturing and process control for predicting effects of change upon complex systems.[4] Closer to home, simulation is being used for operations management of other areas of the hospital such as pharmacy and intensive care units.[5,6]

A good model of a laboratory system would be a computer program that behaves like a real lab and could be used to predict the impact of changes to any part of it, for example, the change in turnaround time caused by an increase in specimens or the improvement in throughput due to acquisition of a new analyzer that had twice the speed of the old, or required half the maintenance.

5.2. PROCEDURE AND TYPES OF SIMULATION MODELING

The steps in creation of a computer simulation model are

1. Define the objectives and plan the project.
2. Build and verify a conceptual model.
3. Collect data.
4. Fit data to theoretical distributions.
5. Write the simulation and animation code.
6. Validate the model.
7. Ask "what if?" questions.

Not many people in the typical laboratory setting understand what simulation modeling means. They may think it is like the training simulators, such as flight simulators. A flight simulator has a predictable outcome for all inputs; it is not an experimental tool. The kind of simulation model we are talking about for the lab will yield surprises and inexact outcomes as we use it to explore both the existence and degree of relationships.

The major benefits of simulation are that

1. It allows us to comprehend how a whole system works. It helps us to see "the big picture" and to see the relative importance of the components.

2. It provides a means for communication. It permits workers and managers and theorists to discuss the whole system—for example, while viewing an animation. It also provides quantitative performance indicators that can be used to describe how the system behaves under different circumstances.

3. It improves insight. We are permitted to see or synthesize relationships we have not noticed before and to ask questions we had not thought of before.

5.2.1. Define the Objectives and Plan the Project

This is too obviously important. The newcomer will need help. In academic circles the expertise is most often found in engineering and business faculties. Large manufacturing concerns and the fast-food service industry are sectors that use pertinent simulation techniques. Journals such as *Simulation* and *Industrial Engineering* are important publications for relevant papers.

Time and money will be wasted by the creation of a model that is either insufficient or more than sufficient to meet the need. There is no point in modelling the flies in the lab. There are often processes that are not critical to the overall flow or that vary little with changes in the rest of the system—it is a waste of time to model them with precision. On the other hand, if the questions to be answered require minor changes or if many questions about different but integrated parts of the system are to be asked then the model may have to be quite detailed.[7,8] Modeling is a statistical process and like any other is much better at interpolation than extrapolation. Models should be used to guide and assist an understanding, not substitute for it.

Modeling in a typical clinical laboratory is a little different from modeling, say, a factory floor. Usually the people in the lab have a lot more autonomy in their choice of how to proceed. Their tasks are frequently interrupted by higher priority tasks and they exercise more personal choice in what to do next. Laboratories are changing and the roles of the personnel may be threatened. In such an atmosphere it is difficult to get the front-line worker to cooperate. Yet cooperation is needed for the modeller to collect good data.

Our solution to this problem is to begin to ask the front-line people what they see as being some of the systems or workflow problems. That is, to involve them from the earliest possible time in the business of defining the "what if?" questions that the model might be asked. Work studies, especially time and motion studies, have received a lot of bad publicity. The kind of detailed observation and questioning that is required to prepare a useful model may seem suspiciously like a management ploy to increase efficiency by forcing the workers to greater productivity. Such problems can be avoided if the workers are partners in the enterprise and realize the model is a tool that they, too, can use.

A recommended prerequisite for a simulation project or at least something to be done early is: educate yourself. You should have at least a basic understanding of statistics. Specifically the notions of different kinds of distributions, random-number generation, sampling theory, confidence limits, truncation and analysis of variance. This can be obtained through basic statistics courses or by reading the introductory part of a textbook on simulation, or by going to a course on simulation (such as those often offered in conjunction with vendor software support or a conference on simulation. If you work with someone who is conversant with simulation, and this is certainly to be recommended, then they must be taught about the process of the lab. Good simulation requires an in-depth knowledge of the process, the products, the decision rules and the relative significance or importance of these to the overall system.

5.2.1.1. SIMULATION TOOLS: LANGUAGES AND SIMULATORS.

Our experience is with discrete-event simulation languages. The oldest, and still one of the most widely used examples of these is GPSS. In discrete event simulation the changes in state of the physical system are represented by a series of events that occur at discrete points in the simulation time. So, for example, a patient (event) may "seize" a phlebotomist (resource) and change the phlebotomist's "state" from idle to busy. If another patient appears (another event occurs) before the phlebotomist is "released" by the first, then the new one may enter a queue (which changes the state of the queue from having no one in it to having one person in it). The appearance of the patients (the events) is generated by a random-number generator selected to produce a distribution of events in time that is the same as reality. Likewise, the particular steps undertaken by the phlebotomist in servicing a patient can be broken down into events that cause a change in state. An encounter then can be modelled as a single event and change in state or as a whole series of component steps.

Programming in a simulation language is similar to writing code in any other language such as C, or Fortran, or Basic. It requires a fair knowledge of the logic and syntax of the language. Simulators or simulation packages, on the other hand, are usually designed with a user-friendly interface and built-in models. These can be modified to a degree by the user but generally are aimed at modeling of a specific class of applications such as manufacturing, transportation. The hidden assumptions inherent to a simulator or package may yield models with important limitations in flexibility and validity. However, they are much easier to program, usually look prettier and will yield demonstrable models more quickly. Some claim to require no programming at all. The appropriate choice between language and simulator will depend upon what you want to do with the model and resources available (time, money, expertise).

5.2.1.2. OUTLINE OF A PROPOSAL FOR A SIMULATION PROJECT

1. Objectives of the study
2. Scope of the study
3. Level of detail to be modelled
4. Questions to be answered
5. Description (layout and flow diagram) of the base model
6. Description of desired models (to answer questions)

7. Verification and validation procedures (including goals and acceptability criteria)
8. Model input and output (including animation)
9. Simulation software and hardware
10. People: principals, collaborators, and consultants
11. Time and effort estimates

5.2.2. Build and Verify a Conceptual Model

This is usually a flow diagram of the system. It is probably best created in a *top–down* fashion. Activities and flow of the real situation should be sufficiently well understood to draw a comprehensive and accurate block diagram and establish all rules by which various operations are controlled. This is accomplished by observation and questioning the people whose activities are to be modelled. Sources of information are direct observation, procedure manuals, and informants.

In our experience, like the other steps of the overall process of model building, this will be iterative. Often there are discrepancies between what you think you see happening, what the procedures manuals prescribe, and what workers say they are doing. It seems logical that the workers version will be the best, but that is not necessarily true. Sometimes they may characterize a process as consisting of two or more separate tasks, whereas the best model treats them as one (and vice versa).

5.2.2.1. TASK AND PRIORITY DEFINITION. Knowledge of the system necessary to develop a structured conceptual model was gained by interviews with lab staff about their duties and priorities, reviews of written procedural manuals, and observation of the laboratory in action. A fixed set of detailed tasks was specified for each staff member before data collection began. In some experiments we imposed a few simple rules of behaviour on the staff for data collection periods when we encountered flexible operations (e.g., racks of specimens were moved from one station to another by no consistent rule or person).

The specification of technologists' task sets for efficient simulation is nonintuitive and these methods have evolved through trial and error. Complex activities were broken down into specific tasks, each of which is usually performed in one chunk of time. For example, activities to produce an analyzer sample list from the laboratory information system (LIS) might not be performed sequentially, so three distinct tasks were specified: (1) view the sample queue in the LIS computer and download a sample list to an analyzer, (2) confirm and print the sample list at the analyzer, and (3) collect and carry the printed list and empty analyzer sample rack to the proper workspace. On the other hand, two or more distinct activities that are usually performed consecutively are best simulated as a single task, for example, the computer log-in and transfer of specimens to the next station.

Task lists must be prioritized for each staff member once individual tasks are defined. This involves educated guess work so models are coded in a manner that permits the priority ranking of tasks to be easily changed during debugging.

5.2.3. Collect Data

Data collection usually takes place during the busiest times of the laboratory operation because one is usually interested in understanding performance when the system is stressed and workflow approaches full capacity.

The data collected consists of event frequencies at each step of the process. These will eventually be turned into distributions to be used to select and control the pseudoevents created by the computer model. It is, of course, possible to make educated guesses about these distributions, or in some simulation packages to simply select a distribution from a list and insert some near-guess parameters. However, as for any other kind of computer program "garbage in, garbage out" (GIGO). For quick reviews to focus on bottlenecks (a sort of sensitivity analysis), such an initial approach may be satisfactory but is unlikely to produce a valid model useful for exploration of the system. Existing laboratory records that document the receipt and processing of specimens may be examined to provide such preliminary data.

We have used three methods to collect data by observation:

1. A hand tally was kept by trained observers who timed specific events and recorded the number of specimens.

2. A videorecording was made of activities in small, select areas of the lab. Either a regular TV camera was set on a tripod at a specific workstation or the surveillance camera with wide-angle lens was mounted overhead. The programmable time-lapse videocassette recorder (VCR) records time and date stamps on the image, and can record as much as 6 h on a 120-min tape. The variable speed playback and rewind features facilitated review of the videotapes. During playback review the data was entered directly into the computer spreadsheet.

3. The lab staff were asked to record times and specimen counts for selected activities. They were also asked to maintain a record, in greater detail, of information they already collect such as a tally of specimen arrivals in 15-min intervals instead of the usual 3-h intervals. We also asked staff to track and record the timing of their own activities.

5.2.4. Fit Data to Theoretical Distributions

If the model is to correctly simulate reality, the generation of events (by random-number generator) must follow the same pattern as reality. The "fitting" of the data to a theoretical pattern (distribution) may be done by inspection or by algorithms (as computer programs). Typical distributions are normal (gaussian), log-normal, exponential, and gamma.[9]

5.2.5. Write Simulation and Animation Code

Creation of the model is performed by writing code in a simulation language or by use of a simulator program. An animation package permits the creation of a moving "cartoon" of the model that can be run in fast-forward mode. This is often helpful, especially to involve and get feedback from the laboratory personnel.

5.2.6. Validate

Validation is achieved by comparing output of the model with real data. Characteristics such as turnaround time, total throughput, length of queues, and staff utilization should closely match reality if the model is valid. We generally accept a model if output is within 10% of reality.

5.2.7. Ask Questions

As with most experimental systems, a simulation model works best or is most useful if the experimenters have clearly formulated hypotheses to test. A discrete-event simulation is not capable of directly answering a question such as "What is the optimum throughput for this device?" Such a question would usually be answered by running the simulation with the modeled device set to various throughput, followed by careful examination of the consequences. In other words, the usefulness of a good model is dependent mostly on the insight and imagination of the experimenter.

5.2.8. Examples of Simulation Projects

5.2.8.1. CONTINUOUS SERIAL PROCESSING IN A LARGE HOSPITAL LABORATORY: CONVENTIONAL BATCH CENTRIFUGE VERSUS SERIAL CENTRIFUGE. Typical batch centrifuges as used for isolating serum have a large capacity and are at least theoretically capable of handling 120–480 tubes per hour; whereas the serial centrifuge,[10] at one tube per load, even though the spin time is only 1 min, can process only 60 tubes per hour. However, because of the limitations of variable input flow, time to load and balance, and time to resort after unloading, this comparison becomes rather more difficult than simply contrasting the theoretical capacity.

Simulation of these systems permitted a better comparison that accounted for the variability in rate of supply and the time spent by technologists in loading, unloading and sorting. This analysis showed the unexpected result that the average specimen time in the serial centrifuge station would be about one-third that in the batch station.[11]

5.2.8.2. SERIAL CENTRIFUGATION IN AN OUTPATIENT LAB. When an outpatient phlebotomy station was modeled, another example of unexpected results occurred. In this outpatient setting the whole process from appearance of the patient to readiness of the serum specimen for courier pickup was modeled. After phlebotomy the specimens were placed into a darkened "clot box" to allow time for clotting to take place. In the conventional system the usual residence time here was about 29 mins, although only 15 were specified by procedural rules. Study of the actual behaviour and the simulation showed that much of this extra time was due to the technologists leaving specimens in the clot box longer than necessary because there were not enough specimens in the box the last time they looked to make it worth while to start the centrifuge. Modeling this behavior with the serial centrifuge showed that, since there was no advantage to batching, they would attend to the waiting specimens "in passing," thus reducing the "hurry up and wait" time.

Anyone familiar with the typical laboratory will be familiar with the amount of time spent in such "hurry up and wait" jobs—if a centrifuge is checked a few minutes before it is ready, the technologist will either wait, idle, for it to complete or go on with another job and return long after. Good simulation modeling permits the randomness of this behavior to be studied and accounted for both in the redesign of existing workflow and the implementation of new technology that facilitates or demands new patterns. The "clot and wait to spin" time was shown to decrease by 30%, when the serial centrifuge was introduced, even though that part of the process preceded centrifugation and was technically unchanged.[12]

5.2.8.3. STAFFING FOR AN INCREASED WORKLOAD IN AN OUTPATIENT LAB. Data from modeling studies will include figures such as turnaround time for processes, throughput, queue lengths, wait times, and resource utilization. In general, we have found that when staff utilization approaches 80% (that is, the operator is busy with identifiable assigned tasks 80% of the time), in the real situation they are very busy, indeed. Utilization figures indicate potential labour bottlenecks just as long queues indicate material bottlenecks.

In a study where two outpatient phlebotomy stations were to be combined, it had been originally proposed to increase most of the services such as clerks, phlebotomists, and technologists. A simulation model of the existing lab showed the somewhat surprising result that the simple addition of one receptionist could easily absorb a one-third increase in customers and that the consequent more rapid servicing of patients would reduce the amount of waiting-room seating (input queue) required, thus providing space for the additional receptionist and not requiring the major physical renovations previously planned for this amalgamation. This result was predictable because the simulation model could be used to test the impact on staff utilization of various changes in workload—in this case, the high utilization of the receptionist compared to other workers.

Similar experiments also showed, in numerical terms, the potential gains of "job sharing" if the workers had a broader range of skills and could do whatever job was required if not busy with a usual assignment. The utilization of five staff members, each dedicated to particular tasks, ranged from 28 to 53% (during peak workload), whereas a balanced and average utilization of 54% would be required of only four staff members who could perform or assist with all functions.[13]

5.2.8.4. OPTIMIZATION OF FREE-TIME.

A detailed study of mode output permits visualization of the flow. For example, in the outpatient bleeding station with a conventional centrifuge, it could be seen that the free times for the technologist were more evenly broken up by busy times, whereas with the serial centrifuge the free times tended to be longer and the busy times more concentrated. These longer free times are then potentially available for other tasks.[12]

This effect and potential was seen also in a simulation of an operator of automated aliquotting devices.[14] If one operator tended two aliquotters on demand, that is, whenever a machine needed loading or unloading of various materials or other servicing, then the operator was utilized 52% of the time but the free time was mostly in short bursts of < 5 mins. However, if the operator was scheduled to tend the machines, then these free-time periods could be made 15 min long, sufficient time to do some other significant task. The throughput of the aliquotters was predicted to decline by about 20%, but if the rest of the process did not demand this full capacity, this tradeoff might yield the more important benefit of increased overall productivity.[15]

5.2.8.5. MACHINE DESIGN.

Generally, the more mechanical the system, the easier it is to simulate. Modeling of the input mechanism of an automated aliquotter was useful to optimize the design of a sample transport station that was the focus of several other inputs (primary tubes, secondary tubes, labels, etc.). Since there is a randomness to the number of aliquots that may have to be produced for any one primary tube, the optimal design is not intuitive or easily determined, although the purely mechanical operation of the machine is easily modeled. Such a model permitted a study of various mechanical configurations with the more random typical laboratory primary tube flow—without the expense of actually building several different designs.[15]

5.2.8.6. REAL-TIME MODELING IN A CONTINUOUS-PROCESS LAB AND PRE-PURCHASE ASSESSMENT OF ALTERNATIVE AUTOMATION.

In an assembly line laboratory, a real-time expert system can be used to simulate the expected impact of changes in workload and changes in system configuration, such as replacement of one type of analyzer with another or use of alternative analyzers with daily fluctuations of workload. This can take into consideration differences in throughput, maintenance time, dwell time, all of which can be built into a simulation model of that device and simply "plugged" into the model of the overall system.[16]

Modeling has been used to evaluate alternative automation proposals for a complete workflow redesign of a major operation.[17]

5.2.8.7. GENERALIZED MODEL CONSTRUCTION. Experience with development of a simulation model of a clinical laboratory, based on a "workcell" concept has resulted in production of a construction set of models.[18] A typology of instruments was developed that results in 12 basic modules. Operator hands-on time and priority assignments were made for the technologists, and assignments were made for tubes to tests and tests to instruments. A Windows (Microsoft)-based data entry program was designed to collect data. A laboratory model is thus built by assembling these modules and collecting data from the ongoing data entry of the laboratory. This approach to laboratory modeling provides the possibility of fairly rapidly and easily generating a useful model of many different laboratories, real and imaginary, from a basic set of generalized instruments ("workcells") and priority rules that reflect the behaviour of technologists.[19]

5.3. CONCLUSION

Simulation modeling is a mathematical technique and, in general, mathematics is cheaper than physics or engineering. Faced with the need to redesign laboratory operations, the modern lab manager needs better tools than intuition and vendor claims to make the best decisions. Modeling experience in the lab is presently very limited (although begun more than a decade ago[20]), but the tools are rapidly becoming more accessible, and the seminal work has been done. These techniques, now routinely used and proven in many other analogous sectors of manufacturing and service industry, have the potential to play a major role in the present coming of age of the clinical laboratory as an automated system.

REFERENCES

1. De Cresce RP, Lifshitz MS: Integrating automation into the clinical laboratory. *Clin Lab Med* 8:759–774, 1988.
2. Winkelman JW, Woo J, Tirabassi CP, O'Connell M: Centralization and decentralization of the hospital clinical laboratory. In Vonderschmitt J, ed. *Laboratory Organization—Automation*. Berlin: Walter de Gruyter, 1991, pp. 81–98.
3. Godolphin W: Robotics and automation in diagnostics. In Singh P, Sharma BP, Tyle P, eds: *Diagnostics in the Year 2000*. New York: Van Nostrand, 1993, pp. 427–456.
4. Schriber TJ: *An Introduction to Simulation Using GPSS/H*. New York: Wiley, 1991.
5. Mukherjee AK: A simulation model for management of operations in the pharmacy of a hospital. *Simulation* 56:91–103, 1991.
6. Mahachek AR: Cardiac surgical intensive care unit (SICU) design by dynamic simulation. *Proc SCS Multiconference on Simulation in Emergency Management and Engineering and Simulation in Health Care* (Anaheim, CA, Jan 23–25). San Diego: Society for Computer Simulation, 1991, pp. 213–220.

7. Keller L, Harrell C, Leavy J: The three reasons why simulation fails. *Indust Eng* 23:27–31, 1991.

8. Dietz M: Outline of a successful simulation project. *Indust Eng* 24:50–53, 1992.

9. Law AM, Kelton WD: *Simulation Modelling and Analysis.* New York: McGraw-Hill, 1991.

10. McEwen JA, Godolphin WJ, Bohl RM, et al: Apparatus and method for separating phases of blood. US Patent 4, 828, 716, 1989.

11. Godolphin W, Bodtker K, Uyeno D, Goh L-O: Automated blood sample-handling in the clinical laboratory. *Clin Chem* 36:1551–1555, 1990.

12. Godolphin W, Bodtker K, Wilson L: Simulation modeling: a tool to help predict the impact of automation in clinical laboratories. *Lab Robot Auto* 4:249–255, 1992.

13. Bodtker K, Wilson L, Godolphin W: Simulation modeling to assist operational management and planning in clinical laboratories. *Simulation* 60:247–255, 1993.

14. Godolphin WJ, Cordua-von Specht WF, Pires DP, et al: Improved apparatus and method for aliquotting blood serum or blood plasma. US Patent 5, 163, 582, 1992.

15. Godolphin W, Bodtker K: Automation and simulation of central processing in clinical laboratories. Chemometrics and intelligent laboratory systems. *Lab Info Management.* 21:181–188, 1993.

16. Mountain PJ, Middleton SR: People, information, & automation—a fully integrated approach. In Eggert AA, Ross PJ, Sobocinski PZ, et al, eds: *Proc Clinical Laboratory Automation Workshop,* June 6–8, 1993. Madison: University of Wisconsin, 1993, pp. 121–125.

17. Bennet KE, Scheetz KJ, O'Sullivan MB, Moyer TP: Automation strategies of the Mayo clinic. In Eggert AA, Ross PJ, Sobocinski PZ, et al, eds: *Proc Clinical Laboratory Automation Workshop,* June 6–8, 1993. Madison: University of Wisconsin, 1993, pp. 59–66.

18. Vogt W, Braun SL, Hanssmann F, et al: Realistic modeling of clinical laboratory operation by computer simulation. *Clin Chem* 40:922–928, 1994.

19. Berchtold G, Blaschke H, Hanssmann F, et al: Simulation modeling as a tool to evaluate alternative configurations of clinical laboratories. *Simulation* 63:108–120, 1994.

20. Winkel P: Operational research and cost containment: a general mathematical model of a workstation. *Clin Chem* 30:1758–1764, 1984.

CHAPTER

6

Model-Based Reasoning

SERDAR UCKUN

CONTENTS

6.1. INTRODUCTION

Model-based reasoning (MBR) has been one of the more active branches of artificial intelligence (AI) during the past decade. MBR aims to predict, diagnose, or explain the behavior of a physical or physiological system based on prior knowledge of its structure, behavior, or function. Qualitative modeling techniques with inherent tolerance for uncertainty and ambiguity provide excellent platforms for the simulation of biological systems that may be difficult to model

Handbook of Clinical Automation, Robotics, and Optimization, Edited by Gerald J. Kost with the collaboration of Judith Welsh.
ISBN 0-471-03179-8 © 1996 John Wiley & Sons, Inc.

quantitatively. Unfortunately, biomedical sciences have not been a major area of interest in MBR and consequently not much has been achieved in terms of fielded systems in neither laboratory medicine nor clinical practice. However, dramatic changes are taking place in methods for acquisition, interpretation, and communication of information in healthcare settings. The vastly different information infrastructure of tomorrow will impose heavy demands on the clinical laboratory in terms of intelligent information processing. In this context, we envision a larger role for MBR in the information processing toolbox of laboratory medicine in the near future.

6.2. Classifying Knowledge-Based Systems

Knowledge-based systems are the typical delivery platforms for AI research. Knowledge-based systems may be categorized using different perspectives such as form, content, and use. Several types may be listed under each category, and model-based systems form a subset of all knowledge-based systems:

- *Form of knowledge.* Rules, frames, causal and associational networks, case histories, influence diagrams, decision trees, and so on.
- *Knowledge content.* Structure, behavior, function, association, causal relations, and so forth.
- *Principal use.* Automated diagnosis, explanation, tutoring, critiquing, planning, monitoring, and so on.

In this chapter, we adopt a four-level classification scheme originally presented by Chandrasekaran and Milne.[1] We will illustrate knowledge at each level using arterial blood-gas regulation as an example:

1. *Structure Level.* Systems with structural knowledge reason with structural or connectivity descriptions. Knowledge at this level may be organized either functionally or physically. For example, structure-level knowledge of blood-gas regulation may describe the connectivity of various organs (lungs, O_2 and CO_2 chemoreceptors, the kidneys, etc.), the flow relations between these organs (e.g., blood flow, gas exchange in the lungs, O_2 consumption in tissues), and the various chemical equations of blood-gas equilibrium. An AI system that reasons at the structure level (for example, performing diagnosis or explaining blood-gas results) is a "model-based system."

2. *Behavior Level.* Knowledge in the behavior level can be derived from knowledge in the structural level through qualitative or numerical simulation (note that numerical simulation tools may not be as powerful as qualitative methods in predicting alternative behaviors or explaining generated behaviors). The appropriate input at this level is a qualitative or numerical model, and a system that reasons at this level is also a model-based system. Behavior commonly represents the "blackbox" description of a component. For example, behav-

ioral knowledge of blood-gas regulation captures complex relations such as oxyhemoglobin dissociation curve, the reaction of chemoreceptors to varying levels of blood gases, and the effect of various factors such as the absence of surfactants or a leaky respiratory membrane on arterial blood-gas levels.

3. *Function Level.* Using additional information related to the structure or design of the particular system, knowledge of behavior can be related to functional knowledge. As discussed in Table 6.1, the "function" of a device is a high-level relationship between the structure and the behavior of the device that enables it to fulfill its overall purpose. For example, the behavior of CO_2 chemoreceptors is a parametric relationship between changes in CO_2 concentration and chemoreceptor output (and hence respiratory stimuli), and their purpose is to help control blood pH. The function of the chemoreceptors, therefore, is to maintain arterial blood CO_2 concentration within a narrow range around normal so that blood pH may be kept at physiological levels at all times.

4. *Association Level.* The most superficial level is the association or pattern matching level. Reasoning at this level is typical of rule-based expert systems based on empirical associations, and of case-based systems. A knowledge base at this level can be obtained by abstracting the knowledge in the functional level. Table 6.1 defines some of the important concepts in knowledge-based systems that relate to MBR.[2]

6.3. MODEL-BASED REASONING

Humans reason well even in the presence of uncertain, incomplete, and inexact knowledge. Cognitive psychologists postulate that people base their understanding of concepts in a given domain on a set of mental models.[8] However, some claim that expert diagnosticians do not use detailed domain models as often as they use associational knowledge.[9] Associational knowledge consists of "heuristic" information relating to problem solving situations, and empirical observations abstracted as *rules of thumb*. It is reasonable to conclude that human experts perform most of their reasoning using associational knowledge, resorting to more detailed domain models when the empirical knowledge proves inadequate for solving complicated problems.[10]

What constitutes a model, and what is the scope of MBR? Some claim that all knowledge bases are in fact qualitative models because they describe what is happening in the world and thus provide a basis for action.[11] However, this does not mean that all knowledge-based systems are, indeed, MBR systems. The distinction between different approaches to reasoning should be made on the basis of knowledge content and reasoning strategies, as opposed to differences in the form of knowledge representation.

In this chapter, we describe MBR as the use of structural, behavioral, and/or functional knowledge of a system in order to diagnose, predict, and/or explain

TABLE 6.1. Model-Based Reasoning Terminology

Structure: The set of components that constitute a system and the connections between these components are generally referred to as the *structure* of a system.[3] However, in qualitative reasoning, structure is also defined in terms of more abstract notions such as sets of constraint equations which collectively define the possible behaviors of a physical structure.[4]

Behavior: *Behavior* refers to the time course of observable changes of state of the components and of the system as a whole.[3]

Function: The *function* of a component is the relationship between the structure of the system and the behavior of the component that enables the component to fulfill its overall purpose in the system. In other words, structure is what a system is, behavior is what a system does, and function is what a system is for.[5] The same definitions apply to biological systems and engineered artifacts alike.

Model-based reasoning: *Model-based reasoning* is the use of structural, behavioral, and/or functional knowledge of a system in order to diagnose, predict, and/or explain its behavior and function in time.

Causal reasoning: The term *causal reasoning* is typically used to denote a more detailed level of reasoning based on cause–effect relations as opposed to simple associations and correlations.[6] Unfortunately, the distinction between association and causation is at times quite subtle and controversial. More appropriately, causal reasoning reflects the derivation of causal arguments of function from the knowledge of structure and behavior, or from other causal arguments.

Qualitative reasoning: *Qualitative reasoning* is the type of reasoning that focuses on the interesting qualitative states that a system may exhibit rather than complete numerical accounts of behavior. Qualitative reasoning, in the strict sense, is based on discrete qualitative values. This is justified by the observation that people tend to reason using discrete quantities rather than continuous variables.

Qualitative simulation: The process of determining a likely course of future behavior starting with a qualitative structural description of a system and an initial state is called *qualitative simulation.*[3] Qualitative simulations differ from numeric simulations in two respects: (1) time is individuated by the occurrence of interesting events rather than fixed increments, and (2) the reduced precision often necessitates branching to represent alternate possible futures.[7]

its behavior and function in time. Similarly, a model is considered as the structural, behavioral, and/or functional knowledge about a system which defines the system at a finer level of detail than of empirical associations. While most examples of case-based reasoning and rule-based expert systems fall outside the range of these descriptions, no distinction is made on the basis of the form of knowledge. A reasoning system based on production rule inferences may as well be categorized as model-based provided it captures domain knowledge at a level deeper than empirical associations.

6.3.1. Advantages and Disadvantages

Domain models that represent structure, behavior, or function enhance the reasoning of knowledge-based computer programs in several ways. These advantages include:[9,12–15]

- Better handling of the problems in the periphery of the knowledge base (i.e., robustness and graceful degradation)
- Better explanation of reasoning processes
- Prediction of future states
- Easier truth maintenance and consistency checking
- Verifiability
- Ability to determine what is happening in a situation at a particular time

Mainly because of the robustness of their knowledge bases, model-based systems are typically expected to outperform associational systems in complicated problem-solving situations. However, disadvantages of model-based systems are also commonly quoted:[9,16–19]

- Increased knowledge acquisition load
- Lack of detailed domain knowledge (an argument especially valid for many medical domains)
- Computational overhead of simulating complex domain models and introduction of undue complexity in solving simple problems.

6.3.2. Qualitative Reasoning

A common misconception is to equate MBR with qualitative reasoning methods. Although there is significant overlap between the two fields, not all MBR systems are qualitative in nature, and not all research on qualitative reasoning applies to MBR. In this chapter, we reserve the term *qualitative reasoning* for computer programs that simulate or analyze the behavior of a device or a system over a sequence of qualitatively distinct states.

Qualitative reasoning was introduced as an attempt to provide artificial intelligence (AI) programs with commonsense knowledge. In 1978, Hayes suggested that the commonsense knowledge about the everyday physical world should be formalized in a framework called "naive physics."[20] The term "qualitative physics" was coined later to avoid negative connotations associated with the word "naive."

Qualitative reasoning is concerned with the development of a theoretical framework for understanding the behavior of physical systems for the purposes of prediction, diagnosis, and explanation.[21] In qualitative reasoning, continuous properties of the world are abstracted into discrete systems of symbols. The lack of precision brings along the problem of ambiguity, namely, the tendency to predict several alternative sequences of behaviors. Ambiguity originates from the lack of the knowledge of precise relationships and quantitative information required to eliminate branching.[7] Although this sounds like a disadvantage, ambiguity may be exploited by a qualitative reasoning system to indicate when detailed knowledge is needed. Ambiguity provides a more skeptical look at a problem, since it helps generate all possible behaviors of a system as opposed to a single behavior as dictated by a fixed domain model. In contrast, numerical simulations have no room for ambiguity and hence may miss possible behaviors because of overprecision. Consequently, qualitative reasoning is an appropriate paradigm for domains such as medicine where complete information is not available or otherwise imprecise.

6.3.3. Causality

Causality is central to qualitative reasoning. Prediction and explanation tasks depend heavily on causal relations between parameters and on causal orders that exist among states and events. MBR derives causal accounts of system behavior and function using descriptions of component behavior and connectivity information. Unfortunately, causality is a widely debated philosophical topic and there is no agreement on what causality means and how it should be utilized by AI programs.

There are several ways to represent different types of causal relations. Some researchers have used multiple levels of causal implications such as causation, enabling, precipitation, and cooccurrence.[19,22,23] Others have experimented with multivariate relation formats.[24,25] Other formalisms make use of simple causal connections with associated likelihoods[26,27] or the more rigorous probabilistic methods such as bayesian belief networks.[28] Since not even philosophers tend to agree on what causality entails, development and use of further formalisms, each covering another significant aspect of causality, seem inevitable. The trick is usually in determining the "right" formalism for the reasoning task in hand.

The issue of appropriate level of detail or granularity is a significant concern for builders of knowledge-based systems. Although finer levels of detail will typically allow more refined reasoning, the computational complexity of reaching a solution may preclude the use of extensively detailed domain models. Detailed models are also more time consuming to compose. Besides, there is the issue of relevance:[29] the most appropriate level of granularity is the coarsest level where all the detail relevant to the current problem is captured. When pragmatic considerations preclude the development (or execution) of a model at an appropriate level of granularity, some simplifications have to be made.[17,29]

These simplifications usually take the form of simplifying assumptions or abstractions.

6.3.4. Multiple Levels of Reasoning

Models for MBR may be based on structure, behavior, function, and/or causation. Note that the use of the term "causal" may be deceptive since causal models may be developed in different grain sizes corresponding to different reasoning levels. For example, a causal reasoning system that uses causal associations such as "meningitis causes stiff neck" is no different from a rule-based expert system that may have a rule that reads "IF stiff neck and high fever THEN consider meningitis."[30] The causal pathways by which meningitis causes a stiff neck, in reality, are much more complicated. A simple causal association fails to observe (and verify) the validity of the inference in varying situations. ABEL, a system that reasons about acid–base and electrolyte disturbances, provides a good example of different levels of causal modeling in the same framework.[24] Most human expertise is based on empirical observations, enabling human reasoners to access diagnostic knowledge quickly. Patil admits that causal reasoning is computationally expensive, and that straightforward cases may be solved more efficiently by means of pattern matching systems such as CADUCEUS.[10] Yet, there are times when empirical knowledge will not suffice. In these cases, human reasoners promptly utilize detailed domain models. It is in this vein that a number of systems have been proposed to incorporate multiple levels of reasoning.[10,30]

6.4. MODEL-BASED REASONING IN LABORATORY MEDICINE

Several model-based computer programs have been devised in medical AI in recent years.[2] Examples of structure-level reasoning are not prevalent in the medical AI literature since it is difficult to use anatomic structure to directly derive behavior or function: behavior and function of most tissues and organs are context-dependent. For example, we can reason about kidney function from different perspectives (blood pressure regulation, acid–base balance, excretion of catabolic waste, etc.). Further, anatomical connections are not an adequate way of representing functional connections in the human body where anatomically distant systems such as the kidney and the pituitary are linked through a common circulatory connection. However, it is still possible to develop structure-level definitions of physiology by appropriate abstractions of physiology and anatomical connectivity within limited contexts.

Most examples of MBR in medicine use behavioral or functional reasoning (causal reasoning may be classified in either category depending on the knowledge content of the particular system in question). Note that some systems use causality as a form of association for pattern matching and as such they should not be considered as examples of MBR. These systems include some early work in medical AI such as PIP,[31] INTERNIST,[26] and QMR.[32]

A number of knowledge-based systems are introduced in the problem domains of laboratory medicine in recent years.[33-40] Most of these systems, however, are based on associational knowledge and thus cannot be regarded as examples of MBR. In this section, we will illustrate the potential use of MBR on three case studies, one taken from the "classic" medical AI literature and two examples representing more recent efforts. In the last section, we will speculate on how MBR can facilitate the expanding role of laboratory medicine in modern medical practice.

6.4.1. Case studies

6.4.1.1. ABEL. ABEL is a model-based diagnostic system developed in the late 1970s for the acid–base and electrolyte disorders domain.[24,41] In ABEL, the basic knowledge structure is a multilevel causal model that is instantiated from the causal knowledge of the domain using patient-specific data. The model represents the current interpretation of patient status during diagnosis.

ABEL uses a hierarchical multilevel representation scheme that consists of five levels of detail. Figure 6.1 shows the three most significant levels of this representation. The lowest level of description consists of pathophysiological knowledge about diseases, which is successively aggregated into higher-level concepts and relations, gradually shifting the content of the description from pathophysiological to syndromic knowledge. Each level of description can be viewed as a semantic network describing relations between diseases and findings. The causal links in ABEL specify multivariate relations between various

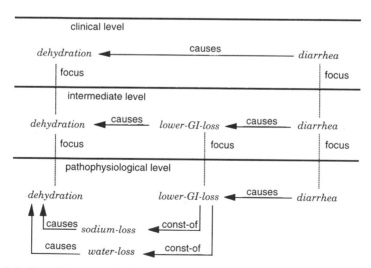

Figure 6.1. Describing causal relations between diarrhea and dehydration in ABEL. (From WJ Clancey and EH Shortliffe, eds: *Readings in Medical Artificial Intelligence: The First Decade,* 1984, p 347. Copyright © 1984 by Addison-Wesley Publishing. Reprinted by permission of Ramesh S. Patil.)

aspects of the cause and the effect. Furthermore, causal relations may be described at several levels of detail. The reasoner can switch between levels using *aggregation* and *elaboration* operations. A *projection* operator is used for hypothesizing states that are not supported by the current set of findings.

ABEL is designed for diagnosis tasks, including the diagnosis of multiple concurrent disorders. Diagnosis is guided by *parsimony*, which is the inference to the smallest possible hypothesis set that explains all observations. ABEL has component summation and component decomposition mechanisms which enable the system to reason about causes that add up or mask each other when inflicted upon an entity. The same mechanisms are used to partially account for observations, allowing ABEL to hypothesize disorders that may induce the effects that are left unaccounted for. When multiple disorders are hypothesized, or when there are a number of models to support different pathophysiological explanations of current observations, ABEL provides a ranking of possible explanations according to Occam's razor. In other words, simpler hypotheses are considered first.

6.4.1.2. NEOANEMIA.

NEOANEMIA is a diagnostic system based on abduction, deduction, and eliminative induction.[42] The application area is iron metabolism and the diagnosis of anemias. Once possible disease hypotheses are identified by means of abduction, a qualitative simulation is performed to predict future values of related parameters. The result of this simulation and future observations guide the inductive refinement of diagnostic hypotheses. The metabolic processes represented in the NEOANEMIA knowledge base include iron metabolism (intestinal absorption, plasma levels, parenchymal cell levels), erythropoiesis, and erythropoietin metabolism. The qualitative model contains approximately 30 variables and 30 qualitative constraint equations. It can simulate and reason about several pathophysiologic states such as sudden or chronic blood loss, hemolysis, failure of erythropoietin production, and defective iron absorption.

An earlier version, ANEMIA, was evaluated in blind tests as to the quality of its diagnoses. In these tests, the diagnostic performance of the system was found to be comparable to human experts' (87% acceptable results for ANEMIA vs. 90% for human experts).[43]

6.4.1.3. SIMON.

The SIMON system aims to assist clinicians with respiratory management tasks in a neonatal intensive care unit.[44,45] SIMON integrates a numerical signal interpretation module (for the analysis of raw data from monitors and laboratory measurements) with a MBR system based on a behavior model of ventilation, oxygenation, and acid–base balance. The knowledge base consists of over 40 parameters (observable and nonobservable) that relate to respiration and over 40 views and processes that define various physiologic and pathophysiologic states. The inference engine uses a qualitative simulation method for prediction purposes.

In SIMON, MBR is primarily used for diagnosis. For this purpose, SIMON

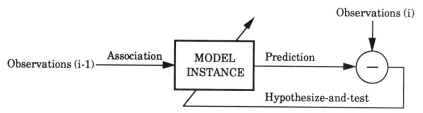

Figure 6.2. *Diagnosis by model revision in SIMON.*

constructs a patient model based on current observations and predicts future course based on this model. Any deviations from the predicted behavior are interpreted as model failures (e.g., an unexpected fault had changed the active model). SIMON then conducts a search for a fault model that explains the current observations. If such a fault model is found, the current patient model is revised to reflect the current fault and the process continues. If no fault model could explain the observations, the observations are flagged as potentially erroneous readings and are subjected to further verification. Figure 6.2 illustrates diagnosis by model revision.

In addition to the model-based diagnosis feature, SIMON is also used to generate alerts based on observations of potentially dangerous ventilator settings or suboptimal oxygenation and ventilation states.[44]

6.5. STATE-OF-THE-ART MEDICAL AI SYSTEMS

6.5.1. Consultation Systems versus "Intelligent Agents"

In earlier days, the common model for medical AI systems used to be the "consultation system" paradigm. This paradigm was based on the premise that medical expertise is a scarce and expensive entity and that computer systems may simulate expert behavior with relative ease. Consultation systems were developed to serve a variety of tasks such as the interpretation of a single test result or a number of test results and offering possible diagnostic hypotheses, guiding a primary-care physician in acquiring information about the present illness of a patient and making therapy recommendations, and simulating the role of an expert in diagnosing and managing complex cases in relatively narrow fields of expertise.

However, the consultation system paradigm failed to make an impact on healthcare delivery. Most consultation systems were not regarded very highly by medical professionals, and consequently very few systems actually saw the light of day in healthcare environments. The reasons for the demise of the consultation system paradigm are manyfold, and a discussion of the topic is beyond the scope of this chapter.

A similar trend may be recognized in model-based systems. Earlier research projects conformed to the consultation system paradigm and were generally designed for diagnostic applications. However, many recent systems are developed for a wider variety of purposes including monitoring, explanation of function and behavior, therapy planning, and prediction. Today's state-of-the-art medical AI systems typically keep low profiles in sharp contrast with the "Greek oracle" posture of older consultation systems. A typical modern system is an "intelligent agent" which would quietly monitor large volumes of data and offer its advice only when it observes conditions worthy of an alert or concern. Given the chance, the agent could also explain its findings and offer suggestions as to the management of the problem. Such a lower profile increases the chances for clinical acceptance since medical professionals would not regard the system as a potential threat or mere nuisance. In addition, today's systems typically focus on narrower areas of expertise at greater depth, thus preventing the illusion of omniscience and handling difficult problems more gracefully.

6.5.2. Inference Types

MBR methods are used for four general types of inference as listed in Table 6.2.[2,46] All four types of inference are routinely performed in relation to laboratory medicine. Diagnosis and explanation tasks relate to the interpretation of physiologic findings, whereas prediction and control tasks imply the grounding of treatment decisions on laboratory measurements. A number of knowledge-based systems have already been fielded in laboratory medicine in areas such as validation of biochemical[40] and clinical chemistry[37] data, diagnosis of thyroid function tests,[39] interpretive reporting of laboratory results and alarming,[36,38] optimization of forensic toxicology procedures,[34] tracking of nosocomial infections,[47] and quality control and fault diagnosis for laboratory instruments.[35]

The rapid evolution of clinical information systems and the enthusiasm for computer-based patient records place the clinical laboratory right on the "information superhighway" of medical care. Suddenly, there will be a capability for two-way communication of information between the patient bedside and the labs. Not only this communication capability will result in a relative knowledge explosion in the clinical laboratory, it also will pose additional demands on the validity and quality of interpretation and reporting of data. The demonstrated need for controlling the knowledge explosion in the clinical laboratory[33] strengthens the case for knowledge-based support of laboratory operations. Although traditional rule-based expert systems, fuzzy logic, and neural networks will be sufficient in many focused reasoning tasks, there is a large potential for

TABLE 6.2. Typical Inference Tasks for MBR

Diagnosis: estimating current state from the knowledge of input and manifestations
Prediction: estimating manifestations from the knowledge of input and current state
Control: estimating required input (perturbation) from the knowledge of current state and desired manifestations
Explanation: tracing and explaining a deductive inference from input to manifestations, or from input to current state

the introduction of model-based systems in the clinical laboratory. MBR systems have an edge over traditional AI systems in many complex reasoning tasks since they generally reason on the basis of models of physiology (providing breadth and depth) that are individualized for specific patients (providing specificity). In the clinical laboratory, such tasks include

- Interpretation and validation of laboratory measurements in the context of other relevant information such as diagnoses, history of prior test results, results of related tests, and physical findings
- Data reduction, or suppression of irrelevant reports
- Generation of clinical alerts for abnormal test results in specific disease and treatment contexts
- Explanation of test results in context (e.g., test–drug interactions)
- Prediction of patient progress based on history of physiologic findings and treatment information
- Assisting with treatment decisions using prediction capabilities

6.5.3. Embedded Systems

In contrast with earlier standalone expert systems, today's AI systems in health care tend to be embedded in larger information management architectures. The prototypical examples of embedded reasoning facilities can be found in the HELP system. HELP is a large-scale hospital information management system in current use at the LDS Hospital in Salt Lake City, Utah.[48] HELP embodies problem solving modules such as CORE, which is a respiratory therapy planning module for ARDS (acute respiratory distress syndrome) patients.[49] The migration toward embedded reasoning systems is also evident in recent academic research where MBR systems are often used as reasoning components of larger information management systems.[45,50,51]

6.5.4. Future Prospects

In this chapter, we described MBR and discussed its applicability in clinical laboratory environment. Given the increasing computer literacy of healthcare professionals, the availability of more sophisticated equipment for information acquisition and processing, and the increasing demand for information management in healthcare fields, the future of biomedical computing is bright. Although the potential impact of AI technology in medical environments cannot be predicted with certainty, there are reasons to be optimistic. Today's AI systems are more sophisticated than their predecessors, and they are also far more accessible to intended end users due to the proliferation of high-powered, low-cost personal computers and workstations. Thanks to advances in hardware platforms and software techniques, more complicated problems may be tackled without the need for simplifying assumptions. A current trend is toward the integration of information management tasks in healthcare, and intelligent problem-solving modules may be integrated into existing and new healthcare information management systems. The key issue is to design decision support systems for accessibility and ease of use. The advice given by these systems should be fast, sound, explainable, and sensible. Furthermore, these decision support systems should operate as intelligent agents or assistants, and the final decision making should rest with healthcare professionals who are ultimately responsible for the well-being of patients. Given these foundations, MBR systems can play an important role in keeping the clinical laboratory at the cutting edge of the information age.

REFERENCES

1. Chandrasekaran B, Milne R: Reasoning about structure, behavior, and function. *SIGART Newslett* (93):4–59, July 1985.
2. Uckun S: Model-based reasoning in biomedicine. *CRC Crit Rev Biomed Eng* 19:261–292, 1992.
3. Bobrow DG: Qualitative reasoning about physical systems: an introduction. *Artif Intell* 24:1–5, 1984.
4. Kuipers B: Commonsense reasoning about causality: deriving behavior from structure. *Artif Intell* 24:169–203, 1984.
5. de Kleer J: How circuits work. In Bobrow DG, ed: *Qualitative Reasoning about Physical Systems.* Cambridge, MA: MIT Press, 1985, pp 205–280.
6. Kuipers B: Causal reasoning. In Shapiro SC ed; *Encyclopedia of Artificial Intelligence.* Wiley-Interscience, New York, 1987, pp 827–832.
7. Forbus KD: Qualitative physics: past, present, and future. In Shrobe HE, ed: *Exploring Artificial Intelligence.* San Mateo, CA: Morgan Kaufmann, pp 239–296.
8. Gentner D, Stevens AL: *Mental Models.* Hillsdale, NJ: Lawrence Erlbaum, 1983.
9. Swartout WR, Smoliar SW: Explaining the link between causal reasoning and expert behavior. In Miller PL, ed: *Selected Topics in Medical Artificial Intelligence.* New York: Springer-Verlag, 1988, pp 71–84.
10. Patil RS, Senyk O: Compiling causal knowledge for diagnostic reasoning. In Miller PL, ed: *Selected Topics in Medical Artificial Intelligence.* New York: Springer-Verlag, 1988, pp 25–39.
11. Clancey WJ: Viewing knowledge bases as qualitative models. *IEEE Expert,* 9–23, 1989.
12. Widman LE, Lee YB, and Pao Y-H: Toward the diagnosis of medical causal models by semiquantitative reasoning. In Miller PL, ed: *Selected Topics in Medical Artificial Intelligence.* New York: Springer-Verlag, 1988, pp 55–70.
13. Bonissone PP, Valavanis KP: A comparative study of different approaches to qualitative physics theories. In *Proc 2nd Conf Artificial Intelligence Applications,* Miami Beach, FL, 1985, pp 236–243.
14. Kulikowski C, Weiss SM: Representation of expert knowledge for consultation: the CASNET and EXPERT projects. In Szolovits P, ed: *Artificial Intelligence in Medicine.* Boulder, CO: Westview Press, 1982, pp 21–55.
15. Forbus KD: Qualitative Process Theory. PhD dissertation, MIT, Cambridge, MA, 1984.

16. Parker RC, Miller RA: Using causal knowledge to create simulated patient cases: CPCS project as an extension of INTERNIST-1. In Miller PL, ed: *Selected Topics in Medical Artificial Intelligence.* New York: Springer-Verlag, 1988, pp 99–115.

17. Falkenhainer B, Forbus KD: Setting up large-scale qualitative models. In *Proc 7th National Conf Artificial Intelligence,* St Paul, MN, 1988, pp 301–306.

18. Senyk, O: The integration of compiled and explicit causal knowledge for diagnostic reasoning. In *Proc 12th Annual Symp Comput Appl Med Care,* Washington, DC, 1988, pp 106–109.

19. Miller PL, Fisher PR: Causal models for medical artificial intelligence. In Miller PL, ed: *Selected Topics in Medical Artificial Intelligence.* New York: Springer-Verlag, 1988, pp 11–24.

20. Hayes PJ: The second naive physics manifesto. In Hobbs J, Moore B, eds: *Formal Theories of the Commonsense World.* Norwood, NJ: Ablex, 1985, pp 1–36.

21. de Kleer J, Brown JS: A qualitative physics based on confluences. *Artif Intell* 24:7–83, 1984.

22. Rieger C, Grinberg M: The declarative representation and procedural simulation of causality in physical mechanisms. In *Proc 5th Internatl Joint Conf Artificial Intelligence,* Cambridge, MA, 1977, pp 250–256.

23. Long WJ, Naimi S, Criscitiello, MG, Jayes R: Development and use of a causal model for reasoning about heart failure. In Miller PL, ed: *Selected Topics in Medical Artificial Intelligence.* New York: Springer-Verlag, 1988, pp 40–54.

24. Patil RS, Szolovits P, Schwartz WB: Causal understanding of patient illness in medical diagnosis. In *Proc 7th Internatl Joint Conf Artificial Intelligence,* Vancouver, BC, 1981, pp 893–899.

25. Blum RL: Induction of causal relationships from a time-oriented clinical database: an overview of the RX project. In *Proc 2nd Natl Conf Artificial Intelligence,* 1982, Pittsburgh, PA, pp 355–357.

26. Miller RA, Pople HE Jr, Myers JD: INTERNIST-1, an experimental computer-based diagnostic consultant for general internal medicine. In Clancey WJ, Shortliffe EH, eds: *Readings in Medical Artificial Intelligence: The First Decade.* Reading, MA: Addison-Wesley, 1984, pp 190–209.

27. Weiss SM, Kulikowski CA, Amarel S, Safir A: A model-based method for computer-aided medical decision making. In Clancey WJ, Shortliffe EH, eds: *Readings in Medical Artificial Intelligence: The First Decade.* Reading, MA: Addison-Wesley, 1984, pp 160–189.

28. Middleton BF, Shwe MA: Probabilistic diagnosis using a reformulation of the Internist-1/QMR knowledge base-II. Evaluation of diagnostic performance. *Meth Info Med* 30:256–267, 1991.

29. Hobbs JR: Granularity. In *Proc 9th Internatl Joint Conf Artificial Intelligence,* Los Angeles, CA, 1985, pp 432–435.

30. Sticklen JH: MDX2: an integrated medical diagnostic system. PhD dissertation, Ohio State University, Columbus, OH, 1987.

31. Pauker SG, Gorry A, Kassirer JP, Schwartz WB: Towards the simulation of clinical cognition: taking a present illness by computer. *Am J Med* 60:981–996, 1976.

32. Miller RA, McNeil MA, Chalinor SM, Masarie FE Jr, et al: The INTERNIST-1/QUICK MEDICAL REFERENCE project—status report. *West J Med* 145:816–822, 1986.

33. Winkel P: The application of expert systems in the clinical laboratory. *Clin Chem* 35:1595–1600, 1989.

34. Cechner RL, Sutheimer CA: Automated rule-based decision systems in forensic toxicology using expert knowledge: basic principles and practical applications. *J Anal Toxicol* 14:280–284, 1990.

35. Groth T, Moden H: A knowledge-based system for real-time quality control and fault diagnosis of multitest analyzers. *Comput Meth Programs Biomed* 34:175–190, 1991.

36. Tate KE, Gardner RM, Weaver LK: A computerized laboratory alerting system. *MD Comput* 7:296–301, 1990.

37. Johansson B, Bergvin L: Arden Syntax as a standard for knowledge bases in the clinical chemistry laboratory. *Clin Chim Acta* 222:123–128, 1993.

38. Nykanen P, Boran G, Pince H, Clarke K, et al: Interpretative reporting and alarming based on laboratory data. *Clin Chim Acta* 222:37–48, 1993.

39. Saarinen K, Nykanen P, Irjala K, Viikari J, et al: Design and development of the THYROID system. *Comput Meth Programs Biomed* 34:211–218, 1991.

40. Valdiguie PM, Rogari E, Philippe H; VALAB: expert system for validation of biochemical data. *Clin Chem* 38:83–87, 1992.

41. Patil RS, Szolovits P, Schwartz WB: Modeling knowledge of the patient in acid-base and electrolyte disorders. In Szolovits P, ed: *Artificial Intelligence in Medicine.* Boulder, CO: Westview Press, 1982, pp 191–226.

42. Quaglini S, Bellazzi, R, Berzuini C, Stefanelli M, et al: Hybrid knowledge-based systems for therapy planning. *Artif Intell Med* 4:207–226, 1992.

43. Quaglini S, Stefanelli M: ANEMIA: an expert consultation system. *Comput Biomed Res* 19:23–27, 1986.

44. Uckun S, Dawant BM: Qualitative modeling as a paradigm for diagnosis and prediction in critical care environments. *Artif Intell Med* 4:127–144, 1992.

45. Uckun S, Dawant BM, Lindstrom DP: Model-based reasoning in intensive care monitoring: the YAQ approach. *Artif Intell Med* 5:31–48, 1993.

46. Bratko I, Mozetic I, Lavrac N: *KARDIO: A Study in Deep and Qualitative Knowledge for Expert Systems.* Cambridge, MA: MIT Press, 1989.

47. Kahn MG, Steib SA, Fraser VJ, Dunagan WC: An expert system for culture-based infection control surveillance. In *Proc 17th Annu Symp Comput Appl Medical Care,* Baltimore, 1993, pp 171–175.

48. East TD, Henderson S, Morris AH, Gardner RM: Implementation issues and challenges for computerized clinical protocols for management of mechanical ventilation in ARDS patients. In *Proc 13th Annu Symp Comput Appl Med Care,* Washington, DC, 1989, pp 583–587.

49. East TD, Bohm SH, Wallace CJ, Clemmer TP, et al: A successful computerized protocol for clinical management of pressure control inverse ratio ventilation in ARDS patients. *Chest* 101:696–710, 1992.

50. Rutledge G, Thomsen G, Farr B, Tovar M, et al: The design and implementation of a ventilator-management advisor. *Artif Intell Med* 5(1):67–82, 1993.

51. Hayes-Roth B, Washington R, Ash D, Hewett R, et al: Guardian: a prototype intelligent agent for intensive-care monitoring. *Artif Intell Med* 4(2):165–185, 1992.

CHAPTER

7

Fuzzy Logic Expert Systems

JACK C. MARTIN AND LAWRENCE C. MAGUIRE

The truth is rarely pure and never simple.

Oscar Wilde

CONTENTS

Handbook of Clinical Automation, Robotics, and Optimization, Edited by Gerald J. Kost with the collaboration of Judith Welsh.
ISBN 0-471-03179-8 © 1996 John Wiley & Sons, Inc.

Fuzzy logic is an exciting technology that is being used increasingly to implement and control complex systems in many applications. The foundations of fuzzy logic were developed in the mid-1960s by Lotfi Zadeh at the University of California, Berkeley as a better way of approaching imprecision. Although Zadeh was a believer in precision, he observed that many complex systems couldn't be represented with exactness. This bothered him, and led to the conception of a new mathematics of vagueness that was better suited to modeling the complex systems that surround us—and ultimately the ways in which we think.

The fundamental problem is that most of the systems we deal with are so complex that exactitude is not feasible. It is clear that biological, social, economic, and many similar sciences are fraught with imprecision. But likewise, descriptions in the physical sciences must forever be imprecise. It is not feasible to depict a weather pattern at the molecular level, and even if one could the description isn't complete unless the molecules are broken down into atoms, the atoms decomposed to subatomic particles and so on. Very little useful science can be done without making simplifying assumptions and approximations, and this is as much true in the clinical sciences as anywhere else.

As humans, we find it very natural to deal with vagueness. "It's hot today" is imprecise. There is no magic number at which everyone agrees that it is "hot." We cannot say that 90°F is "hot" and 89°F is "not-hot." Instead, we deal with an imprecise usage of the term, and add modifiers ("very hot," "not too hot") to indicate degrees of "hotness." Similarly, we have less than precise definitions of what constitutes a "long time," what "large" means, when a person is "sick," and virtually every term that we use in our daily communications. If we had to control our body's every motion with absolute precision we would find it impossible to walk across the room; similarly, if our cognitive processes did not deal in approximations, we would find it impossible to complete a train of thought. It turns out that this capacity for dealing with vagueness is a crucial factor in our ability to comprehend our world.

The contribution of fuzzy logic is that it allows systems (e.g., computer programs) to be built that deal with our world in a very natural fashion. Expert systems* that are built on fuzzy logic can outperform conventional techniques in many applications, and have proven successful in domains where other artificial intelligence techniques have failed. From automated subways to better vacuum cleaners, fuzzy systems have established a solid record of effectiveness.

Acceptance of fuzzy logic technology has been slow in the United States. Zadeh's seminal work was done three decades ago, yet fuzzy systems have just recently begun to gain acceptance in this country. However in Japan fuzzy logic was readily embraced, and has become a mainstay technology in applications ranging from science to consumer products.

Today, fuzzy systems can be found in complex applications like recognizing handwriting, manipulating aircraft control surfaces, running steam plants, de-

---

*Computer systems that capture knowledge from human experts and mimic, at some level, their expertise.

tecting credit-card fraud, and forecasting weather. They are used in products such as copiers, cameras, check scanners, elevators and automobiles, and in household appliances such as washers, microwave ovens, refrigerators, and televisions. In the healthcare industry, fuzzy systems are directing drug research, directing treatment of diabetes and rheumatology, providing clinical instrument control, and performing hospital management. There are few limits to the potential applications of fuzzy logic.

7.1. FUZZY SYSTEM THEORY CONCEPTS

This is not a treatise on fuzzy system theory—rather, it is an overview of the basic concepts and terms. In this abbreviated venue it is possible to introduce the principles only so that the reader may grasp the fundamentals. A fuzzy system developer should consult one of the references on fuzzy theory.[1-5] After an introduction to fuzzy sets and operations on them, fuzzy reasoning—the foundation for fuzzy models—will be described. The section will conclude with an outline of the development of fuzzy expert systems.

7.1.1. Fuzzy Sets

Fuzzy set theory is a mathematics for encoding the lexicon of our everyday reasoning. We don't think in terms of absolute precision—rather, we rely heavily on concepts such as around, some, about, not too, almost, somewhat, near, and so forth. Fuzzy sets provide a rigorous description of these imprecise terms that are pervasive in our communications and fundamental to our thought patterns.

It is our nature to categorize things. Our languages are build around classifications of the objects and concepts of our world. However, conventional set theory does not model the way we approach the real world very well. Classical set theory as developed by mathematician Georg Cantor in the late 1800s is very precise. A set is defined by the criteria necessary for membership. Something is either a member of a set or not a member—the boundary of the set is very crisp. Mathematicians and logicians have built an entire field on Cantor's definitions of sets and operations on them.

For most of the things we deal with in real life, however, crisp sets offer a poor model. Membership in categories is not crisp, it comes in degrees. The world does not divide neatly into hot and not-hot, risky and not-risky, tall and not-tall, strong and not-strong, expensive and inexpensive. To pick a number x and say that any house costing x or more is expensive seems very unrealistic to us. Suppose your house cost x and your neighbor's house cost one dollar less than x—does it seem reasonable to call your house expensive and your neighbor's house inexpensive? Yet crisp sets require such a precise criterion for membership. In contrast, fuzzy sets are defined in terms of *degree of membership*. Figures 7.1 and 7.2 contrast the crisp set approach with the fuzzy set approach.

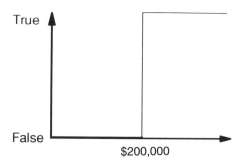

Figure 7.1. Membership in the "Expensive House" crisp set.

Fuzzy sets come in varied styles. Several useful types are the linear fuzzy set, the *S*-curve fuzzy set, the bell-shaped fuzzy set, and the geometric fuzzy set. There are a number of other types of fuzzy sets. Fuzzy sets also can be irregularly shaped.

The *linear* fuzzy set is represented by a straight line. It can be *increasing* (as in Fig. 7.2) or *decreasing*. The membership function for an increasing linear fuzzy set is defined by

$$
\begin{aligned}
\mu(x, a, b) &= \frac{x - a}{b - a} &&\text{for} \quad a < x < b \\
&= 0 &&\text{for} \quad x <= a \\
&= 1 &&\text{for} \quad x >= b
\end{aligned}
$$

where μ is the degree of membership for value x, ranging from zero (not a member) to one (full membership), and a and b are the left and right endpoints of the set. A decreasing linear fuzzy set is similarly defined.

The *S-curve* fuzzy set (see Fig. 7.3) and the bell-shaped fuzzy set (see Fig. 7.4) are particularly useful in modeling experts' perception of classifications. The *S*-curve fuzzy set, which can be either increasing (as in Fig. 7.3) or decreasing, is

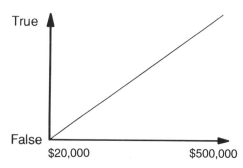

Figure 7.2. Degrees of membership in the "Expensive House" fuzzy set.

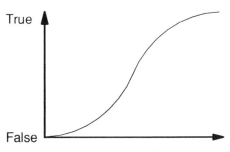

Figure 7.3. An S-curve fuzzy set.

defined by three parameters—the two endpoints (zero membership and full membership) and an inflection point. The increasing S-curve fuzzy set membership function is

$$\mu(x, a, b, i) = 2\left(\frac{x - a}{b - a}\right)^2 \qquad \text{for} \quad a < x < i$$
$$= 1 - 2\left(\frac{x - b}{b - a}\right)^2 \qquad \text{for} \quad i < x < b$$
$$= 0 \qquad \text{for} \quad x <= a$$
$$= 1 \qquad \text{for} \quad x >= b$$

where i is the point of inflection and μ, a, and b are as before. The decreasing S-curve fuzzy set is similarly defined.

Bell-shaped fuzzy sets can be defined by several different curves. Two useful ones are the *beta curve* and the *gaussian curve*. The beta curve tends to be rather broad, admitting some degree of membership to the fuzzy set over a wide range. The gaussian curve is much more narrow, falling to zero membership very quickly. The formula for the gaussian curve is

$$\mu(x, c, k) = e^{-k(c - x)^2}$$

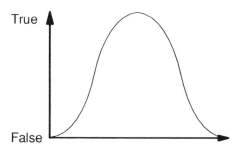

Figure 7.4. A bell-shaped fuzzy set.

where c is the center of the domain and k is a factor controlling the width of the curve. The formula for the beta curve is

$$\mu(x, c, \beta) = \frac{1}{1 + ((x - c)/\beta)^2}$$

where c is the center of the domain and β is a factor controlling the width of the curve.

7.1.2. Fuzzy Set Operations

In order to accomplish nontrivial reasoning using fuzzy logic, it is necessary to operate on fuzzy sets—to combine them, restrict them, transform them. The basic fuzzy set operations defined by Zadeh correspond to the fundamental operations for classic set theory. However, the definitions are based on degree of membership (the membership function), and the resulting operations are at the heart of fuzzy logic. The operations are

$$\text{Intersection, } A \cap B = \min(\mu_A[x], \mu_B[x])$$
$$\text{Union, } A \cup B = \max(\mu_A[x], \mu_B[x])$$
$$\text{Complement, } \bar{A} = 1 - \mu_A[x]$$

In the years since Zadeh defined these basic operations, alternative forms have been devised that are better for the construction of complex fuzzy models. These are referred to as *compensatory operators* since they are designed to compensate for the strict nature of Zadeh's rules, avoiding the tendency of a very restrictive (or very unrestrictive) fuzzy assertion to dominate the results of fuzzy reasoning. A number of alternative forms are in common use. There are simple compensatory operators that rely on calculations of mean values, products, and so on. And there are operators of considerable complexity that are "tunable" to produce desired effects when combining fuzzy assertions. The selection of a particular form is a heuristic part of the modeling effort—the modeler may try several different forms and select the one that works.

7.1.2.1. HEDGES. Hedges are important operations performed on fuzzy sets. Hedges have a purpose similar to the role played by adjectives in our natural language—they modify fuzzy sets by qualifying, limiting or intensifying requirements for membership. Hedges are extremely useful in building fuzzy expert systems because they map very well to ordinary semantics used by experts. For instance, there is a *very* hedge that can be applied to a fuzzy set such as *expensive* to intensify the requirements for membership. Zadeh defined the *very* hedge to be μ^2, which results in a more restrictive membership requirement. Since the membership value ranges from 0 (no membership) to 1.0 (full membership), the hedge has the effect of making the membership value less true throughout the range (see Fig. 7.5).

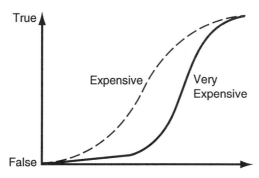

Figure 7.5. A hedged fuzzy set.

It turns out that using μ^2 closely mimics the subjective effect most people give to the adjective *very.* Similarly, using the square root of the membership function as a hedge for the adjective *somewhat* maps well to common usage of that word to dilute the strength of a statement (contrast the notions of *somewhat hot, hot,* and *very hot*). In addition to intensification/dilution hedges (such as *very* and *somewhat*), there are approximation hedges (*around, about*), restriction hedges (*above, below*), and others. The application of hedges to fuzzy sets is fundamental to encoding experts' common descriptions of things for use in modeling.

7.1.3. Fuzzy Propositions

The basis for fuzzy modeling is *fuzzy reasoning.* Fuzzy reasoning combines fuzzy set membership with "fuzzy rules" and, making use of fuzzy set operations, forms a conclusion. These rules are called *fuzzy propositions,* and take two forms:

$$a \text{ is } b \quad \text{(unconditional proposition)}$$
$$\text{If } c \text{ is } d, \text{ then } a \text{ is } b \quad \text{(conditional proposition)}$$

For instance,

The patient is infected
If the patient's temperature is high, the patient is infected

Propositions are in effect approximate statements. We say that a proposition is true to the extent of membership in the underlying fuzzy set. In other words, *a is b* is true to the degree that *a* is a member of fuzzy set *b.* Unconditional propositions are used for describing boundary conditions for a problem and for setting default action when other propositions have little or no effect.

A conditional proposition is actually two propositions connected by a conditional (if . . . then). It states that the second proposition (the *consequent*) is true to the extent that the first proposition (the *antecedent*) is true. In other words, *a is b* will be true to the same degree that *c is d* is true. The antecedent may actually be a compound proposition—that is, a series of propositions connected by fuzzy operators. For instance,

If *c* is *d* and *e* is *f,* then *a* is *b*

where "and" is a fuzzy operator (e.g., a Zadeh intersection). In this case, the membership of *a* in fuzzy set *b* is

$$\mu_b(a) = \min(\mu_d(c), \mu_f(e))$$

That is, *a*'s membership in *b* is the same strength as the weakest of *c*'s membership in *d* and *e*'s membership in *f*.

7.1.3.1. PROPORTIONAL REASONING. A simple and straightforward type of fuzzy reasoning is *proportional* reasoning (also called *monotonic* reasoning). This type of reasoning works when one proposition is sufficient to describe the relationship between the input variable(s) and the (single) output variable of interest, and the membership function of the fuzzy set underlying the output variable is monotonically increasing. The proposition may have either a simple or compound antecedent. In practice, most models are more complex than this, but proportional reasoning is a useful building block. A simple estimator may be created based on proportional reasoning, using the following steps:

> Given an input variable *x,* determine the membership value of *x* in F_1
> Select the output variable *y* that has the same membership value in F_2

where F_1 and F_2 are the underlying fuzzy sets. For instance, consider a body surface estimator based on the fuzzy proposition

If height if TALL, then body surface is LARGE

Given a person's height, by determining the person's membership in the TALL fuzzy set and selecting the body surface in the LARGE fuzzy set at the same membership level, we can estimate the person's body surface. Figure 7.6 shows how the estimator works for a given height *h,* yielding a body surface estimate of *s*.

7.1.3.2. COMPOSITIONAL INFERENCE RULES. When there are multiple propositions and it doesn't make sense to chain them together serially, then conclusions must be formed by considering the propositions in parallel. There are ways to do this so that the effects of several propositions are combined to infer a conclusion. Combining propositions relies on the basic tenant that the truth of the result cannot be any greater than the truth of the premises. Thus, the task is

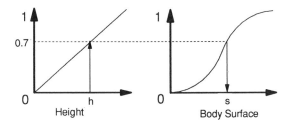

Figure 7.6. Body surface estimator using proportional reasoning.

to determine how much to restrict the truth of the inference based on the proposition truths, and how to go about accomplishing the restrictions.

There are two principal ways of determining how much to restrict the truth of the conclusion (i.e., how much to limit the membership values of the consequent fuzzy set)—the *min–max* implication rule and the *fuzzy additive* implication rule. The min–max method truncates the consequent fuzzy region using each predicate truth value, whereas the fuzzy additive method adds a contribution for each predicate truth value. There are also two popular ways of applying the restrictions—the *correlation minimum* method and the *correlation product* method. The correlation minimum method truncates the predicate fuzzy sets at the limit value, whereas the correlation product method scales the consequent fuzzy region using the limit value. For example, in Fig. 7.7 the min-max rule and the correlation minimum method have been used to combine the following predicates:

$$P_1: \text{If } a \text{ is } A \text{ and } b \text{ is } B, \text{ then } s \text{ is } S_1$$
$$P_2: \text{If } c \text{ is } C \text{ and } d \text{ is } D, \text{ then } s \text{ is } S_2$$

Assume that we start with four fuzzy sets: linear set A, triangular set B, linear set C, and triangular set D, and two bell-shaped sets S1 and S2 for the solution variable s. We will use the min-max rule and the correlation minimum restriction method. The composition is a three step process:

Step 1: A and B are combined to restrict S_1 by using a restriction level of 0.7 (the minimum of 0.7 and 0.9)

Step 2: C and D are combined to restrict S2 by using a restriction level of 0.4 (the minimum of 0.7 and 0.4)

Step 3: The solution set S is computed by taking the union of S_1 and S_2.

A real-life problem that fits this pattern is a fuzzy model for determining the correct dosage of, say, an antibiotic in a patient with some degree of renal failure. In this case, sets A and B might represent the patient's weight and renal

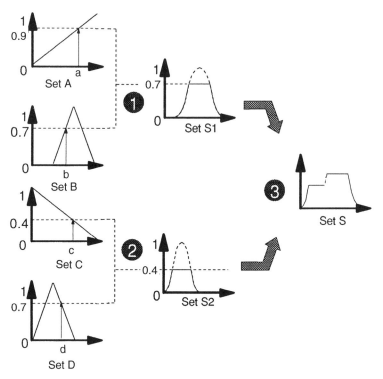

Figure 7.7. Compositional inference.

function, and sets C and D might represent the characteristics of the drug and the desired normalized dosage. The solution variable for the model would be the actual dosage to prescribe. The compositional process outlined above yields a fuzzy solution set, rather than an exact number of the solution variable. There is one more step in the process.

7.1.4. Defuzzifying

The steps outlined so far yield a fuzzy set representing the solution variable. Although this is interesting, it is not generally useful as a final result; rather, a scalar value for the solution is what is needed. The final step in fuzzy reasoning is *defuzzifying* the solution fuzzy set. Simply put, this means picking one number that is representative of the solution set. There are several different methods of doing this. These approaches rely on heuristic rather than theoretical principles. The two most frequently used defuzzification methods are the *centroid* method and the *composite maximum* method.

The centroid method is the best general-purpose defuzzification method because it yields reliably smooth changes in response to input variations, and it is rather easy to compute. This method seeks to determine the "center of gravity"

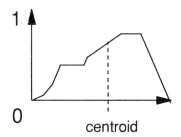

Figure 7.8. Centroid of a fuzzy solution set.

of the solution fuzzy set. To visualize this, consider the fuzzy set in Fig. 7.8. The dotted line crosses the fuzzy set at a point such that equal areas of the fuzzy set are on each side of the line. The point at which the line crosses the domain axis (*x* axis), then, is the scalar output used to represent the solution. The centroid is the weighted mean of the fuzzy set. This is calculated by taking the mean after weighting each point of the domain by its membership value. The result is an equal area under the membership curve above and below the centroid point of the domain. The exact arithmetic for calculating this point depends on the representation of the domain.

The composite maximum method seeks to find a point that represents the maximum truthfulness of the solution fuzzy set. Whereas the centroid method takes into account contributions from all the propositions weighted according to their truthfulness, the composite maximum method is sensitive to the single proposition that is most true. This results in less smooth response characteristics (which can be accentuated if the correlation product (scaling) method is also used). However, composite maximum is used in many models where it is important to base the results on the "most likely scenario."

Figure 7.9 shows the composite maximum method used to defuzzify the same solution set as in Fig. 7.8. Note that since there was an entire region with maximum truth value, the average point (center) of this region was selected. There are other more esoteric defuzzification methods, but one of these two methods will suffice in most applications.

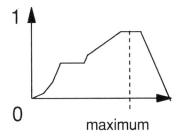

Figure 7.9. Composite maximum of a fuzzy solution set.

7.2. MODELING WITH FUZZY LOGIC

Computers are used for many things—one of the most intriguing uses is for modeling. A *model* is a computer program that represents something in the real world and, through some level of understanding, provides a useful function such as control, decision support, simulation, or analysis. Models are among the most sophisticated uses of computer technology, and are found in applications ranging from economics (e.g. Wall Street) to outer space.

Fuzzy models—models based on fuzzy reasoning—have become very popular in the last few years, most notably in Japan. They have been used for consumer applications ranging from cameras to dishwashers, and industrial applications from kilns to subways. One of the most promising areas is expert systems—computer systems for encapsulating and applying the knowledge of experts. Human experts possess domain knowledge consisting of a theoretical understanding coupled with experience in problem solving. Expert systems seek to capture knowledge from human experts and encode it in a way that permits one to apply it to solve a class of similar problems. Traditional expert systems are based on crisp rules—but human experts don't think that way. Fuzzy logic provides a technology for modeling the expert's knowledge in a more direct fashion.

The synergy between expert knowledge and fuzzy technology exists on two levels. First, the vocabulary of fuzzy logic is very close to the human vocabulary. Experiments dating back 20 years[6] confirm that humans think with a "fuzzy" vocabulary. Thus, it is straightforward for an expert to describe domain knowledge to a fuzzy model. Second, the methodology with which a fuzzy model develops a conclusion closely mimics the human thought process (but of course on a very primitive level). This leads to model decisions that can approach the accuracy and consistency of a human expert. Fuzzy logic also presents an excellent methodology for synthesizing the knowledge of multiple experts, including apparently contradictory rules.

Usually, expert systems are developed by a domain expert and a model designer ("knowledge engineer") working as a team. This applies to fuzzy expert systems as well, but the synergy of vocabulary greatly strengthens the teamwork. The domain expert provides the description of the problem domain and the rules for reaching conclusions. These are usually demonstrated with examples, which may become test cases for the model. The domain expert's involvement continues even after the expert system is developed, in the form of tuning and validation of the model's actions.

7.2.1. Developing Fuzzy Expert Systems

In general, fuzzy expert systems can be developed substantially quicker than conventional models, since fuzzy set theory provides a much more efficient knowledge encapsulation mechanism. Indeed, although academic debates abound over whether fuzzy modeling actually yields results that are significantly better than methods based on crisp mathematics, it is generally accepted that fuzzy models have much shorter development times.

Most good software development methods are applicable to writing models. However, object technology[7]—object-oriented design[8] and programming—is particularly well suited to modeling, since the object-oriented paradigm maps so naturally to real-world phenomena. This is equally true for fuzzy models, which are our focus. Object technology provides significant gains in software development productivity also, and the combination of using object technology and fuzzy theory for modeling is ideal for rapid model development.

There are many ways to develop models, just as with any software. Some ways are better than others for specific types of model developments. One can argue that some methods are better in the general case—and computer scientists frequently do so. In truth, there are many good methods, and the most important thing is to follow *some* method of design and development rather than building the model in an ad hoc fashion.

We present here a four phase description of the process for building a fuzzy model that presumes an object-oriented method of design and development. The first phase is the *assessment,* in which the problem at hand is assessed along with the resources to solve it. Then in the *design* phase the look and feel of the model and the solution approach are determined, and the model architecture is designed. In the *construction* phase, the fuzzy sets and the propositions are built and code is written to fuzzify, combine and defuzzify, as well as for all the model support structure. The code is tested and the model is tuned and validated in the *verification* phase. It should be noted that this process is not rigorously sequential—the different phases are actually overlapped, and, for a significantly complex model, development is an iterative process of incremental refinement.

7.2.1.1. ASSESSMENT. The first thing to do in writing a model is to carefully formulate a problem statement. Although this seems self-evident, many developers have started building models without knowing exactly what it is that the model should do. Needless to say, the success of such models is serendipitous at best. A good problem statement leads directly to selecting the output variables of the model.

The next step is to assess the resources available to the model. From the spectrum of domain information available, determine what is important and germane to the problem. From this, input variables can be selected.

The last step is to search for pertinent relationships between the input and output variables. These may exist as direct or indirect relationships. It is these relationships that will lead to formal propositions. This step puts a premium on domain expertise (knowledge of the problem domain being modeled).

7.2.1.2. DESIGN. Design is best accomplished as an iterative process. The process entails making incremental refinements at progressively lower levels of abstraction until the design is complete at a sufficient level of granularity for implementation. Actually, good designers work simultaneously at several levels of abstraction, and the design isn't completely finished until the implementation is well in hand. Particularly with an object-oriented design, many iterations may be appropriate before the design is finalized.

The first step is to design the output representation. The saying "if you don't know where you're going, you'll wind up somewhere else" applies equally well to model development. It is crucial to get the output of the model designed correctly or the rest of the model design is in jeopardy of being driven to the wrong purpose. Define objects that can represent the desired output from the model by seeking out key abstractions of the problem solution space and identifying characteristics or relationships that typify the solution. Then decide how the solution should be presented. To determine the best presentation, carefully think about the use of the result.

For instance, if the model's purpose is to select "safe" research projects, then the important objects in the solution space (as well as throughout the model in this case) would be projects and a key characteristic would be risk. Any measure of risk is obviously fuzzy, so a good output would be the *project* with the lowest membership in the *risk* fuzzy set. Assuming that this model is part of a decision support system, it would seem appropriate to present not only the winning project but also some indication of the level of discrimination of this solution over the nearest competitors (perhaps by showing the top three projects).

For models with human interfaces, there is an output consideration which is very important and almost always overlooked—a model should indicate to the user *how* it arrived at the conclusion. Not only is this crucial during the tuning and verification of the model by the developer and domain experts; it is important to end users that they be able to follow the model's reasoning in order to have faith in the model's results.

Having established the output at a relatively high level of abstraction, we know what the model must produce and this will guide us in the next steps of model design. Without this knowledge, the rest of the model design in the best-case scenario will require additional iterations, and in the worst-case scenario will be seriously flawed. Next is the input design. The input may come from a user interface if appropriate (for instance, in a decision support model), from sensors (in a control application), or perhaps from an upstream system (if the fuzzy model is a subsystem of a larger system). The input may be either fuzzy or crisp.

Having defined the output and input objects, the next step is to select the appropriate fuzzy set topologies for representing the key characteristics of the objects. Domain knowledge is the critical ingredient here, and the modeler must work closely with the domain expert to decide which types of fuzzy sets (linear, S-curve, etc.) best describe the characteristics of the objects. Likewise, the applicable types of hedges must be selected. Once the types of fuzzy sets and hedges have been picked, the vocabulary for the model is established (subject, of course, to subsequent refinement in future design iterations). The terms are available with which to describe things in the problem space. At this stage, the developer should have a good mental image of the problem, and be able to converse with the domain expert with considerable fluency. We've established the vocabulary; next we build sentences.

Descriptions are embodied in the fuzzy set definitions, including appropriate hedges. But facts describing something are only one part of the knowledge. It is the understanding of the thing that is crucial to a useful model. In a fuzzy system model, that understanding is embodied in the key relationships between the objects of the model. These take the form of propositions.* A good starting point is to write down all the relationships that the domain expert can think of, using the vocabulary of the input and output variables, the fuzzy sets and the hedges. Then, go back and consider each of them, asking which relationships the expert would use in trying to solve the problem. Then restate these key relationships as formal propositions. It is likely that in developing the propositions, the need to expand the model's vocabulary will arise (e.g., a new hedge may be needed to adequately express a relationship).

The next step is to decide how to put the propositions together—that is, to select the fuzzy compositional method(s) to use. A good choice for the compositional inference rule is the min–max rule coupled with the correlation minimum restriction method. However, the characteristics of the problem or solution domain may indicate a different selection.

The transition from the fuzzy solution set to a specific answer is the next step. Although there are numerous defuzzification methods, the two most likely candidates are the centroid method and the composite maximum method. The better choice for control applications is the centroid method since it yields a smooth output. For a selection application (picking the "best" of something), the composite maximum is the better choice.

Knowledge of the thing being modeled is generally separated from the mechanism for applying that knowledge. We can think in terms of an "engine" that takes knowledge and applies it to yield conclusions. The engine may be general purpose and possess little if any awareness of the thing being modeled. Good software design dictates separation and encapsulation of tasks according to purpose, and this division of knowledge from the engine follows this premise. Separating the engine from the knowledge also makes the design reusable in other models. Indeed there are fuzzy system shells available that provide the engine and execution logic, and one must only provide the fuzzy set descriptions, propositions, and so on—specifically, the "knowledge." A similar approach can be taken using object technology. A *framework* can be built which implements at an abstract level the mechanism of a fuzzy model.

7.2.1.3. CONSTRUCTION. Construction has two primary facets: encoding information about the model domain (e.g., fuzzy set parameters, proposition wording) and coding the program which will accept and process the information and yield a result.

The first thing to do in the construction phase is to pick an implementation

---

*In a pure object-oriented design, propositions could be objects of classes called *SimpleConditionalProposition, CompoundConditionalProposition,* or *UnconditionalProposition,* which could be subclasses of a *Proposition* base class. They can act as transform objects with the capability of altering the working solution set (which might be an object of a type-specific subclass of *FuzzySet.*

language. The dominant object-oriented programming languages today are C++ and SmallTalk. Either of these languages is an excellent choice for developing models, including fuzzy models. By selecting one of these languages, the developer has available various class libraries that can significantly enhance model creation. Good libraries exist for collection classes, for communication classes and for constructing graphical user interfaces in both languages. Major vendors like IBM, Borland and Microsoft provide extensive class libraries with their language products. Code libraries are also becoming available for fuzzy systems development. One example of a library that can speed development of fuzzy systems is included in Reference 9; although not really object-oriented, this library is written in C++ and can be used effectively for an object-oriented model written in C++. Additionally, this reference is an excellent guide to developing fuzzy systems.

Next, the input phase is written. If the input is via a human interface, the most usable approach has proven to be a graphical user interface (GUI).* Extensive class libraries exist for developing GUIs. Some are portable across different hardware and operating system platforms, providing an added incentive to developers of multiplatform models. As in all human-interactive software, human factors testing using real subjects is important in getting the interface correct.

The next step is to code the internal representation of the model information. Using object technology, this involves writing the appropriate class definitions; with conventional programming techniques the information will be represented in arrays, structures, lists, and the like. In either case, careful consideration of performance issues must be made here. Many developers fail to appreciate the importance of the data representation in the overall performance characteristics of a model. This step frequently leads to design iteration (not a bad thing). Closely tied to the representation of the data is the method of loading the data into the model. For this there are several alternative approaches. The most straightforward way (but least desirable, unless speed is of paramount importance) is to encode this information directly into the source code of the model. The most usable approach (but also the most time-consuming from a code development standpoint) is to design a special human interface for inputting the model information into a file that is loaded by the model at execution time. A middle-ground approach is to provide for the loadable information file, but rely on using a standard editor for file creation. The choice will depend on how much information must be entered, how frequently the information will be changed, how valuable is the time of the domain expert, and how much reuse can be anticipated.

For the next (and most crucial) step of construction—building the fuzzy sets and hedges and writing the propositions—the expert's knowledge must be translated to the formalisms of the model's vocabulary. This involves selecting the parameters of the fuzzy sets to match the expert's perception of the real

---

*This is not specific to models—rather, it is a generally held tenant for software that interacts with humans that GUIs are more intuitive, easier to learn, and more powerful than other approaches.

world, developing the hedges with which to transform the fuzzy sets, and encoding the propositions in the vernacular of the model. During the verification phase, this activity will be revisited to accomplish the model tuning.

The next step is to code the composition logic. The mathematics of composition are rigorous, and the focus in coding the composition logic is to make it right and make it fast—in that order. Likewise, the defuzzification logic is an echo of the relevant mathematics describing the chosen defuzzification method. Whether the selected design is object-oriented or not, the predominant effort in this step will be in data handling and transform encoding.

Building the output phase of the model is a highly variable activity, depending heavily on the model design. In general, there are building blocks in the form of class libraries (e.g., GUI, communications) that will make the task much easier. If the model is part of a larger system (e.g., a mechanism controller), the environment in which it operates—its *connectivity*—will be the dominant force in how the code is written for this phase.

The final step of construction is integration—putting all the pieces together. However, this is best done incrementally rather than waiting until all parts are complete. Incremental integration benefits the developer in a couple of ways. First, it provides a growing scaffold for checking out pieces of the model as they are ready, and ensures testing of the pieces *in situ.* Second, coding problems (as well as design problems) become apparent earlier, rendering them easier to deal with. So each part should be hooked into the system as soon as it has basic functionality. Then the final integration occurs when the last piece falls into place.

7.2.1.4. VERIFICATION. There are three principal activities in the verification phase, and each is crucially important to the success of the model development effort. First, the software must be tested to ensure quality. Second, the model must be tuned—that is, calibrated for the environment in which it will operate. Third, the accuracy of the model must be verified.

Testing the software is done standalone and then integrally with the system or device in which the model will be embedded. Testing should follow a formal test plan that provides for an exhaustive number of written test cases as well as ad hoc testing by both the developer and someone not involved in the development. The formal test cases should consist of execution scenarios and expected responses. They should be codified and repeatable. They should be designed to provide complete coverage of the code—all functions should be exercised, including error paths. By recording the effort spent on testing over time and the results of testing (number of defects found), statistical projections about the quality of the model may be made. These projections can be compared to predetermined quality criteria to decide when the model is ready to be put into production.

The model is tuned by adjusting the domain information encoded in the fuzzy set descriptions and the hedges. In some cases it also may be appropriate to alter the working of the propositions or even add or delete propositions as part of the tuning process. The goal is to make the model behave as closely to expectations as possible. In many cases, models will be routinely tuned when they are moved between environments. Thus, a model may be reused essentially intact for similar but not identical applications.

The final step is to verify the model. This, the most important step of all, is the *acceptance test* for the model. The way in which this is accomplished will be highly dependent on the model and its application. In many cases, the test will boil down to whether the model will perform as well as an expert doing the same task.

7.2.2. Process Summary

Here is a step-by-step outline of the approach described above:

1. Assessment
    a. What do you want the model to decide?
    . . . chose output variable(s)
    b. What do you have to work with? What is important?
    . . . discover input variables
    c. What pertinent relationships exist?
    . . . requires domain expertise
2. Design
    a. Design output presentation
    b. Design input phase (e.g., user interface)
    c. Choose fuzzy set topology for output and input variables
    d. Choose hedge types and applications
    e. Determine propositional structure
    f. Select fuzzy compositional method(s)
    . . . implication and correlation
    g. Select defuzzification method
3. Construction
    a. Build input phase
    b. Construct fuzzy sets
    c. Construct hedges
    d. Build propositions
    e. Code composition logic
    f. Code defuzzification logic
    g. Build output phase
    h. Integrate
4. Verification
    a. Tune the model
    b. Standalone and integral testing
    c. Verify the model

7.3. FUZZY SYSTEMS IN THE CLINICAL LABORATORY

Healthcare, like much of American industry, is under extreme pressure to be better, faster, and less expensive. Quality is assumed and added value is required. As a result, effort to improve and optimize the healthcare system is a requirement at all levels.

We as humans are not 100% reliable, accurate and untiring. Our customers, however, require us, their suppliers, to be ever closer to these ideals. In order to achieve this, the development and use of automation methods can help. Of particular interest are computer-based expert systems that can combine the expert knowledge of the best human in a field and the untiring, rapid and absolutely consistent features of a computer. The concept is a very appealing one. However, in many applications of such systems using earlier programming methods, the systems have often been too rigid and inflexible for the successful replacements of human judgment. Fuzzy logic expert systems, however, are better able to match the decision making capability of technical experts.

7.3.1. Fuzzy Systems Application Domains

Not all problems in the clinical laboratory are ideal candidates for fuzzy systems solutions. Further, there aren't hard and fast rules that determine whether a problem is amenable to a fuzzy solution. Indeed, deciding whether to use a fuzzy system is itself a fuzzy problem! Some characteristics which indicate use of fuzzy system technology are

Control Parameters That Are "Fuzzy." Experts' description of parameters used for control are imprecise and couched in fuzzy terms, such as "somewhat," "moderately," and "very."

Multiple Experts. A decision must be synthesized from conflicting opinions of multiple experts.

Complex Problem. The problem or the problem domain is complex or quite large and does not admit to a straightforward description.

Lack of Complete Problem Domain Knowledge. Even though articulate domain experts may exist, the problem domain knowledge is incomplete or conflicting, or characterized by uncertainty.

Incomplete or Flawed Data. The input to the system lacks precision or accuracy, or the system must yield results even when some important data is missing.

Nonlinear Relationships Abound. Relationships between given input and desired output are highly nonlinear and thus not amenable to other modeling techniques.

Fast Performance Is Essential. A real-time system with demanding performance constraints is required.

Fast Development Is Desirable. The system must be developed more quickly or less expensively than other techniques (e.g., conventional expert systems) permit, yet give reasonably accurate results.

Smooth Response Required. The application of the system is intolerant of "aberrant" behavior (small changes in input producing large or unexpected variations in model results).

Naturally, these are just guidelines and the list is not complete. But if a clinical laboratory problem has several of these characteristics, a fuzzy system approach has a better chance of success than conventional methods.

7.3.2. Synopses of Clinical Applications

There have already been a number of applications of fuzzy logic based expert systems in the healthcare industry. These have included applications in clinical psychology to evaluate such problems as driver fatigue,[10] memory function and cognition evaluation,[11] and evaluation of depth perception.[12] Similar systems have been used to evaluate the ability of medical students to solve clinical problems.[13]

In the clinical medicine setting, interesting applications of this type of expert system have been used in the monitoring and adjustment of medications to patients in very complex clinical situations. To date, such systems have been used to (1) control and adjust the administration of anesthesia during surgery,[14] (2) monitor and adjust continuous infusions of medications to control blood pressure in an intensive care environment,[15,16] and (3) monitor and evaluate cardiac rhythms.[17,18]

Fuzzy expert systems are also being used in the interpretation of diagnostic imaging of CT (computed tomography) scans, MRI (magnetic resonance imaging) scans,[19] and regular x-rays,[20] particularly since the advent of digital recording with these imaging modalities, as digital recording lends itself better to computer interpretation than traditional images on hard copy.

Fuzzy systems have been used in the evaluation of devices to monitor and adjust pain medication delivery in the post operative setting.[21] A very exciting application has been in the evaluation, diagnosis, and treatment of osteoporosis.[22] This latter example represents the first in a large number of similar clinical situations where this type of expert system can help physicians directly in caring for patients.

The laboratory has begun to see the application of this technology as well. In addition to our example outlined below (see Section 7.4), fuzzy systems have been used in quantitative cytologic examinations[23] and in the automation of protein 2D proton NMR (nuclear magnetic resonance) assignment.[24] Although the use of such systems in the laboratory is as yet limited, the flexibility and the much closer to human decision making ability of these systems allow not only the evaluation of blood collection tubes but also a wide spectrum of other possibilities. These can include (1) interpretation of complex test results, (2) choosing the correct testing sequence and follow-up tests for given clinical problems, (3) monitoring all instruments and their results as well as maintenance and calibration, (4) resource and supply monitoring and management in the laboratory, and (5) management of data flow within the lab and to the client through many paths. These applications do not address by any means all the possible applications of fuzzy logic expert systems in the clinical laboratory. We can expect to see this technology becoming increasingly a part of our everyday life. It will make our lives easier and our work more efficient, rapid and of the highest quality.

7.4. A CASE STUDY

The preparation of clinical medical samples for testing is a time-consuming, labor-intensive, expensive, and potentially hazardous process. Although robots and other manipulators can accomplish a number of steps in specimen processing, the majority of specimens require human intervention because of the need to externally evaluate clinical samples, make correct judgments and direct the automation. We describe a fuzzy logic based expert system (SEDEX[25]) used to mimic technologists' judgments about clinical chemistry samples, which was developed as a component of the Medical Robotics Serumax II closed-tube serum processor. *The description presented here is a simplification of the actual system, which employed additional variables and fuzzy rules, and more complex compositional inference techniques and fuzzy set topology.*

In manual aliquoting, the external evaluation of samples made by experienced technologists defines the locality, quality, quantity and adequacy of the sample, and this information then drives sample triage, handling, manipulation, and preparation for analysis. Bar coded samples can capture some of the demographic data needed for correct triaging, but an objective evaluation of the sample itself is usually required. In the automated SEDEX system, computer vision is employed to view the contents of a sample tube and fuzzy logic is used to understand it.

Prototype work using a deterministic algorithm established that serum detection was a limiting factor to instrument throughput. It also exhibited other shortcomings—it failed to achieve an acceptable success rate in detecting the serum, it had low tolerance for marginal samples, and it had failure modes that could damage the instrument. Thus, we looked for better technologies. After studying the problem domain and working with experienced laboratory technicians to understand their thought processes, fuzzy logic was selected for building an expert system for serum detection. We felt that this approach promised faster and more accurate detection, less aberrant behavior, and easier tuning. And, importantly, we believed that it would allow us to closely model the experts who could reliably perform the task manually.

7.4.1. Model Input and Output

The SEDEX subsystem's output is used in controlling the automated sample aliquoting. SEDEX informs the downstream head transfer station of the suitability of the sample, the physical location of the top and bottom if the serum in the sample tube, and the volume present. This information is used to control the positioning of the transfer needle and the withdrawal and transfer of serum. So the required output from the expert system is a boolean variable indicating the presence (or absence) of serum of sufficient quality, and displacements in the tube where the upper and lower serum interfaces are located. (The volume can be calculated from the interface displacements, based on known sample tube diameter).

The model's input comes from a scanner that looks at the sample tube. A linear reflectance profile is obtained by scanning the tube with a moving white-light source and detector, and compiling a series of reflectance measurements. The resulting data scan is used by the expert system to make serum presence, location and quality determinations. The detector is electrically calibrated to ensure that the usable reflectance measurement range encompasses the typical reflectance of the major constituents of the sample tubes—serum, red blood cells, gel clot, and the air-filled portion of tubes. The reflectance data are captured and stored as detector output values versus vertical detector displacement values (see Fig. 7.10 for a plot of a sample scan). Normalization of the reflectance

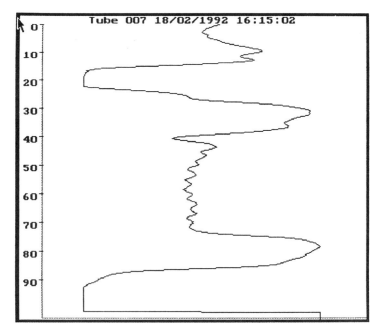

Figure 7.10. Reflectance (x axis) versus displacement from top of tube.

data, resulting in values ranging from 0.0 to 1.0, is performed before the information is input to the fuzzy logic portion of the model.

7.4.2. Expert Knowledge Assimilation

In manual aliquoting, of course, the laboratory technician can readily detect the location of the serum by looking at the sample tube. What we discovered in working with the vision system was that experienced technologists are able to reliably detect serum location by looking at a plot of the normalized reflectance data from the vision system (similar to that of Fig. 7.10). This was a learned ability, based on experience with thousands of samples processed through the system. Therefore, we were encouraged with the prospects of developing an expert system that could approximate this ability in software.

We examined the decision factors employed by the experienced technologists in making the serum location determination. The first observation was that when they looked at the reflectance plots, they mentally decomposed the curve into regions with distinctive features. This gave a set of segments that were the "candidates" for selection as the serum area. We selected a data reduction technique (discussed in Section 7.4.3) that accurately reproduced this visual segmentation performed by the experts.

Development of the decision factors required definition of a set of parameters used by experienced technologists in their evaluation process. The parameters were evaluated in groups of two and then larger collections to further define the most important characteristics for clinical judgments. Note that it was apparent that the human decision process was not based on absolute determinations. Rather, it was a synthesis of less precise factors into a selection of the segment that most probably represented the serum. It is also important to note that the experts tended to rely on all the key accumulated evidence about a segment, not just the dominant feature of a segment.

We studied the factors used in the human determination of which segment represents the serum. Three factors were selected as the primary discriminators:

1. The size of the segment—of the many components of the sample tube (stopper, air, meniscus, serum, gel clot, red blood cells, tube bottom, etc), the serum was among the larger segments.
2. The location of the segment—the serum was generally in the middle or just above the middle of the sample tube.
3. The reflectance of the segment—the serum's reflectance was midrange; less bright than the gel clot, noticeably brighter than red blood cells.

Note that in these descriptions, some less-than-precise terms are used ("generally," "among," "noticeably," etc.). It was apparent that the human decision process was not based on absolute determinations (e.g., normalized reflectance value between 0.6 and 0.7). Rather, it represented a synthesis of less precise factors into a selection of the segment that most probably represented the serum. This discovery reinforced our selection of a fuzzy logic approach.

7.4.3. Data Reduction

The selected data reduction technique yielded a segmentation of the data into regions (line segments) that closely matched the human experts' decomposition of the scan plots. Subsequent testing confirmed that the segmentation performed by the data reduction methods would reliably contain exactly one segment whose endpoints closely matched the top and bottom of the serum. This is an effect of the distinct interfaces between the serum and surrounding material in the sample tube.

The data reduction is performed by fitting a *polycurve* to the data, yielding a set of segments that approximates the original curve. Figure 7.11 shows the polycurve for a sample tube. The polycurve algorithm[26] replaces the hundreds of data points with a set of connected line segments approximating the original data. This facilitates the decision process since fewer data imply faster operation, while each segment contains more information than the points it replaced.

7.4.4. Fuzzy Sets and Propositions

Each parameter was evaluated for its characteristic values in an ideal sample, based on input from the experts. A curve was created that related each possible

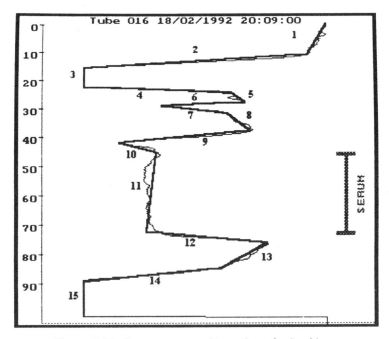

Figure 7.11. Segments created by polycurve algorithm.

value of the parameter with the likelihood of occurrence in an ideal sample. These curves were used to select types of fuzzy sets for encoding in the model. The topology chosen for "relative volume is large" is a *linear* fuzzy set. Membership is qualified with a *somewhat* hedge (see proposition P_1 below). For "position is middle of the tube," a fuzzy set with a *Gaussian* membership function is used and a *slightly above* hedge is applied. A *beta* curve gives the topology for "reflectance is midrange."

As noted, the goal of the model is to find the segment that represents the serum. Therefore, the consequent of each of the fuzzy propositions is "segment is serum." The propositions that represent the experts' deductive reasoning are

P_1: If relative volume is somewhat large, segment is serum
P_2: If position is slightly above middle of the tube, segment is serum
P_3: If reflectance is midrange, segment is serum

It is important to note that although the initial propositions were selected on the basis of extensive dialog between the modeler and the domain experts, several design iterations and considerable "tuning" in the verification phase yielded the final form of the propositions and the underlying fuzzy set definitions as shown above. This is quite normal and to be expected in the development of expert systems. However, many projects fail to allow time in the schedule for these iterations.

7.4.5. Inference and Defuzzification

The *fuzzy additive* implication rule and the *correlation product* method of correlation were chosen to combine the propositions, since, in the expert's opinion, it was important for each of the propositions to contribute to the solution set. For instance, if, for a given segment, P_1 and P_2 had high truth but P_3 was largely false, the expert would conclude that the segment was *not* serum. These inference methods best accommodate this behavior.

The domain of the solution set "segment is serum" is the set of segments derived from the polycurve data reduction process. The membership value for a given segment is, of course, the degree to which the model thinks the segment represents serum. Since the goal of the model is to select the one segment that best represents the serum, the logical choice for defuzzification is the *composite maximum* technique, as this method finds the point (segment) which represents the maximum truthfulness of the solution fuzzy set.

7.4.5. Decision Discrimination

Of equal importance to making the right selection was the ability to decide that the selection was not sufficiently discriminating. In practice, it is far more desirable to reject a sample tube (thus necessitating recycling of the tube or manual aliquoting) than to make an erroneous serum location determination that could lead to sample contamination or even machine downtime (e.g., needle clogging by driving into a gel clot). Two discriminators are used to determine whether the segment with the highest membership value should be selected, or if a "no-match" situation should be declared. First, the membership value for the candidate segment must be above a certain (programmable) threshold. If not, it is likely that the tube does not contain any serum. Second, the difference between the membership values for the best segment and the next-best segment must be larger than a predetermined delta (also programmable). By performing these two tests, the model exhibits an ability to report that it can't find the serum or that it's not sure about the selection. The machine then takes the appropriate action to elicit manual intervention.

7.4.6. Model Construction

The model framework was built, and input and output capabilities were coded. Data reduction routines were written next. Then the coding of the fuzzy logic proper was undertaken. After the correct mix of parameters was selected and their underlying fuzzy sets and attendant hedges were created, code was written to read in the fuzzy set definitions from an editable file. Routines were written to evaluate each parameter of an actual sample and assign its membership value. Some special processing is done for one factor—volume—that yields a normalized index for that factor. (The volume function transforms absolute volume measurements into relative volume values. For instance, it yields 1.0 for the segment representing the domain with the largest volume in the sample, and 0.5 for a segment representing a domain with half the volume of the largest). Routines were written to encode the propositions and perform the compositional inference. Defuzzification logic was straightforward, and the decision discriminator was incorporated into the defuzzification code.

After integrating the parts of the model and testing the code, model tuning was undertaken. The fuzzy set definitions and the propositions represent the principal infusion of expert judgment. By adjusting a fuzzy set's membership function or adding a hedge, the human expert may fine-tune the characteristics of a particular factor that make the corresponding segment a likely match. This was an iterative process. Initially, a small set of samples were carefully selected to give a wide range of characteristics. After tuning the model to reliably detect serum in these samples, the model was exposed to a broader set. After several iterations in tuning, the model was judged ready for clinical validation.

7.4.7. Clinical Validation

Over 500 clinical samples were used to validate the SEDEX Expert System.* Modifications of the fuzzy sets and hedges, and thresholds for sample acceptance were adjusted based on the results. Subsequent clinical testing indicated a 98% plus concordance level with results obtained by experienced instrument tech-

---

*Large-scale clinical testing will begin in the near future.

nologists. This substantially exceeded the success rate of the prototype deterministic detection algorithm.

There are three possible failure modes: the evaluation is indeterminate (manual aliquoting required), the evaluation picks a region higher in the tube (air is drawn), and the evaluation picks a region lower in the tube (sample contaminated with gel, fibrin or red blood cells, and possible instrument damage from gel clot). The failures seen were predominantly of the first type. No failures of the third types were experienced, in contrast with the prototype.

The speed of SEDEX exceeds that of the prototype by an order of magnitude. It runs on a 80486 PC-based system and is able to detect serum in less than one second (< 1 s) per sample evaluation. This ensures that serum detection will not be on the critical timing path for high-speed sample processing.

The algorithm yields very good discrimination on most samples. An example of the resulting solution set for the sample plotted in Figure 7.11 is shown in Figure 7.12. As can be seen, segment 11 is the clear choice as the segment that represents the serum. In Figure 7.13, we see the robustness of the algorithm displayed. With a completely different sample profile, it still reliably detects the location of the serum. The membership value for the selected segment is 0.661. Since the two closest rivals are 0.092 and 0.034, we see excellent discrimination by the model.

7.4.8. Summary

The SEDEX system has 98% concordance rate with experienced technologists. Where earlier algorithms were limited by slow speed, the SEDEX system is able to make total evaluation of specimen location, quality, quantity and appropriateness for testing within one second. This allows potential instrument throughput

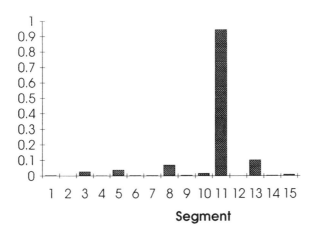

Figure 7.12. "Segment is serum" solution set.

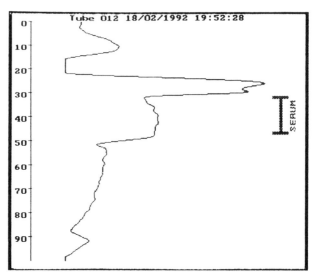

Figure 7.13. Another sample.

of over 1500 samples per hour. Reliability of decisions is excellent, with only "safe" failure modes exhibited. This expert system can now be integrated with other pieces of laboratory automation to produce fully automated integrated clinical sample processing systems that will greatly improve the economics, speed, and safety of the clinical medical laboratory.

The SEDEX fuzzy-logic-based expert system is fast, accurate and captures the decision making knowledge of the best trained medical technologists, providing consistent evaluation of samples for automated systems. The use of fuzzy logic in this application has succeeded where a deterministic approach failed.

REFERENCES

1. Yager RE, Zadeh LA, eds: *An Introduction of Fuzzy Logic Applications in Intelligent Systems.* Norwell, MA: Kluwer Academic Publishers, 1992.

2. Klir GJ, Folger TA: *Fuzzy Sets, Uncertainty, and Information.* Englewood Cliffs, NJ: Prentice-Hall, 1988.

3. Terano T, Asai K, Sugeno M: *Fuzzy Systems Theory and Its Applications.* San Diego, CA: Academic Press, 1991.

4. Sugeno M, ed: *Industrial Applications of Fuzzy Control.* Amsterdam: North-Holland, 1985.

5. Zimmerman HJ: *Fuzzy Set Theory and Its Applications,* 2nd ed. Boston: Kluwer Academic Publishers, 1991.

6. Rosch E: On the internal structure of perceptual and semantic categories. In Moore T

ed: *Cognitive Development and the Acquisition of Language.* New York: Academic Press, 1973, pp 111–144.

7. Lorenz M: *Object Oriented Software Development—A Practical Guide.* Englewood Cliffs, NJ: Prentice-Hall, 1993.

8. Booch G: *Object Oriented Design with Applications.* Redwood City, CA: Benjamin/Cummings, 1991.

9. Cox E: *The Fuzzy Systems Handbook.* Boston: AP Professional, 1994.

10. He C, Zhao C: Evaluation of the critical value of driving fatigue based on the fuzzy sets theory. *Environ Res* 61:150–156, 1993.

11. Brainerd CJ, Reyna VF: Memory independence and memory interface in cognitive development. *Psychol Rev* 100:42–67, 1993.

12. Massaro DW, Cohen MM: The paradigm and the fuzzy logic model of perception are alive and well. *J Exp Psychol Gen* 122:115–124, 1993.

13. Stevens RH, Najafi K: Artificial neural networks as adjuncts for assessing medical students' problem solving performances on computer-based simulations. *Comput Biomed Res* 26:172–187, 1993.

14. Tsutsui T, Arita S: Fuzzy-logic control of blood pressure through enflurane anesthesia. *J Clin Monit* 10:110–117, 1994.

15. Ruiz R, Borches D, Gonzalez A, et al: A new socium-nitroprusside-infusion controller for the regulation of arterial blood pressure. *Biomed Instrum Technol* 27:244–251, 1993.

16. Ying H, McEachern M, Eddleman DW, et al: Fuzzy control of mean arterial pressure in postsurgical patients with sodium nitroprusside infusion. *IEEE Trans Biomed Eng* 39:1060–1070, 1992.

17. Ruttkay-Nedecky I, Riecansky I: Dipolar electrocardiotopographic evaluation of ventricular activation in patients with various degrees of coronary artery disease. *J Electrocardio* 27:149–155, 1994.

18. Sittig DF, Cheung KH, Berman L: Fuzzy classification of hemodynamic trends and artifacts: experiments with the heart rate. *Internatl J Monit Comput* 9:251–257, 1992.

19. Brandt ME, Bohan TP, Kramer LA, et al: Estimation of CSF, white and gray matter volumes in hydrocephalic children using fuzzy clustering or MR images. *Comput Med Imag Graph* 18:25–34, 1994.

20. Lin JS, Ligomenides PA, Freeman MT, et al: Application of artificial neural networks for reduction of false-positive detection in digital chest radiographs. *Proc Annu Symp Comput Appl Med Care* 434–438, 1993.

21. Carollo A, Tobar A, Hernandez C: A rule-based postoperative pain controller: simulation results. *Int J Biomed Comput* 33:267–276, 1993.

22. Binaghi E, DeGiorgi O, Maggi G, et al: Computer-assisted diagnosis of postmenopausal osteoporosis using a fuzzy expert system shell. *Comput Biomed Res* 26:498–516, 1993.

23. Molnar B, Szentirmay Z, Bodo M, et al: Application of multivariate, fuzzy set and neural network analysis in quantitative cytological examinations. *Anal Cell Pathol* 5:161–175, 1993.

24. Xu J, Straus SK, Santuary BC, et al: Automation of protein 2D proton NMR assignment

by means of fuzzy mathematics and graph theory. *J Chem Info Comput Sci* 33:668–682, 1993.

25. Maguire LC, Martin JC: Fuzzy logic based expert system for clinical sample triaging and evaluation. In *Laboratory Information Management*. Amsterdam: Elsevier Science Publishers, in press.

26. Ballard DH, Brown CM: *Computer Vision*. Englewood Cliffs, NJ: Prentice-Hall, 1982.

CHAPTER

8

Artificial Intelligence and New Knowledge Structures

GERALD J. KOST

CONTENTS

8.1. OBJECTIVE AND DEFINITIONS

The objectives of this chapter are to (1) provide an overview of the recent applications of artificial intelligence and expert systems in laboratory and diagnostic medicine, (2) summarize the current status of temporal optimization and new knowledge structures used to optimize critical care, and (3) assess which of these approaches might be effective in the future. *Artificial intelligence* can be defined succinctly as "the study of ideas that enable computers to be intelligent"[414] or "the study of the computations that make it possible to perceive, reason, and act."[414] Alternately, artificial intelligence is "the collective attributes of a computer, robot, or other mechanical device programmed to perform

Handbook of Clinical Automation, Robotics, and Optimization, Edited by Gerald J. Kost with the collaboration of Judith Welsh.
ISBN 0-471-03179-8 © 1996 John Wiley & Sons, Inc.

functions analogous to learning and decision making."[404] Artificial intelligence also can be defined as "the discipline devoted to producing computing systems that perform tasks which would require intelligence if done by a human being"[39] or more abstractly as "the study of mental faculties through the use of computational models"[57] and finally as "a new research area that combines sophisticated representations and computing techniques with the insights of expert physicians to produce tools for improving health care."[375,387] An *expert system* is "a computer system that achieves high levels of performance in areas that for human beings require large amounts of expertise."[39] An expert system also should be capable of explaining its reasoning.[413]

A *knowledge structure* is defined here as a new pattern of intelligence, created, generated, or devised through the integration, synthesis, and optimization of interrelated conceptual, strategic, or factual components. A knowledge structure focuses on human reasoning, intellectual content, and problem solving and is not limited by its organization or connectivity. Additionally, it may include beliefs, hybrid sets, and "real world" components. This differs from *knowledge representation,* which is "the process of mapping the knowledge of some domain into a computational medium."[39] A *knowledge-based system* is defined as "a system containing knowledge which can perform tasks that require intelligence if done by human beings."[39] Procedural knowledge is knowledge about procedures, and declarative knowledge is knowledge about logical and empirical relationships[413] or about the meaning of objects.[39] These are relatively straightforward definitions, each with a slightly different twist or practical implication. These definitions will be used throughout this chapter, since works cited are drawn from a variety of sources in basic science, clinical medicine, and this book.

8.2. INTRODUCTION, THE LITERATURE, AND A BRIEF EXAMPLE

There are important new factors motivating and justifying innovative applications of artificial intelligence and expert systems in medicine. These factors include the increasing use of robotics and integrated systems in the clinical laboratory and the pressing need for optimization of critical, medical, and surgical patient care under the fiscal constraints imposed by managed care and capitation. However, after 20 years of development, artificial intelligence and expert systems must still fulfill the goal of fielding completed systems, and therefore, the practical uses in health care are incomplete.[376,387] The National Library of Medicine (NLM) Medline databases classify literature into artificial intelligence, expert systems, and related subject headings. Figure 8.1 shows the annual volume of references in the NLM Medline databases. The apparent falloff in annual volume volume is due in part to branching of the categorization of research into three new subject headings: (1) natural language programming in 1991, (2) neural networks in 1992, and (3) fuzzy logic in 1993. *Neural networks* represent a class of techniques where a machine learns from examples; Vertosick discusses neural networks in detail in Chapter 4.[396] *Fuzzy logic,* the "new mathematics of vagueness,"[243] is discussed in Chapter 7. Figure 8.2 illustrates the growth in the annual

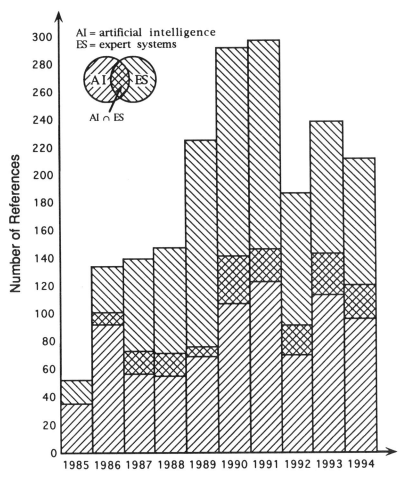

Figure 8.1. Growth of artificial intelligence in medicine. The graph shows the annual volume of references in the National Library of Medicine Medline databases over the past decade. The subject heading, artificial intelligence, started in 1986. Expert systems started in 1987. The numbers of publications plotted in the first two years are based in part on title word searches and are approximate.

volume of references in the new subject headings. Overall, the annual volume of publications has increased progressively, although there was some apparent leveling in 1993 and 1994, when the total annual volume was 524 and 500 references, respectively.

The list of references in this chapter was compiled selectively from these NLM databases and other sources. It covers a large portion of the publications relevant to laboratory medicine, diagnostic testing, or critical care from the past 5 years. Many references are cited individually. The others listed provide a compact resource for the reader to explore. However, this set of references repre-

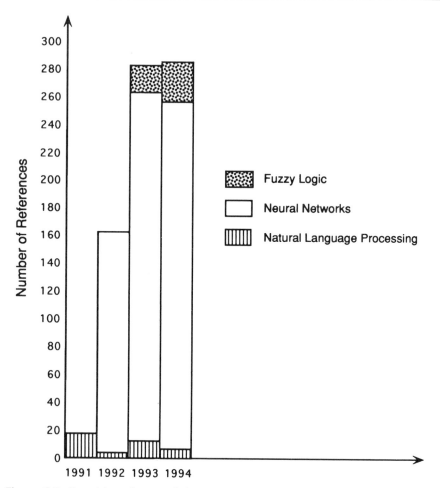

Figure 8.2. Branching of research into new areas. Branching into natural language programming, neural networks, and fuzzy logic explains the apparent decrease in annual volume after 1991 in Figure 8.1. The total volume in the Medline database for the ten year period was 2687 references (52 in 1985; 134, 1986; 141, 1987; 148, 1988; 226, 1989; 293, 1990; 317, 1991; 352, 1992; 524, 1993; and 500, 1994). By 1994, references were categorized into five subject headings.

sents only a fraction of the total number of medically relevant references in the NLM databases. For example, the total 10-year volume included in Figures 8.1 and 8.2 is 2687 references! An additional subject heading, robotics, includes 275 references from the year of inception, 1987, through 1994. The use of robotics will accelerate as hospitals streamline personnel and also strive to provide high-quality and inexpensive diagnostic services in order to compete medically and financially. Please see chapters 11, 12, and 24 by Markin[241a] and Felder,[113,114] who discuss the current applications of robotics and remote review in laboratory medicine.

Before reviewing the clinical role of artificial intelligence, a brief example of the use of an expert system will demonstrate the concept.[61–64] A nuclear magnetic resonance expert system (NMRES) was developed to capture and formalize [31]Phosphorus NMR spectroscopists' expert knowledge, and to provide a reliable, efficient, and automated system for the interpretation of biological spectra.[64] Expert knowledge was acquired from NMR spectroscopists and represented as production rules in the knowledge base (Fig. 8.3). The inference engine contains the programming needed to generate solutions and explanations for the user from the production rules. A feedback loop allows updating of the fact base. Data derived from previously identified peaks were used to guide subsequent peak processing, a form of progressive learning. A heuristic weights method was employed to determine the confidence levels of potential peaks in the ^{31}P NMR spectra (Fig. 8.4). Statistical and numerical methods were used to facilitate processing decisions.

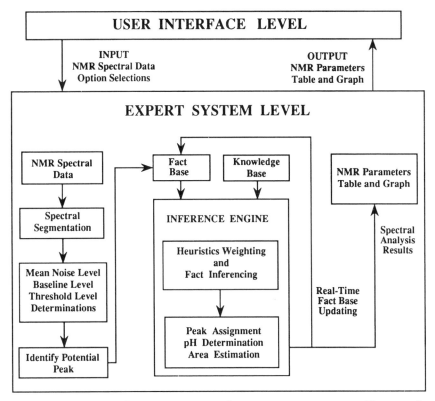

Figure 8.3. Schematic of the nuclear magnetic resonance expert system. The organization of the expert system and its modular structure emulate the logical steps that NMRES pursues, similar to the human expert analyzing NMR biological spectra. Note that newly identified peak characteristics are updated in real-time to the fact base, which can be used to guide subsequent reasoning. (Reproduced, with permission of the *Annals of Biomedical Engineering*, from Ref. 64.)

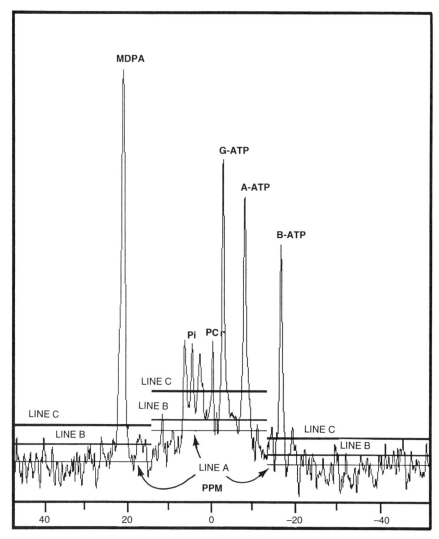

Figure 8.4. A ^{31}Phosphorus NMR spectrum obtained from the neonatal heart during control perfusion. Six phosphorus resonances, namely the MDPA standard, inorganic phosphate (Pi), phosphocreatine (PCr), and the three ATP peaks (γ, α, and β) were the major chemical species of interest that NMRES interpreted. The mean noise level (line A), baseline level (line B), and threshold level (line C) are determined by NMRES. The baseline level generally is approximated by the mean noise level. They are separated here to facilitate their illustration. (Reproduced, with permission of the *Annals of Biomedical Engineering*, From Ref. 64.)

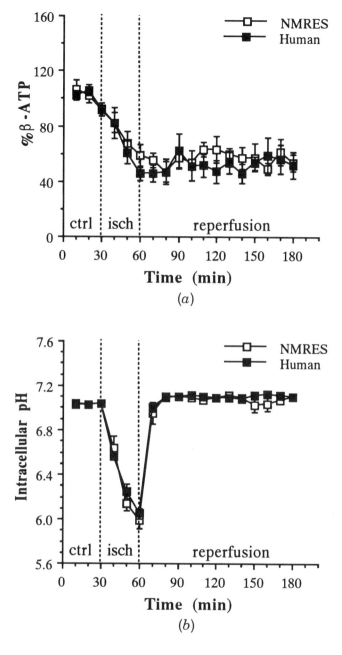

Figure 8.5. Performance of NMR expert system. The figures compare the performance of (a) normalized β-ATP peak area estimations and (b) intracellular pH determinations by NMRES and the human expert from five immature heart experiments. Determination of intracellular pH is based on the chemical shift of the Pi peak referenced to the PCr peak position. The experimental protocol is represented as ctrl = control, isch = ischemia, and reperfusion phases. Results shown as mean ± standard error (SE). (Reproduced, with permission of the *Annals of Biomedical Engineering,* From Ref. 64.)

The expert system performed signal extraction, noise treatment, resonance assignment, intracellular pH determination, algorithmic peak fitting, and metabolite intensity quantitation in about 10 s per (4 kbyte) ^{31}P NMR spectrum. Inferencing typically required about 80% of the total processing time. NMR spectra obtained from studies of ischemic neonatal and immature hearts were used to assess the performance of the expert system in cardiovascular research. The peak identification success rate was 98.2%. Peak areas and pH estimation by the expert system compared favorably with those determined by human experts (Fig. 8.5). This "snapshot" of an expert system illustrates how satisfactory performance could be achieved in a laboratory setting where procedural knowledge and uncertainty can be dealt with in a relatively straightforward manner. Now, we will discuss laboratory medicine and clinical pathology, where several tasks potentially could be performed more efficiently with the aid of artificial intelligence. Following a discussion of artificial intelligence in laboratory medicine, we will conclude with critical care, where the necessity for immediate action, temporal optimization, and outcomes improvement calls for innovation and flexibility.

8.3. ARTIFICIAL INTELLIGENCE IN LABORATORY MEDICINE

Reviews of artificial intelligence in laboratory medicine and clinical pathology published most recently include those by Gendler,[133a] Place et al.,[289a] and Roseman[312] in 1994, Winkel in 1994[413] and 1989,[412] Marquardt in 1993,[242] Makino in 1992,[238] Laemmle and Wolterman in 1991,[213] Connelly[76] and Isenhour and Marshall[174] in 1990, Armas in 1989,[13] Sher[337] and Trendelenburg[383] in 1988, Spackman and Connelly[361] in 1987, and Castellani et al.[52] in 1986. In addition, Liscouski[228] recently outlined strategic approaches to laboratory and scientific computing and provided valuable guidance on planning, evaluating, and implementing, including data archival, electronic records, hyperinformation systems, networks, and communications. His monograph[228] is useful because it can help bridge the gap between traditional clinical laboratory information systems and discrete workstations where artificial intelligence, expert systems, neural network, and other software programs often reside. Next, we will consider the suggestions found in these sources, the historical context, and future directions for clinical applications.

Marquardt[242] suggested major and minor objectives for development. The major objectives encompass systems that can reason about a patient's symptoms and clinical findings, produce a diagnosis, and recommend treatment. The approaches suggested to achieve these objectives include causal models, reasoning from statistics, case-based reasoning, learning algorithms, neural networks, and expert systems. The minor objectives target practical decision-making tasks and include speech recognition,[415] laboratory test selection, entry of test requisition information, classification of cells, validation of test results, critical results reporting, interpretative reporting of test results, automatic coding of findings and diagnosis, drug-dosage regulation, quality control and quality assurance, selection and interpretation of statistical tests, education, interpretation of instrument output, and instrument maintenance. Roseman[312] added troubleshooting, supplies purchasing, and personnel scheduling to the list of practical objectives. Armas et al.[13] suggested using expert systems to replace manual data handling, control inappropriate test ordering, address textural test results, formulate numerical test results, perform quality improvement functions, facilitate database communications, decentralize laboratory infomatics, and provide computer-aided instruction; they cited several examples of expert systems that have been developed [e.g., ABEL,[281,282] (see Uckun—Chapter 6[390]) EXPERT,[407] LIVER,[55] MYCIN,[340a] and others[7a,358] in laboratory medicine; and INTERNIST-1,[254–256] ONCOCIN,[160] and PUFF[6a] in internal medicine, cancer therapy, and pulmonary disease, respectively].

Realization of these objectives, many of which would directly improve clinical laboratory operations and the ability to use and interpret diagnostic information, will require that software developers become more familiar with artificial intelligence and expert systems, and that programs are embedded in hospital and laboratory information systems, as well as in patient-focused care workstations[206] or wireless personal digital assistants, both of which are easily accessible to laboratory professionals and physicians. Gendler[133a] compared features (architecture, validation, capacities, premises, conclusions, and applications) of expert systems offered with laboratory information systems. He found that system architectures included traditional logic (e.g., Boolean operators), but only rarely included nontraditional logic or neural networks. Similarly, validation features (rule version control, internal documentation, preactive state, tracing, and statistical reports), capacities (premise limit, conclusion limit, and chaining), and areas of application (e.g., general laboratory, microbiology, and blood bank) were not provided consistently by the four commercial vendors that he compared. Premises features (demographics, orders, collections, results, species, calculations, and ad hoc inquiries) delineate what information the expert system can evaluate. Conclusions features (terminal message, order/cancel order, create/cancel charge, result creation, result verification, interpretative phrase, flag for retrieval, ad hoc inquiry, facsimile, electronic mail, calculation, and work queue routing) determine the actions that the laboratory information system can execute following the evaluation of premises. Gendler's analysis shows that laboratory information systems must incorporate many more of these expert system features to assure, for example, laboratory process simplification with optimization, validation of interpretation of complex test results, and interactive medical/economic outcomes decisions.

Connelly[76] recognized the importance of embedding expert system capabilities in the laboratory information system[73] to facilitate order entry, specimen distribution, processing, and results reporting, and earlier[13,74] described one of the initial applications of an expert system in laboratory medicine. Isenhour and Marshall[174] promoted the use of expert systems to supervise laboratory robots with the objectives of standardizing robot methods and of assuring that complex analytical procedures give reproducible results in different laboratories. Winkel[412,413] offered a list of 13 expert systems that emphasize the interpretation of laboratory data. Generally, these focus on diagnosis and include domains such as, specific diseases,[7a,55] test ordering,[394] acid–base and electrolyte physiology,[281] chemistry pathophysiology,[251,382,407] and hematologic disorders (e.g., RED for the diagnosis of erythrocyte antibodies[358] and ANEMIA for the diagnosis of anemia[302,303]—Uckun discusses ANEMIA and the sequel, NEOANEMIA in Chapter 6[390]). Spackman and Connelly[361] identified areas in which knowledge-based systems promised to be useful, for example, to generate interpretive reporting of patterns of laboratory values, assist in the classification and diagnosis of difficult cases, facilitate more effective involvement in consultation on laboratory utilization, advance results communications, monitor requests for expensive or overused tests or blood products, adapt computers to individual knowledge and style, provide easy and powerful database query capability, and help in the control of instrumentation. Knowledge-based systems could improve the cost-effectiveness of test ordering[52] and the clinical use of probabilistic reasoning using sensitivity, specificity, and prevalence.[382,383] Sher[337] envisioned a hospital network of decentralized workstations that would allow access to computer-facilitated analysis of laboratory results for rapid, consistent, and more cost-effective decision making.

Recently published literature provides us with an appreciation of the current status of AI applications in laboratory medicine and clinical pathology. Table 8.1 categorizes the topics of publications that appeared from 1990 through 1995 by the area of application. Often, these represent developmental research used effectively in individual laboratories. Not many enjoy commercial dissemination. The practical application of artificial intelligence and expert systems is not yet widespread in laboratory medicine, despite the fact that several of these published methods represent innovative and creative solutions to important laboratory and clinical problems, such as decreasing turnaround time[85a,335a] in order to reduce the patient's length of stay. As Uckun notes,[390] there now is a switch from consultative systems to "intelligent agents" embedded in information systems (e.g., the HELP expert system for antibiotic selection[37]). Recently, Winkel[413] suggested that expert systems be combined with methods such as mathematical models of biochemical systems, time series analysis, and machine learning, which may be used to extract knowledge at a high level of abstraction. Table 8.1 and Figure 8.2 reveal an increasing emphasis on research involving neural networks. Neural networks, as well as computer-facilitated methods such as rule-based efficiency systems,[85] performance maps and quality paths,[206] and Winkel's[413] interesting pattern declaration–action monitors should prove useful and cost-effective in laboratory medicine niches by increasing the efficiency of diagnostic processes and improving clinical services.

Consistent with the progress of automation and robotization in the clinical laboratory and with the evolution and branching of artificial intelligence, several research and commercial innovations described in this book are emerging and in some cases, are ready for implementation. For example, in Chapter 4 Ver-

TABLE 8.1. AI Applications in Laboratory Medicine and Clinical Pathology, 1990–1995[a]

Category	Topic
Alerting	Computerized system (378), reporting and alarming (272)
Cost-effectiveness	Hematology (85)
Data analysis	Autoverification of peripheral blood count (84a), chromogenic interferents (48a), clinical assessment of knowledge base (268), output (47a), validation (392)
Diagnosis	Computer-aided (348), computer-assisted principles (245), qualitative models (173)
Informatics	Expert systems (73,76) and feature evaluation (133a)
Interpretation	Hepatitis tests (2,3), pancreatic enzymes (187), reports (105), tumor markers (365), urinary calculi (415a)
Monitoring	Pattern declarations and actions (412a)
Neural networks	Cytology (260), diagnosis (65), electrophoresis (208), enzyme-linked immunoassay (395), evaluation (329), immunoelectrophoresis (360), information utilization (306), interpretation (18,19), monoclonal gammopathy detection (239), polygenic trait analysis (225), quantitation (100), rheumatic diagnosis (18a), serial cardiac enzymes (130), thyroid diagnosis (335a)
Quality	Culture-based infection control surveillance (183), multitest analyzer fault diagnosis (145), quality assurance and quality improvement (14,15)
Robotics	Artificial intelligence and expert system applications (174)
Specialization	Blood banking (68,179,362), clinical chemistry (177,416a), genetics (41,364), hematology workstation (94), oncology (85a,240), toxicology (54)
Systems	Decision support (242), expert systems support (213,238,289a,353), object-oriented design (407a)
Test ordering	Improving clinician requesting patterns (287), management system (267), stats (311e)
Utilization	Optimizing resource use (41), platelet request evaluation (75,347), sample triaging (236), time and resources (264a)

[a]The figures in parentheses are reference numbers (listed at the end of this chapter). For publications prior to 1990, please see the list of references. For recent reviews since 1986, see References 13, 52, 76, 133a, 174, 213, 238, 242, 312, 337, 361, 383, 412, and 413, and the text. For a summary of current applications described in the other chapters in this book, please refer to the text.

tosick[396] details several useful practical applications[19,187,329,395] of neural networks and also notes that neural network software is relatively accessible. Because of the ability of neural networks to extract knowledge from patient case examples, recognize patterns or classes, identify important quantities, and optimize critical decision thresholds,[413] it is predictable that neural networks will contribute substantially to clinical laboratory science. For example, they could be used to identify clinically important tests or to eliminate tests that are either useless or redundant.[413] Felder lists simulation modeling products (see Table 1.2) that could be used in the clinical laboratory.[114] In Chapter 5 Goldophin describes the salient features of simulation modeling.[139] In Chapter 6 Uckun analyzes the potential role of model-based reasoning in laboratory medicine.[390] In Chapter 7 Martin and Maguire present a case study of a fuzzy logic expert system that "mimic(s) technologists' judgments about clinical chemistry samples"[243] and is integrated with automated sample processing equipment to improve speed, safety, and cost-effectiveness.

Markin states that "the software controlling the laboratory automation platform is the most significant system component"[241] and adds that rules (expert system—see Fig. 10.9) are used in the system he describes to facilitate clinical laboratory workflow, diagnostic testing, and test utilization options for managed care. Computer processing and analysis are pivotal to the image processing techniques described by Wells and Memoli[408] in Chapter 14. In some cases, software–enabled sophistication eventually will supersede, if not exceed, human talents. For instance, Agapakis and Krishnaswamy[4] predict that "the use of machine vision and vision guided robotics to meet (the) demands on speed, quantity, and quality will sharply increase over the next few years," and that "computer vision sensing and processing (will become) an indispensable part of laboratory procedure as positioning and measurement tolerances fall beyond the limits of human capabilities" (see Chapter 13). It is clear from these examples that artificial intelligence, expert systems, and neural networks will continue to increase in use as they become embedded in highly automated and roboticized laboratory systems and more accessible to laboratory and medical professionals. This may result in one of the most useful, productive, and cost-effective applications in medicine. Overall, the trend can be viewed as an evolving paradigm shift in clinical laboratory strategies and operations.[240a] In essence, diagnostic testing must become a user-friendly core process (e.g., an icon on a screen) in an information architecture designed for and capable of facilitating knowledge creation.[206] Given the burgeoning knowledge base in laboratory medicine, knowledge itself will be the primary product of the future!

8.4. AI-FACILITATED DIAGNOSIS AND CLINICAL DECISION SUPPORT SYSTEMS

Medical reasoning strives to modify the current state of the patient, and in this endeavor, artificial intelligence can amplify the cognitive skills of the physician in the immediate tasks of diagnosis, therapy, and monitoring.[368] Given a limited body of observational data, the clinician needs some means of deciding which hypotheses to pursue and which to ignore. Selected hypotheses become working hypotheses that are submitted to detailed exploration and testing. Historically, strategies have been developed to simultaneously limit the breadth of hypotheses and incorporate pathophysiological reasoning in order to make artificial intelligence more clinically relevant.[376] Table 8.2 summarizes several

TABLE 8.2. Recent Clinical Applications of AI and Computer-Based Systems, 1992–1995[a]

Category	Topic
Cost-effectiveness	Test ordering in low prevalence conditions (36), workload (142)
Decision support	Computer-enhanced (117), connectionist expert systems (30), management of abdominal pain (408a), pharmacokinetics (22a), physician-based architecture (223), probabilistic systems (79), reminders for vaccination (312a), rheumatology hypothesis testing (164), septicemia management (99), support program (401), symbolic (169), uremic patients (175)
Diagnosis—methods	Clinical care (151), consistency-based (97), differential diagnosis (158), efficiency (263), graphical knowledge (132), histories (71), influence diagram (266), outcomes and quality parameters (269), probabilistic knowledge (226,230), qualitative models (173)
Diagnosis—specific	Acute appendicitis (286), dysmorphic syndromes (136), emergency room (354), iron deficiency (53), neuromuscular (417)
Education	Inductive learning (192), learning system (47)
Neural networks	Coronary artery disease (128), diagnostic tasks (96), multiple disorder diagnosis (59,374), student problem-solving performance (369)
Outcomes	Performance of computer-based decision support (181)
Prediction	Immune dysfunction (237)
Specialty areas	Cardiology (132a,218), hepatology (81,232), nephrology (5), nuclear medicine (84), rheumatology (409)
Therapeutics	Antibiotic selection (37), fluid and electrolyte (143), gestational diabetes (159), hybrid knowledge-based systems for planning (301)
Transplantation	Selection and management of patients (259)

[a]The figures in parentheses are reference numbers. For publications prior to 1992, please see the list of references. References related to temporal optimization, critical care, and new knowledge structures used in these areas are not included in this table. Please refer to the text for these references.

recent (1992–1995) innovations in AI-facilitated diagnosis and clinical decision support systems that are designed to assist physician reasoning, hypothesis testing, and decision making. Realization of the power of these techniques clinically and in medical education[110,111] will depend in part on the integration of communications with computing in order to merge knowledge-based systems, medical informatics,[344] and decision support.[22a,147,202,343a] Belkora et al.[32] and Kroll[210] explain the value of decision analysis (see Chapters 29 and 30). Kroll also discusses the clinical value of automated–facilitated causal reasoning[209] (see Chapter 31). Algorithmic diagnosis, which should play an increasingly important role in the economical use of diagnostic tests in managed care, is described by Yang et al.[418] (see Chapter 32).

The dissemination of artificial intelligence and expert systems in clinical medicine has been sluggish. Potential reasons for this include[13] (1) medical decision making often exceeds the capacity of the knowledge representation schemes, or the schemes may not resemble professional traditions; (2) output from the expert system may lack detailed rationales, ranked alternatives, or full explanations of why some alternatives are selected and others are not; (3) input or output may be erroneous,[22a] difficult to automate, temporally dyssynchronized, awkward, user-unfriendly,[80] tedious, or too slow, in view of competing demands for the clinician's time; (4) uncertainty and tradeoffs involving risks may be unclear, and error checking may be inadequate; (5) there may be little or no provision for software updating and continuous quality improvement; (6) expert systems may not emulate important problem-solving talents for diagnosis, such as common sense, creativity, intuition, and perception; (7) inadequate flexibility for learning from experience may inhibit integration, synthesis, and optimization in clinical settings, particularly when practice patterns change; (8) an emphasis on the physician rather than collaborative practice may miss important opportunities to facilitate team-supportive tasks; and generally (9) there may be no improvement in patient outcomes.

The area of greatest concern is whether computer-assisted decision support and artificial intelligence actually improve patient outcomes. Johnston et al.[181] recently provided an extensive critical review of the impact of decision support systems on patient outcome and documented, for 28 controlled trials that met predefined criteria, a track record of variable performance from 1974 to 1992. They found that "three of four studies of computer-assisted dosing, one of five studies of computer-aided diagnosis, four of six studies of preventative care reminder systems, and seven of nine studies of computer-aided quality assurance for active medical care that assessed clinical performance showed improvements," and that "three of ten studies that assessed patient outcomes reported significant improvements."[181] The lack of improvement in patient outcomes may have been due to small sample size, inappropriate study design, failure to measure responsive outcomes, or a limited focus on just improving physician efficiency in some of the studies.[181] Johnston et al.[181] cautioned that computer-based decision support systems "have the potential for not only good but also harm and waste," that clinical trials "should be reserved for mature systems," and that "the accepted standard (should) be randomized controlled trials showing unequivocal benefits for important clinical outcomes."

In regard to artificial intelligence techniques, a possible line of explanation for suboptimal performance relates to whether the systems used are "deep."[190,390] To assess whether a system is deep, one asks questions such as[402]

Does the expert system represent factual and strategic knowledge explicitly?

Can it cover exceptions?

Can it also retract conclusions in the light of new facts?

These are challenging performance criteria, nearly comparable to human thinking! Fortunately, innovative research is tackling many of these dilemmas. (See a recent special issue of *Artificial Intelligence in Medicine*.[387]) For example, second-generation knowledge acquisition methods[218] help emulate human medical experts by incorporating pathophysiological reasoning and machine learning.[137,280,280a] In addition, interesting computer-assisted approaches are becoming available for critical care, one of the most challenging clinical settings, where the ability to accommodate sudden and unanticipated change is essential.

8.5. TEMPORAL OPTIMIZATION AND CRITICAL CARE

As increasing competition for resources restricts allocations for critical care patients, temporal optimization potentially can help physicians to balance the demands for simultaneously increased time efficiency, enhanced decision making, improved patient outcomes, and documented cost-effectiveness. Investigators have drawn heavily from artificial intelligence,[307] expert systems, and related areas in computer science to develop new techniques appropriate for temporal reasoning,[26,154,196,314] temporal domains, and time-dependent data.[6b,45a,55a,76a,104a,396a] For example, Das and Musen[83] recently described an algebra that allows temporal queries needed for protocol-directed decision support used to screen patients for clinical trials. Wade et al.[399] described an inference engine and query language for finding temporal patterns represented by using temporally ordered sets of data objects. They applied this approach to the identification of inappropriate use of prescription drugs. Burke and Madison[48] used artificial intelligence for patient triage in the emergency department. Several novel approaches, many with temporal modeling or prediction, exist to assist diabetics in the management of glucose levels and insulin therapy.[38,92,93,168,224,334,335] Deutsch and colleagues[93] used symbolic representation and time series analysis to devise decision support systems that combine data processing, a glucose–insulin dynamic simulator, interpretation, qualitative algebra,[92] and quantitative[220,221] advice for the management of insulin-dependent diabetic patients. They also designed an insulin dosage optimizer with a feedback loop for use in education and clinical research.[221] Hovorka et al.[166] devised a system that predicts blood glucose levels for diabetics using insulin pumps in the hospital. The inclusion of temporal information, processing, and optimization in software programs such as these is necessary to closely simulate medical expert performance[196] and to provide results that are relevant to ongoing patient care, particularly for the critically ill patient.

Innovative intelligent facilitators for patient monitoring can improve on simple alarms, alerts, and advisories, such as those commonly found on automated instruments[131,182,203–205,272,322] and monitoring devices,[17,125,207,215] and eventually, could be widely accessible on communications networks.[31,107,123,165,176,206] Applications to monitoring include fuzzy logic,[350] expert systems,[397] and influence diagrams.[6] Coiera[70] conceptualized the construction of an intelligent monitoring and control system that spans the range from patient signals to control decisions. Uckun[386,388,389] and colleagues[152,153] designed intelligent monitoring systems for the intensive care unit. One[388] (discussed in Chapter 6[390]) focused on the diagnosis of clinical conditions, alerts for abnormalities, prediction of the effects of therapy, and therapy management assistance. Coleman et al.[72] used computational logic to help identify linkages in different levels of critical care decision-making processes. Other authors[262] have used expert systems for the symbolic classification of numeric variables in the intensive care unit, or for decision support during anesthesia or postoperatively.[323,384,419] Timcenko and Reich[380] described a distributed real-time expert system with continuous automated patient data acquisition that provided differential diagnoses and treatment recommendations during cardiac surgery. Ursino et al.[391] used an expert system to integrate qualitative and numerical reasoning involving the relationships between hemodynamic and metabolic quantities following cardiac surgery.

New software programs are becoming available for outcomes management and include, for example, AccuBase,[1] Project IMPACT,[300] and QuIC (Quality Intensive Care System).[303a] Formal outcomes optimization soon will become the norm.[206] This is essential in order to improve patient care while simultaneously addressing the requirements of the changed criteria for fiscal reimbursement. Emphasis on improving the cost-effectiveness of procedures associated with clinical problems that incur large healthcare expenditures would be valuable. For example, algorithmic evaluation performed quickly in the emergency room when a patient presents with chest pain would conserve expensive critical care resources. Computer-facilitated diagnosis[406] and management of patients with acute myocardial infarction[132a] is an important area for future research. Ebell[103] used neural networks to predict outcome following cardiopulmonary resuscitation. Koski et al.[201,372] designed a knowledge-based alarm system for postoperative monitoring of four pathological states (e.g., left ventricular failure) in cardiac surgery patients. Seiver[330,331] designed decision systems with sequential two-stage models and knowledge maps to capture medical knowledge in critical care. Lau[216] described a decision-support system with physiologic pattern matching, therapeutic protocols, drug-dosage response modeling, and expert reasoning that recommended preferred interventions for intensive care unit patients with hypovolemic hypotension. Sitting et al.[351] developed a computerized management system from detailed physician care protocols for intensive care unit patients with acute respiratory distress syndrome. Russ[315] used reasoning modules in a system capable of handling time-dependent data for patient management. The decision support system of Zarkadakis et al.[419] assists clinicians in the interpretation of blood gases and provides a trace that reflects the line of reasoning used. Fruitiger and Branner[126] also developed computerized blood gas interpretation. Tong[381] showed that a knowledge-based system for weaning a patient from mechanical ventilation[16,101,102,124,217,316,405] can reduce the number of arterial blood gases needed. Roberts et al.[311] addressed the cost-effectiveness of intensive care. Real-time knowledge-based systems[21] and knowledge-based decision support[323,326] are promising areas for investigation and application in critical care. Documentation of *impact on patient outcomes* is necessary to assess which of these techniques will be most effective in the future.

8.6. CONCLUSIONS

Managed care and restructuring are increasing the value of computer-assisted efficiency in the clinical laboratory. Reengineering of diagnostic services is promoting new thinking about how physicians and patients utilize diagnostic testing. Table 8.3 suggests future directions worthy of at least exploration, if not financial investment. Commercial distribution of instruments, robotics, and integrated systems that carry along embedded intelligent software modules will help

TABLE 8.3. Future Directions for Artificial Intelligence and New Knowledge Structures

---

Microeconomic Strategies for Restructuring and Reengineering Patient Care

Computer-assisted optimization of workflow and response time for tests performed in intramural, regional, and reference laboratories

Remote automated review, robotic testing sites, and connectivity to improve resource utilization and informatics coordination with a continuum to the point of care

Computer-facilitated differential diagnosis and algorithmic protocols to assure cost-effective patient evaluation

Decision support for conservative diagnostic testing, economical laboratory ordering (e.g., blood products), and continuous quality improvement

Embedded Intelligent Components

Incorporation of accessible artificial intelligence techniques, machine learning, and computer-facilitated decision support in professional practice and teaching

Use with instruments, robotics, and fully integrated diagnostic testing and monitoring systems including advanced process control

Translation of procedural tasks and monitoring to automated solutions and practice actions, clinically and for total laboratory automation

Dissemination of intelligent software modules in laboratory, hospital, and portable ("ubiquitous") computer systems and universal workstations

Accelertion of medical reasoning and care team tasking with "smart" patient-focused workstations, wireless communications, virtual databases, and data warehousing

Knowledge Optimization

New knowledge structures incorporating temporal optimization and diagnostic-therapeutic process optimization

Computer-assisted analysis of diagnostic–therapeutic processes for the critically ill patient

Enhanced learning and performance of hybrid teams focused on collaborative care

Improved Outcomes

Software for the analysis, prediction, and management of patient outcomes, and marriage of the outcomes programs to artificial intelligence techniques

Integrated efficiency among the emergency department, operating room, intensive care unit, patient-focused care center, and healthcare system sites

Improved utilization of medical resources based on optimized medical and economic outcomes

---

alleviate the "cottage industry" hurdles experienced in the past decade. Accessible techniques (e.g., neural networks) should prove efficient, timely, and cost-effective in laboratory medicine. Connectivity in the forms of networks and wireless communications will be a powerful computational resource and an indispensable infrastructure as these trends mature. It is advantageous, and possibly even essential to survival, for laboratory professionals to implement artificial intelligence techniques, as well as robotics, at this time. Proof of benefits and validation of efficacy must be documented as milestones in development are achieved. The clinical laboratory has an advantage since significant cost savings can accrue from internal efficiencies alone. However, the most significant goal is clinical benefit.

We can expect increasing use of artificial intelligence and new knowledge structures in clinical tasks, such as differential diagnosis, algorithmic test selection, conservation of blood products, procedural problem solving, and patient monitoring in the laboratory or at the point of care. Decentralizing intelligent software modules will foster the transcription, translation, and creation of knowledge, as well as a better appreciation of how to design dynamic systems that can learn and adapt to changing practice patterns. Customization will convey a sense of ownership and empowerment. Improved physician efficiency is a worthy objective by itself. Accelerated medical reasoning at the point of care should fulfill vital physician, nurse, and care team needs. The parallel development of temporal optimization, diagnostic–therapeutic processes optimization, and software systems for outcomes analysis and management should help improve the effectiveness of critical care. Collaborative performance teams will be better equipped and better able to focus their attention, efforts, and actions on improving and optimizing medical and economic outcomes as well as patient well-being.

ACKNOWLEDGMENTS

I am indebted to Dr. John Chow for creating and validating the NMR expert system. Ms. Julia Barry provided valuable assistance with library research. Ms. Kate Maney prepared the illustrations. The staff of the Interlibrary Loan Department of the Health Sciences Library at the University of California, Davis, helped extensively with literature retrieval. I thank them for their efforts with this and the other chapters. I also thank Ms. Judith Welsh for her numerous contributions to this chapter and for her expert assistance rendered to the other authors.

REFERENCES

1. *AcuBase.* Seattle: Clinical Information Systems, Inc.
1a. Adlassing KP, Kolarz G, Scheithauer W, Effenberger H, Grabner G: CADIAG: approaches to computer-assisted medical diagnosis. *Comput Biol Med* 15:315–335, 1985.

2. Adlassnig KP, Horak W. Hepaxpert-1: Automatic interpretation of tests for hepatitis A and B. *MD Comput* 8:118–119, 1991.

3. Adlassnig KP, Horak W: The knowledge base of the Hepaxpert I System: automatic interpretation of Hepatitis A and B serology. *Leber Magen Darm* 23:251–267, 1993.

4. Agapakis JE, Krishnaswamy S. Machine vision in laboratory automation. In Kost GJ, ed. *Handbook of Clinical Automation, Robotics, and Optimization.* New York, NY: John Wiley and Sons, Inc., 1996: Chapter 13.

5. Agar JW, Webb GI: Application of machine learning to a renal biopsy database. *Nephrol Dial Transplant* 7:472–478, 1992.

6. Agogino AM, Ramamurthi K: Real time influence diagrams for monitoring and controlling mechanical systems. In Oliver RM, Smith JQ, eds: *Influence Diagrams, Belief Nets and Decision Analysis.* New York: Wiley, 1990, pp 199–228.

6a. Aikins JS, Kunz JC, Shortliffe EH, Fallar RJ: PUFF: An expert system for interpretation of pulmonary function data. *Comput Biomed Res* 16:199–208, 1983.

6b. Albert A, Chapelle JP, Bourguignat A: Dynamic outcome prediction from repeated laboratory measurements made on intensive care unit patients. I. Statistical aspects and logistic models. *Scand J Clin Lab Invest* 44 (Suppl 171):259–268, 1984.

7. Aller RD: New directions in interpretive test reporting. *Med Lab Observer* 21:27–33, 1989.

7a. Alvey P, Myers C, Greaves M: High performance for expert systems: escaping from the demonstrator class. *Med Info* 12:85–95, 1987.

8. Aminzadeh F, Jamshidi M, eds: *Soft Computing: Fuzzy Logic, Neural Networks, and Distributed Artificial Intelligence.* Englewood Cliffs, NJ: PTR Prentice-Hall, 1994.

9. Anderson J: Medical knowledge—its relationship to medical informatics and information systems. In Kohout L, Baldler W, eds: *Knowledge Representation in Medicine and Clinical Behavioural Science.* Cambridge, MA: Abacus Press, 1986, pp 11–18.

10. Andreassen S: Knowledge representation by extended linear models. In Keravnou E, ed: *Deep Models for Medical Knowledge Engineering.* New York: Elsevier, 1992, pp 129–146.

11. Arbib MA: *Brains, Machines and Mathematics.* New York: McGraw-Hill, 1987.

12. Arbib MA: *The Metaphorical Brain. An Introduction to Cybernetics as Artificial Intelligence and Brain Theory.* New York: Wiley-Interscience, 1972.

12a. Arbib MA: *The Metaphorical Brain 2: Neural Networks and Beyond.* New York: Wiley, 1989.

13. Armas SE, Warkentin ME, Armas OA: Expert systems in laboratory medicine and pathology. *Artif Intell Med* 1:79–85, 1989.

14. Aronow DB: Information technology applications in quality assurance and quality improvement. *Jt Comm J Qual Improv* 19:403–415, 1993.

15. Aronow DB: Information technology applications in quality assurance and quality improvement. Part II. *Jt Comm J Qual Improv* 19:465–478, 1993.

16. Arroe M: A computerized aid in ventilating neonates. *Comput Biol Med* 21:15–21, 1991.

17. Ash D, Gold G, Seiver A, Hayes-Roth B: Guaranteeing real-time response with limited resources. *Artif Intell Med* 5:49–66, 1993.

18. Astion ML, Wener MH, Thomas RG, Hunder GG, Bloch DA: Overtraining in neural networks that interpret clinical data. *Clin Chem* 39:1998–2004, 1993.

18a. Astion ML, Bloch DA, Werner MH: Neural networks as expert systems in rheumatic disease diagnosis: artificial intelligence or intelligence artifice? *J Rheumatol* 20:1465–1468, 1993.

19. Astion ML, Wilding P: Application of neural networks to the interpretation of laboratory data in cancer diagnosis. *Clin Chem* 38:34–38, 1992.

20. Autio K, Kari A, Tikka H: Integration of knowledge-based system and database for identification of disturbances in fluid and electrolyte balance. *Comput Meth Programs Biomed* 34:201–209, 1991.

21. Aynsley M, Hofland A, Morris AJ, Montague GA, Di Massimo C: Artificial intelligence and the supervision of bioprocesses (real-time knowledge-based systems and neural networks). *Adv Biochem Eng Biotechnol* 48:1–27, 1993.

22. B Pereira CA de: Influence diagrams and medical diagnosis. In Oliver RM, Smith JQ, eds: *Influence Diagrams, Belief Nets and Decision Analysis.* New York: Wiley, 1990, pp 351–358.

22a. Baer DM, Kotschi ML: On-line computer pharmacokinetics program: lessons learned from its failure. *Clin Chem* 41:491–494, 1995.

23. Bagwell CB: New horizons: expert systems for flow cytometry. *Cytometry Suppl.* 3:89–93, 1988.

24. Bandler W, Kohout L: A survey of fuzzy relational products in their applicability to medicine and clinical psychology. In Kohout L, Baldler W, eds: *Knowledge Representation in Medicine and Clinical Behavioural Science.* Cambridge, MA: Abacus Press, 1986, pp 107–118.

25. Banks G: Artificial intelligence in medical diagnosis: the INTERNIST/CADUCEUS approach. *Crit Rev Med Inf* 1:23–54, 1986.

26. Barahona P: A causal and temporal reasoning model and its use in drug therapy applications. *Artif Intell Med* 6:1–27, 1994.

27. Barahona P: A causal-functional model for medical knowledge representation. In Keravnou E, ed: *Deep Models for Medical Knowledge Engineering.* New York: Elsevier, 1992, pp 101–128.

28. Barlow RE, Irony TZ, Shor SWW: Informative sampling methods: the influence of experimental design on decision. In Oliver RM, Smith JQ, eds: *Influence Diagrams, Belief Nets and Decision Analysis.* New York: Wiley, 1990, pp 177–197.

29. Barnett GO, Cimino JJ, Hupp JA, et al: DXplain: an evolving diagnostic decision-support system. *JAMA* 258:67–74, 1987.

29a. Barnett GO, Winickoff RN, Morgan MM, Zielstorff RD: A computer-based monitoring system for follow-up of elevated blood pressure. *Med Care* 21:400–409, 1983.

30. Barreto JM, de Azevedo FM: Connectionist expert systems as medical decision aid. *Artif Intell Med* 5:515–523, 1993.

31. Bauer S: A blood gas network: using blood gas and electrolyte analyzers at the point of care. *Med Lab Observer* 26(9S):2–9, 1994.

32. Belkora JK, Fehling MR, Esserman LJ. Assuring medical decision quality through decision analysis for patients and physicians. In Kost GJ, ed. *Handbook of Clinical Automation, Robotics, and Optimization.* New York, NY: John Wiley and Sons, Inc., 1996: Chapter 29.

33. Bellazzi R, Quaglini S, Berzuini C, Stefanelli M: GAMEES: a probabilistic environment for expert systems. *Comput Meth Programs Biomed* 35:177–191, 1991.

33a. Benson ES: Decision analysis and the clinical laboratory. In Kerhof PJ, van Dieijen-Visser MP, eds: *Laboratory Data and Patient Care.* New York: Plenum Press, 1988, pp 59–66.

34. Berger-Hershkowitz H, Neuhauser D: Artificial intelligence in the clinical laboratory. *Cleveland Clin J Med* 54:165–166, 1987.

35. Berner ES, Brooks CM, Miller RA, Masarie FE, Jackson JR: Evaluation issues in the development of expert systems in medicine. *Eval Health Prof* 12:270–281, 1989.

36. Bernstein RM, Hollingworth GR, Wood WE: Prompting physicians for cost-effective test ordering in the low prevalence conditions of family medicine. *Proc Annu Symp Comput Appl Med Care* 824–828, 1994.

37. Betts M: Doctors get HELP to fight infections; expert system at LDS Hospital assists doctors with selection of best antibiotics for patients. *Computerworld* 28:67, 1994.

38. Beyer J, Schulz G, Strack T, Kustner E, Schrezenmeir J: Computer-assisted diabetes therapy—a challenge for modern medicine. *Z Gesamte Inn Med* 45:673–677, 1990.

39. Beynon-Davies P. *Expert Database Systems: A Gentle Introduction.* New York: McGraw-Hill, 1991.

40. Beynon-Davies P: *Knowledge Engineering for Information Systems.* New York: McGraw-Hill, 1993.

41. Bickel AS, Bickel RW: Determination of near-optimum use of hospital diagnostic resources using the GENES genetic algorithm and shell. *Comput Biol Med* 20:1–13, 1990.

42. Blomberg DJ, Guth JL, Fattu JM, Patrick EA: Evaluation of a new classification system for anemias using Consult Learning System. *Comput Meth Programs Biomed* 22:119–125, 1986.

43. Blum BI: Artificial intelligence and medical informatics. *Med Info* 11:3–18, 1986.

44. Blum RL: Induction of causal relationships from a time-oriented clinical database: an overview of the RX project. In *Proc. 2nd Natl Conf Artificial Intelligence,* Pittsburgh, PA, 1982, pp 335–357.

45. Bobrow DG, ed: *Artificial Intelligence in Perspective.* Cambridge, MA: MIT Press, 1994.

45a. Bourguignat A, Albert A, Chapelle JP: Dynamic outcome prediction from repeated laboratory measurements made on intensive care unit patients. III. Application to severe head injury. *Scand J Clin Lab Invest* 44 (Suppl 171):279–287, 1984.

46. Bradshaw KE, Gardner RM, Pryor TA: Development of a computerized laboratory alerting system. *Comput Biomed Res,* 22:575–587, 1989.

46a. Bratko I, Mozelic I, Lavrac N: *KARDIO: A Study in Deep and Qualitative Knowledge for Expert Systems.* Cambridge, MA: MIT Press, 1989.

46b. Brownbridge G, Evans A, Fitter M, Platts M: An interactive computerized protocol for the management of hypertension: effects on the general practitioner's clinical behavior. *J R Coll Gen Pract* 36:198–202, 1986.

47. Bruha T, Kockova S: A support for decision-making: cost-sensitive learning system. *Artif Intell Med* 6:67–82, 1994.

47a. Burgess PR, Kershaw GW, Coleman RH et al: A computerized expert system for handling the output of the Technicon H1 haematology analyser. *Clin Lab Haemat* 15:21–32, 1993.

48. Burke MD, Madison DE: Artificial intelligence in emergency department triage. *J Ambulatory Care Management* 13:50–54, 1990.

48a. Burtner K, Huber M, Frye S: Use of serum blank information to quantify chromogenic interferents and correct sensitive analyses. *Clin Chem* 36:1584–1586, 1990.

49. Bylander T: Some causal models are deeper than other. In Keravnou E, ed: *Deep Models for Medical Knowledge Engineering.* New York: Elsevier, 1992, pp 169–176.

50. Campbell JA, Wolstencroft J: Cases and the elucidation of deep knowledge. In Keravnou E, ed: *Deep Models for Medical Knowledge Engineering.* New York: Elsevier, 1992, pp 219–230.

51. Campbell JA, Wolstencroft J: Structure and significance of analogical reasoning. In Keravnou E, ed: *Deep Models for Medical Knowledge Engineering.* New York: Elsevier, 1992, pp 199–218.

52. Castellani W, Chou D, Van Lente F, Galen RS: Use of artificial intelligence for the optimization of laboratory test selection. In Salamon R, Blum B, Jorgensen M. *Medinfo 86, Proc 5th Conf Medical Informatics,* Washington, DC, Oct 26–30, 1986. New York: North-Holland, 1986, pp 82–86.

53. Causer MB, Findlay GA, Hawes CR, Boswell DR: Assessment of a computerized system for the diagnosis of iron deficiency. *Pathology* 26:37–39, 1994.

54. Cechner RL, Sutheimer CA: Automated rule-based decision systems in forensic toxicology using expert knowledge: basic principles and practical applications. *J Anal Toxicol* 14:280–284, 1990.

55. Chang E, McNeely M, Gamble K: Strategies for choosing the next test in an expert system. In *Proc Am Assoc Med Syst Informatics Congress 1984.* Bethesda, MD: American Association of Medical Systems and Informatics, 1984, pp 198–202.

55a. Chapelle JP, Albert A, Bourguignat A: Dynamic outcome prediction from repeated laboratory measurements made on intensive care unit patients. II. Application to acute myocardial infarction. *Scand J Clin Lab Invest* 44 (Suppl 171):269–278, 1984.

56. Chard T, Chard DT, Macintosh M: Prediction of future outcome using Bayesian logic. *Baillieres Clin Obstet Gynaecol* 8:607–624, 1994.

57. Charniak E, McDermott D: *Introduction to Artificial Intelligence.* Reading, MA: Addison-Wesley, 1986.

57a. Chase CR, Vacek PM, Shinozaki T, Giard AM, Ashikaga T: Medical information management: improving the transfer of research results to presurgical evaluation. *Med Care* 21:410–424, 1983.

58. Cheeseman P, Oldford RW, eds: *Selecting Models from Data: Artificial Intelligence and Statistics IV.* New York: Springer-Verlag, 1994.

59. Cho S, Reggia JA: Multiple disorder diagnosis with adaptive competitive neural networks. *Artif Intell Med* 5:469–487, 1993.

60. Chou D, Naito H, Castellani W, Berger-Hershkowitz H: Development of a microcomputer lipid/lipoprotein profile interpretive report using Rutgers EXPERT artificial intelligence consultation system. *Clin Chem* 32:1179, 1986.

61. Chow JL, Olsen DR, Anderson SE, VanderWerf QM, Kost GJ: A microcomputer-based system for processing 31-phosphorus nuclear magnetic resonance spectra from studies of cardiac metabolism in immature hearts. *Comput Meth Programs Biomed* 25:39–46, 1987.

62. Chow JLH: An expert system for 31-phosphorus nuclear magnetic resonance spectral analysis and interpretation. Davis, CA: biomedical engineering thesis; 1988, 189 pp.

63. Chow JL, Levitt KN, Kost GJ: Biological NMR spectral analysis by an expert system. *IEEE Eng Med Biol* 10:1391–1392, 1988.

64. Chow JL, Levitt KN, Kost GJ: NMRES: an artificial intelligence expert system for quantification of cardiac metabolites from 31-phosphorus nuclear magnetic resonance spectroscopy. *Ann Biomed Eng* 21:247–258, 1993.

65. Cicchetti DV: Neural networks and diagnosis in the clinical laboratory: state of the art. *Clin Chem* 38:9–10, 1992.

66. Clancy WJ, Shortliffe EH, eds: *Readings in Medical Artificial Intelligence: The First Decade.* Reading, MA: Addison-Wesley, 1984.

67. Clancy WJ, Smolian SW, Stefik MJ, eds: *Contemplating Minds: A Forum for Artificial Intelligence.* Cambridge, MA: MIT Press, 1994.

68. Clark BD, Leong SW: Crossmatch prediction of highly sensitized patients. *Clin Transpl* 435–455, 1992.

69. Clark K, O'Moore R, Smeets R, et al: A methodology for evaluation of knowledge-based systems in medicine. *Artif Intell Med* 6:107–121, 1994.

69a. Coe FL, Norton E, Oparil S, Tatar A, Pullman TN: Treatment of hypertension by computer and physician—a prospective controlled study. *J Chron Dis* 30:81–92, 1977.

70. Coiera E. Intelligent monitoring and control of dynamic physiological systems. *Artif Intell Med* 5:1–8, 1993.

71. Coiera E. Monitoring diseases with empirical and model generated histories. In Keravnou E, ed: *Deep Models for Medical Knowledge Engineering.* New York: Elsevier, 1992, pp 71–88.

72. Coleman WP, Siegel JH, Giovannini I, et al: Computational logic: a method for formal analysis of the ICU knowledge base. *Int J Clin Monit Comput* 20:67–79, 1993.

73. Connelly DP, Bennet ST: Expert systems and the clinical laboratory information system. *Clin Lab Med* 11:135–151, 1991.

74. Connelly DP, Holt T: Expert systems and clinical operations. US Healthcare 5:38–40, 1988.

75. Connelly DP, Sielaff BH, Scott EP: ESPRE—expert system for platelet request evaluation. *Am J Clin Pathol* 94:S19–S24, 1990.

76. Connelly DP: Embedding expert systems in laboratory information systems. *Am J Clin Pathol* 94:S7–S14, 1990.

76a. Connelly DP, Rhodes JB: Decision making in clinical monitoring: Experts, expert systems and statistics. In Kerkhof PLM, van Dieijen-Visser MP, eds: *Laboratory Data and Patient Care.* New York: Plenum Press, 1988, pp 171–176.

77. Connolly JH, Edmonds EA, eds: *CSCW and Artificial Intelligence.* New York: Springer-Verlag, 1994.

78. Connolly MB: Bedside data entry using portable RF terminals. In Salamon R, Blum B, Jorgensen M, eds: *Medinfo 86, Proc 5th Conf Medical Informatics,* Washington, DC, Oct 26–30, 1986. New York: North-Holland, 1986, pp 996–998.

79. Cooper G: Probabilistic and decision-theoretic systems in medicine [editorial]. *Artif Intell Med* 5:289–292, 1993.

80. Cramp DG, Nicolosi E, Leaning MS, Carson ER: Design requirements for a user-friendly computer-aided decision support system in laboratory medicine. In Salamon R, Blum B, Jorgensen M, eds: *Medinfo 86, Proc 5th Conf Medical Informatics,* Washington, DC, Oct 26–30, 1986. New York: North-Holland, 1986, pp 204–208.

81. Darmoni SJ, Poynard T: Computer-aided decision support in hepatology. *Scand J Gastroenterol* 27:889–896, 1992.

82. Dartnall T, ed: *Artificial Intelligence and Creativity: An Interdisciplinary Approach.* Boston, MA: Kluwer Academic, 1994.

83. Das AK, Musen MA: A temporal query system for protocol-directed decision support. *Meth Info Med* 33:358–370, 1994.

84. Datz FL, Rosenberg C, Gavor FV, et al: The use of computer-assisted diagnosis in cardiac perfusion nuclear medicine studies: a review (part 3). *J Digit Imag* 6:67–80, 1993.

84a. Davis GM: Autoverification of the peripheral blood count. *Lab Med* 25:528–531, 1994.

85. Davis GM: A rule-based system for cost savings in hematology. *Med Lab Observer* 26:44–46, 1994.

85a. Dawson AE, Austin RE, Weinberg DS: Nuclear grading of breast carcinoma by image analysis classification by multivariate and neural network analysis. *Am J Clin Pathol* 95 (Suppl 1):29–37, 1991.

85b. De Dombal FT, Leaper DJ, Horrocks JC, Staniland JR, McCann AP: Human and computer-aided diagnosis of abdominal pain: further report with emphasis on performance of clinicians. *Br Med J* 1:376–380, 1974.

86. De Mantaras RL, Poole D, eds: *Uncertainty in Artificial Intelligence: Proc 10th Conf,* July 29–31, 1994, University of Washington, Seattle; San Francisco: Morgan Kaufmann, 1994.

87. Dean TL, Allen J, Aloimonos J: *Artificial Intelligence: Theory and Practice.* Redwood City, CA: Benjamin/Cummings, 1995.

88. Debenham JK: *Knowledge Systems Design.* New York: Prentice-Hall; 1989.

89. Dechter R, Dechter A, Pearl J: Optimization in constraint networks. In Oliver RM, Smith JQ, eds: *Influence Diagrams, Belief Nets and Decision Analysis.* New York: Wiley, 1990, pp 411–425.

90. Degoulet P: Artificial intelligence—its use in nephrology. *Boll Soc Ital Biol Sper* 64:161–173, 1988.

91. Dempster AP: Construction and local computation aspects of network belief functions. In Oliver RM, Smith JQ, eds: *Influence Diagrams, Belief Nets and Decision Analysis.* New York: Wiley, 1990, pp 121–141.

92. Deutsch T, Boroujerdi MA, Carson ER, et al: The principles and prototyping of a knowledge-based diabetes management system. *Comput Meth Programs Biomed* 29:75–88, 1989.

93. Deutsch T, Lehmann ED, Carson ER, Roudsari AV, Hopkins KD, Sonksen PH: Time series analysis and control of blood glucose levels in diabetic patients. *Comput Meth Programs Biomed* 41:167–182, 1994.

94. Diamond LW, Mishka VG, Seal AH, Nguyen DT: A clinical database as a component of a diagnostic hematology workstation. *Proc Annu Symp Comput Appl Med Care* 298–302, 1994.

95. Dong Z, ed: *Artificial Intelligence in Optimal Design and Manufacturing.* Englewood Cliffs, NJ: Prentice-Hall, 1994.

96. Dorffner G, Porenta G: On using feedforward neural networks for clinical diagnostic tasks. *Artif Intell Med* 6:417–435, 1994.

97. Downing KL: Physiological applications of consistency-based diagnosis. *Artif Intell Med* 5:9–30, 1993.

98. Durkin J: *Expert Systems: Design and Development.* New York: Macmillan, 1994.

99. Dybowski R, Gransden WR, Phillips I: Towards a statistically oriented decision support system for the management of septicaemia. *Artif Intell Med* 5:489–502, 1993.

100. Dytch HE, Wied GL: Artificial neural networks and their use in quantitative pathology. *Anal Quant Cytol Histol* 12:379–393, 1990.

101. East TD, Bohm SH, Wallace CJ, et al: A successful computerized protocol for clinical management of pressure control inverse ratio ventilation in ARDS patients. *Chest* 101:696–710, 1992.

102. East TD, Henderson S, Morris AH, Gardner RM: Implementation issues and challenges for computerized clinical protocols for management of mechanical ventilation in ARDS patients. In *Proc 13th Annu Symp Comput Appl Med Care.* Washington, DC, 1989, pp 583–587.

103. Ebell MH. Artificial neural networks for predicting failure to survive following in-hospital cardiopulmonary resuscitation. *J Fam Pract* 36:297–303, 1993.

104. Eddy DM, Hasselblad V, Shachter R: *Meta-analysis by the Confidence Profile Method. The Statistical Synthesis of Evidence.* Boston: Academic Press, 1992.

104a. Eddy DM: Timing of repeated monitoring tests. *Scand J Clin Lab Invest* 44 (Suppl 171):131–152, 1984.

105. Edwards G, Compton P, Malor R, Srinivasan A, Lazarus L: PEIRS: a pathologist-maintained expert system for the interpretation of chemical pathology reports. *Pathology* 25:27–34, 1993.

106. Edwards M, Cooley RE: Expertise in expert systems: knowledge acquisition for biological expert systems. *Comput Appl Biosci* 9:657–665, 1993.

107. Elevitch FR: Multimedia communications networks: patient care through interactive point-of-care testing. *Clin Lab Med* 14:559–568, 1994.

108. Elliman AD: Medical data base management. In Kohout L, Baldler W, eds: *Knowledge Representation in Medicine and Clinical Behavioural Science.* Cambridge, MA: Abacus Press, 1986, pp 51–68.

109. Epton J, ed: *Expert Systems and Optimisation.* Brookfield, VT: Ashgate, 1994.

110. Evans DA, Patel VL, eds: *Advanced Models of Cognition for Medical Training and Practice.* New York: Springer-Verlag, 1992.

111. Evans DA, Patel VL, eds: *Cognitive Science in Medicine: Biomedical Modeling.* Cambridge, MA: MIT Press, 1989.

112. Evans S. PACE/CPC (Patient Care Expert Systems/Clinical Protocol Consultant): nursing care planning and decision support for the 1990s. *Healthcare Info* 7:26–28, 1990.

113. Felder RA. Automation of Pre-Analytical Processing and Mobile Robots. In Kost GJ, ed. *Handbook of Clinical Automation, Robotics, and Optimization.* New York, NY: John Wiley and Sons, Inc., 1996: Chapter 12.

114. Felder RA. Robotic automation of near-patient laboratory testing. In Kost GJ, ed. *Handbook of Clinical Automation, Robotics, and Optimization.* New York: John Wiley and Sons, Inc., 1996: Chapter 24.

115. Feldman MJ, Barnett GO: An approach to evaluating the accuracy of DXplain. *Comput Meth Programs Biomed* 35:261–266, 1991.

116. Fieschi M: Expert systems for medical consultation. *Health Policy* 6:159–173, 1986.

117. Fitzpatrick K: Computer-enhanced medical decision making. *Physician Assist* 18:67,70–72,74–75, 1994.

118. Flood RL, Cramp DG, Leaning MS, Carson ER: Mathematical modeling of fluid-electrolyte, acid-base balance for clinical application. In Salamon R, Blum B, Jorgensen M, eds: *Medinfo 86, Proc 5th Conf Medical Informatics,* Washington, DC, Oct 26–30, 1986. New York: North-Holland, 1986, pp 133–137.

119. Forastrom J, Nuutila P, Irjala K: Using the ID3 algorithm to find discrepant diagnoses from laboratory databases of thyroid patients. *Med Decision Making* 11:171–175, 1991.

120. Fox J, Fieschi M, Engelbrecht R, eds: *AIME 87: Proc European Conf Artificial Intelligence in Medicine* (Marseilles, France). New York: Springer-Verlag, 1987.

121. Fox J, Myers CD, Greaves MF, et al: Knowledge acquisition for expert systems: experience in leukemia diagnosis. *Meth Info Med* 24:65–72, 1985.

122. Fox J: On the soundness and safety of expert systems. *Artif Intell Med* 5:159–179, 1993.

123. Friedman BA, Mitchell W: Integrating information from decentralized laboratory testing sites: the creation of a value-added network. *Am J Clin Pathol* 99:637–642, 1993.

124. Friesdorf W, Gross-Alltag F, Konichezky S, Schwilk B, Fattroth A, Fett P: Lessons learned while building an integrated ICU workstation. *Int J Clin Monit Comput* 11:89–97, 1994.

125. Friesdorf W, Konichezky S, Gross-Alltag F, Fattroth A, Schwilk B: Data quality of bedside monitoring in an intensive care unit. *Internatl J Clin Monitor Comput* 11:123–128, 1994.

126. Frutiger A, Brunner JX: Computerized blood gas interpretation as a tool for class-room and ICU. *Intensive Care Med* 19:209–214, 1993.

127. Fu L: Polygenic trait analysis by neural network learning. *Artif Intell Med* 6:51–65, 1994.

128. Fujita H, Katafuchi T, Uehara T, Nishimura T: Application of artificial neural networks to computer-aided diagnosis of coronary artery disease in myocardial SPECT bull's eye images. *J Nucl Med* 33:272–276, 1992.

129. Funck-Bretano JL: The clinical practitioner and expert systems. *Contrib Nephrol* 78:166–173, 1990.

130. Furlong JW, Dupuy ME, Heinsimer JA: Neural network analysis of serial cardiac enzyme data: a clinical application of artificial machine intelligence. *Am J Clin Pathol* 96:134–141, 1991.

131. Furukawa T: Revolution of paradigm in clinical diagnosis—from the mechanization to the intelligent being. *Rinsho Byori* 39:1044–1048, 1991.

132. Gappa U, Puppe F, Schewe S: Graphical knowledge acquisition for medical diagnostic expert systems. *Artif Intell Med* 5:185–211, 1993.

132a. Gardner B. Using artificial intelligence to predict myocardial infarction. *Healthcare Informatics* 12:40–42, 44, 1995.

133. Gardner RM: Computerized management of intensive care patients. *MD Comput* 3:36–51, 1986.

133a. Gendler SM: LIS expert system: Feature evaluation. *Amer Clin Lab* April: 12–13, 1995.

134. Gero JS, Sudweeks F, eds: *Artificial Intelligence in Design '94*. Boston: Kluwer Academic Publishers, 1994.

135. Gibilisco S, ed: *The McGraw-Hill Illustrated Encyclopedia of Robotics and Artificial Intelligence*. New York: McGraw-Hill, 1994.

136. Gierl L, Stengel-Rutkowski S: Integrating consultation and semi-automatic knowledge acquisition in a prototype-based architecture: experiences with dysmorphic syndromes. *Artif Intell Med* 6:29–49, 1994.

137. Gilhooly KJ, Simpson S: Deep knowledge in human medical expertise. In Keravnou E, ed: *Deep Models for Medical Knowledge Engineering*. New York: Elsevier 1992, pp 273–285.

138. Giuse DA, Guise NB, Miller RA: Consistency enforcement in medical knowledge base construction. *Artif Intell Med* 5:245–252, 1993.

139. Godolphin WJ. Simulation modeling. In Kost GJ, ed. *Handbook of Clinical Automation, Robotics, and Optimization*. New York, NY: John Wiley and Sons, Inc., 1996: Chapter 5.

140. Goldschmidt HMJ, Vuysters FAM, Leijten JF: Costs of laboratory monitoring tests evaluated with regard to the medical information present. In Salamon R, Blum B, Jorgensen M, eds: *Medinfo 86, Proc 5th Conf Medical Informatics,* Washington, DC: Oct 26–30, 1986. New York: North-Holland, 1986, pp 266–270.

141. Goldstein M: Influence and belief adjustment. In Oliver RM, Smith JQ, eds: *Influence Diagrams, Belief Nets and Decision Analysis*. New York: Wiley, 1990, pp 133–174.

141a. Gonzalez ER, Vanderheyden BA, Ornato JP, Comstock TG: Computer-assisted optimization of aminophylline therapy in the emergency department. *Am J Emerg Med* 7:395–401, 1989.

142. Grossi EA, Steinberg BM, LeBoutillier M, Coppa GF, Roses DF: The use of artificial intelligence to analyze clinical database reduces workload on surgical house staff. *Surgery* 116:250–254, 1994.

143. Groth T, Collison PO: Strategies for decision support for fluid and electrolyte therapy in the intensive care unit—approaches and problems. *Internatl J Clin Monitr Comput* 10:3–15, 1993.

144. Groth T, Hakman M: A PC-workstation supporting interpretation of clinical chemistry laboratory data. In Kerkhof PLM, van Dieijen-Visser MP, eds: *Laboratory Data and Patient Care*. New York: Plenum Press, 1988, pp 147–157.

145. Groth T, Moden H: A knowledge-based system for real-time quality control and fault diagnosis of multitest analyzers. *Comput Meth Programs Biomed* 34:175–190, 1991.

146. Groth T: Data base management and knowledge-based systems in clinical laboratory medicine. In Kerkhof PLM, van Dieijen-Visser MP, eds: *Laboratory Data and Patient Care*. New York: Plenum Press, 1988, pp 101–108.

146a. Groth T, De Verdier CH, Benson ES, eds. *Optimized Use of Clinical Laboratory Data.* Oxford: Blackwell Scientific Publications, 1984.

147. Haight SA, Connelly DP, Gatewood LC, Burke MD: Decision making and laboratory test utilization: the effects of decision support. In Salamon R, Blum B, Jorgensen M, eds: *Medinfo 86, Proc 5th Conf Medical Informatics,* Washington, DC, Oct 26–30, 1986. New York: North-Holland, 1986, pp 271–274.

148. Harber P, McCoy JM, Shimozaki S, Coffman P, Bailey K: The structure of expert diagnostic knowledge in occupational medicine. *Am J Indust Med* 19:109–120, 1991.

149. Harrington PB, Isenhour TL: TORTS: an expert system for temporal optimization of robotic procedures. *J Chem Inf Comput Sci* 28:215–221, 1988.

150. Hatcher M: Uniqueness of group decision support systems (GDSS) in medicine and health applications. *J Med Syst* 14:351–364, 1990.

151. Haug PJ: Uses of diagnostic expert systems in clinical care. *Proc Annu Symp Comput Appl Med Care* 379–383, 1993.

152. Hayes-Roth B, Uckun S, Larsson JE, et al: Guardian: an experimental system for intelligent ICU monitoring. *Proc Annu Symp Comput Appl Med Care* 1004, 1994.

153. Hayes-Roth B, Washington D, Ash R, et al: Guardian: a prototype intelligent agent for intensive-care monitoring. *Artif Intell Med* 4:165–185, 1992.

153a. Haynes RB, Walker CJ: Computer-aided quality assurance. A critical appraisal. *Arch Intern Med* 147:1297–1303, 1987.

154. Hazen GB: Factored stochastic trees: a tool for solving complex temporal medical decision models. *Med Decision Making* 13:227–236, 1993.

155. Healy JC, Spackman KA, Beck JR: Small expert systems in clinical pathology. Are they useful? *Arch Pathol Lab Med* 113:981–983, 1989.

156. Hefley D, Hefley T: Scheduling personnel with an artificial intelligence program. *Med Lab Observer* 21:85–88, 1989.

157. Henrion M: Towards efficient probabilistic diagnosis in multiply connected belief networks. In Oliver RM, Smith JQ, eds: *Influence Diagrams, Belief Nets and Decision Analysis.* New York: Wiley, 1990, pp 385–409.

158. Henson-Mack K, Chen HC, Wester DC: Integrating probabilistic and rule-based systems for clinical differential diagnosis. *Proc IEEE Southeast Conf* 2:699–702, 1992.

159. Hernando ME, Gomez EJ, Corcoy R, del Pozo F, Arredondo MT: A hybrid knowledge based system for therapy adjustment in gestational diabetes. *Proc Annu Symp Comput Appl Med Care* 973, 1994.

160. Hickman DH, Shortliffe EH, Bischoff MB, Scott CA, Jacobs CD: The treatment advice of a computer-based cancer chemotherapy protocol advisor. *Ann Intern Med* 103:928–936, 1985.

160a. Holman JG, Cookson MJ: Expert systems for medical applications. *J Med Eng Technol* 11:151–159, 1987.

161. Holtzman S: *Intelligent Decision Systems.* Reading MA: Addison-Wesley, 1989.

162. Honavar V, ed: *Artificial Intelligence and Neural Networks: Steps Toward Principled Integration.* Boston: Academic Press, 1994.

163. Hopcroft JE, Ullman JD: *Introduction to Automata Theory, Languages, and Computation.* Reading, MA: Addison-Wesley, 1979.

164. Horn W: Utilizing detailed anatomical knowledge for hypothesis formation and

hypothesis testing in rheumatological decision support. In Keravnou E, ed: *Deep Models for Medical Knowledge Engineering*. New York: Elsevier, 1992, pp 27–50.

165. Hortin GL, Utz C, Gibson C: Managing information from bedside testing. *Med Lab Observer* 27:28–32, 1995.

166. Hovorka R, Svacina S, Carson ER, Williams CD, Sonksen PH: A consultation system for insulin therapy. *Comput Meth Programs Biomed* 32:303–310, 1990.

167. Howard RA: From influence to relevance to knowledge. In Oliver RM, Smith JQ, eds: *Influence Diagrams, Belief Nets and Decision Analysis*. New York: Wiley, 1990, pp 3–24.

168. Howorka K, Thoma H, Grillmayr H, Kitzler E: Phases of functional, near-normoglycaemic insulin substitution: what are computers good for in the rehabilitation process in type I (insulin-dependent) diabetes mellitus? *Comput Meth Programs Biomed* 32:319–323, 1990.

169. Huang J, Fox J, Gordon C, Jackson-Smale A: Symbolic decision support in medical care. *Artif Intell Med* 5:415–430, 1993.

170. Hughes C: The representation of uncertainty in medical expert systems. *Med Info* 11:367–374, 1989.

171. Hunter J, Cookson J, Wyatt J, eds: *AIME 89: Proc 2nd European Conf Artificial Intelligence in Medicine* (London). New York: Springer-Verlag, 1989.

172. Interpretive reporting to improve the effectiveness of clinical laboratory test results. An ECRI technology assessment. *J Health Care Technol* 2:269–282, 1986.

173. Ironi L, Stefanelli M, Lazola G: Qualitative models in medical diagnosis. In Keravnou E, ed: *Deep Models for Medical Knowledge Engineering*. New York: Elsevier 1992, pp 51–70.

174. Isenhour TL, Marshall JC: Laboratory robotics and artificial intelligence. *Clin Chem* 36:1561–1566, 1990.

175. Jablonski G, Nordahl K, Halse J, et al: PTH-stimulated adenylate cyclase activity and bone histomorphometry in iliac crest biopsies in the evaluation of uremic patients: a pilot study with the use of artificial intelligence. *Miner Electrolyte Metab* 19:351–361, 1993.

176. Jacobs E. Information integration for point-of-care and satellite testing. In Kost GJ, ed. *Handbook of Clinical Automation, Robotics, and Optimization*. New York: John Wiley and Sons, Inc., 1996: Chapter 25.

177. Johansson B, Bergvin L: Arden Syntax as a standard for knowledge bases in the clinical chemistry laboratory. *Clin Chim Acta* 222:123–128, 1993.

178. Johnson J, McKee S, Vella A, eds: *Artificial Intelligence in Mathematics*. New York: Clarendon Press, 1994.

179. Johnson KA, Johnson TR, Smith JW, et al: RedSoar—a system for red blood cell antibody identification. *Proc Annu Symp Comput Appl Med Care* 664–668, 1991.

180. Johnson L: Medical concepts. In Kohout L, Baldler W, eds: *Knowledge Representation in Medicine and Clinical Behavioural Science*. Cambridge, MA: Abacus Press, 1986, pp 27–36.

181. Johnston ME, Langton KB, Haynes RB, Mathieu A: Effects of computer-based clinical decision support systems on clinician performance and patient outcome: a critical appraisal of research. *Ann Intern Med* 120:135–142, 1994.

181a. Jorgens J: FDA medical device software regulation. In Salamon R, Blum B, Jorgensen M, eds: *Medinfo 86, Proc 5th Conf Medical Informatics,* Washington, DC, Oct 26–30, 1986. New York: North-Holland, 1986, pp 1072–1073.

182. Joshi MJ, Omand KL, Kost GJ: Current status and automation of radioimmunoassay (RIA). *Lab Robot Auto* 4:269–275, 1992.

183. Kahn MG, Steib SA, Fraser VJ, Dunagan WC: An expert system for culture-based infection control surveillance. In *Proc. 17th Annu Symp Comput Appl Med Care.* Baltimore: 171–175, 1993.

184. Kanal L, ed: *Parallel Processing for Artificial Intelligence.* New York: North-Holland, 1994, Vols 1, 2.

185. Karagiannis D, ed: *Database and Expert Systems Applications: Proc 5th Internatl Conf, DEXA '94,* Athens, Greece, Sept 7–9, 1994. New York: Springer-Verlag, 1994.

186. Kassirer JP: Diagnostic reasoning. *Ann Intern Med* 110:893–900, 1989.

187. Kazmierczak SC, Catrou PG, Van Lente F: Diagnostic accuracy of pancreatic enzymes evaluated by use of multivariate data analysis. *Clin Chem* 39:1960–1965, 1993.

188. Kelemen J: Evaluation of rationality of diagnostics (the problem space approach). In Salamon R, Blum B, Jorgensen M, eds: *Medinfo 86, Proc 5th Conf Medical Informatics,* Washington, DC, Oct 26–30, 1986. New York: North-Holland, 1986, pp 190–193.

188a. Keller LS, McDermott S, Alt-White A. Effects of computerized nurse careplanning on selected health care effectiveness measures. In Clayton PD, ed: *Proc 15th Annual Symposium on Computer Applications in Medical Care.* Washington, DC: American Medical Informatics Association, 1991, pp 38–42.

189. Kenley CR, Casaletto TR: Multi-target tracking using influence diagram models. In Oliver RM, Smith JQ, eds: *Influence Diagrams, Belief Nets and Decision Analysis.* New York: Wiley, 1990, pp 229–251.

190. Keravnou E, ed: *Deep Models for Medical Knowledge Engineering.* New York: Elsevier 1992.

191. Keravnou ET: Computer representation of fuzzy data structures. In Kohout L, Baldler W, eds: *Knowledge Representation in Medicine and Clinical Behavioural Science.* Cambridge, MA: Abacus Press, 1986, pp 129–140.

191a. Kerkhof PLM: Laboratory, patient and expert system as a triad in patient care. In Kerkhof PLM, van Dieijen-Visser MP, eds: *Laboratory Data and Patient Care.* New York: Plenum Press, 1988, pp 141–146.

192. Kern J, Dezelic G, Durrigl T, Vuletic S: Medical decision making based on inductive learning method. *Artif Intell Med* 5:213–223, 1993.

193. Kitano H, Hendler JA: *Massively Parallel Artificial Intelligence.* Menlo Park, CA: AAAI Press, 1994.

194. Klar R, Bayer U: Computer-assisted teaching and learning in medicine. *Internatl J Biomed Comput* 26:7–27, 1990.

195. Kleinmuntz B, Elstein AS: Computer modeling of clinical judgment. *Crit Rev Med Info* 1:209–228, 1987.

196. Kohane IS: Temporal reasoning in medical expert systems. In Salamon R, Blum B, Jorgensen M, eds: *Medinfo 86, Proc 5th Conf Medical Informatics,* Washington, DC, Oct 26–30, 1986. New York: North-Holland, 1986, pp 170–174.

197. Kohout L, Bandler W, eds: *Knowledge representation in Medicine and Clinical Behavioral Science.* Cambridge MA: Abacus Press, 1986.

198. Kohout LJ, Bandler W: Knowledge representation, clinical action and expert systems. In Kohout L, Baldler W, eds: *Knowledge Representation in Medicine and Clinical Behavioural Science.* Cambridge, MA: Abacus Press, 1986, pp 1–10.

199. Kohout LJ: On functional structures of behavior. In Kohout L, Baldler W, eds: *Knowledge Representation in Medicine and Clinical Behavioural Science.* Cambridge, MA: Abacus Press, 1986, pp 69–94.

200. Korsan RJ: Towards better assessment and sensitivity procedures. In Oliver RM, Smith JQ, eds: *Influence Diagrams, Belief Nets and Decision Analysis.* New York: Wiley, 1990, pp 427–455.

201. Koski EM, Sukuvaara T, Makivirta A, Kari A: A knowledge-based alarm system for monitoring cardiac operated patients—assessment of clinical performance. *Internatl J Clin Monit Comput* 11:79–83, 1994.

202. Kost GJ: *Generalized Models of Pharmacokinetic Action.* School of Medicine. University of California, San Francisco, CA, 1970.

203. Kost GJ. *State of the Art, Computer-Controlled Automation of the Clinical Immunoassay Laboratory and New Automated Non-Isotopic Immunoassay Systems.* Clinical Chemistry, School of Medicine, University of California, Davis, 1987.

204. Kost GJ, Vogelsang PJ, Reeder BL, Omand KL, Leach CS: Future trends in automation of non-isotopic immunoassay. *Laboratory Robotics and Automation* 1:275–284, 1990.

205. Kost GJ, Omand KL: Automation of the clinical laboratory: cancer markers and challenges for the 1990's. *Laboratory Robotics and Automation* 4:235–239, 1992.

206. Kost GJ. Point-of-Care Testing $\Rightarrow$ The Hybrid Laboratory $\Rightarrow$ Knowledge Optimization. In Kost GJ, ed. *Handbook of Clinical Automation, Robotics, and Optimization.* New York, NY: John Wiley and Sons, Inc., 1996: Chapter 28.

207. Kost GJ, Hague C: *In Vitro, Ex Vivo* and *In Vivo* Biosensor Systems. In Kost GJ, ed: *Handbook of Clinical Automation, Robotics, and Optimization.* New York, NY: John Wiley and Sons, Inc., 1996: Chapter 27.

208. Kratzer MA, Ivandic B, Fateh-Moghadam A: Neuronal network analysis of serum electrophoresis. *J Clin Pathol* 45:612–615, 1992.

209. Kroll MH. Automated-facilitated causal reasoning in diagnosis and management. In Kost GJ, ed. *Handbook of Clinical Automation, Robotics, and Optimization.* New York, NY: John Wiley and Sons, Inc., 1996: Chapter 31.

210. Kroll MH. Medical decision analysis. In Kost GJ, ed. *Handbook of Clinical Automation, Robotics, and Optimization.* New York, NY: John Wiley and Sons, Inc., 1996: Chapter 30.

211. Kulikowski CA, Weiss SM, Galen RS, Neuhauser D, Brennan P, Safran C: Evaluation and testing of decision models with data bases: laboratory and clinical medicine/nursing applications. In Barber B, Cao D, Qin D, Wagner G, eds: *Medinfo 89. Proc 6th Conf Medical Informatics.* Amsterdam: North-Holland, 1989, pp 1182.

212. Kumar AA, Vasudevan C: Artificial intelligence for medical decision making. *J Assoc Physicians India* 38:475–478, 1990.

213. Laemmle P, Wolterman D: Expert systems: a new dimension for the lab. *Healthcare Info* 8:62,64, 1991.

214. Lanzola G, Stefanelli M: Inferential knowledge acquisition. *Artif Intell Med* 5:253–268, 1993.

215. Lass M, Paulat K, Brucher R, et al: A new experimental approach for monitoring postoperative bypass patency after coronary artery bypass grafting. *Internatl J Clin Monit Comput* 11:49-55, 1994.

216. Lau F: A clinical decision support system prototype for cardiovascular intensive care. *Internatl J Clin Monit Comput* 11:157–169, 1994.

217. Laubscher TP, Frutiger A, Fanconi S, Jutzi H, Brunner JX: Automatic selection of tidal volume, respiratory frequency and minute ventilation in intubated ICU patients as start up procedure for closed-loop controlled ventilation. *Internatl J Clin Monit Comput* 11:19–30, 1994.

218. Lavrac N, Mozetic I: Second generation knowledge acquisition methods and their application to medicine. In Keravnou E, ed: *Deep Models for Medical Knowledge Engineering.* New York: Elsevier 1992, pp 177–198.

219. Leaning MS, Summerfield JA: Microcomputer-based management of fluid and electrolyte balance in hospitalized patients. In Salamon R, Blum B, Jorgensen M, eds: *Medinfo 86, Proc 5th Conf Medical Informatics,* Washington, DC, Oct 26–30, 1986. New York: North-Holland, 1986, pp 138–141.

220. Lehmann ED, Deutsch T, Carson ER, Sonksen PH: AIDA: an interactive diabetes advisor. *Comput Meth Programs Biomed* 41:183–203, 1994.

221. Lehmann ED, Deutsch T, Carson ER, Sonksen PH: Combining rule-based reasoning and mathematical modeling in diabetes care. *Artif Intell Med* 6:137–160, 1994.

222. Lehmann HP, Shortliffe EH: Thomas: building Bayesian statistical expert systems to aid in clinical decision making. *Comput Method Prog Biomed* 35:251–260, 1991.

223. Lehmann HP, Shachter RD: A physician-based architecture for the construction and use of statistical models. *Meth Info Med* 33:423–432, 1994.

224. Leicester HJ, Roudsari AV, Lehmann ED, Carson ER: Methodological issues in validating decision-support systems for insulin dosage adjustment. *Artif Intell Med* 6:161–173, 1994.

225. Li Min Fu: Polygenic trait analysis by neural network learning. *Artif Intell Med* 6:51–65, 1994.

226. Li YC, Haug PJ, Warner HR: Automated transformation of probabilistic knowledge for a medical diagnostic system. *Proc Annu Symp Comput Appl Med Care* 765–769, 1994.

227. Lilford RJ: Limitations of expert systems: intuition versus analysis. *Baillieres Clin Obstet Gynaecol.* 4:851–856, 1990.

228. Liscouski J: *Laboratory and Scientific Computing: A Strategic Approach.* New York: Wiley, 1995.

229. Lochmuller CH, Lung KR, Meiseles B: An application of expert system software in laboratory robotics. In *Advances in Laboratory Automation—Robotics.* Zymark Center, Hopkinton, MA: Zymark Corp, 1986, Vol 2, p 339.

230. Long WJ, Naimi S, Criscitiello MG, Adusumuilli RK: Validation of a causal probabilistic medical knowledge base for diagnostic reasoning. In Keravnou E, ed: *Deep Models for Medical Knowledge Engineering.* New York: Elsevier, 1992, pp 147–160.

231. Lotto ID, Stefanelli M: *Proc Internal Conf Artificial Intelligence in Medicine,* Pavia, Italy. New York: Elsevier, 1985.

232. Lucas P: Refinement of the HEPAR expert system: tools and techniques. *Artif Intell Med* 6:175–188, 1994.

233. Lucas P: The representation of medical reasoning models in resolution-based theorem provers. *Artif Intell Med* 5:395–414, 1993.

234. Maceratini R, Rafanelli M, Pisanelli KM, Crollari S: Expert systems and the pancreatic cancer problem: decision support in the pre-operative diagnosis. *J Biomed Eng* 11:487–510, 1989.

235. MacNish C, Pearce D, Pereira LM, eds: *Logics in Artificial Intelligence: Proc European Workshop JELIA '94,* York, UK, Sept 5–8, 1994. New York: Springer-Verlag, 1994.

236. Maguire LC, Martin JC: Fuzzy logic based expert system for clinical sample triaging and evaluation. In *Laboratory Information Management.* Amsterdam: Elsevier, in press.

237. Mahler EM, Schmidt RM, Kvitash VI: An artificial intelligence system to predict progression of immune dysfunction in healthy older patients. *J Med Syst* 17:173–181, 1993.

238. Makino M: Clinical laboratory and expert system. *Rinsho Byori* 40:333–338, 1992.

239. Manner GA, Schweiger CR, Soregi G, Pohl AL: Detection of monoclonal gammopathies in serum electrophoresis by neural networks. *Clin Chem* 39:1984–1985, 1993.

240. Marchevsky AM, Coons G: Expert systems as an aid for the pathologist's role of clinical consultant: CANCER-STAGE. *Mod Pathol* 6:265–269, 1993.

240a. Markin RS: Historical perspectives and critical issues. In Kost GJ, ed. *Handbook of Clinical Automation, Robotics, and Optimization.* New York, NY: John Wiley and Sons, Inc., 1996: Chapter 2.

241. Markin RS: Laboratory automation platform. In Kost GJ, ed. *Handbook of Clinical Automation, Robotics, and Optimization.* New York, NY: John Wiley and Sons, Inc., 1996: Chapter 10.

241a. Markin RS: Robotics, interfaces, and the docking device. In Kost GJ, ed. *Handbook of Clinical Automation, Robotics, and Optimization.* New York, NY: John Wiley and Sons, Inc., 1996: Chapter 11.

242. Marquardt VC: Artificial intelligence and decision-support technology in the clinical laboratory. *Lab Med* 24:777–782, 1993.

243. Martin JC, Maguire LC.: Fuzzy logic expert systems. In Kost GJ, ed. *Handbook of Clinical Automation, Robotics, and Optimization.* New York, NY: John Wiley and Sons, Inc., 1996: Chapter 7.

244. Matheson JE: Using influence diagrams to value information and control. In Oliver RM, Smith JQ, eds.: *Influence Diagrams, Belief Nets and Decision Analysis.* New York: Wiley, 1990, pp 25–48.

245. Matsuda N: Computer-assisted laboratory diagnosis—principles and clinical application. *Rinsho Byori Jpn J Clin Pathol* 39:1028–1034, 1991.

246. Mazoue JG: Diagnosis without doctors. *J Med Philos* 15:559–579, 1990.

247. McAdam WA, Brock BM, Armitage T, et al: Twelve years' experience of computer-aided diagnosis in a district general hospital. *Ann R Coll Surg Eng* 72:140–146, 1990.

247a. McAlister NH, Covvey HD, Tong C, Lee A, Wigle ED: Randomised controlled trial of computer assisted management of hypertension in primary care. *Br Med J (Clin Res Ed)* 293:670–674, 1986.

247b. McDonald CJ: Use of a computer to detect and respond to clinical events: its effect on clinician behavior. *Ann Intern Med* 84:162–167, 1976.

247c. McDonald CJ: Protocol-based computer reminders, the quality of care and the nonperfectability of man. *N Engl J Med* 295:1351–1355, 1976.

247d. McDonald CJ, Wilson GA, McCabe GP Jr: Physician response to computer reminders. *JAMA* 244:1579–1581, 1980.

247e. McDonald CJ, Hui SL, Smith DM, et al: Reminders to physicians from an introspective computer medical record. A two-year randomized trial. *Ann Intern Med* 100:130–138, 1984.

247f. McDowell I, Newell C, Rosser W: Comparison of three methods of recalling patients for influenza vaccination. *Can Med Assoc J* 135:991–997, 1986.

247g. McDowell I, Newell C, Rosser W: A randomized trial of computerized reminders for blood pressure screening in primary care. *Med Care* 27:297–305, 1989.

247h. McDowell I, Newell C, Rosser W: Computerized reminders to encourage cervical screening in family practice. *J Fam Pract* 28:420–424, 1989.

248. Medsker L, Liebowitz J: *Design and Development of Expert Systems and Neural Networks.* New York: Macmillan, 1994.

249. Merkhofer MW: Using influence diagrams in multiattribute utility analysis— improving effectiveness through improving communication. In Oliver RM, Smith JQ, eds: *Influence Diagrams, Belief Nets and Decision Analysis.* New York: Wiley, 1990, pp 297–317.

250. Middleton BF, Shwe MA: Probabilistic diagnosis using a reformulation of the Internist-1/QMR knowledge base-II. Evaluation of diagnostic performance. *Meth Info Med* 30:256–267, 1991.

251. Miller PL, Blumenfrucht SJ, Black HR: An expert system which critiques patient workup: modeling conflicting expertise. *Comput Biomed Res* 17:554–569, 1984.

252. Miller PL: *Expert Critiquing Systems: Practice-Based Medical Consultation by Computer.* New York: Springer-Verlag, 1986.

252a. Miller PL: The evaluation of artificial intelligence systems in medicine. *Comput Meth Programs Biomed* 22:5–11, 1986.

253. Miller PL: *Selected Topics in Medical Artificial Intelligence.* New York: Springer-Verlag, 1988.

254. Miller RA, Pople HE, Myers JD: INTERNIST-I, an experimental computer-based diagnostic consultant for general internal medicine. *N Engl J Med* 307:468–476, 1982.

255. Miller RA, Pople HE, Myers JD: INTERNIST-1, an experimental computer-based diagnostic consultant for general internal medicine. In Clancey WJ, Shortliffe EH, eds: *Readings in Medical Artificial Intelligence: The First Decade.* Reading, MA: Addison-Wesley, 1984, pp 190–209.

256. Miller RA, McNeil MA, Chalinor SM, Masarie FE, et al: The INTERNIST-1/QUICK MEDICAL REFERENCE PROJECT—status report. *West J Med* 145:816–822, 1986.

257. Miller RA: From automated medical records to expert system knowledge bases: common problems in representing and processing patient data. *Top Health Rec Management* 7:23–26, 1987.

258. Moens HJ, van der Korst JK: Computer-assisted diagnosis of rheumatic disorders. *Semin Arthritis Rheum* 21:156–169, 1991.

258a. Molino G, Ballare M, Aurucci PE, Di Meana VR. Application of artificial intelligence techniques to a well defined clinical problem: jaundice diagnosis. *Internatl J Biomed Comput* 26:189–202, 1990.

259. Molino G, Arrigoni A: Design of a computer-assisted programme supporting the selection and clinical management of patients referred for liver transplantation. *Ital J Gastroenterol* 26:31–43, 1994.

260. Molnar B, Szentirmay Z, Bodo M, et al: Application of multivariate, fuzzy set and neural network analysis in quantitative cytological examinations. *Anal Cell Pathol* 5:161–175, 1993.

261. Moore JE: Artificial intelligence approaches to rapid estimation of network flow. *Intellimotion* 4(1):6–13, 1994.

262. Moret-Bonillo V, Alonso-Betanzos A: Uncertainty based approach for symbolic classification of numeric variables in intensive care units. *J Clin Eng* 15:361–369, 1990.

263. Mozetic I, Pfahringer B: Improving diagnostic efficiency in KARDIO: Abstractions, constraint propagation and model compilation. In Keravnou E, ed: *Deep Models for Medical Knowledge Engineering.* New York: Elsevier, 1992, pp 1–26.

264. Murphy GC, Friedman CP: Automated medical knowledge acquisition: a study of consistency. *Proc Annu Symp Comput Appl Med Care* 725–729, 1994.

264a. Mutimer D, McCauley B, Nightingale P, Ryan M, Peters M, Neuberger J. Computerized protocols for laboratory investigation and their effect on use of medical time and resources. *J Clin Pathol* 45:572–574, 1992.

265. Myers JD: The computer as a diagnostic consultant, with emphasis on the use of laboratory data. *Clin Chem* 32:1714–1718, 1986.

266. Neopolitan RE: Computing the confidence in a medical decision obtained from an influence diagram. *Artif Intell Med* 5:341–363, 1992.

267. Nightingale PG, Peters M, Mutimer D, Neuberger JM: Effects of a computerized protocol management system on ordering of clinical tests. *Qual Health Care* 3:23–28, 1994.

268. Nishibori M: Clinical assessment of the knowledge base of an expert system for data analysis in laboratory medicine. *Bull Tokyo Med Dent Univ* 39:35–42, 1992.

269. Nohr C. The evaluation of expert diagnostic systems. How to assess outcomes and quality parameters? *Artif Intell Med* 6:123–135, 1994.

270. Novakowska M: Perception of time: a new theory. In Kohout L, Baldler W, eds: *Knowledge Representation in Medicine and Clinical Behavioural Science.* Cambridge, MA: Abacus Press, 1986, pp 95–106.

271. Nycum SN. Legal liability for expert systems. In Salamon R, Blum B, Jorgensen M, eds: *Medinfo 86, Proc 5th Conf Medical Informatics,* Washington DC, Oct 26–30, 1986. New York: North-Holland, 1986, pp 1069–1073.

272. Nykanen P, Boran G, Pince H, et al: Interpretative reporting and alarming based on laboratory data. *Clin Chim Acta* 222:37–48, 1993.

273. O'Connor ML, McKinney T: The diagnosis of microcytic anemia by a rule-based expert system using VP-Expert. *Arch Pathol Lab Med* 113:985–988, 1989.

274. Oberholzer M, Feichter G, Dalquen P, Ettlin R, Christen H, Buser M: A simple "expert system" for morphometric evaluation of cells in pleural effusions. *Pathol Res Practice* 185:647–651, 1989.

275. Olesen KG, Andreassen S: Specification of models in large expert systems based on causal probabilistic networks. *Artif Intell Med* 5:269–281, 1993.

276. Oliver RM, Smith JQ, eds: *Influence Diagrams, Belief Nets and Decision Analysis.* New York: Wiley, 1990.

277. Oliver RM, Yang HJ: Bayesian updating of event tree parameters to predict high risk incidents. In Oliver RM, Smith JQ, eds: *Influence Diagrams, Belief Nets and Decision Analysis.* New York: Wiley, 1990, pp 277–296.

278. Pal SK. X-ray pattern recognition: a fuzzy set theoretic approach. In Kohout L, Baldler W, eds: *Knowledge Representation in Medicine and Clinical Behavioural Science.* Cambridge, MA: Abacus Press, 1986, pp 153–182.

279. Parker RC, Miller RA: Using causal knowledge to create simulated patient cases: CPCS project as an extension of INTERNIST-1. In Miller PL, ed: *Selected Topics in Medical Artificial Intelligence.* New York: Springer-Verlag, 1988, pp 99–115.

280. Patel VL, Groen GJ, Ramoni MF, Kaufman DR: Machine depth versus psychological depth: a lack of equivalence. In Keravnou E, ed: *Deep Models for Medical Knowledge Engineering.* New York: Elsevier, 1992, pp 249–272.

280a. Patel VL, Groen GJ, Arocha JF: Medical expertise as a function of task difficulty. *Memory Cognition* 18:394–406, 1990.

280b. Paterson-Brown S, Vipond MN. Modern aids to clinical decision-making in the acute abdomen. *Br J Surg* 77:13–18, 1990.

281. Patil RS, Szollovits P, Schwartz WB: Modeling knowledge of the patient in acid-base and electrolyte disorders. In Szolovits P, ed: *Artificial Intelligence in Medicine.* Boulder, CO: Westview Press, 1982, pp 191–226.

282. Patil RS, Szolovits P, Schwartz WB: Causal understanding of patient illness in medical diagnosis. In *Proc 7th Internatl Joint Conf Artificial Intelligence,* Vancouver, BC, 1981, pp 893–899.

283. Pearl J, Geiger D, Verma T: The logic of influence diagrams. In Oliver RM, Smith JQ, eds: *Influence Diagrams, Belief Nets and Decision Analysis.* New York: Wiley, 1990, pp 67–87.

284. Pearl J: *Probabilistic Reasoning in Intelligent Systems: Networks of Plausible Inference.* San Mateo, CA: Morgan Kaufmann Publishers, 1988.

285. Perry CA: Knowledge bases in medicine: a review. *Bull Med Libr Assoc* 78:271–282, 1990.

286. Pesonen E, Ikonen J, Juhola M, Eskelinen M: Parameters for a knowledge base for acute appendicitis. *Meth Info Med* 33:220–226, 1994.

287. Peters M, Broughton PM: The role of expert systems in improving the test requesting patterns of clinicians. *Ann Clin Biochem* 30:52–59, 1993.

287a. Petrucci K, Petrucci P, Canfield K, McCormick KA, Kjerulff K, Parks P: Evaluation of UNIS: Urological Nursing Information Systems. In Clayton PD, ed: *Proc 15th Annu Symp Computer Applications in Medical Care.* Washington, DC: American Medical Association, 1991, pp 43–47.

288. Philips LD, Humphreys P, Embrey D, Selby DL: A socio-technical approach to assessing human reliability. In Oliver RM, Smith JQ, eds: *Influence Diagrams, Belief Nets and Decision Analysis.* New York: Wiley, 1990, pp 253–276.

289. Pinkava V: Classification and diagnostics. In Kohout L, Baldler W, eds: *Knowledge Representation in Medicine and Clinical Behavioural Science.* Cambridge, MA: Abacus Press, 1986, pp 37–50.

289a. Place JF, Truchaud, A, Uzawa K, Pardue H, Schnipelsky P. Use of artificial intelligence in analytical systems for the clinical laboratory. *Clin Chim Acta* 231:S5–34, 1994, and *Ann Biol Clin* 52:729–743, 1994.

290. Popovic D, Bhatkar VP: *Methods and Tools for Applied Artificial Intelligence.* New York: Marcel Dekker, 1994.

291. Porter JF, Kingsland LC III, Lindberg DA, et al: The AI/RHEUM knowledge-based computer consultant system in rheumatology: performance in the diagnosis of 59 connective tissue disease patients from Japan. *Arthritis Rheum* 31:219–226, 1988.

291a. Pozen MW, D'Agostino RB, Mitchell JB, et al: The usefulness of a predictive instrument to reduce inappropriate admissions to the coronary care unit. *Ann Intern Med* 92:238–242, 1980.

291b. Pozen MW, D'Agostine RB, Selker HP, Sytkowski PA, Hood WB Jr: A predictive instrument to improve coronary-care admission practices in acute ischemic heart disease. A prospective multicentre clinical trial. *N Engl J Med* 310:1273–1278, 1984.

292. Pratt IE: *Artificial Intelligence.* Basingstoke, UK: Macmillan, 1994.

293. Pribor HC: Expert systems in laboratory medicine: a practical consultative application. *J Med Systems* 13:103–109, 1989.

294. *Proc 6th Internatl Conf Artificial Intelligence and Information-Control Systems of Robots.* River Edge, NY: World Scientific, 1994.

295. *Proc 12th National Conf Artificial Intelligence,* July 31–Aug 4, 1994, Seattle, WA. Menlo Park, CA: AAAI Press, 1994.

296. *Proc 1994 IEEE 7th Symp Computer-Based Medical Systems.* Winston-Salem, NC. Los Alamitos, CA: IEEE Computer Society Press, 1994.

297. *Proc 6th Internatl Conf Tools with Artificial Intelligence:* Nov 6–9, 1994, New Orleans, LA. Los Alamitos, CA: IEEE Computer Society Press, 1994.

298. *Proc Symp Engineering of Computer-Based Medical Systems.* Minneapolis, MN. Sponsors: The Computer Society, IEEE Engineering in Medicine and Biology Society. Los Angeles, CA: Computer Society Press, 1988.

299. *Proc 10th Conf Artificial Intelligence Applications,* March 1–4, 1994, San Antonio, TX. Los Alamitos, CA: IEEE Computer Society Press, 1994.

300. *Project IMPACT. A National Critical Care Database Developed by the Society of Critical Care Medicine (SCCM) and Tri-Analytics, Inc.* Anaheim, CA: SCCM, 1995.

300a. Puppe B, Puppe F: Standardized forward and hypothetico-deductive reasoning in medical diagnosis. In Salamon R, Blum B, Jorgensen M, eds: *Medinfo 86, Proc 5th Conf Medical Informatics,* Washington, DC, Oct 26–30, 1986. New York: North-Holland, 1986, pp 199–203.

301. Quaglini S, Bellazi R, Berzuini M, et al: Hybrid knowledge-based systems for therapy planning. *Artif Intell Med* 4:207–226, 1992.

302. Quaglini S, Stefanelli M: A performance evaluation of the expert system ANEMIA. *Comp Biomed Res* 21:307–323, 1988.

303. Quaglini S, Stefanelli M: ANEMIA: An expert consultation system. *Comput Biomed Res* 19:23–27, 1986.

303a. *Quality Intensive Care (QuIC) System.* Redmond, WA: SpaceLabs Medical.

304. Ralescu A, ed: *Fuzzy Logic in Artificial Intelligence: Proc IJCAI '93 Workshop,* Chambery, France, Aug 28, 1993. New York: Springer-Verlag, 1994.

305. Reggia JA: Neural computation in medicine. *Artif Intell Med* 5:143–157, 1993.

306. Reibnegger G, Weiss G, Werner-Felmayer G, Judmaier G, Wachter H: Neural networks as a tool for utilizing laboratory information: comparison with linear discriminant analysis and with classification and regression trees. *Proc Natl Acad Sci* (USA) 88:11426–11430, 1991.

307. Rennels GD, Miller PL: Artificial intelligence research in anesthesia and intensive care. *J Clin Monit* 4:274–289, 1988.

308. Reynolds CF: A personal information system for doctors. In Kohout L, Baldler W, eds: *Knowledge Representation in Medicine and Clinical Behavioural Science.* Cambridge, MA: Abacus Press, 1986, pp 183–191.

309. Rich E: *Artificial Intelligence.* New York: McGraw-Hill, 1991.

310. Rienhoff O, Piccolo U, et al: Peter L. Reichertz Memorial Conference (1988: Hannover, Germany). Expert systems and decision support in medicine, 33rd Annual Meeting of the GMDS, EFMI Special Topic Meeting. New York: Springer-Verlag, 1988.

311. Roberts DE, Bell DD, Ostryznuik T, et al: Eliminating needless testing in intensive care—an information-based team management approach. *Crit Care Med* 21:1452–1458, 1993.

311a. Rodman JH, Jelliffe RW, Kolb E, et al: Clinical studies with computer-assisted initial lidocaine therapy. *Arch Intern Med* 144:703–709, 1984.

311b. Rogers JL, Haring OM: The impact of a computerized medical record summary system on incidence and length of hospitalization. *Med Care* 17:618–630, 1979.

311c. Rogers JL, Haring OM, Goetz JP: Changes in patient attitudes following the implementation of a medical information system. *QRB* 10:65–74, 1984.

311d. Rogers JL, Haring OM, Wortman PM, Watson RA, Goetz JP: Medical information systems: assessing impact in the areas of hypertension, obesity and renal disease. *Med Care* 20:63–74, 1982.

311e. Rollo JL, Fauser BA: Computers in total quality management. Statistical process control to expedite stats. *Arch Pathol Lab Med* 117:900–905, 1993.

312. Roseman E: Using artificial intelligence in the laboratory. *Medi Lab Observer* 26:57–58,60, 1994.

312a. Rosser WW, Hutchison BG, McDowell I, Newell C: Use of reminders to increase compliance with tetanus booster vaccination. *Can Med Assoc J* 146:911–917, 1992.

313. Roszak T: *The Cult of Information: A Neo-Luddite Treatise on High Tech, Artificial Intelligence, and the True Art of Thinking.* Berkeley, CA: University of California Press, 1994.

314. Rucker DW, Maron DJ, Shortliffe EH: Temporal representation of clinical algorithms using expert-system and database tools. *Comput Biomed Res* 23:222–239, 1990.

315. Russ TA: A system for using time dependent data in patient management. In Salamon R, Blum B, Jorgensen M, eds: *Medinfo 86, Proc 5th Conf Medical Informatics.* Washington, DC, Oct 26–30, 1986. New York: 1986, pp 165–169.

316. Rutledge G, Thomsen B, Farr M, et al: The design and implementation of a ventilator-management advisor. *Artif Intell Med* 5:67–82, 1993.

317. Saarinen E, Nykanen P, Irjala J, et al: Design and development of the THYROID system. *Comp Meth Programs Biomed* 34:211–218, 1991.

318. Sadegh-Zadeh K: Fundamentals of clinical methodology: 1. Differential indication. *Artif Intell Med* 6:83–102, 1994.

319. Salamon R, Blum B, Jorgensen M: *Medinfo 86: Proc 5th Conf Medical Informatics,* Washington, DC, Oct 26–30, 1986. New York: North-Holland, 1986.

320. Sanchez E: Possibility distributions, fuzzy intervals and possibility measures in a linguistic approach to pattern classification in medicine. In Kohout L, Baldler W, eds: *Knowledge Representation in Medicine and Clinical Behavioural Science.* Cambridge, MA: Abacus Press, 1986, pp 141–152.

321. Sandell HSH, Bourne JR: Expert systems in medicine: a biomedical engineering perspective. *Crit Rev Biomed Eng* 12:95–129, 1985.

322. Sasaki M, Ogura K, Kataoka H, Imamura J. Automated Handbook of Clinical systems. In Kost GJ, ed. *Handbook of Clinical Automation, Robotics, and Optimization.* New York, NY: John Wiley and Sons, Inc., 1996: Chapter 17.

323. Schecke T, Langen M, Popp HJ, Rau G, Kasmacher H, Kalff G: Knowledge-based decision support for patient monitoring in cardioanesthesia. *Internatl J Clin Monit Comput* 9:1–11, 1992.

324. Schioler T, Talmon J, Nolan J, McNair P: Information technology factors in trans-ferability of knowledge based systems in medicine. *Artif Intell Med* 6:189–201, 1994.

325. Schmidt HG, Boshuizen HPA, Norman GR: Reflections on the nature of expertise in medicine. In Keravnou E, ed: *Deep Models for Medical Knowledge Engineering.* New York: Elsevier, 1992, pp 231–248.

326. Schwaiger J, Haller M, Finsterer U: A framework for the knowledge-based inter-pretation of laboratory data in intensive care units using deductive database tech-nology. *Proc Annu Symp Comput Appl Med Care* 13–17, 1992.

327. Schwartz S, Griffin T, Fox J: Clinical expert systems versus linear models: do we really have to choose. *Behav Sci* 34:305–311, 1989.

328. Schwartz WB, Patil RS, Szolovits P: Artificial intelligence in medicine: where do we stand? *N Engl J Med* 316:685–688, 1987.

329. Schweiger CR, Soeregi G, Spitzauer S, Maenner G, Pohl AL: Evaluation of laboratory data by conventional statistics and by three types of neural networks. *Clin Chem.* 39:1966–1971, 1993.

330. Siever A, Holtzman S: Decision analysis: a framework for critical care decision assistance. *Internatl J Clin Monit Comput* 6:137–156, 1989.

331. Seiver A: A decision class analysis of critical life-support decision-making. *Internatl J Clin Monit Comput* 10:31–66, 1993.

332. Senyk O: The integration of compiled and explicit causal knowledge for diagnostic reasoning. In *Proc 12th Annual Symp Comput Appl Med Care,* Los Angeles: IEEE Computer Society Press, Washington, DC, 1988, pp 106–109.

333. Shacter RD, Eddy DM, Hasselblad V: An influence diagram approach to medical technology assessment. In Oliver RM, Smith JQ, eds: *Influence Diagrams, Belief Nets and Decision Analysis.* New York: Wiley, 1990, pp 321–350.

334. Shahar Y, Das AK, Tu SW, Kraemer FB, Musen MA: Knowledge-based temporal abstraction for diabetic monitoring. *Proc Annu Symp Comput Appl Med Care* 697–701, 1994.

335. Shahar Y, Musen MA: A temporal-abstraction system for patient monitoring. *Proc Annu Symp Comput Appl Med Care* 121–127, 1992.

335a. Sharpe PK, Solberg HE, Rootwelt K, Yearworth M. Artificial neural networks in diagnosis of thyroid function from in vitro laboratory tests. *Clin Chem* 39:2248–2253, 1993.

336. Sher PP: Graphics utilization in the clinical laboratory. In Zinder O, ed: *Optimal Use of the Clinical Laboratory. Proc 5th Internatl Meeting Clinical Laboratory Organization and Management.* Basel: Karger, 1985, pp 84–91.

337. Sher PP: Knowledge-based automation. *Clin Lab Med* 8:713–722, 1988.

338. Sher PP: Microcomputer workstations for laboratory data management. In Harris EK, Yasaka T, eds: *Maintaining a Healthy State within the Individual.* Elsevier: North-Holland, 1987, pp 203.

339. Sher PP: Present and future status of computer-based graphics and interpretive systems. *Scand J Clin Lab Invest* 44(Suppl 171):375–382, 1984.

340. Sherwood CG: Towards a design for clinical data analysis. In Kohout L, Baldler W, eds: *Knowledge Representation in Medicine and Clinical Behavioural Science.* Cambridge, MA: Abacus Press, 1986, pp 119–128.

340a. Shortliffe EH: *Computer-Bsed Medical Consultations: MYCIN.* New York: Elsevier, 1976.

341. Shortliffe EH: Computer programs to support clinical decision making. *JAMA* 258:61–66, 1987.

342. Shortliffe EH: Medical knowledge and decision making. *Methods Info Med* 27:209–218, 1988.

343. Shortliffe EH: Medical informatics and clinical decision making: the science and the pragmatics. *Med Decision Making* 11(Suppl 4):S2–S14, 1991.

343a. Shortliffe EH: AI meets decision science: emerging synergies for decision support. In Evans DA, Patel VL, eds: *Advanced Models of Cognition for Medical Training and Practice.* New York: Springer-Verlag, 1992, pp 71–89.

344. Shortliffe EH: The adolescence of AI in medicine: will the field come of age in the '90s? *Artif Intell Med* 5:93–106, 1993.

344a. Shortliffe EH, Buchanan BG, Feigenbaum EA: Knowledge engineering for medical decision making: a review of computer-based clinical decision aids. In Clancy WJ, Shortliffe EH, eds: *Readings in Medical Artificial Intelligence.* Reading, MA: Addison-Wesley, 1984, pp 35–71.

345. Sielaff BH, Connelly DP, Scott EP: ESPRE: a knowledge-based system to support platelet transfusion decisions. *Trans Biomed Eng* 36:541–546, 1989.

346. Sielaff BH, Scott E, Connelley DP: ESPRE: Expert system for platelet request evaluation. In Stead WW, ed: *Proc 11th Annu Symp Computer Applications in Medical Care.* IEEE Computer Society Press, Washington, DC, 1987, p 237.

347. Sielaff BH, Scott EP, Connelly DP: Design and preliminary evaluation of an expert system for platelet request evaluation. *Transfusion* 31:600–606, 1991.

348. Siguel EN: The future of computer-aided diagnosis in the laboratory. *Med Lab Observer* 23:71–73, 1991.

349. Singh MG, Cook R: A new class of intelligent knowledge-based systems with an optimisation-based inference engine. *Decision Support Syst* 1:299-312, 1985.

350. Sittig DF, Cheung KH, Berman L: Fuzzy classification of hemodynamic trends and artifacts: experiments with the heart rate. *Internatl J Monit Comput* 9:251–257, 1992.

351. Sittig DF, Gardner RM, Pace NL, Morris AH, Beck E: Computerized management of patient care in a complex, controlled clinical trial in the intensive care unit. *Comput Meth Programs Biomed* 30:77–84, 1989.

352. Sittig DF, Pace NL, Gardner RM, Beck E, Morris AH: Implementation of a computerized patient advice system using the HELP clinical information system. *Comput Biomed Res* 22:474–487, 1989.

353. Slickers K: The application of expert systems to the support of a clinical laboratory systems. *Proc Oak Ridge Conf Clinical Laboratory Information Highway,* 1995, p 2.

354. Smith JL: Computer assisted E.R. diagnosis. *Health Syst Rev* 27:58,60,62, 1994.

355. Smith JQ: Statistical principals on graphs. In Oliver RM, Smith JQ, eds: *Influence Diagrams, Belief Nets and Decision Analysis.* New York: Wiley, 1990, pp 89–120.

356. Smith JW, Bayazitoglu A: Exploring the relationship between rationality and bounded rationality in medical knowledge-based systems. *Artif Intell Med* 5:125–142, 1993.

357. Smith JW, Spreicher CE, Chandrasekaran B: Expert systems as aids for interpretive reporting. *J Med Syst* 8:373–388, 1984.

358. Smith JW, Sviebely JR, Evans CA, et al: RED: a red-cell antibody identification expert module. *J Med Syst* 9:121–138, 1985.

359. Smith JW, Svirbely J, Fannin E: A gentle introduction to knowledge-based systems in medicine. *Top Health Rec Management* 9:36–54, 1988.

360. Sondergaard I, Krath BN, Hagerup M: Classification of crossed immu-noelectrophoretic patterns using digital image processing and artificial neural networks. *Electrophoresis* 13:411–415, 1992.

361. Spackman KA, Connelly DP: Knowledge-based systems in laboratory medicine and pathology: a review and survey of the field. *Arch Pathol Lab Med* 111:116–119, 1987.

362. Spackman KA: A knowledge-based system for transfusion advice. *Am J Clin Pathol* 94:S25–S29, 1990.

363. Speed TP: Complexity, calibration and causality in influence diagrams. In Oliver RM, Smith JQ, eds: *Influence Diagrams, Belief Nets and Decision Analysis.* New York: Wiley, 1990, pp 49–63.

364. Spiegelhalter DJ: Fast algorithms for probabilistic reasoning in influence diagrams, with applications in genetics and expert systems. In Oliver RM, Smith JQ, eds: *Influence Diagrams, Belief Nets and Decision Analysis.* New York: Wiley, 1990, pp 361–384.

365. Stajic A, Novakovic R, Bosnjakovic V: An expert system approach for the objective interpretation of serum tumour marker levels. *Nucl Med Commun* 15:298–304, 1994.

366. Steels L, McDermott J: *The Knowledge Level in Expert Systems: Conversations and Commentary.* Boston: Academic Press, 1994.

367. Stefanelli M et al, eds: *AIME 91: 3rd Conf Artificial Intelligence in Medicine* (Maastrict, Netherlands). New York: Springer-Verlag, 1991.

368. Stefanelli M, Ramoni M: Epistemological constraints on medical knowledge-based systems. In Evans DA, Patel VL, eds: *Advanced Models of Cognition for Medical Training and Practice.* New York: Springer-Verlag, 1992, pp 3–20.

368a. Stefanelli M: European research efforts in medical knowledge-based systems. *Artif Intell Med* 5:107–124, 1993.

369. Stevens RH, Najafi K: Artificial neural networks as adjuncts for assessing medical students' problem solving performances on computer-based simulations. *Comput Biomed Res* 26:172–187, 1993.

370. Sticklen JH: MDX2: an integrated medical diagnostic system. Ph.D. dissertation, Ohio State University, 1987.

371. Sturman MF, Perez M: Computer-assisted diagnosis of acute abdominal pain. *Compr Ther* 15:26–35, 1989.

372. Sukuvaara T, Koski EM, Makivirta A, Kari A: A knowledge-based alarm system for monitoring cardiac operated patients-technical construction and evaluation. *Internatl J Clin Monit Comput* 10:117–126, 1993.

373. Sultan C, Imbert M, Priolet G: Decision-making system (DMS) applied to hematology. Diagnosis of 180 cases of anemia secondary to a variety of hematologic disorders. *Hematol Pathol* 2:221–228, 1988.

374. Sungzoon Cho, Reggia JA: Multiple disorder diagnosis with adaptive competitive neural networks. *Artif Intell Med* 5:469–487, 1993.

374a. Sutton GC: Computer-aided diagnosis: a review. *Br J Surg* 76:82–85, 1989.

375. Szolovits P, ed: *Artificial Intelligence in Medicine*. AAAS Selected Symposia Series. Boulder, CO: Westview Press, 1982.

376. Szolovits P, Patil RS, Schwartz WB: Artificial intelligence in medical diagnosis. *Ann Intern Med* 108:80–87, 1988.

377. Talman JL, Fox J. eds: *Knowledge Based Systems in Medicine: Methods, Applications, and Evaluation: Proc Workshop System Engineering in Medicine*. New York: Springer-Verlag, 1991.

378. Tate KE, Gardner RM, Weaver LK: A computerized laboratory alerting system. *MD Comput* 7:296–301, 1990.

379. Taylor MC: Logical optimisation of distributed knowledge base queries. *Comput J* 33:49–60, 1990.

379a. Tierney WM, Hui SL, McDonald CJ: Delayed feedback of physician performance versus immediate reminders to perform preventive care. Effects on physician compliance. *Med Care* 24:659–666, 1986.

379b. Tierney WM, McDonald CJ, Hui SL, Martin DK: Computer predictions of abnormal test results. Effects on outpatient testing. *JAMA* 259:1194–1198, 1988.

380. Timcenko A, Reich DL: Real-time expert system for advising anesthesiologists in the cardiac operating room. *Proc Annu Symp Comput Appl Med Care* 1005, 1994.

381. Tong DA: Weaning patients from mechanical ventilation. A knowledge-based system approach. *Comput Meth Programs Biomed* 35:267–278, 1991.

382. Trendelenburg C: Routine application of the expert system PRO.M.D. In Kerkhof PLM, Dieijen-Visser MP, eds: *Laboratory data and patient care*. New York: Plenum Press, 1988.

383. Trendelenburg C: Expert systems in clinical chemistry. In Okuda K, ed: *Automation and New Technology in the Clinical Laboratory*. Oxford: Blackwell Scientific Publications, 1988, pp 13–17.

384. Tsutsui T, Arita S: Fuzzy-logic control of blood pressure through enflurane anesthesia. *J Clin Monit* 10:110–117, 1994.

385. Uckun S: Model-based reasoning in biomedicine. *CRC Crit Rev Biomed Eng* 19:261–292, 1992.

386. Uckun S, Dawant BM: Qualitative modeling as a paradigm for diagnosis and prediction in critical care environments. *Artif Intell Med* 4:127–144, 1992.

387. Uckun S: Artificial intelligence in medicine: state-of-the-art and future prospects. *Artif Intell Med* 5:89–91, 1993.

388. Uckun S, Dawant BM, Lindstrom DP: Model-based diagnosis in intensive care monitoring: the YAQ approach. *Artif Intell Med* 5:31–48, 1993.

389. Uckun S: Instantiating and monitoring treatment protocols. *Proc Ann Symp Comput Appl Med Care* 689–693, 1994.

390. Uckun S. Model-based reasoning. In Kost GJ, ed. *Handbook of Clinical Automation, Robotics, and Optimization.* New York, NY: John Wiley and Sons, Inc., 1996: Chapter 6.

391. Ursino M, Artioli E, Avanzolini G, Potuto V: Integration of quantitative and qualitative reasoning: an expert system for cardiosurgical patients. *Artif Intell Med.* 61:9–10, 1994; Suppl 1:229–247.

392. Valdiguie PM, Rogari E, Philippe H. VALAB: expert system for validation of biochemical data. *Clin Chem* 38:83–87, 1992.

393. Van Denneheuvel S, Van Emde Boas P, De Geus F, Rotterdam E: Reduced constraint models. In Keravnou E, ed: *Deep Models for Medical Knowledge Engineering.* New York: Elsevier, 1992, pp 89–100.

394. Van Lente F, Castellani W, Chou D, Matzan RN, Galen RS: Application of the EXPERT consultation system to accelerated laboratory testing and interpretation. *Clin Chem* 32:1719–1725, 1986.

395. Vertosick FT, Rehn T: Predicting behavior of an enzyme-linked immunoassay model by using commercially available neural network software. *Clin Chem* 39:2478–2482, 1993.

396. Vertosick FT. Neural networks. In Kost GJ, ed. *Handbook of Clinical Automation, Robotics, and Optimization.* New York, NY: John Wiley and Sons, Inc., 1996: Chapter 4.

396a. Vitek PJ, Lennard-Jones P: Disciplining time-related clinical and laboratory data. In Kerkhof PLM, van Dieijen-Visser MP, eds: *Laboratory Data and Patient Care.* New York: Plenum Press, 1988, pp 165–170.

397. Volkov VIa, Gladkov IuM, Zavadskii VK, Ivanov VP: Enhancing the reliability and accuracy of pulse oximetry using a built in expert system. *Med Tekh* 14–18, May–June 1993.

398. Von Luck K, Margurger H, eds: *Management and Processing of Complex Data Structures: Proc 3rd Workshop on Information Systems and Artificial Intelligence.* Hamburg, Germany, Feb 28–March 2, 1994. New York: Springer-Verlag, 1994.

399. Wade TD, Byrns PJ, Steiner JF, Bondy J: Finding temporal patterns—a set-based approach. *Artif Intell Med* 6:263–271, 1994.

400. Ward CD: Meditations on uncertainty. In Kohout L, Baldler W, eds: *Knowledge Representation in Medicine and Clinical Behavioural Science.* Cambridge, MA: Abacus Press, 1986, pp 19–26.

401. Warner HR, Bouhaddou O: Innovation review: Iliad—a medical diagnostic support program. *Top Health Info Management* 14:51–58, 1994.

402. Washbrook J, Keravnou E: Making deepness explicit. In Keravnou E, ed: *Deep Models for Medical Knowledge Engineering.* New York: Elsevier, 1992, pp 161–168.

403. Waxman HS, Worley WE: Computer-assisted adult medical diagnosis: subject review and evaluation of a new microcomputer-based system. *Medicine* 69:125–136, 1990.

404. *Webster's Electronic Dictionary and Thesaurus.* New York: Random House, 1993.

405. Weiler N, Heinrichs W, Kessler W: The AUL-mode: a safe closed loop algorithm for ventilation during total intravenous anesthesia. *Internal J Clin Monitor Comput* 11:85–88, 1994.

406. Weiss SM, Galen RS: An expert system for diagnosis of myocardial infarction. In Salamon R, Blum B, Jorgensen M: *Medinfo 86, Proc 5th Conf Medical Informatics.* Washington, DC, Oct 26–30, 1986. New York: North-Holland, 1986, pp 219–221.

407. Weiss SM, Kulikowski CA, Galen RS: Representing expertise in a computer program: the serum protein diagnostic program. *J Clin Lab Auto* 3:383–387, 1983.

407a. Wells IG, Cartwright RY, Farnan LP: Practical experience with graphical user interfaces and object-oriented design in the clinical laboratory. *Clin Chim Acta* 222:13–18, 1993.

408. Wells WA, Memoli VA. Image analysis. In Kost GJ, ed. *Handbook of Clinical Automation, Robotics, and Optimization.* New York, NY: John Wiley and Sons, Inc., 1996: Chapter 14.

408a. Wellwood J, Johannessen S, Spiegelhalter DJ: How does computer-aided diagnosis improve the management of acute abdominal pain? *Ann R Coll Surg Engl* 74:40–46, 1992.

408b. Wexler JR, Swender PT, Tunnessen WW Jr, Oski FA: Impact of a system of computer-assisted diagnosis. Initial evaluation of the hospitalized patient. *Am J Dis Child* 129:203–205, 1975.

408c. White KS, Lindsey A, Pryor TA, Brown WF, Walsh K: Application of a computerized medical decision-making process to the problem of digoxin intoxication. *J Am Coll Cardiol* 4:571–576, 1984.

408d. White RH, Hong R, Venook AP, et al: Initiation of warfarin therapy: comparison of physician dosing with computer-assisted dosing. *J Gen Intern Med* 2:141–148, 1987.

408e. White RH, Mungall D: Outpatient management of warfarin therapy: comparison of computer-predicted dosage adjustment to skilled professional care. *Ther Drug Monit* 13:46–50, 1991.

409. Widmer G, Horn W, Nagele B: Automatic knowledge base refinements: learning from examples and deep knowledge in rheumatology. *Artif Intell Med* 5:225–243, 1993.

410. Wieland H, Trendelenburg C: Expert system for the evaluation of disturbances of lipid metabolism and assessment of risk for coronary heart disease. In Okuda K, ed: *Automation and New Technology in the Clinical Laboratory.* Oxford: Blackwell Scientific Publications, 1988, pp 19–21.

410a. Wiener FM: A system for medical reasoning (SMR) in the clinical laboratory. In Kerkhof PLM, van Dieijen-Visser MP, eds: *Laboratory Data and Patient Care.* New York: Plenum Press, 1988, pp 135–140.

411. Williams BT, Yoder JW, Littel E: Probability graphics support for medical reasoning. *Methods Info Med* 32:229–232, 1993.

412. Winkel P: The application of expert systems in the clinical laboratory. *Clin Chem* 35:1595–1600, 1989.

412a. Winkel P, Ravn NH: A laboratory protocol language. *Lab Robotics Auto* 4:213–225, 1992.

413. Winkel P: Artificial intelligence within the chemical laboratory. *Ann Biol Clin* 52:277–282, 1994.

414. Winston PH: *Artificial Intelligence.* Reading, MA: Addison-Wesley, 1984 and 1992.

414a. Woodbury WF: The development of a PC-based expert system to aid in the troubleshooting of clinical laboratory instrumentation. *Lab Med* 20:176–182, 1989.

415. Wulfman CE, Rua M, Lane CD, Shortliffe EH, Fagan LM: Graphical access to medical expert systems: integration with continuous speech recognition. *Meth Info Med* 32:33–46, 1993.

415a. Wulkan RW, Zwang L, Liem TL, Blijenberg BG, Leijnse B: Renal stone analysis: LITHOS, an expert system for evaluation or X-ray diffractograms of urinary calculi. *Clin Chem Clin Biochem* 25:719–722, 1987.

416. Wulkan RW, Leijnse B: Experience with expert systems in clinical chemistry. In Kerkhof PLM, van Dieijen-Visser MP, eds: *Laboratory Data and Patient Care.* New York: Plenum Press, 1988, pp 117–124.

416a. Wulkan RW: Expert systems and multivariate analysis in clinical chemistry. Thesis. Dordrecht: ICG Printing, 1992.

416b. Wyatt J: Lessons learnt from the field trial of ACORN, an expert system to advise on chest pain. In Barber B, Cao D, Quin D, Wagner G, eds: *Proc 6th World Conf Medical Informatics,* Singapore, New York, Amsterdam, 1989, pp 111–115.

416c. Wyatt J, Spiegelhalter D: Field trials of medical decision-aids: potential problems and solutions. In Clayton PD, ed: *Proc 5th Annu Symp Computer Applications in Medical Care.* Washington, DC: American Medical Informatics Assoc, 1991, pp 3–7.

416d. Wyatt J, Spiegelhalter D: Evaluating medical expert systems: what to test and how? *Medical Informatics* 15:205–217, 1990.

417. Xiang Y, Eisen R, Beddoes MP, Poole D: Multiply sectioned Bayesian networks for neuromuscular diagnosis. *Artif Intell Med* 5:293–314, 1993.

418. Yang JM, Lewandrowski KB, and Laposata M: Algorithmic diagnosis. In Kost GJ, ed. *Handbook of Clinical Automation, Robotics, and Optimization.* New York, NY: John Wiley and Sons, Inc., 1996: Chapter 32.

419. Ying H, McEachern M, Eddleman DW, et al: Fuzzy control of mean arterial pressure in postsurgical patients with sodium nitroprusside infusion. *IEEE Trans Biomed Eng* 39:1060–1070, 1992.

420. Zarkadakis G, Carson ER, Cramp DG, Finkelstein L: ANABEL: intelligent blood-gas analysis in the intensive care unit. *Internatl J Clin Monit Comput* 6:167–171, 1989.

421. Young DW: Improving the consistency with which investigations are requested. *Med Informatics* 6:13–17, 1981.

ROBOTICS, VISUAL PROCESSING, AND INTEGRATED SYSTEMS

CHAPTER

9

Logistics and Transport

DONNA S. WEBER

CONTENTS

Handbook of Clinical Automation, Robotics, and Optimization, Edited by Gerald J. Kost with the collaboration of Judith Welsh.
ISBN 0-471-03179-8 © 1996 John Wiley & Sons, Inc.

9.1. INTRODUCTION

The purpose of this chapter is to acquaint the reader with the various technologies available to solve the problems associated with the movement of materials throughout a healthcare or laboratory facility. Literally thousands of items must be transported daily in a busy hospital to meet the needs of the patients and the staff. Logistics become especially complex when many items are needed or tests are ordered on a stat basis. Automated material transport systems eliminate the manual labor required to perform this function and give thousands of non-productive hours back to the medical professionals.[1]

System selection depends on a variety of factors such as payload size, speed requirements, and installation space available. The following chapter discusses the various systems available to laboratories and healthcare facilities and the key functions that they serve.

9.2. COMPUTERIZED TUBE SYSTEM (CTS)

9.2.1. General System Definition

A computerized tube system (CTS) provides a cost-effective solution for transporting thousands of small items essential to the day-to-day operations of a healthcare facility. The system consists of a network of tubing intertwined throughout a facility that enables any department with a station on the system to transport small materials to any other department on the system. Materials are packaged in polycarbonate plastic carriers before being placed into the system. Carriers are moved through the system by airflow generated by blowers and are switched between routes of tubing by transfer units. The carriers travel at approximately 20–25 ft/s or, an average of 1500 ft/min, making the CTS the fastest transport system available.

System payloads range according to the diameter size of the system installed. The smallest diameter is the 4-in. system (referring to the outside diameter of the pipe). The system will support payloads of ≤7 lb. The 6-in.-diameter system can support payloads of ≤15 lb. Most hospital applications rarely exceed 3-lb loads. For instance, a 1-liter IV bag weighs only 2.5 lb.

Multistation systems, generally with greater than 10 stations, are laid out in interconnected zones, or clusters of stations, to facilitate the handling of multiple carriers simultaneously. The system traffic is microprocessor controlled to track and ensure delivery of the carriers and provide managers with system usage data.

9.2.2. System Control Center and System Software

9.2.2.1. CONTROL CENTER. The central control, or "brain" of the system, directs, monitors, and records all system operations. Closed-loop control and route verification confirm that a dispatch request can be accepted and delivered by the system. System diagnostics assist maintenance in identifying potential problems, helping to keep downtime to a minimum. The control center is usually located in the maintenance or plant operations department of a hospital so that maintenance personnel can care for the system.

Systems are controlled by modern microcomputer technology. The control center includes a color videodisplay terminal, UPS (uninterrupted power supply), and a printer. The computer must be outfitted with a proprietary board that communicates with the zone control boards, transfer units, blowers, and stations.

9.2.2.2. SOFTWARE. The system operating software has historically been a DOS (disk-operating-system) based system, but some manufacturers have recently developed OS/2 versions. The control center's primary function is to operate the system components to ultimately route a carrier from point A to point B by the shortest route possible. The software offers many different functions to accomplish this goal. In addition to routing and traffic management functions, the system tracks each transaction and archives the associated data from the transaction. This event information can be used for analysis. From the printed transaction record, the source station, receiving station, and transaction times can be determined.

A secondary function of the software is to constantly monitor the entire system for malfunctions and alert the appropriate personnel of problems should they occur. Software diagnostics details a problem and suggests corrective action to be taken by maintenance. In some cases, the system software will attempt to correct a problem before taking the situation to an alarm status. Malfunctions that do not disable the system, such as an isolated sensor failure, will be posted as an advisory for future attention rather than an alarm that needs to be tended immediately.

The system software also incorporates scheduling functions that allow the user to schedule events, such as automatic shutdown of a station, at certain times of the day. This is important for remote areas such as ambulatory care clinics that operate on a <24-h/day basis. Carriers cannot be sent to shut down stations or closed departments thus avoiding "lost" materials. The schedule will also automatically turn stations back on at the preprogrammed time.

Station priorities can be scheduled such that at peak times certain stations have a higher sending or receiving priority to meet the departmental traffic needs. The system has an automatic empty carrier distribution function that lets the user put empty carriers back into the system and essentially gives them to the computer for determination of the stations in need of carriers.

The software is designed such that component additions to the system are added to the system configuration. The program accepts the new additions and downloads information to the components, putting them on line. Software changes are not generally required with station and zone additions.

In addition to control center software features, there are special functions that can be initiated at the individual stations by the user. One special function, stat transaction, allows the user, through use of a security code, to give a carrier the highest send priority. This instructs the computer to transact that carrier above all others. Another special function, called "secure transaction," allows a carrier to be sent and locked above the receiving station until an authority code is entered by the receiver. One application of this function is its use in the handling of chain of custody specimens.

A user who is sending a particularly sensitive material such as a cerebral spinal fluid can also choose to track a carrier from the sending station until it is received at its destination using the carrier tracking special function. Additionally, the users can program their station to alert them with a series of beeps of carrier arrivals and full receiver bins.

Another special function at the station allows the user to initiate an "emergency off" action. This function will shut down the entire system. This function is important when a spill has been detected in the laboratory due to improper packaging of a specimen. System shutdown contains the spread of a spill to a limited area of the system. The affected part of the system can be identified by maintenance through the control center and a cleanout procedure initiated. Unaffected zones can be put back into use right away.

9.2.2.3. INTEGRATION WITH HOST COMPUTERS. It is possible on some systems to interface with a higher-level host computer for purposes of exchanging information. One example is the marrying of bar-code information from the contents in the carrier to the carrier itself. This would enable an exact record of transaction data.

9.2.3. Transfer Units

Transfer units (TUs) are switching devices used at branching points in the system to direct the path of a carrier from a single tube at one end of the TU to any one of two, four, or six tubes at the other end of the TU. The computer sets the appropriate route depending on the destination selected by the user before the carrier passes through the transfer unit. Carriers are routed to their destination via the shortest path possible. A sensor is contained within each unit to detect the passage of a carrier. Verification is sent to the central control as part of the carrier tracking process.

9.2.4. Blowers

The blower unit provides the vacuum or pressure that moves carriers through the system. A regenerative type centrifugal blower is used to provide the best combination of flow characteristics for pneumatic systems. This type of blower has a linear pressure–flow characteristic resulting in a more stable carrier velocity at the low pressures normally required [typically 0.5 psi (lb/in.^{2})] and yet is capable of increased pressure necessary for heavily loaded carriers. Most units have an automatic shutoff if idle for a designated period of time. Blowers are typically located in a mechanical space but can be sound deadened and placed above ceiling tiles if necessary.

9.2.5. Stations

Recessed, console or desktop stations are combined sending and receiving units. The dispatcher and receiver share the same transmission tube in most systems. Carriers arriving at a station are decelerated on an air cushion to minimize impact and sound and are then deposited gently into a receiving bin. Desktop box-type units may be limited in their receive capability if the arriving carrier remains in the receiving station. Optic sensors are used to sense the departure and arrival of the carriers. Most stations utilize LCD (liquid crystal display) displays to provide messages to the operator of the station. Directories provide stations addresses and a keypad is typically the mode of interface for the operator. Stations may have storage bins for extra carriers and packaging products.

9.2.6. Carriers

Carriers are designed to carry a diverse set of materials ranging from single vials of blood to 1000-mL IV bags to medical records. They are molded of high-impact-resistant thermoplastic (generally, polycarbonate). Many carriers are transparent for easy recognition of contents. Carriers may be side-opening or end-opening. End opening carriers are less common as there is the potential to deposit contents into the system should the end latch or lid dislodge. Side opening carriers are held intact by the diameter of the steel tubing.

9.2.7. System Options

9.2.7.1. TRAFFIC ANALYSIS SOFTWARE. Some systems include software which enables users to analyze the traffic volumes and patterns on their system. Particularly in larger systems with multiple zones, system layout is key to optimal traffic flow and analysis software can help pinpoint bottlenecks. System parameters can be changed to adjust the traffic flows once the patterns are known. Transactions between stations or zones or within the entire system can be evaluated, as well as carrier wait and travel times (see Fig. 9.1).

9.2.7.2. MODEM SUPPORT PACKAGE. A modem support package allows system maintenance personnel to access the control center from remote locations within the same building or from other locations. A typical application would involve access from home on weekends on third shift by the technical expert on the system. Modems also enable technical contact via phone by system service personnel to assist customers in system diagnostics.

9.2.7.3. CARRIER LINERS AND SPECIMEN PACKAGING PRODUCTS. It is necessary to package most items placed in a carrier before being sent in the system.

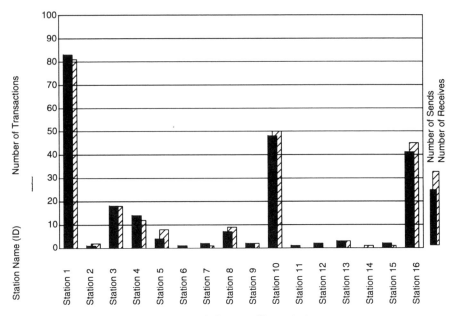

Figure 9.1. *Sample graph from traffic analysis program.*

Key reasons for packaging include immobilization to prevent jostling of contents within the carrier and secondary containment of liquids to prevent leakage into the system. The primary reasons for containing liquids are to protect workers from potentially harmful materials and to protect susceptible parts of the system from damage. Immobilization products range from heavy vinyl pouches to various types of foam liners. Containment products may consist of vinyl pouches or a variety of Ziplock-type bags. Biohazard carrying bags should be labeled as such.

9.2.8. General Hospital Applications

The CTS system increases the efficiency of medical professionals charged with the primary responsibility of patient care. Today's systems are able to transport even the most fragile of pharmacy syringes or laboratory specimens due to soft handling capabilities and high reliability. Items as large as 1000-mL IV bags can be transported at will.

Since patient care personnel must continually interface with ancillary departments for supplies, drugs, tests, and records, a constant demand is placed on the nursing staff to assure that the materials are transported in a timely manner.

The CTS is the fastest of systems in the automated transport arena and reduces turnaround time significantly. In a study conducted at The Bryn Mawr Hospital, Bryn Mawr, Pennsylvania, the laboratory participated in a survey administered by the College of American Pathology that examined turnaround time between the laboratory and the emergency department. Turnaround time was measured from the time of phlebotomy to result reporting. The survey was conducted both before and after the installation of a CTS. For the 90th percentile turnaround times, the laboratory improved from the 52nd to the 86th percentiles among all hospitals for potassium and from the 30th to the 82nd percentiles for hemoglobin. The improvement was determined to be a direct result of using the CTS to transport specimens rather than manual transport.[2]

With current emphasis on patient centered care, the CTS assists laboratories in bringing service closer to the patient care areas without the added cost of decentralizing the physical location of the laboratory.

9.2.8.1. CRITICAL RESPONSE SYSTEMS. Because of the modular nature of the pneumatic tube systems, it is feasible to start with a system that serves a few key areas and to expand the system over time as needed. A common application is the critical response system that generally ranges from 2 to 10 stations is size (see Fig. 9.2).

This system configuration is designed to connect the patient care areas that are responsible for generating the majority of critical stats in a hospital to the laboratory and pharmacy. Typical patient care areas include the emergency department, surgery, and critical-care units. Some facilities start with as few as two departments, usually laboratory and emergency, and expand to other areas later. It is key to install a system that can be added to in a modular fashion when future expansion is a possibility. The initial system is generally designed on a single zone and can be expected to handle a minimum of 50–60 transactions per station per day from a typical nursing unit.

Items moved by nursing are predominately specimens for stat testing and pharmaceutical orders. Pharmacy uses the system to transport IVs with admixtures, drugs that must be stored in the pharmacy, first doses, change orders, and stat pharmaceuticals.

9.2.8.2. HOSPITALWIDE SYSTEMS. Hospitalwide systems are generally laid out in multiple zones to handle a significant amount of traffic. Each zone, or cluster of stations, is operated by a separate blower. Zones are connected by interzone pipes that allow transactions to go between zones. In a multizone system, carriers can be moving simultaneously within each zone and within each interzone pipe. For example, in a three-zone system, six carriers can be in transit at any given time, one in each of the three zones and one in each of the three connecting interzone pipes. The diagram below represents a three-zone 27-station system. In most hospital multizone systems it is generally recommended that no more than about 10 stations be placed on a zone (see Fig. 9.3).

Hospitalwide systems include routine nursing units in addition to the critical-care areas contained in the critical response systems. Ambulatory-care areas and

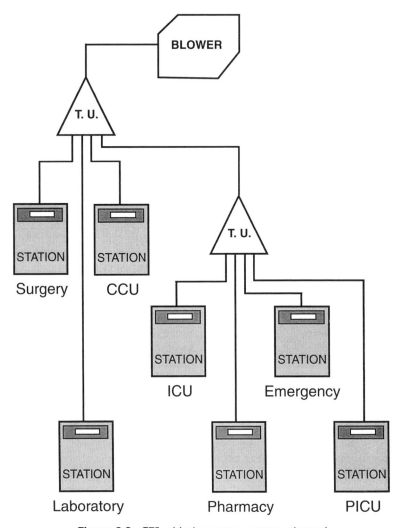

Figure 9.2. CTS critical response system schematic.

clinics are other common station locations. The presence of a CTS transport station in these areas eliminates the need for satellite pharmacies and laboratories and the costs associated with each.

Many facilities implementing patient centered care initiatives have opted to utilize a CTS system to provide better service to the units, thereby reducing the high cost associated with total decentralization. In many cases, the patient care teams assume the responsibility of the phlebotomy function. Pharmacists on the floor are able to spend a majority of their time in a clinical capacity rather than

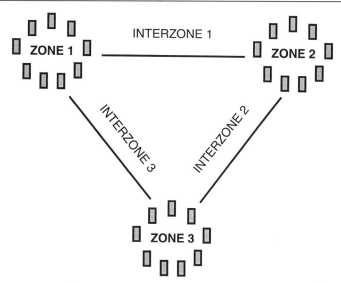

Figure 9.3. Multizone system configuration.

distribution and dispensing functions in this modified patient-centered care setting.

Other departments found on a hospitalwide system typically include medical records, central supply, maintenance, administration, admissions, dietary, and radiology. On occasion, laboratories will equip each floor of a medical office building, located on the same campus, with a CTS station. This enables physician office personnel to collect and send specimens to the laboratory for testing. The goal is to provide better service to the physicians and their patients. In addition, the system is helping to keep the outpatient laboratory test revenue in the hospital laboratory rather than it being diverted to a competing reference laboratory.

9.2.8.3. SPECIMEN TRANSPORT ISSUES. It is imperative that the automated transport system not affect the specimen such that the test results are altered. This applies particularly to blood specimens. The tests that are the most sensitive to agitation of the sample due to hemolysis are lactate dehydrogenase, potassium, and hemoglobin. Several studies have been published confirming the capability of sending specimens in a reliable, properly designed, soft handling system.[2-3]

Insured-specimen integrity should be the first concern of a laboratory in evaluating the use of a CTS system. The first step in evaluating a system for specimen integrity is to confirm that the system is a soft handling system by design. This essentially means that the carrier rides and coasts to a halt on an air cushion throughout its transport in the system. This is particularly crucial at turnaround points.

Second, vendors should be able to supply studies done on the system model being considered prior to purchase that demonstrate that specimen integrity is maintained. In addition, it is recommended that samples be tested, after installation of a system, since each system is configured differently. One sample of a twin sample pair, should be hand-walked to the lab while the second of the set is tubed. All other steps should occur together and the results statistically compared. It is up to the laboratory to determine the amount of deviation that is acceptable and whether there is clinical significance.

As mentioned previously, specimens should be both immobilized and secondarily contained within the carrier when being transported in a CTS. These actions are a necessary part of the soft handling of the specimens.

A key issue of controversy centers around the need to see the contents of the carrier prior to opening. Two arguments for visual inspection are as follows: (1) if the specimen condition can be inspected prior to opening the carrier (i.e., has leaked into the secondary containment bag), it is possible to open the carrier and handle the contents in a hooded environment; and (2) if the carrier is accidentally sent to the wrong department, personnel unprepared to handle biohazard contents can identify the carrier as containing a specimen prior to opening the carrier and redirect it to the laboratory. Most foam packaging materials are opaque and do not allow viewing of contents.

Infection control is a key topic in the use of the CTS system. Advancements in design and reliability enable the CTS to transport laboratory specimens with integrity. However, no system is absolutely foolproof and infection control procedures should be followed to protect the worker and the environment from potentially hazardous situations.

The primary concern in the transportation of clinical specimens is leakage of the specimen into the carrier and potentially into the system tubing. This action could expose workers to hazardous material if not properly handled. It should be noted that breakage, as a cause of leakage, has been virtually eliminated with the use of carrier packaging devices and the soft handling features of the system. Leakage more commonly results from improper packaging and/or the use of primary containers that have not been shown to be leakproof. Containers should be tested to be leak tight prior to being used for specimen transport.

The key elements that should be included in infection control procedures to comply with OSHA standards are as follows:

1. Training of the employee on the use of the CTS as it pertains to specimen transport and infection control
2. Documentation of the training
3. Secondary containment of the specimens
4. Proper biohazard labeling
5. The wearing of the appropriate barrier protection (universal precautions) by the employees handling specimens

6. Cleaning procedures for the carriers and the packaging (if reusable)
7. Procedures for decontaminating and cleaning the system
8. Barrier protection (universal precautions) for the maintenance personnel performing system cleanout procedures[4-8]

9.3. ELECTRIC TRACK VEHICLE SYSTEM (ETV)

9.3.1. General System Description

The electric track vehicle (ETV) system features self-propelled vehicles that independently and simultaneously traverse a network of modular aluminum track and switches under the direction of a central controller. The system, generally speaking, is similar to a miniature train set. Reliable transport of payloads of ≤ 50 lb is accomplished at speeds of ≤ 200 ft/min. The system is energy-efficient and provides on-demand delivery directly between any two stations in a system containing from two to hundreds of stations (see Fig. 9.4).

9.3.2. System Control Center

The system control center utilizes modern microcomputer technology for supervising and monitoring system functions and information. The control center includes a color videodisplay terminal, UPS, and a printer. The control center utilizes plug-in proprietary printed-circuit boards (PCBs).

Traffic management is optimized by the control center, regulating the constantly changing traffic patterns through communications with stations, transfer units, and cars. Closed-loop control prohibits dispatch of a car if it cannot reach its destination. Further, should an in-transit car's destination become unavailable, the car will return to its source after a programmable number of delivery attempts.

Computer control flexibility permits easy modification to the operating program when alterations occur to the layout configuration. An interactive, diagnostic, and troubleshooting program prompts immediate corrective action to minimize equipment downtime.

The software provides information on status of the system and the means to set up schedules for user-desired station operation. All displays and transactions can be routed to the printer for a permanent record. Service and preventive maintenance is supported with display of accumulated equipment cycles and car run times and reporting of alarm information.

It is possible to interface the ETV control center to a host computer. Information concerning the load can be transmitted to the host, and work commands can be downloaded from the host to the system central control. In highly automated environments, special adaptations to the system can enable the system to automatically load and unload its material or cargo.

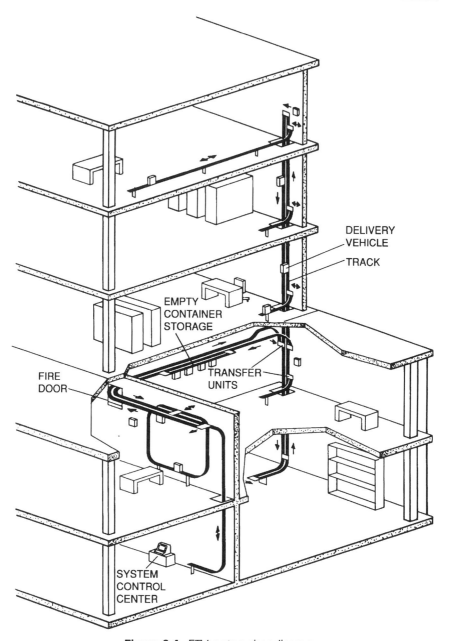

Figure 9.4. ETV system riser diagram.

9.3.3. Track

Lightweight, aluminum track is provided in preassembled, quick-connecting sections that permit easy future expansion or re-routing of the system. Modular track components include bends, curves and straight sections that can be connected in any combination to allow both vertical and horizontal transport. Track networks can be floor mounted to present loads at work level or suspended overhead to relieve floor congestion.

The aluminum track contains groove strips used to drive the car in vertical sections, bends, and curves. In addition, the track houses brass contact rails for communication with the central control center.

9.3.4. Transfer Units

Transfer units, which comprise mounted, short, movable sections of track, move cars between two parallel track sections. Transfer units are used for cars to enter and exist stations and to transfer cars from one track to another. A microprocessor controller on the unit provides a communication link with the central computer, serves as control for nearby power supplies, and monitors nearby fire dampers.

9.3.5. Fire and Air Dampers

Because of the right-of-way required for cars and track, it is necessary to install fire dampers in walls and floors as required to meet fire protection regulations. Fire dampers are normally closed but held open by a fuse link or electromagnet for connection to building fire and smoke alarm systems. A motor operator can be installed to automatically reopen a fire damper following a test.

Air dampers or flaps can be installed at wall or floor penetrations to separate air-conditioned or regulated air sections of a building.

9.3.6. Stations

Electric track vehicle stations, which are made up of a section of track and a control panel, can be configured in three ways. The three station types are through stations, reversing stations, and in-line stations. High-vehicle-volume locations require the use of through stations, which consists of a loop of track that handles vehicles on a first-in/first-out (FIFO) basis. Lower volume locations are able to use reversing stations that handle traffic on a last in/first out manner. The length of the section of track that makes up the station can vary in length to accommodate more cars, or parking places.

The third configuration, the in-line station, is used in situations where an application requires very sequential, routine delivery patterns. Cars basically stop on the mainline track segment for a period of time and then continue on to the next in-line stop.

Station control panels consist of a set of dials or a keypad to address cars for dispatch, arrival chimes to alert users of incoming vehicles, and other information such as system operational status. A directory of stations on the system provides other user addresses.

9.3.7. Cars

ETV vehicles are generally referred to as "cars." The cars house a microprocessor board that communicates its location to the central control center through a brass rail located on the aluminum track. In addition, information such as run time on the motor and other maintenance data is relayed.

The cars can be likened to flat bed train cars with attached containers for carrying payload. Containers can be custom designed to meet certain payload requirements. It is common in laboratory applications that the containers be mounted on a pivot arm so that the contents are always carried in an upright position. Because of this feature, test tube racks for example can be easily transported (see Fig. 9.5).

9.3.8. Hospital Applications

The ETV can be used exclusively within the laboratory or externally to connect laboratories together. Within the lab, overhead track delivers cars containing specimens to the various departments. All areas may be connected to central processing or only those areas that are the farthest away and require better response. Because the ETV can travel vertically as well as horizontally, the connection of laboratory departments on multiple floors is a key benefit.

A second application involves the use of the ETV to connect remote areas that have the need to send larger volumes or payloads to or from the laboratory. The system can be used to transport blood units to the emergency department or surgery, or volumes of specimens from outpatient collection areas (such as in clinics) to central processing.

Hospitalwide or clinic systems serve other departments' needs as well as those of the laboratory. Central supplies, radiology film packets, medical records, surgical kits, and pharmaceutical supplies are a few of the materials able to be transported in a hospitalwide system. Clinics have a key interest in the transport of medical records from archives to the various clinic locations that a patient must visit.

9.3.8.1. SPECIMEN TRANSPORT ISSUES. Because pivoting containers can be adapted to the flatbed cars for the transport of specimens and the vehicles travel at a slower speed than the carriers in the high-speed computerized pneumatic-tube systems, specimen integrity is not as key of an issue in the ETV system.

The car container provides a closed environment for the transport of the specimens and can be supplied with a lock if so desired. The key elements that should be included in infection control procedures that comply to OSHA standards are as follows:

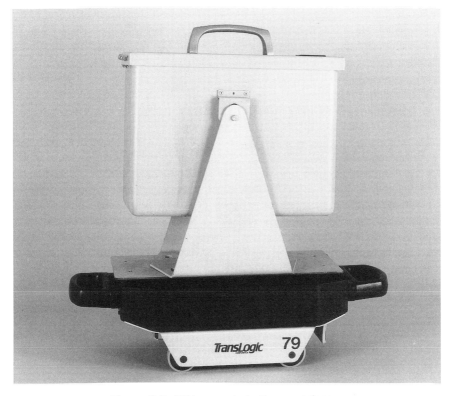

Figure 9.5. ETV car and pivoting container.

1. Training of the employee on the use of the ETV as it pertains to specimen transport and infection control
2. Documentation of the training
3. Secondary containment of the specimens
4. Proper biohazard labeling when appropriate
5. Wearing of appropriate barrier protection (universal precautions) by the employees handling specimens
6. Cleaning procedures for the cars and the containers
7. Procedures for decontaminating and cleaning the system
8. Barrier protection (universal precautions) for the maintenance personnel performing system cleanout procedures[4–8]

9.3.9. System Restrictions

The ETV system requires approximately a 2 × 2-ft right-of-way for the track and the car combined. It can be difficult in older buildings to find or free available space in either the interstitial or ceiling space. It is possible in some restricted environments to suspend the track below the ceiling. Another restriction to the system concerns the car's speed of travel. Faster systems, such as the CTS, may be more appropriate if time is of the essence and the distance to be traveled is significant.

9.4. AUTOMATED GUIDED VEHICLES (AGV)

9.4.1. General System Definition

Automated guided vehicle (AGV) systems feature battery-powered, rechargeable vehicles that travel along the floor at speeds of ≤120 ft/min and carry loads of ≤800 lb. Vehicles are dispatched on preprogrammed routes that can be changed as required. Systems are available featuring automatic door and elevator interfaces. Most AGVs follow passive guidepaths. Systems are available with both single- and bidirectional travel vehicles. A wide variety of carrier modules or trolleys have been designed to meet the needs of the laboratory and healthcare facility.

9.4.2. System Control Center

Most AGV systems have a microprocessor control that communicates with the vehicles via infrared (IR) or radiofrequency (RF) communications. The control center is responsible for dispatching, traffic control at intersections, and automatic interface with elevators, doors, and other equipment, such as sorters.

The central control monitors the location and status of all vehicles as they execute their routes. Should a malfunction occur, the control center identifies the problem area and activates an alarm. Diagnostic information helps minimize downtime. System activities can be printed and archived to provide history for system management. In cases where a single vehicle exists in a system or individual vehicles are not expected to share or cross paths, local vehicle control may be feasible.

9.4.3. Guidance Systems

Automated guided vehicles may be path-guided or self-guided (the latter are often referred to as *mobile robots* or *self-guided vehicles*). The primary difference between the two is the method of navigation used by the vehicle in reaching its destination. Path-guided vehicles follow either a passive or active path that has been physically installed along the route. Passive paths may be made of metal tape, magnetic tape, retroreflective tape, or fluorescent sprays. The tapes can generally be placed under floor surfaces such as tile or carpet if desired. Active paths are embedded wires that carry signals from the control center to direct the vehicles.

Self-guided vehicles utilize all or some combination of various navigation methods. The key techniques are dead reckoning (counting wheel revolutions and translating these into distance), ultrasonic wall mapping (bouncing ultrasonic signals off of walls to create an image of the environment and then comparing this to a map in its software), camera vision (using infrared signals to map the environment similarly to the ultrasonic mapping), and odometry (using complex x and y coordinate calculations based on a set reference point to plot a location). These vehicles essentially use the walls, hallways, and other landmarks as their physical route.

Changing or extending pathways with path-guided vehicles involves the laying of additional tape or path and instructing the controller of its presence. Changing paths in self-guided vehicles involves laying additional routes in the computer software, or mapping an area. This is usually accomplished with the assistance of a CAD/CAM (computer-aided design/manufacturing) program, which is part of the mapping program in the vehicle control.

Because automated guided vehicles are larger than other systems and share physical space with humans, most are equipped with obstacle detection devices. Once an object or human is spotted by the vehicle, it stops. Vehicles are usually touch sensitive as well. Most vehicles have bells, buzzers, lights, or the like to alert humans of their approach.

Vehicles are available in many shapes and sizes. In some systems, the vehicle is separate from the payload-carrying trolley. In this configuration, the vehicle drives under the trolley, either lifts it or attaches to it by some means and in essence carries the load. It can also tow additional payload behind it if so required. This naturally limits the vehicles ability to maneuver and turn around.

The trolley may be integral to the vehicle in other systems. This is generally the case with self-guided vehicles. Size may vary from trolley and vehicle combinations measuring 4 ft long by 2 ft wide by 4 ft high, with an 800-lb load-carrying capacity, to units no larger than a human and able to carry only 50 lb. As an aside, keep in mind that larger AGVs are sometimes used by other departments for transporting linens, dietary carts, and the like (see Fig. 9.6).

In all cases, the vehicles are battery-operated and must be recharged periodically. A full battery charge is generally able to run a vehicle continuously for an 8–12-h period. Vehicles can stay in service for longer periods of time if the system uses opportunity charging. This is a quick-charge method whereby the vehicle docks itself to a charger for short charges during idle times of the day.

9.4.4. General Laboratory Applications

The primary application within the laboratory is the delivery of specimens, reagents, and supplies between laboratory departments. The home base for the vehicle(s) is generally the central processing area. In most cases, the path layout is such that the vehicle will travel a standard route on a timed interval. Most systems will allow random dispatch of a vehicle to a single location on the route.

In high-volume applications, specimens are processed and sorted into racks

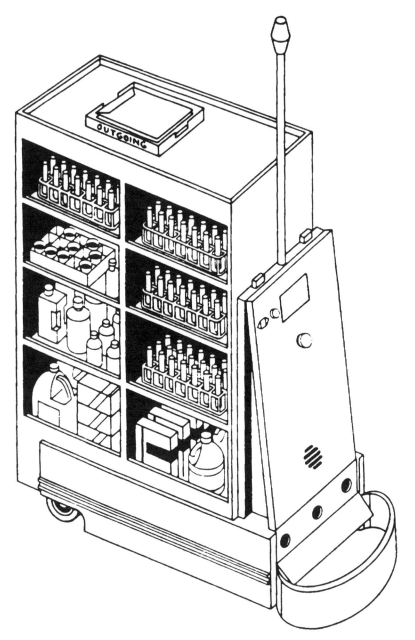

Figure 9.6. Sample automated guided vehicle and trolley.

by department, placed on bins on the AGV, and dispatched for delivery. Vehicles can be programmed to pass a location as frequently as necessary. Frequency of delivery is based on the length of the route and the number of AGVs in service.

In one application, a reference laboratory utilizes AGVs to deliver to the various test departments every 15 mins. Two vehicles are en route at any given time in order to accomplish the 15-min goal. In this scenario, the trolleys are separate from the vehicles so that the specimen processors can be loading additional empty trolleys while vehicles are delivering full trolleys.[9]

A second application involves the transport of specimens from remote laboratories to the main site. This is feasible provided there is a continuous hallway or tunnel system in which the vehicle can travel.

9.4.5. System Restrictions

Primary restrictions in an application are based on the right-of-way requirements of the vehicle. A turning radius and turnaround space is required depending on the size of the vehicle and whether it is bidirectional. Hallways must be sufficiently wide to permit the presence and passage of humans at the same time as the vehicle. This is mandated by safety rules and fire codes.

In addition, the vehicle may not be ideal for the handling of stats depending on the layout and size of the laboratory. It may be disruptive to the delivery of the routine specimens if the vehicles is constantly being redeployed for stat deliveries, interrupting its routine job. The use of multiple vehicles may be a solution to this problem, however.

Travel in public hallways can be disruptive to the duties of the AGV. Personnel unfamiliar with the technology and enamored with its uniqueness may impede its journey. This problem can been resolved in part by an on-board enunciator that asks the obstacle to "please step away from the vehicle" so that it can continue on its way.

REFERENCES

1. Weber D: Calculating pneumatic systems' productivity. *Health Fac Management* 5:12–13, 1992.
2. Keshgegian A, Albert, Bull E, Glenn: Evaluation of a soft-handling computerized pneumatic tube specimen delivery system: effects on analytical results and turnaround time. *Clin Chem* 4:535–540, 1992.
3. Hardin G, Quick G, Ladd DJ: Emergency transport of AS-1 red cell units by pneumatic tube system. *J Trauma* 30.3:346–248, 1990.
4. Weber D, Welss B: *Infection Control Procedure for the Transport of Specimens in a Pneumatic Tube System.* TransLogic Brochure, 1993.
5. USCDC: Recommendations for preventing transmission of infection with T-lymphotrophic virus type III/lymphadenopathy-associated virus in the workplace. *MMWR* 34:681–684,691–695, 1985.

6. OSHA Instruction CPL-2-2.44C, March 6, 1992, Office of Health Compliance.

7. NCCLS Document M29-T: *Protection of Laboratory Workers from Infectious Disease Transmitted by Blood, Body Fluids and Tissue,* 1989, Vol 9, No 1.

8. *Biosafety in the Laboratory.* National Research Council (U.S.) Committee on Hazardous Biological Substances in the Laboratory. Washington DC: National Academy Press, 1989.

9. Keuhn-Kelly, Christine: *Robotics Assist Staff at Largest Clinical Lab Under One Roof.* Advance 2:1–2, 1990.

10. *Computerized Pneumatic Tube System CTS-30.* TransLogic System Planning Guide, 1994.

11. *Electric Track Vehicle System.* TransLogic System Planning Guide, 1994.

10

Laboratory Automation Platform

RODNEY S. MARKIN

CONTENTS

10.1. INTRODUCTION

The laboratory automation platform (LAP) is a concept originally proposed in 1990 by my research group at the University of Nebraska Medical Center.[1-4] The concept parallels the paradigm of automated flexible light manufacturing in that a variety of options are available in a fixed period for movement of processing components or units through a series of steps. This compares to the current manual laboratory operation where automation has matured at the level of the "workbench" with the development of automated analyzers such as the Kodak Ektachem clinical chemistry analyzer and the Coulter counter hematology analyzer. The transportation of specimens, the order in which they are transported, and the unique requirements of each specimen are currently under the control

Handbook of Clinical Automation, Robotics, and Optimization, Edited by Gerald J. Kost with the collaboration of Judith Welsh.
ISBN 0-471-03179-8 © 1996 John Wiley & Sons, Inc.

of human transportation and the recognition of feedback by instrument operators (technologists) and other laboratory workers.

Most industrial manufacturing operations have become more cost-effective in
the last three decades by implementing increased levels of automation. They
have changed the work or paradigm operations in their environment to enable
them to receive the benefits of automation. For the purposes of this discussion,
the concept of a laboratory automation platform will include the software, hardware, and transportation components necessary to interconnect different workstations or workbenches in the clinical laboratory.

10.2. THE ENVIRONMENT AND THE APPROACH

In order to build and design a system to accommodate a variety of different
laboratories, operations, including methodologies, instrumentation, and business requirements, the laboratory operation must be viewed in two different
ways: (1) from a global perspective and (2) from the perspective of the patient.

10.2.1. Global and Enterprise Perspectives

The global perspective in this context means the evaluation of the laboratory
operation as it fits into the enterprise, specifically the entire patient-care operation. We as laboratorians are not necessarily accustomed to viewing the world
from a global perspective based on historical events. For us to succeed as the
laboratorians of the future, our thoughts and observations from the point of view
of the enterprise, and with respect to how the laboratory fits into the enterprise,
will be very important. The role of the laboratory and the delivery of results and
interpretations in managed care will be pivotal to successful operation of the
enterprise. The two important issues currently facing the clinical laboratory are
(1) the financial performance of the clinical laboratory and (2) laboratory resources management.

In the current laboratory paradigm, approximately 50% of the operating
budget of a clinical laboratory in the United States is used to pay salaries and
benefits. The remaining 50% is used to pay for instrument rental and leases,
reagents, supplies, and other overhead costs. Altering the equation for the
bottom-line or financial performance in the laboratory could be an alteration in
the combination of all components that are used in the final calculation. Labor,
however, is the only component that can be significantly impacted. The cost of
reagents and supplies continues to increase at a rate that varies between 4 and
12% per year and does not appear to be declining. In application of industrial
automation solutions in the past, the greatest cost savings were possible in the
labor component.

The second issue related to the operation of the clinical laboratory revolves around utilization management. Utilization management issues are becoming increasingly important as more strict peer review and financial constraints are applied to the enterprise or organization. The goal of both the enterprise and the clinical laboratory is to provide the same or better patient outcome with fewer laboratory tests performed. This is necessary because laboratorians are now through the enterprise sharing the risks for laboratory operations as well as those for the enterprise as a whole.

Reducing tests performed can be accomplished only by implementing complex algorithms and methods to reflexly or automatically order tests, cancel tests, or spawn a different set of procedures related to the care of the patient and laboratory testing. Applying these algorithms can be enabled through two mechanisms: (1) people and (2) automated transportation. The application of personnel resources to solve this problem would require a greater number of employees and a much higher payroll. A transportation system to provide the same or a similar function would require significant capital outlay at the time of purchase but would allow for reduction in laboratory staff and recapture of unexpended salary dollars. The hardware and software described in this chapter follows from these concepts.

10.2.2. Patient Perspectives

The second important approach in dealing with the application of laboratory automation platform are the issues surrounding the patient. Hospitals and other medical service organizations define their first priority as patient care. The issue of patient care, with respect to design of a laboratory automation system, means that patient factors be taken into account when the system is designed. The most important issue regarding patients is the size and shape of the containers in which patient specimens are delivered. There are a variety of blood collection containers used in the clinical laboratory environment today, most of which are produced by Becton Dickinson Vacutainer Systems (Franklin Lakes, NJ). Becton Dickinson and other companies manufacture a variety of containers based on the requirements for collection of specimens from patients, including blood volume, matrix requirements for testing, and some issues regarding transportation. This makes the issue of transportation very complex; however, anyone who has been involved in the application of patient care will realize that the process is not one of an assembly line or manufacturing operation but one of individualized care and timely application of appropriate therapies.

From the standpoint of the engineer, a unifying concept is the approach of choice. Those intimately involved in patient care, however, realize that the application of therapy is patient-dependent, and therefore, an exception-based operation as opposed to a well-defined operation applied across all treated patients. The needs of the patient and the requirements of the enterprise as a whole to serve the patient necessitates accepting the approach from a patient perspective as opposed to an engineering perspective.

10.3. THE LABORATORY AUTOMATION PLATFORM

10.3.1. Hardware

10.3.1.1. ANALYSIS OF LABORATORY SPECIMEN VOLUME. In our approach to developing the laboratory automation platform, we analyzed the volumes and types of specimens received in our clinical laboratory operation. Our analysis revealed that approximately 95% of the specimens that were received in our laboratory were blood collection tubes of varying sizes and shapes. The remainder of the specimens, which accounted for approximately 5% of the total specimens, were a variety of sizes and shapes, including glass slides, swabs, blood culture bottles, sputum cups, histology specimens, and the other specimens usually delivered to the laboratory.

After analyzing these specimens, it was clear that we had to develop two

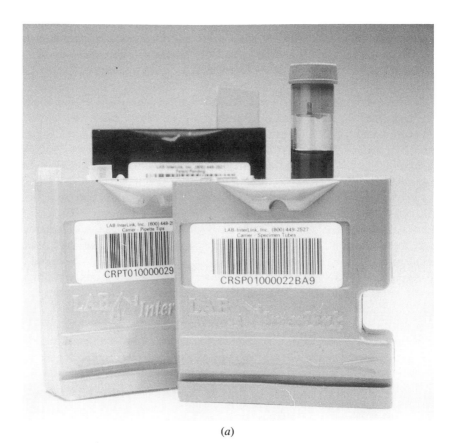

(*a*)

Figure 10.1. A LAB-*InterLink,* Inc. specimen carrier carries all sizes of evacuated blood collection containers, pediatric blood collection devices and glass slides: (*a*) side view; (*b*) top view showing payload configuration. (Photographs courtesy of LAB-*InterLink,* Inc.).

different modes of transportation for specimens that fell into each of the two groups: tubes and nontubes. That realization spawned the development of the specimen carrier (described in the next section) and the implementation of automated guided vehicle (AGV) technology (described later in this chapter and in more detail in Chapters 9 and 11).

10.3.1.2. SPECIMEN TRANSPORTATION CARRIER. The previous discussion regarding the approach to development of an automation platform is paramount to the design of a carrier to transport specimens throughout the laboratory.

Through our research program at the University of Nebraska Medical Center, we devised a specimen transportation carrier that holds different sizes of evacuated blood collection tubes, pediatric specimen collection containers, and a glass slide. The final design is shown in Figures 10.1*a* and 10.1*b*. The specimen

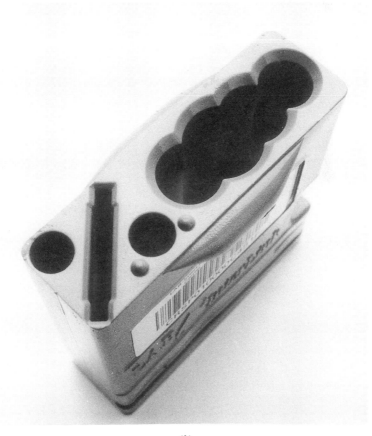

(*b*)

Figure 10.1. (*Continued*)

container is approximately $3 \times 3 \times 1$ in. in greatest dimensions and is produced using a mold injection process. Figure 10.1b shows the payload configuration from the top view. The overlapping holes for holding specimens form a 20-mL well that can serve as a secondary specimen container to comply with OSHA specimen transportation requirements (the OSHA requirement is usually satisfied by using a sealable plastic bag).

One of the most important issues that we were confronted with very early in the design process was the application of computer integrating manufacturing (CIM) principles to the clinical laboratory operation. In order to track and route specimens through the laboratory, each specimen must have a unique specimen identification number. Most of the laboratory information systems (LISs) that are sold by vendors in the United States use an archaic method of specimen grouping known as the *accession number*. The accession number may represent one or many specimens (tubes, blood culture bottles, urine containers, etc.). It is, therefore, not unique in terms of the individual specimens and the containers in which they are received. This design is based upon the concept of a patient encounter and has been carried through in laboratory operations for the past 30 years. In retrospect, the adoption of this methodology by the LIS vendors is a failure on their part to evaluate the laboratory process prior to developing their product.

In order to uniquely identify each specimen, we labeled the individual carriers with a unique and reusable identification number. The carrier identification number can then be electronically linked to the accession number and a tube subnumber, a cap color, or some other unique attribute of the specimen to produce a unique representation in specimen tracking and trafficking. Figure 10.2 demonstrates the flexibility of the specimen carrier design. The specimen carrier may be configured to carry multiple different specimen types including glass slides and pipette tips. Specialized transportation needs, such as tranporting a urine sediment tube, can be accomplished by changing the mold.

10.3.1.3. CONVEYOR SYSTEM. In our search for components to develop the laboratory automation platform, we preferred to purchase rather than construct our own components. At the outset of the project, the defined criteria for a specimen transportation system included the following: (1) the transportation system should be designed to mount in any configuration and be placed on the floor, on the wall, or suspended from the ceiling; (2) it must be modular in design to enable easy installation and on-site service; (3) it should have a sleek design and be "lablike" in its appearance; (4) it must be virtually noiseless during operation; and (5) it must conform to or support the OSHA guidelines for the protection of laboratory employees.

We evaluated a variety of different transportation systems, but none provided the solution that we required for a clinical laboratory operation. We, therefore, designed our own modular conveyor system based on the previously defined criteria.

The transportation system is constructed to serve as the enabler for the

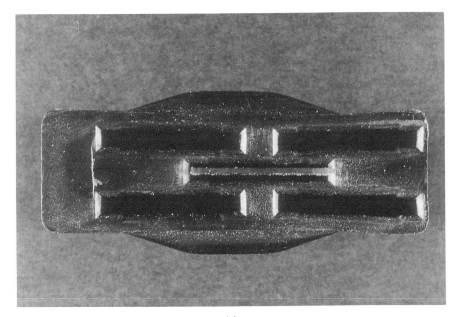

(a)

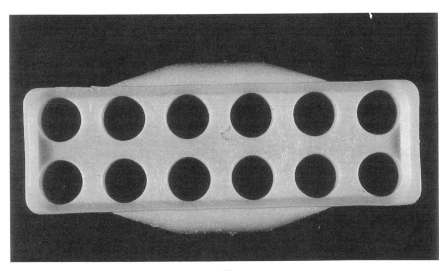

(b)

Figure 10.2. Specimen carrier: (a) top view showing configuration to hold glass slides; (b) top view showing configuration to hold pipette tips. (Photographs courtesy of LAB-*InterLink*, Inc.)

laboratory automation platform. The components are manufactured from extruded aluminum. There are multiple hardware components constituting the hardware component of the LAP, including straight segments of track, diverter/inverter units, corners, elevators, gates with or without a bar-code reader, and gates with or without a camera system to operate a vision system.

10.3.1.4. TRACK SEGMENTS. The track segments are constructed of extruded aluminum and use a roller chain mechanism to transport the specimen in the specimen transportation carrier. (Fig. 10.3). The function of the roller chain is significant in two ways. The roller chain used to construct the segments has a unique property that allows specimens transported across the surface to move at approximately $2\frac{1}{2}$ times the speed of the chain. This is due to a differential in the diameters of the rollers that transport the chain versus the rollers that transport

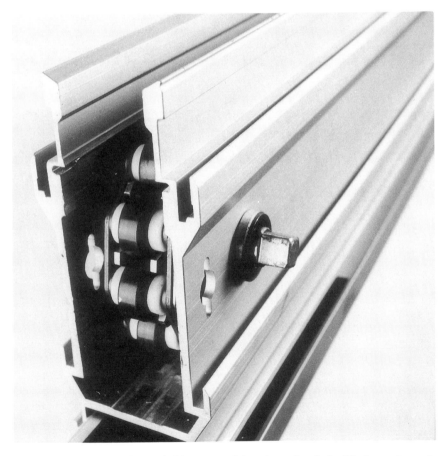

Figure 10.3. Segment of track (without cover) showing roller chain. (Photograph courtesy of LAB-*InterLink*, Inc.)

the specimen. The second important characteristic is the ability of the roller in the chain to act as a "free-wheeling" device to put specimens into a queue on the track segment. This eliminates a significant amount of friction and the need for large "off-track" holding areas for specimens waiting to be tested.

Each track segment is sealed with a plastic end cap to prevent users or operators from becoming entangled in the gear mechanisms or roller chain. Contained within each segment is a well that serves as a well for the internal spill containment. Any spills which may extend outside the body of the specimen carrier are captured in the segment wall. A clip-on plastic cover encloses specimens being transported along the conveyor mechanism. Each track segment may operate as an independent motor-driven unit. Track segments may be connected together with drive boxes (power transfer boxes) so that only a limited number of motors need to be used. Drive boxes also allow segments of track to be connected to diverter/inverter units and carriers.

10.3.1.5. CORNER. One important constraint in the laboratory relates to the availability of space. In most industrial manufacturing operations, conveyor segments are continuous and require wide arcs to move specimens around a corner to transport them in a different direction. Clinical laboratory space is at a premium. In order to provide the same functionality in constrained space, we designed a corner mechanism that moves specimens through a 90° corner without the usual large transportation arc (see Fig. 10.4).

The corner mechanism uses two parallel belts with differential speeds. The incoming belt moves at a speed X. The belt placed at right angles to the incoming belt moves at speed $1.25 X$. The initial incoming belt pushes the specimen into the perpendicular belt making contact with the front edge of the carrier, pulling it around the corner. The mechanism is highly reliable and facilitates specimen transportation throughout the laboratory.

One of the more interesting problems in developing a laboratory automation platform is the issue of installation of components without a customized solution. In order to handle differences in lengths, we designed the corner so that the lengths of the corner arms are adjustable. With two corners in place, this allows up to 13 in of adjustability in one dimension.

10.3.1.6. DIVERTER/INVERTER. The diverter/inverter component is similar to a switch on a model railroad (Fig. 10.5). Within the body of a diverter a solenoid actuates an arm. Specimens move straight through the diverter when the arm is in a neutral position. When the arm is moved, specimens are diverted onto a side track. The diverter may also be used to invert specimens bringing two parallel tracks together with the inverter providing the junction.

10.3.1.7. GATE MECHANISM. The gate mechanism is designed as a system module to stop a specimen transportation carrier at a location where the bar code on the carrier is read (Fig. 10.6). The gate mechanism is operated by solenoids, electronic devices that produce linear motion when energized. The

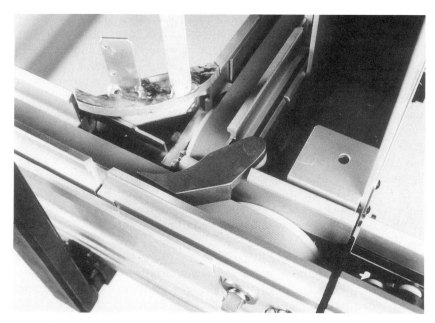

Figure 10.4. Top view of corner mechanism. (Photograph courtesy of LAB-*InterLink,* Inc.)

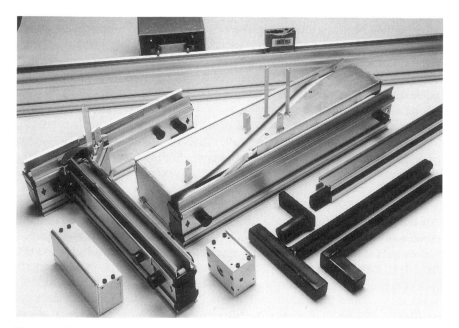

Figure 10.5. Top view of a diverter (center) which allows carriers from one track to be diverted to multiple other tracks or conversely allows two tracks to converge into one track. (Photograph courtesy of LAB-*InterLink,* Inc.)

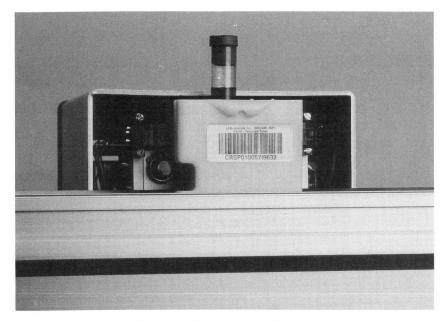

Figure 10.6. Modular gating mechanism may be configured with or without a bar-code reader and for vision system operations, with or without a camera. (Photograph courtesy of LAB-*InterLink*, Inc.)

solenoids are driven by a programmable logic controller that controls the movement of the gates and the firing of the bar-code reader. The logic controller also processes the signal from the bar-code reader and passes it on to the automation platform software. The gate mechanism may also be configured with a camera to capture an image of the specimen carrier payload. The image analysis subsystem evaluates the position of the carrier payload, and the cap color of the tube in the carrier. The gate may be used without either bar-code reader or camera to control the flow of specimens to an elevator or to form a queue.

10.3.1.8. ELEVATOR. In order to move specimens from the work level to an elevated level above the operational envelope of the people working in the laboratory, an elevator mechanism needed to be designed. Our original attempts at working with elevator mechanisms produced a serial operation that was a rate-limiting step in high volume scenarios. We, therefore, redesigned the system to provide a continuous-flow, discrete vertical elevator that operates on a principle similar to a carousel. Referring to the carrier in Figure 10.1*a,* you will see a set of wings or plastic extensions on each side at the top of the carrier. These plastic extensions function as the "handles" that allow the elevator to function. The pins from the chains on the elevator move into position underneath the wings on the carrier, make contact, and vertically elevate the carrier to the next level. The specimens are moved through an arc and gently placed onto the next layer of conveyor mechanism. At that moment, the pins are disengaged from the carrier wings and the specimen moves in a horizontal plane.

10.3.1.9. MOUNTING SYSTEM. In order to implement our system using the concept of modularity, it was necessary to develop a mounting system or infrastructure to support the components. We developed a mounting rail: a piece of extruded aluminum produced in 7- and 13-ft lengths (Fig. 10.7). This lightweight aluminum channel contains three compartments that are integral to its function. The top compartment is a "drip tray" to catch any spillage from track segments or carriers. This spillage containment system is of the utmost importance since the specimen transportation system would most likely be installed from the ceiling. Compliance with OSHA regulations for the protection of laboratory employees is of paramount importance. The drip tray supports the secondary specimen container concept encouraged by OSHA. The other two channels in the lower half of the mounting rail may be used as trays for power and communication cables.

All of the component parts including motors, gates, and power supplies clip onto the side of the track. The mounting bar is attached to the floor or the wall, or suspended from the ceiling by using three different mounting struts.

The combination of modularity, lightweight extruded-aluminum components, and sleek look allow the transportation mechanism to fit easily into the existing laboratory environment without significant renovation or modification. In the event that this transportation system would be moved between rooms, an opening approximately 5 in. wide and 15 in. tall would be required for pass through.

10.3.2. Software

The software controlling the laboratory automation platform is the most significant system component. In designing a laboratory automation platform, the issue of flexibility and where it resides is highly significant. After analyzing the situation of our laboratory and many other clinical laboratory operations, it was clear that the flexibility in the system must reside within the software with the hardware used as an enabler to transport specimens. We, therefore, designed the system to meet the requirements of a broad cross section of hospital, private, and commercial laboratory operations. The software also supports the contribution of the laboratory to the enterprise or organization as a whole.

The software system we designed is an application of computer integrated manufacturing specifically adapted for use in the clinical laboratory operation. As with the hardware used for transportation, we evaluated a large number of programs designed to be used with computer integrated manufacturing operations. Our analysis revealed that there were significant limitations in terms of scaleability, flexibility, and response time for processing the steps used for specimen manipulation and testing based on our criteria. We decided to design our laboratory automation platform software using tools to enhance the process

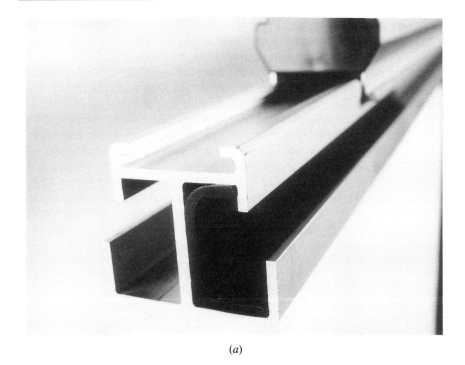

(a)

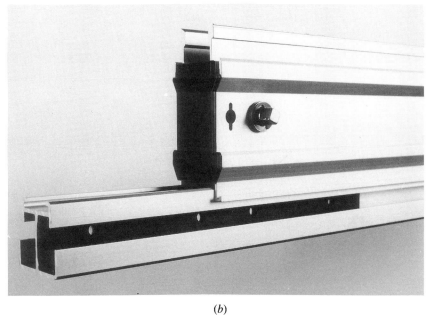

(b)

Figure 10.7. A segment of mounting rail: (a) the mounting rail contains a power and communication cable tray and a drip tray on the top of the rail; (b) track mounted on rail for suspension purposes. (Photographs courtesy of LAB-*InterLink*, Inc.)

and provide the flexibility needed to operate in the clinical laboratory environment. The Oracle® database software and tools were selected to develop our application. We designed the system so that rules for clinical operations could be applied at any level in the database. In Chapter 2, Figure 2.2 shows a representation of the hierarchy constructure relating enterprises, facilities, patient locations, and patient-specific data to physicians who may be ordering tests on that specifically identified patient. The use of such a scheme allows for a rule to be applied at any level in the structure facilitating the application of managed care. This managed care implementation may be facilitated through the application of a rule that would provide a predefined set of laboratory tests based on the patient's healthcare plan (e.g., HMO, PPO, Healthcare Alliance) and the patient's location within the healthcare environment (hospital, clinic, etc.). (See also Table 10.1.)

The patient location as a concept is traditionally used in the nursing arena and for grouping patient draws from a laboratory information system. The use of

TABLE 10.1 Component Data Transferred between the Laboratory Information System and the Laboratory Automation System and Interface

Admission/discharge transfer (ADT)
    Patient name
    Patient number (unique identifier)
    Age
    Sex
    Patient location
    Attending physician
Order entry (OE)
    Accession number
        Test code (unique test identifier)
            Specimen container type (i.e., tube, slide)
            Cap color (if tube)
            Minimum volume
            Workstation
Result reporting (RR)
    Accession number
        Test code
            Results
            Method
            Instrument
Instrument interface information (III)
    Instrument query function
        Reagents
        Operation parameter
    Instrument control
        Operational function control codes

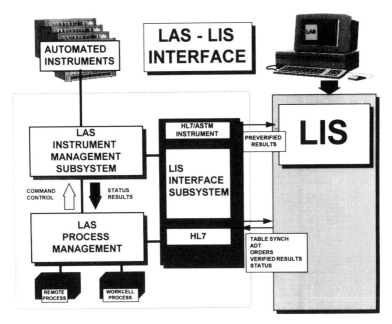

Figure 10.8. Schematic diagram of software architecture relating lab automation platform software to the lab information system and other operations within the hospital or clinic environment. (Photograph courtesy of LAB-*InterLink*, Inc.)

patient location may give a first-pass or low-level estimate of the patient's acuity for the purposes of perspective payment or implementation of rules based on perspective analysis. The current peer review organizations reviewing physician practice and patient outcomes use simple criteria such as the presence or absence of IV during a patient's stay for purposes of defining acuity and appropriate (based on their opinion) reimbursement.

The issue of scaleability in the software was difficult to address. Figure 10.8 shows a schematic diagram of the relationships between the software platform, the laboratory information system, and the remainder of the enterprise. It signifies the relationship between the laboratory information system, the laboratory automation system software, and the potential sources of the original information such as the hospital information system. Figure 10.9 shows a schematic diagram of the internal architecture of the laboratory automation system software. The LIS software was required by design to be scaleable so that the application could be used in a 50-bed hospital or adapted to a large clinical laboratory such as the MedPath Laboratory operation in Teterboro, NJ. In order to do that, specific servers and processes need to be set up to allow the operation to occur with multiple processes running in parallel. The schematic diagram of the software shown in Figure 10.9 demonstrates the parallel servers and the parallel subsystems feeding the servers with information obtained from the

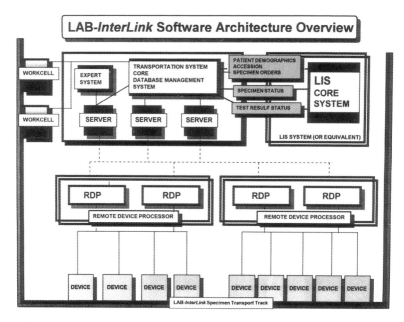

Figure 10.9. Schematic diagram of software architecture of the laboratory automation platform. (Photograph courtesy of LAB-*InterLink,* Inc.)

feedback mechanisms onboard active devices such as gates, divertors, active corners, and elevators.

The front end or entry point into the application is very important. In the past as a user of services, we have been required by vendors of information systems and other applications to use their proprietary or specified frontend or entry point to access the system. Due to the diversity of information systems and a changing environment of desktop workstation applications, we chose to support a PC workstation running Windows, Macintosh using the Macintosh operating system, X-windows using Motif, and a simple VT300 application. Using client/server-based architecture, we can support all of these front-end applications into our software platform and allow users to conserve their current investment in hardware and software.

Two important subcomponents of the software that merit mentioning include the help system and the paging system. The help system built into the software includes a "booklike" manual that contains repair and replacement functions for maintenance of the system in both text and real-time video. The video systems have been designed so that you identify the specific icon related to the part or component needing repair or replacement, click on that icon, and a screen appears. The real-time video is segregated into video and audio tracks. The audio track is tied to the users log-on password and presented in the natural language of the employee requesting assistance; for instance, a Spanish-speaking employee would receive a Spanish soundtrack in the help application.

The paging system is constructed to notify the appropriate operator of a zone system (a group of workcells and track components) of any system errors that occur within that zone. There is an escalation algorithm built into the software to enable the user to define the next several levels of supervision if response times are not met. This allows operators to continue their assigned duties without being required to view the system from an operators console.

10.4. SUMMARY

The laboratory automation platform consists of both hardware and software components. Flexibility is present in different levels within these components. The hardware components are flexible in that they may be reconfigured to meet the immediate transportation needs of the laboratory. System software is designed to provide support functions to the laboratory operating in a managed care environment, including reflex testing, reflex routing, tests, cancellation, and the implementation or rules at the enterprise facility, patient or physician level.

The future of laboratory automation systems is yet to be defined; however, it

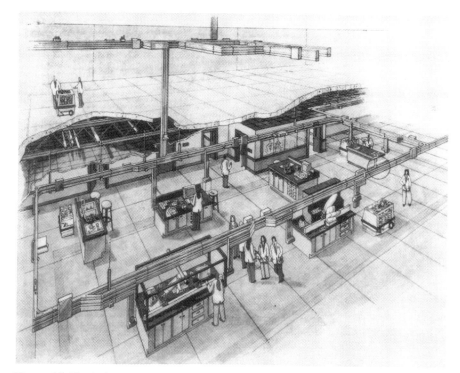

Figure 10.10. Artist rendering of a laboratory automation system in the clinical laboratory. (Photographs courtesy of LAB-*InterLink*, Inc.)

is clear that the comparison between the laboratory and its transition from a cottage industry to a commercial application is parallel to the changes that have occurred over the last 30–60 years in the industrial manufacturing arena. We look forward to seeing spectacular changes in laboratory operation in the future with the introduction of this and similar automation technologies. Figure 10.10 is an artist rendering that represents our vision of the laboratory of the future— the automated laboratory.

REFERENCES

1. Markin RS: Implementing automation in a modern clinical laboratory. *Lab Info Management; Sect Chemometr & Intell Lab Sys* 21:169–179, 1993.
2. Markin RS: Clinical laboratory automation: a paradigm shift. *Clin Lab Management Rev* 7:243–251, May/June 1993.
3. Markin RS: Laboratory automation: an introduction to concepts and terminology. *AJCP, Pathology Patterns,* 98(Suppl 1):S3–S10, Oct 1992.
4. Markin RS, Sasaki M: A laboratory automation platform: The next robotic step. *Med Lab Observ* 24:24–29, Oct 1992.

CHAPTER

11

Robotics, Interfaces, and the Docking Device

RODNEY S. MARKIN

CONTENTS

11.1. INTRODUCTION

The concept of robotics, interfaces, and the docking device brings together the essential elements needed for transforming a manual workstation or manually operated instrument into an automated workcell or island of automation. As noted in Chapter 2, there has been a dramatic change in the workstation of the clinical laboratory over the past 30 years. What once was a manual procedure at the workbench performed in microtiter plates, test tubes, or other reaction vials may now be a manually operated workstation such as the Kodak Ektachem

Handbook of Clinical Automation, Robotics, and Optimization, Edited by Gerald J. Kost with the collaboration of Judith Welsh.
ISBN 0-471-03179-8 © 1996 John Wiley & Sons, Inc.

(Eastman Kodak Corporation, Rochester, NY) or Coulter counter (Coulter Corporation, Kendall, FL) hematology instrument. Introducing robotic devices into the clinical laboratory environment proved to be a pivotal strategy. The use of specialized robotic devices facilitated developing random access analytical instruments.

The next quantum leap in laboratory automation at the instrument level is the modification or introduction of dedicated robotic devices, interfaces, and a "dock" for the introduction and egress of specimens from the instrument. This chapter provides an introduction to robotics, interfaces, and a vision for the future.

11.2. ROBOTICS

The concept of a robot was first described by playwright Carl Capek in his manuscript entitled *Rossum's Universal Robots* (RUR). The word "robot" is derived from the Czechoslovakian word *robota,* which is translated into English as servant, slave, or laborer. Robots were originally envisioned to perform tasks that humans found distasteful, e.g., such as cooking, cleaning, and manual labor. The study of robots and robotic engineering has gradually evolved to produce a discipline and a useful tool.

The Robot Institute of America (RIA) defines a robot as a "reprogrammable multifunctional manipulator capable of moving materials, parts, or tools through variable programmed motions for the performance of a variety of tasks."[1] Several types of robots are described for use in a variety of settings including cartesian robots, cylindrical robots, and jointed robots. These types of robots have been applied to useful applications in the clinical laboratory.

11.2.1. Cartesian Robots

Cartesian robots are currently the most commonly used robot in the clinical laboratory setting. They have three degrees of freedom (xyz) and are usually mounted in the arrangement of a frame (Fig. 11.1). In the industrial setting, the cartesian robot is used to move specimens along a longitudinal workspace. In the clinical laboratory, they are applied to the same task and find their most common application as a pipetting station.

Examples of the application of a cartesian robot in the clinical laboratory include the Tecan sampler 505 (Tecan AG Hombrech, Tecan, Switzerland)[2-4] and the Biomek pipetting station (Beckman Instruments, Brea, CA). The cartesian robot is fitted with a pipet that is used for aliquotting and diluting specimens and dispensing reagents. These pipetting devices can be programmed to handle a variety of liquid handling protocols.

The Biomek pipetting station is unique in that it has a variety of interchangeable manipulators that allow it to perform multiple different pipetting sequences. It also has its own onboard spectrophotometer for specimen evalua-

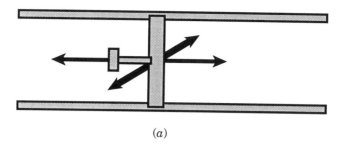

(a)

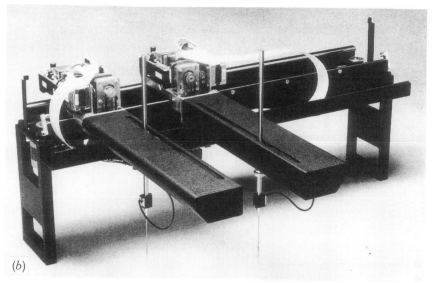

(b)

Figure 11.1. Cartesian robot: (a) schematic diagram; (b) Cavro cartesian robot similar to the mechanism that may be found in an automated pipetting station.

tion. The Biomek system has been used to perform immunoassays for carcinoembryonic antigen (CEA)[5] with good results. The Tecan sampler 505 has been used in the analysis of HTLV-3 antibodies.[4] In these studies, the Tecan instrument is shown to have better precision and throughput equal to or better than its human analog.

11.2.2. Cylindrical Robots

Cylindrical robots are characterized by their basic structure (Fig. 11.2) and their performance envelope (the physical space in which the robot works). The cylindrical robot has four degrees of freedom: rotation at the base and wrist, elevation, and lateral movement. The most common cylindrical robot used in the laboratory setting is the Zymate robot (Zymark Corp., Boston, MA). The Zymate robot may be programmed to perform several different functions to process and

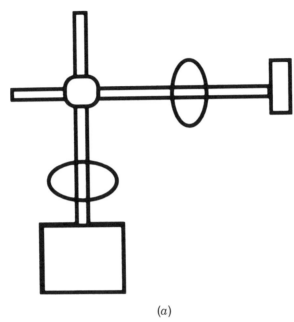

(a)

Figure 11.2. Cylindrical robot: (a) schematic diagram; (b) Zymark cylindrical robot system (top view with peripherals).

analyze clinical specimens. One of the unique aspects of the Zymate robot is its removable interchangeable end actuators (hands). The end actuators are different types, including a unit with "fingers" that utilize pressure sensitive sensors for handling glass tubes containing specimens.

Cylindrical robots have been used in a number of clinical and research settings. Work by Pippinger has described the preparation of HPLC specimen by the Zymark robot in the assay of antidepressants.[6] Other investigators have reported the use of cylindrical robots in the preparation of immunologic precipitates and in loading rotors from the Cobas-Bio Analyzer (Roche Diagnostics, Nutley, NJ).

Cylindrical robots have also been used in the analysis of specimens in the blood bank.[7] A commercially available product, Microbank (Dinatech Laboratories, Chantilly, VA) was the first successful robotic application in the blood bank determining blood groups. Freedman and Severns have also used a Zymate robot to compare samples for the analysis of blood groups in the blood banks.[8] This system utilized the robot to orient specimens prior to being read by a barcode reader and to manipulate a pipetting device.

11.2.3. Articulating Robots

Articulating robots are characterized by yet another degree of freedom. The articulating robot simulates the human forearm including shoulder, elbow, and

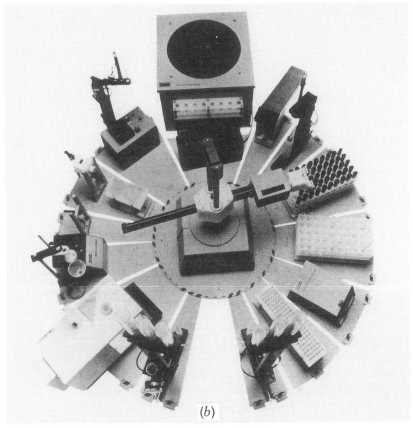

(b)

Figure 11.2. (*Continued*)

wrist rotation (Fig. 11.3). In addition, the "shoulder joint" of the robot is mounted on a base, allowing rotation. The wrist motion has both pitch and roll, allowing the complex, precise movements necessary to access some instruments. Examples of programmable articulating robots include D-TRAN series from Seiko (Seiko Instruments & Electronics, Ltd., Osaka, Japan) and CRS robot from Cyberfluor (Cyberfluor Inc., Toronto, Ontario, Canada). The similarity of the articulating robot to the function of the human arm allows the articulating robot to be integrated into several different laboratory tasks. Dr. Masahide Sasaki, Director of Laboratories, Kochi Medical School, Kochi, Japan, integrated Seiko robots into his clinical laboratory operation.[9,10] He uses articulating robots to automate type-and-cross match analysis for the blood bank, complex immunoassays, microbiology assays, including MIC and MBC analysis and enzyme-linked immunoassays (EIA). His work and the work of others, such as Dr. Robin Felder at the University of Virginia, pioneered the use of the articulating robot in clinical laboratory applications.[11–16]

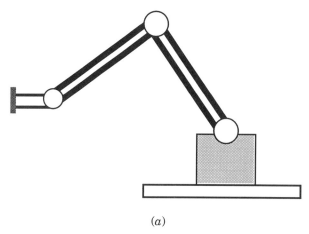

(a)

Figure 11.3. Articulated robot: (a) schematic diagram; (b) Mitsubishi articulated robot with auto encoders.

11.2.4. Automated Guided Vehicle Systems

The term *automated guided vehicle* (AGV), which is used to identify a driverless vehicle guided by a control mechanism, refers to an entire series of vehicles, with guidance mechanisms and traffic control devices as well as peripheral and on-board computer systems. AGV's are generally composed of two subsystems; a transportation system and an information system. The transportation system may have a variety of subcomponents including forward, backward, and sideways motion and additional load-handling systems, up to and including a robotic arm. The onboard information system controls system movement, including timing, distance, and turns. The information system communicates with other computers or devices to signal a change in the programming for determining routing or materials handling (several different AGV manufacturers use infrared signaling as the vehicle passes a transceiver.)

AGVs have found application in industry and are slowly becoming accepted in the healthcare environment. In the industrial environment, the variety of materials-handling functions are performed by different types of AGVs. Some AGVs, such as the type that we are incorporating into our clinical laboratory operation, carry a load on top of the vehicle (Fig. 11.4). Other AGVs operate as a tractor–trailer system where the AGV pulls racks or trucks to different locations. Several AGV options from Panasonic Industrial Systems use wing-shaped AGVs to engage a cart and pull it to a series of preprogrammed locations.

The load-handling systems attached to the AGVs have several potential applications. Simple load-handling units, such as motorized conveyors, may load or unload an item for transport. More complex systems utilize a robotic arm to distribute different components from the same vehicle at different points on its path.

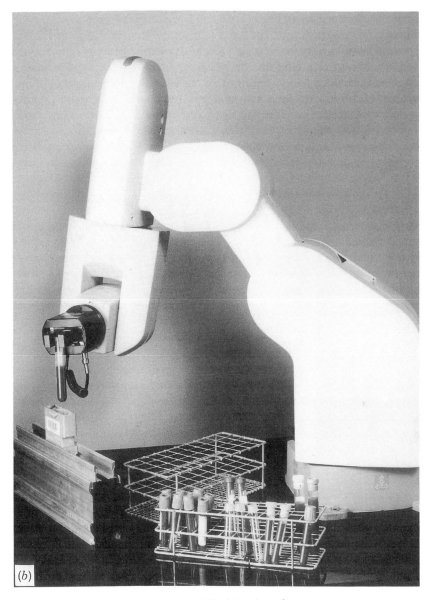

(b)

Figure 11.3. (*Continued*)

AGVs used in the healthcare industry include applications in the clinical laboratory, materials handling, and in some dietary divisions.[17] The clinical laboratory uses AGVs to include transport of both specimens and reagents. In addition to the application currently being installed in our clinical laboratory operation, the Smith-Kline Reference Laboratory in Atlanta, Georgia, uses automated

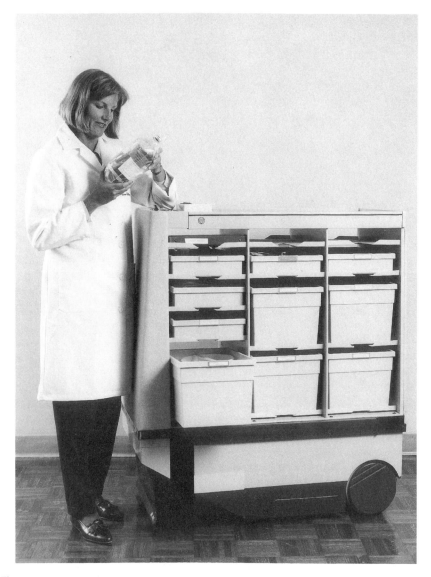

Figure 11.4. Automated guided vehicle in use at the University of Nebraska Medical Center. The rack and buckets positioned on top of the vehicle are used to carry specimens.

guided vehicles to transport all types of specimens throughout the laboratory. Dr. Masahide Sasaki of Kochi, Japan, utilizes AGVs to return specimens after processing and to handle other laboratory related materials.

For the past year, we have implemented an AGV to deliver specimens within the University of Nebraska Medical Center clinical laboratory. A Bell & Howell

Sprint Mailmobile was modified by adding a narrowband RF transmitter to the AGV to drive an enunciator system. The transmitter sends a signal to a receiver (frequency-dependent) located in each laboratory section where the AGV makes a stop for specimen delivery. When a specimen for a specific laboratory section is on the AGV, the corresponding receiver is signaled and the technologists from the laboratory section may retrieve the specimen. The use of the enunciator system reduces the effort of the technologists by signaling them only when a specimen is delivered. The AGV makes deliveries to microbiology, urinalysis, histology, cytology, tissue typing, and surgical pathology transcription.

In the future, the use of AGV's in the clinical laboratory should expand. It is likely that vendors will soon realize the potential market for their product and services.

11.3. INTERFACES:INFORMATION AND CONTROL

The current instrument information interface technology allows us to communicate with clinical laboratory instrumentation as compared to industrial standards, primitive. Current instrument interfaces allow communications to occur in either a unidirectional or bidirectional mode from the instrument to the laboratory information system (LIS). The communications level varies from instrument to instrument, however, generally providing the following functionality.

The *unidirectional interface* allows one-way results transmission. The specimen identification number, which may be a unique patient identification number, an accession number, or a specimen identification number, is entered into the instrument. That number may also be represented by a bar code attached to the specimen. The test performed on the specimen is either preprogrammed by manual entry or a battery of tests performed by an instrument that runs in parallel, such as the Coulter counter. The results are transmitted from the instrument through the interface to the laboratory information system. The results are reviewed by a technologist or by an electronic filtering mechanism and released based on criteria defined on a laboratory-by-laboratory basis back to the patient's record in the laboratory information system. The results are distributed through either a paper or electronic distribution mechanism or both, depending on the needs of the customers at that particular hospital.

The *bidirectional interface* allows the laboratory information system to download specimen identification numbers, patient identification numbers, or accession numbers coupled with orders to specific instruments. The instruments usually receiving these types of transmissions are random-access chemistry analyzers and some random-access immunoassay analyzers. The instrument either reads the bar code on the specimen container or has a unique relationship, predefined by the operator, between the unique specimen and a cup or tray identification on the instrument's sampling mechanism. The results are transmitted back to the laboratory information system and handled in a fashion similar to the method described previously for the unidirectional interface.

By applying the concepts of computer integrated manufacturing (CIM) to the clinical laboratory, it is imperative that there is a well-defined electronic communications system that allows the CIM software to control the process up to the level of the analyzer. The current CIM workcell automation existing in industry uses standardized protocols to transmit information back and forth between the workcell, its operating parameters or characteristics, and the CIM software. The industrial workcell technology uses various communication protocols; *machine automation protocol* (MAP) and *distributed data exchange* (DDE) are examples. Feedback from the workcell is transmitted back to the information system to allow the CIM software to understand the state of the machine and its operating characteristics.

Current clinical laboratory instrumentation lacks this type of automation interface. In order to promote the development of this type of automation interface, the laboratory automation research group at the University of Nebraska Medical Center, in conjunction with Eastman Kodak's clinical products division and Real Time Enterprises (Pittsford, NY), developed a control interface for the Kodak Ektachem 700 Series that works through the serial communications port on the back of the instrument. This automation control software allows the basic operation of the Kodak Ektachem 700 Series analyzer through a remote terminal by sending commands for operations usually performed at the touch screen on the instrument. The software developed by the University of Nebraska Medical Center was licensed back to Eastman Kodak in an attempt to jump-start the introduction of technology for the application of automation into the clinical laboratory arena.

11.3.1 Mechanical Interfaces

The mechanical interface to the current clinical laboratory instrument is designed for manual pick–place operations. The current designs were constructed around the manual–human operator paradigm.

Evaluation of the current technology is best performed by attending an equipment instrument exposition at one of the national meetings, such as the exposition associated with the American Association for Clinical Chemistry (AACC). A low-level evaluation reveals that most instrumentation uses some type of linear or circular specimen arrangement. These modes of manual specimen loadings functionally transform the random-access technology of each instrument into a batch analyzer. The manually loaded queuing stations effectively disable the true random access capabilities of the instruments. The linear or circular loading stations provide the technologist with the ability to utilize multiple instruments simultaneously.

11.3.2. The Docking Device as a Concept

During the past 4 years, our laboratory automation research group has promoted the concept of the "docking device" as a mechanism to produce a stan-

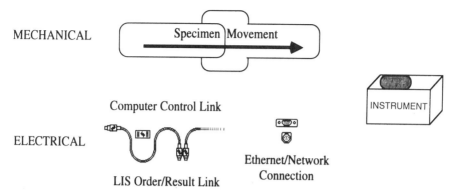

MECHANICAL

Specimen Movement

Computer Control Link

INSTRUMENT

ELECTRICAL

LIS Order/Result Link

Ethernet/Network
Connection

Figure 11.5. Schematic diagram of the "docking device."

dard electronic and mechanical interface between pieces of laboratory automation and clinical instruments configured as workcells.[18–21] Our concept is that the docking device would be as generic as an electric plug for use with a household outlet; for example, any piece of automation equipment could plug into any instrument in a mix–match scenario. The development of the docking device could position the instrument manufacturers who adopt this approach to gain a significant sales advantage over their competitors. If the projected savings in salaries are realized, sales of instruments with a docking device incorporated

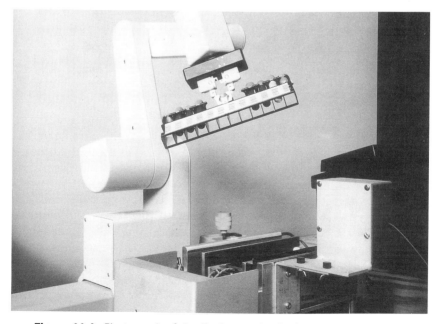

Figure 11.6. Photograph of the Coulter workcell with robotic interface.

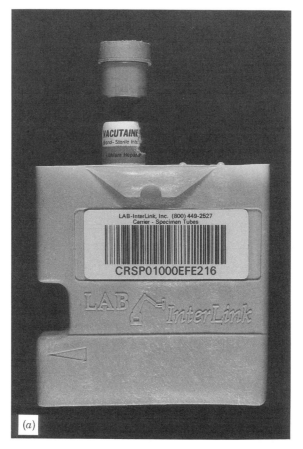

Figure 11.7. Photograph of the current selection of specimen transportation carriers: (a) LAB-*InterLink;* (b) Coulter/IDS; (c) AutoLab/AutoMed; (d) Hitachi.

into their architecture would accelerate rapidly. The concept of a docking device in its early stages, however, may compromise some laboratories since their instrument manufacturer may choose not to participate in the development or implementation of docking technology into their product line.

We divided the concept of the docking device into two components: the electronic interface and the mechanical interface (Fig. 11.5). The electronic interface is described above as the one necessary component to apply CIM concepts to the laboratory operation. The significant difference between the interface itself and the docking device is that the docking device provides the mechanical transportation of specimens integral to the instrument. The interface described in Section 11.3.1 allows an articulated robot to combine with the interface software to form a workcell that simulates the manual operation of the instrument from a mechanical standpoint (Fig. 11.6).

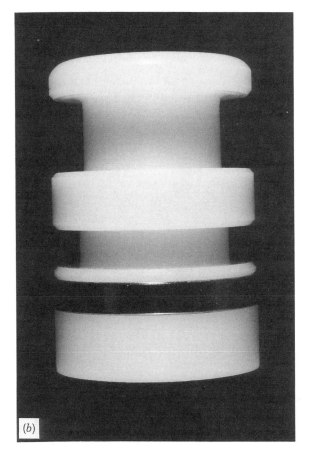

Figure 11.7. (*Continued*)

The mechanical component of the docking device is as simple or as complex as one wishes. One of the significant issues to take under consideration at this point is the diversity of the specimen transportation carriers that have been developed by several different vendors. The specimen transportation carrier developed at the University of Nebraska Medical Center is a patient-based specimen carrier that handles the needs of the clinical laboratory and provides unique specimen identification for routing and trafficking of each individual specimen in the laboratory. Several other vendors have developed specimen transportation carriers, including MDS Laboratories (Toronto, Canada), Coulter/IDS (Kendall, FL), and Hitachi Systems (Japan). Figure 11.7 shows a comparison between the different specimen carriers, including size and shape. When considering a docking device design, all the different specimen transportation carriers currently available need to be addressed. At this stage in the game, none

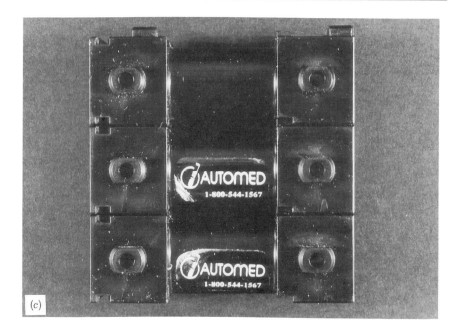

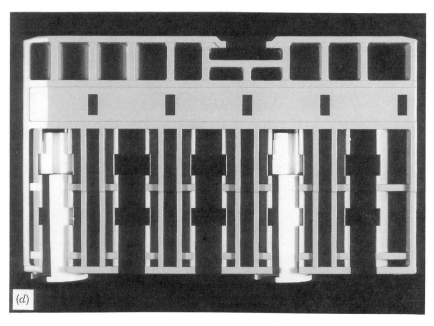

Figure 11.7. (Continued)

of the vendors can logically be eliminated due to a lack of understanding regarding the market for automation systems.

The docking device concept would, therefore, be a mechanism whereby specimens enter the machine at a predefined point with a sleeve or collar specific to the transportation system used (Fig. 11.8). This collar is an interchangeable piece of technology that positions the carrier in the appropriate place, reads the bar code on the tube, and provides feedback to the instrument and to the automation system. The gating mechanism allows specimens to move through one at a time. The gate also allows the random access of individual specimens, which is necessary to implement rules in a computer integrated manufacturing laboratory environment.

11.3.3. The Workcell as a Module

Our goal with respect to laboratory automation is to provide modularity to enable each individual laboratory to meet the needs of its customers using

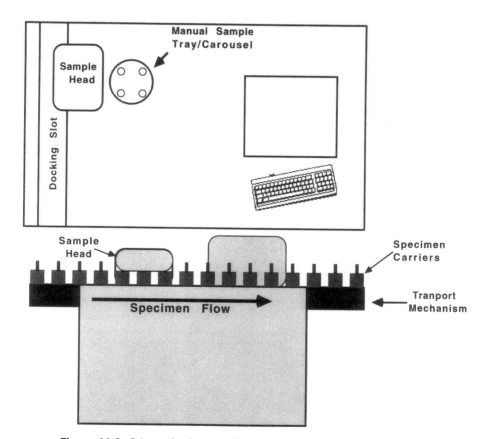

Figure 11.8. Schematic diagram of proposed docking device technology.

available off-the-shelf instrumentation transportation components and software. It is unreasonable to expect that any one vendor is able to serve the needs of all the laboratories across the United States and the rest of North America and the world. Specific instrumentation is purchased for a variety of reasons; however, it is clear that not one instrument serves all environments. The workcell as a module is a piece of "remove and replace" technology. It can be substituted, as needed, by new and improved technology without sacrificing the investment in the interface incorporating instrumentation into a laboratory automation platform.

11.4. CONCLUSION

Our vision is that the laboratory of the future will be equipped with instruments with docking devices containing both mechanical and electronic interfaces. Transportation systems connecting workcells in the laboratory with point-to-point transportation mechanisms allow random access of any specimen through the entire laboratory automation. These laboratories will be scaleable, ranging in size from small to large to fit a variety of different space and laboratory test menu configurations. This vision is not far from being realized. By the turn of the century, we envision fully automated laboratories operated by technologist managers to provide optimized patient care and a reduction in the number of tests performed for a better patient outcome.

REFERENCES

1. Hurst WJ, Mortimer JW: *Laboratory Robotics. A Guide to Planning, Programming, and Applications.* New York, NY: VCH Publishers, 1987.
2. Brennan JE, Severns ML: A robotic system to prepare samples for ABO/Rh testing. *Proc. 37th Annu Conf. Eng Med Biol* 26:253, 1984.
3. Brennan JE, Severns ML, Kline LM: Centralized sample preparation using a laboratory robot. In Strimaitis JR, Hawk GL, eds: *Advances in Laboratory Automation Robotics,* Vol. 2 Hopkinton, MA: Zymark, 1985, pp 481–495.
4. Brennan JE, Severns ML, Kline LM, et al: A robotic system to prepare samples for HTLV-III testing. *Med Instrum* 20:45–47, 1986.
5. Dumont L: Adaptation of the Biomek™ 1000 automated laboratory workstation for performing the Roche® heat-based EIA for carcinoembryonic antigen (CEA). In Strimaitis JR, Hawk GL, eds: *Advances in Laboratory Automation Robotics,* Vol 5. Hopkinton, MA: Zymark, 1988, p 537.
6. Pippinger C: The robots are coming. *Med Lab Observ* (Feb):30–36, 1985.
7. Severns ML, Hawk GL: Medical laboratory automation using robotics. In Michael Brady, Lester A. Gerhardt, Harold F. Davidson, eds: NATO ASI series, Vol F11, *Robotics and Artificial Intelligence.* Berlin: Springer, 633:43, 1984.

8. Friedman LI, Severns ML: Application of robotics in blood banking. *Vox Sang* 51(S1):57–62, 1986.

9. Sasaki M: Newly built automated laboratory system in Kochi Medical School [abstract]. In Kozakai N, ed: *Proc 12th World Congress Pathol, Tokyo;* reprinted in *Jpn J Clin Pathol* 31:518, 1983.

10. Ogura K, Sasaki M, Kataoka H, Nishida M: The innovative robot system for serological examination test and blood transfusion test: using Seiko RT-3000 robot. *Jpn J Clin Lab Auto* 12:613–618, 1987. (In Japanese)

11. Felder RA: Lab researches robotics potential. *Clin Chem News* 12:28–30, 1986.

12. Boyd JC, Felder RA, Margrey KS, et al: Use of a robotic arm for specimen handling in a remote, unmanned clinical chemistry laboratory. *Clin Chem* 33:1560, 1987.

13. Felder RA, Boyd JC, Margrey K, et al: Robotic automation of the intensive care laboratory. In Strimaitis JR, Hawk GL, eds: *Advances in Laboratory Automation: Robotics 4.* Hopkinton, MA: Zymark, 1988, p 533.

14. Felder R, Boyd J, Savory J: Robotics in the clinical laboratory. *Med Lab Prod* 2:18, 1987.

15. Felder RA, Boyd JC, Savory J, et al: Robotics in the clinical laboratory. *Clin Lab Med* 8:699–711, 1988.

16. Felder RA, Boyd JC, Margrey K, et al: Robotics in the medical laboratory. *Clin Chem* 36:1534–1543, 1990.

17. Lob WS: Robotic transportation. *Clin Chem* 36:1544–1550, 1990.

18. Markin RS: Implementing automation in a modern clinical laboratory. *Lab Info Management, Chemometr Intell Lab Sys* 21:169–179, 1993.

19. Markin RS: Clinical laboratory automation: A paradigm shift. *Clin Lab Management Rev* 7:243–251, 1993.

20. Markin RS: Laboratory automation: an introduction to concepts and terminology. *AJCP, Pathol Patterns* 98(Suppl 1):S3–S10, 1992.

21. Markin RS, Sasaki M: A laboratory automation platform: The next robotic step. *Med Lab Observ* 24:24–29, 1992.

12

Automation of Preanalytical Processing and Mobile Robotics

ROBIN A. FELDER

CONTENTS

Handbook of Clinical Automation, Robotics, and Optimization, Edited by Gerald J. Kost with the collaboration of Judith Welsh.
ISBN 0-471-03179-8 © 1996 John Wiley & Sons, Inc.

12.1. SPECIMEN PROCESSING

The rather sudden appearance of pre-analytical specimen processors on the market is a result of fiscal pressures brought on by runaway costs for healthcare delivery.[1] The attention focused on cost containment was also brought on by global recession in the early 1990s. Besides the economic incentives for front-end automation, there are additional benefits of installing advanced automation. Specimen processing is a source of many laboratory errors and consumes a large percentage of the laboratory labor budget. Job satisfaction is often the lowest in this area of the laboratory because of the assembly-line nature of the tasks. There are many opportunities to improve laboratory safety, reduce costs, and improve worker morale by automating central receiving. Furthermore, large reference laboratories must adopt automated systems in order to remain competitive because of the low profit margins. Therefore, many large laboratories such as the Mayo Clinic Commercial Laboratories, Smith Kline Beecham, and MetPath are embarked on multi-million-dollar projects to introduce advanced automation into their laboratories. Fortunately, the recent commercial attention focused on developing automation for this area of the laboratory is improving the number of commercially available systems from which to choose. Instrument manufacturers initially saw this area as a method to maintain customer loyalty by tailoring specimen processing to suit only their analytical instruments. However, the market for robotic specimen processors and sorters has become significant enough in its own right that multivendor platforms will be necessary. Early progress in automating this area of the clinical laboratory has been reviewed and updated in this chapter.[2]

Robotic arms that became available in the early 1980s charmed laboratories into believing that these would provide the solution to laboratory automation. Suddenly, interest has been focused on laboratory automation systems which resemble a factory assembly-line more than the robotic arm.[3,4] In less than 2 years, five commercially available preanalytical processors for the clinical laboratory have become commercially available. An Autolab device is already operational in the Mayo Clinic (Rochester, MN) and two Coulter IDS sample-handling systems are installed in two other sites in the United States (St. Louis, MO and Charlottesville, VA). Following this lead, two Diagnostic companies, Boehringer Mannheim and Olympus America are looking for a first United States installation of advanced clinical laboratory automation systems from Japan. Estimates have projected that up to 40 clinical laboratory sites will have automated systems installed before the end of 1996. Questions most frequently asked by clinical laboratory directors are: What kind of equipment is best for my laboratory, and can I be assured of a successful installation and rapid return on investment. This chapter will focus on this "new wave" technology and attempt to describe the many options that are already commercially available.

Most of the commercially available systems are Japanese in design and manufacture, specifically, the systems offered by Coulter, Hitachi, Olympus America, Toa, Joel, Shimadzu, Nagase, and Aloka. These Japanese systems are modeled after the pioneering work by Masahide Sasaki, M.D. in Kochi, Japan.[3,4] Two other systems, BDC and LAB-*InterLink* are American-made. The LAB-*InterLink* system is also inspired by Dr. Sasaki's work. The Canadian company, Autolab and the German company EFL, have unique preanalytical systems. Individual systems will be described below.

Essential components of a robotic processing system will include a labeling system (see also Section 12.2), vision system (see also Chapter 13), mechanical area (see below) specimen distribution system (see also Section 12.3), centrifugation section, and storage and retrieval. Specimen processing systems will have to deal efficiently with nonstandard containers, leaking specimens, improper labels, stat requests, insufficient quantity, repeat or add-on requests, and fibrin clots, to name only a few. Furthermore, a useful processor will be able to differentiate hemolyzed, icteric, and lipaemic specimens and perform some degree of corrective action early in the accessioning process. The systems that can efficiently handle normal specimen will not be as successful in the market and those that can also deal with the exceptions. As soon as customers get over the initial excitement of watching their first robotic system process all the ideal specimens, they will begin to look carefully at how much of the total workload it will process. Finally, continuous tracking of specimens will be necessary to allow the laboratory to precisely locate any specimen in the system at any time as well as allow physicians to request repeat and additional tests. These features will form the basis of intelligent processing systems of the future.

Mechanical manipulation of specimen containers for sortation and centrifugation can be accompanied by a variety of laboratory robots and/or conveyance systems. Large complex hardware that accomplishes many preanalytical processing and accessioning tasks are available as well as modular devices which will accomplish selected processing steps. Devices are being manufactured to perform specific "laboratory unit operations" (Table 12.1). Accessioning consists of all the processes that take place prior to analysis. Individual components of laboratory automation will be described in the remainder of this chapter.

12.1.1. Carriers

Automation of specimen transportation begins with placing the specimen in a carrier. Most laboratorians can suggest at least two ideal designs for a specimen carrier. Considering the number of laboratorians in the world, the possible configurations of specimen carriers is infinite. Several interesting designs have come to the market as part of analytical instruments or as carriers in large

TABLE 12.1. Laboratory Unit Operations

Unpacking	Unbagging, unboxing, unwrapping, and other steps to actually locate the specimen in the transportation material.
Examination	Checking the medical specimen for breakage, labels, volume, and proper container.
Indentification	Identification of the specimen by reading alphanumeric characters or bar-code label.
Sortation	The process of separating specimens based on analytical method or destination in the laboratory.
Decapping	Removing the cap (Becton Dickinson Vacutainers) or punching the foil (Terumo), or unscrewing the lid (Sarstedt) to gain access to the specimen. this task may also be performed by piercing the cap.
Aliquotting	Creating separate containers with a portion of the original specimen. This is required when the ordered analytical techniques are separated by a geographic distance or on separate analyzers.
Analysis	Performance of hematology, chemistry, microbiology, coagulation, type and cross-match, and other analyses on the specimen.
Storage	Holding the specimen for possible retrieval at refrigerated or frozen temperatures for a specified period according to laboratory policy or government regulations.

automated specimen processors (Fig. 12.1). The Coulter specimen transport carrier or (STC) will carry a test tube of any size upright. The STC is constrained to move within the conveyance system and cannot be removed from the system. This configuration requires the medical specimen to be placed in and removed from the STC. The STC can also carry an insert that will allow it to hold any-size laboratory test tubes in the upright position. The STCs from AutoLab will also carry any size test tubes yet can be removed from the automated system. Furthermore, STCs can be snapped together on either of two sides to form linear or larger two-dimensional (2D) arrays of tubes. LAB-*InterLink* provides a specimen carrier that is individually bar-coded and can carry not only test tubes of many sizes and syringes but also microscope slides, pipette tips, and microtainers. Each carrier is color-coded to indicate the kind of payload it is designed to carry. The specimen carrier configuration has an internal 20-mL geometry that allows the contents of a broken tube to be contained within the carrier. Each rack carries a single specimen, and so the pair become inseparable during the accessing process. The internal geometry of the LAB-*InterLink* carrier allows microscope slides to accompany the original hematology specimen from which it was derived. BDC has created a carrier that holds five tubes. A vertical slot in the carrier provides visual access to the bar code. The primary tube is held in the first position in the BDC carrier while the aliquots are held in the remaining five positions. The flat base prevents tipping on the bench as well as on the conveyor belt.

Two ideological groups are forming in the carrier field: the individualists and

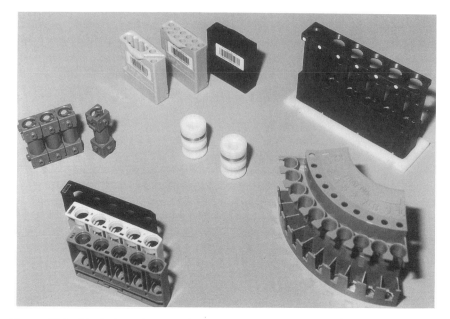

Figure 12.1. Medical specimen carriers come in a variety of shapes and sizes that carry specimens individually, in groups, or options for either. Clockwise from top center: Lab Interlink, BDC, Johnson & Johnson, Hitachi (Boehringer Mannheim), Autolab, Coulter (center of picture). Racks were provided as a courtesy of the manufacturers.

the collectivists. Individualists adhere to the principle that carriers should carry tubes entirely separately, such as the Coulter STC or the LAB-*InterLink* rack. Within this group there are opposing opinions as to whether the rack (LAB-*Inter-Link*) or the tube (Coulter STC) should carry the label. The collectivists, on the other hand, feel that specimens are better carried collectively in groups of five or seven, such as the BDC rack or most analyzer racks. Others play both fields, such as the Autolab Specimen Transport Carriers, which can be used collectively or individually. The best configuration is dependent entirely on the organization of the overall preanalytical, analytical, and postanalytical process.

12.2. BAR CODING

Bar codes have evolved to be the most efficient method to label medical specimens and their daughter aliquot tubes. A variety of bar codes are currently in use in clinical laboratories throughout the United States. Even though bar codes have been used on virtually 100% of products sold in retail stores in the United States, their use on medical specimens is still relatively rare. Estimates provided by Maclin suggest that only 19% of clinical laboratories are employing bar-coded specimens. However, other estimates suggest that over 50% of laboratories use some form of bar code.

The ASTM standard specifies that code 39 or 128 should be used exclusively on medical specimens and that the label should not exceed 60 mm (2.36 in.) in length or 10 mm (0.04 in.) in width. The standard also dictates that all the data contained in the bar code also appear in human readable form except when specially compacted. Furthermore, the alignment zone should be within 62 mm (2.44 in.) measured from the top of the tube.[5] Newer coding schemes are beginning to appear to overcome either the low densities allowed by standard codes or the need for paper labels on tubes. Recently, at the St. Raffaele Hospital in Milan, Italy, Dr. Bonini and Pedrazzinni have developed a laser specimen coding device. One difficulty with bar codes has been consistent automatic application of the label to the tube. The laser labeling device overcomes this difficulty by using a high-powered CO_2 laser to etch the code into the container surface. Users have many choices of bar, dot, or even user-definable codes. Information densities have approached 1 Mbit/cm². Laser codes can be made to be either human-readable at low densities while simultaneously providing higher data density for vision system decoding. Another attractive feature of this proposed system is that the user is not limited by the choice of test tube material. Lasers can etch into glass or a wide variety of plastic containers.

A novel bar code has emerged in recent years that may replace code 39 or 128 as the most common bar code used in the United States. The matrix code (Fig. 12.2) consists of two black bars which intersect at right angles to define the perimeter of the code. Within this boundary, a series of black-and-white squares are written. The pattern of created by the alternating squares can depict very high data densities. Advantages of the matrix code are its ability to be written on curved surfaces, its smaller size relative to code 39 or 128, low-cost printers can be used to print the code, and internal redundancy that allows recovery of data with 20% obliteration of the code. Matrix code has been adopted as a standard by the Japanese Medical Association.

01234567890123456789

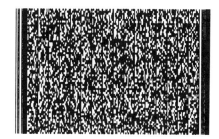

Figure 12.2. Two-dimensional bar codes achieve high data densities in a small surface area. The Matrix code is pictured on the left; on the right, the PDF-427 code.

12.2.1. Bar-Code Reading

Bar-code readers are devices that will interpret the bar-code symbol and communicate the interpreted information to the laboratory system in order to allow an individual or software to make a decision. In their simplest form these devices use a laser or light-emitting diode to illuminate the code and use a light-sensitive diode to receive the reflected pulses of light. Laser or diode readers cannot read bar codes if the bar codes are smudged, torn, or placed incorrectly on the tube (typically 0.5–1% of total specimens). However, bar-code readers are inexpensive devices. More complex devices employing machine vision will check cap color, measure total blood volume, read the bar code in any orientation, and assess quality of the total specimen. In the past, these devices have been too expensive for routine laboratory use; however, reduction in the price of computer power has reduced the price of machine vision systems dramatically, making them more accessible to the clinical laboratory.

Machine vision systems that are designed specifically for clinical laboratory specimens have been developed at LAB-*InterLink* and the University of Virginia. The LAB-*InterLink* device is an integral component to the specimen processing system. The imaging system will determine cap color while a separate laser reads the bar code in 650 ms. Lot-to-lot variation in cap color is accounted for by using a neural network. At the University of Virginia, the Robotics Research Group has developed a device that will function autonomously in the front end of the laboratory to read tubes as they are received in the laboratory. This device is capable of communicating with the LIS to determine whether the specimen has been collected in the proper tube by reading its bar code, cap color, and also determines specimen volume. Postcentrifugation, the UVA vision system will also measure the height of the red cell serum interface.

12.2.2. Sortation

Sortation is the process in which specimens are moved from an input holding area into analytical groups. Sorters usually employ cartesian robots because of their low cost and easy programmability. Either the specimen itself or the specimen in the carrier can also be moved onto the conveyance system with these devices. There are at least three approaches to sorting specimens:

1. The robot can separate specimens into groups according to their destination in the laboratory and then send them down a dedicated line.
2. The conveyance system can make a dynamic sort during the transportation process.
3. The conveyor may be configured as a continuous loop and the analytical instrument will take the appropriate specimens from the conveyor. In the Coulter IDS system (described below) the STCs travel along the conveyor belt taking the appropriate path to their analytical destination.

12.2.3. Centrifugation

With the exception of the spatula, the laboratory centrifuge has undergone less evolution than any other piece of laboratory equipment. Centrifugation has traditionally been a batch process. Several novel concepts in specimen centrifugation have recently been developed to fully automate and/or reduce the time necessary to separate serum or plasma from formed elements.[6-8]. Furthermore, emphasis has been placed on changing the centrifugation into a serial process that is more adaptable to the needs of conveyor belts. William Godolphin, Ph.D, at Vancouver General Hospital, originated the concept of axial separation in which the blood collection tube is spun on its long axis (as if you placed in on a lathe) (Fig. 12.3). Axial separation reduces the time necessary to separate red cells from serum or plasma since they have to traverse only the distance from the center of the tube to the nearest wall. In conventional centrifugation the red cells at the top of the tube have to traverse over half the entire length of the tube before they reach the packed cell layer. Axial separate reduces separation time to one minute and be accomplished in a serial fashion (i.e., one at a time). The axial separation module (centrifuge) can accept up to 10 tubes in its sample introduction tray. Finished tubes accumulate in the output tray. In order to accomplish cell separation on the long axis, a special tube is required which draws blood in through the bottom of the tube. A proprietary phase separator in the tube is pushed down the length of the tube while it is spinning causing the serum to accumulate in the top of the tube and the red cells to remain trapped below the separator. Equivalent chemistries have been demonstrated using this technology. The axial separation module system has been developed by DuPont Canada.

The Kodak PROUD system, developed several years ago, has never been commercialized. The PROUD container is similar in dimension to a Becton Dickinson vacutainer tube, however, it has an internal architecture that allows separation and compartimentalization of erythrocytes and serum. The PROUD container is spun lengthwise, like the axial separation centrifuge, but the axis of spin does not go directly through the middle of the tube. One centrifugation speed is used to separate erythrocytes from serum followed by a higher-speed spin to move the serum into a dedicated and isolated compartment from which the serum can be directly metered onto Kodak chemistry slides.[7]

Nonconventional centrifugation technology that requires proprietary specimen containers will be difficult to sell due to market inertia. Becton Dickinson ™Vacutainers are firmly entrenched in the American medical marketplace. Therefore, much effort has been placed on automating conventional centrifugation. The IDS, Hitachi, and AutoLab automated preanalytical processing systems all have conventional centrifuges with automated loaders and unloaders. The IDS system determines the volume in each vacutainer tube using a scanning device. Specimen tubes are then loaded four at a time into a centrifuge rack. If balancing of a rack is required, a special set of balancing tubes are available to the automated loader. The mass of the centrifugation rotor is sufficient such that precise

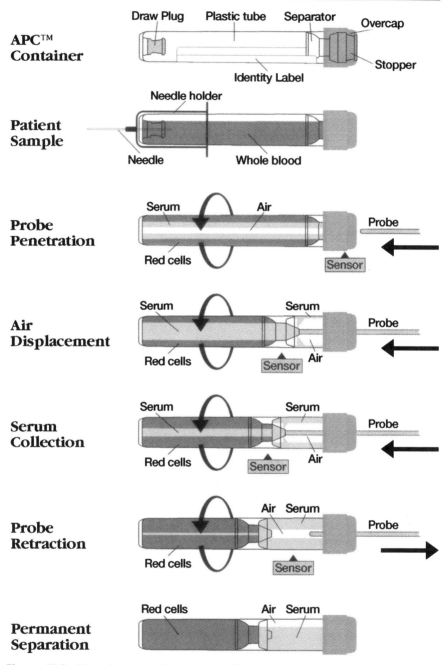

Figure 12.3. The axial separation module offers an efficient new way to obtain and maintain high-quality serum or plasma from whole blood.

balancing is not required. Centrifugation times have been reduced to <2 min because of the large radius of the rotor. After centrifugation the rotor is stopped with a large break to reduce deceleration time. Tubes are than unloaded and placed back on the conveyor belt.

The concept that elimination of the need to balance a centrifuge will reduce the complexity of the task has been the focus of a group of investigators at the Baylor College of Medicine. Dudley and Leu have developed a self balancing centrifuge based on the basic laws of physics described by Archimedes and Pascal.[8] Basically, Archimedes principal demonstrates that a floating object placed in water will displace a volume of water equal to its weight. Pascal's principal demonstrates that when a siphon is created between two buckets of water the water levels will equilibrate between the two buckets. The automatic balancing centrifuge (ABC) uses both principals to cause fluid to flow from one bucket to another on a spinning centrifuge to effectively balance the load. Hitachi Ltd. has also manufactured a dynamic self-balancing centrifuge. Up to 80 specimens may be loaded into the Hitachi Ltd. centrifuge at one time. If an imbalance is created then counterweights are redistributed to balance the load. Rotor radii of 36 inches are used to reduce spin time to approximately 2–5 min.

12.2.4. Electronic Interfacing

Only 50% of laboratories had installed LIS systems in 1993.[9] In order to maximize the efficiency of automated systems, access to patient demographics and tests requests is required through an electronic interface. Using an interface to access patient information, an automated system can decide whether the tube needs centrifugation, how many aliquots are necessary, and the best choice of analytical technique. Interfaces can be unidirectional, bidirectional, or bidirectional with remote control. Unidirectional interfaces simply collect data from the instrument and translates it into a form readable by the LIS. Bidirectional interfaces allow patient identification to be sent to the instrument by the host computer. The instrument usually send back an acknowledgment via an ACK signal or alternately a not acknowledgment signal, NAK. Analytical data is then appended to the patient identification and sent back to the LIS using the same ACK/NAK handshaking protocol. Modern instruments (e.g., the Ciba Corning 850 blood-gas analyzer) will also allow the host computer to control the functions of the instrument. Remote control is essential for instruments which are to be fully incorporated into advanced automation.

12.2.5. Mechanical Interfacing

Rodney Markin proposed a mechanical docking device to provide a consistent mechanical interface between specimen transportation systems and analytical instruments.[10]

12.2.6. Conveyance

Physical movement of specimens around the laboratory can be accomplished in many ways, including human delivery, fixed linear conveyor (conveyor belt), and mobile robot [also called an *automated guided vehicle* or (AGV)]. It has been estimated that the typical medical technologist spends 20% of the day moving specimens around the laboratory. In buildings where laboratories are spread out over a large geographic area, specimen delivery can account for an even larger percentage of technologist time. Laboratory profit originates from the analysis itself, not moving material from one place to another; therefore conveyance should be inexpensive since it does not add value to the data. Conveyor belts are used widely in industry where production schedules are predictable and the time relationship between the input of raw material and output of finished products is calculable. However, many clinical laboratories are not operated like factories because technologists must react to the changing numbers of laboratory requests, additional processing steps, and problem specimens. Furthermore, there are over 80 different types of specimen containers in use in medical facilities and over 250 different analytical tests to be performed. Providing conveyance for a system of this complexity requires flexibility so that specimens can be directed to any point within the laboratory at any time.

When designing conveyance systems the following points should be addressed:

1. Determine accessible pickup and dropoff locations.
2. Map the shortest path between pickup and dropoff points.
3. Determine the method for delivery (conveyors or mobile robots).
4. Program the routing and scheduling of vehicles on the paths and at the pickup and dropoff points.

Many of the commercial systems described later in this chapter have used modified industrial conveyer belts for specimen transportation. Simulation modeling supports this approach as an efficient method to substantially reduce specimen handling. Serial transportation, in which each specimen is treated as a discreet entity, allows specimens to be redirected to their analytical destination. Alternatively, if specimens are sorted into analytical batches in the accessioning section of the laboratory, these batches may be transported to analytical stations. As long as the batches are frequent and keep pace with the analytical instrument, the batch process can resemble serial conveyance. Mobile robots are beginning to be used to provide a flexible transportation scheme for a few laboratories. These flexible devices are particularly useful in laboratories where there is a wide geographic separation between the source and the analytical instrument. Conveyor belts may be too costly to install when distances begin to exceed hundreds of yards or the laboratories are located in another building.

12.3. MOBILE ROBOTS

Several companies offer programmable mobile roots (Table 12.2). Today's mobile robots are capable of riding elevators, opening doors, while not running over patients. Two of the companies listed in Table 12.2 have engineered their robots specifically for the needs of the medical environment.

The TRC Helpmate (Fig. 12.4) is guided through the hospital by following a blueprint of the medical facility that has been downloaded into its computer memory.[11,12] Reflective tape strips are also mounted on the ceiling at selected intervals so that the Helpmate can calibrate its wheel revolutions with the actual location in the building. The orientation of the robot within the hallway is determined by measuring by sonar the distance to both walls, as well as comparing its internal gyroscope with the information obtained by other sensors. The Helpmate is equipped with sensors of various types. Facing forward and to the side are sonar sensors that, like the sonar used by bats, indicate the presence of an object with reflective properties. Patients and inanimate objects can be detected by the sonar sensors. In addition, the robot has a vision system and infrared sensors. If all else fails, the robot has collision bumpers mounted front and rear to prevent the 450-lb device from doing any damage. Emergency stop buttons are also located on either side.

When the Helpmate needs to change floors, it signals a request using a radio transmitter to a modified elevator. The sensor equipped elevator will shut its doors after being vacated and immediately move to the floor occupied by the Helpmate. Humans are prevented from riding the elevator with the robot because it moves very close to the door, effectively blocking entry. As soon as the elevator doors open, the Helpmate warns potential riders to "stand clear." The Helpmate boards the empty elevator, shuts the doors by radio control, and rides to the floor of interest. Once vacated, the elevator is free to return to normal service. Doors are opened by retrofitted mechanical devices that are operated by infrared remote control by the robot. Alternately, the robot can signal an

TABLE 12.2. Mobile Robotics for Laboratories

Company	City/State	App. Cost	Guidance	In Use at
Cyberotocs	Waltham, Massachusetts	$50,000	Ceiling beacons	Layne Clinic
Sauer	Holland, Michigan	$30,000	Clear floor paint	Univ. Nebraska
Denning	Wilmington, Massachusetts	$25,000	Computer/sensor	
Cybermotion	Salem, Virginia	$58,000	Computer/sensors	Kodak
TRC	Danbury, Connecticut	$60,000	Computer/sensors	Univ. Virginia
CCRI	Lake Arrowhead, California	$25,000	Floor tape	Univ. Virginia
Cyberworks	Orillia, Ontario, Canada	$60,000	Sonar	Newtech (Paris)

Contact people: Cybermotion—Ken Stockton CCRI—Don Nagy TRC—John M. Evans.

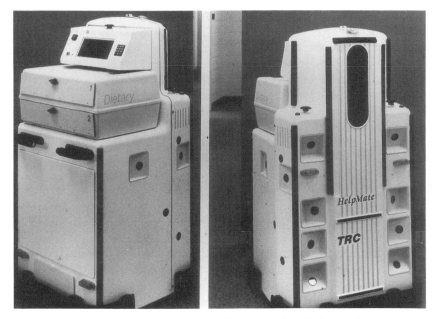

Figure 12.4. The Helpmate mobile robot is pictured as front (left panel) and side views (right panel). Specimens are transported in the box that is accessible through the back. The circular areas on the front and side are sonar sensors. Machine vision and infrared sensors are mounted in the large black oval-shaped areas as well as on top. Collision bumpers and stop buttons are easily accessed to provide safety.

annunciator that will sound an alarm inside a closed door to announce its presence.

If the Helpmate is stranded outside a door (e.g., a hallway door automatically closed during a fire alarm), it will calmly wait while asking for assistance very 15 ss. The Mark I robot offered by TRC has several preprogrammed phrases such as "stand clear" and "please remove obstacle." The next generation robot will allow the users to program their own list of choice phrases. However, the Helpmate makes use of its sophisticated obstacle-avoidance software to do a remarkable job of avoiding getting stuck while en route.

The Helpmate is equipped with a transportation pack with a rear-opening door capable of carrying medical specimens, late food trays, pharmacy orders, and blood transfusion products, to name only a few. The list price of the Helpmate is approximately $70,000. Alternately, the Helpmate may be leased for $6.00 per hour for a minimum of 12 h per day. Nickel cadmium batteries are used to power the Helpmate and usually last 8–10 hs before they must be changed with a fresh set while the original batteries are charged.

At the University of Virginia, the Helpmate was installed to deliver specimens between an outpatient clinic laboratory and a central laboratory. The Helpmate, which spends the night in the basement of the hospital, begins its morning rounds by being loaded with a fresh set of batteries and being sent to its starting point outside the door of the outpatient phlebotomy area. Routine specimens are loaded into the backpack, and the Helpmate is sent on its way via the push of a button. En route it passes through the lines of patients forming at the pharmacy window. Some patients move to a safe distance away when they see it coming; others blankly watch it approach and then move only when the robot tries desperately to chart a path through the line. Although clearly marked on the collision bumpers, "NO STEP," patients watch with amusement as their children climb on to the robot as if it were a ride in an amusement park. Once the Helpmate clears the pharmacy lines, it continues down the hall toward the cafeteria. Helpmate software slows the speed to a crawl as it approaches the bumpy tile floor next to the cafeteria dining area. A group of curious visitors and hospital staff form behind the robot as they observe its progress across the tile floor. An amateur physician–programmer pushes the pause button and attempts in vain to reprogram the on-board computer. After the brief automatic timeout as a result of the pause command, the robot continues down the hall to the elevator lobby. Pulling in close in-front of the elevator, it waits for the elevator software to open the doors. Once the elevator is accessible, the robot sounds a "stand clear" and begins to board. A group of impatient medical students squeeze past the robot and board the elevator at the same time. While in the privacy of the elevator, the medical students push all the buttons, including the emergency stop. Fortunately, they pull the button back out, avoiding total disablement of the robot. At the second floor, the robot exits the elevator, turns down the hall, and proceeds to the main clinical laboratory. After a final pirouette, it announces its presence and awaits further instructions.

For lighter duty applications or for areas where the 450-lb Helpmate cannot fit, the CCRI 2010 mobile cart may be employed (Fig. 12.5). The 2010 carts communicate with a host computer via a wireless local-area network (LAN). Guidance is provided by light sensitive diodes that follow a reflective tape applied to the floor. Drive is provided by two stepper motors attached to independent compliant wheels that can be driven together to propel the cart forward or independently to make the cart rotate on its axis. Even the most crowded laboratories are accessible to the 2010 cart since it has a small footprint and can rotate on its axis. Lead acid batteries are used to power the cart and so perform best when charged frequently after minimal drain. Power pods are therefore provided on the floor so that the robot may dock and charge whenever there is an idle moment. It is estimated that the cart can go for 36 h without a charge; however, the cart will operate continuously for up to 5 years if frequent charges are provided. The wireless LAN technology and scheduling algorithms will allow many 2010 carts to be guided along a maze of intersecting paths.

The $30,000–$40,000 price tag for the 2010 cart is considerably less than that of the TRC Helpmate. However, these two robots have different working domains where they are most comfortable. Buildingwide deliveries are best performed by the TRC because of its autonomous guidance system, ability to ride elevators, and ability to move around obstacles, allowing it to coexist with pa-

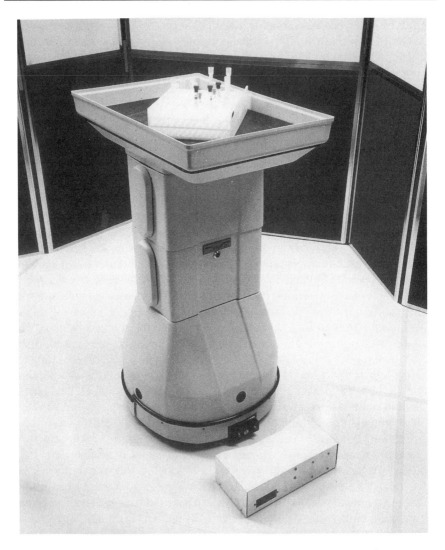

Figure 12.5. The CCRI 2010 cart docks with a power pod mounted on the floor to allow it to operate continuously for years. Its narrow size and height make it ideal for delivering specimens to any area of the laboratory. The 2010 cart operates at a speed similar to that of a briskly moving technologist.

tients with minimal disruption. Intralaboratory deliveries are best performed by the 2010 cart because of its small size; wireless control architecture, which allows it to be called from anywhere in the laboratory; and low cost.

The other commercially available robots have features that are intermediate between the Helpmate and the 2010 cart. Cybermotion has developed a three-wheeled cart (the SR2) that is primarily used for security purposes (Fig. 12.6). It

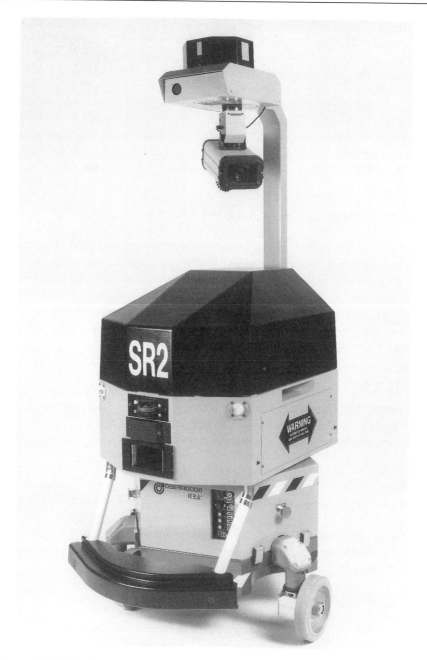

Figure 12.6. The Cybermotion cart is used primarily for security purposes but can also be equipped to deliver specimens.

features a patented SynchroDrive that provides synchronous three-wheeled steering and drive. Cyberworks has also been producing mobile robots for a variety of applications. The G-5 series modular multi-function service robot will travel at 14 in./s (35 cm/s) and weighs approximately 400 lb (185 kg). Panasonic Industrial Systems have a unique feature of a separate cart and drive unit. The Panasonic cart can pull up, hook up a cart, and tow it to a defined location. The Bell & Howell Sprint is being used for clinical specimen delivery by the University of Nebraska Medical Center. This mobile robot follows a clear chemical path on the floor and is also equipped with a collision-avoidance sensor. Its large payload capacity is ideal for long-distance delivery of many specimens.

12.4. COMMERCIALLY AVAILABLE PREANALYTIC SYSTEMS

Eventually, all instrument manufacturers will create standardized docking stations so that their analytical systems will easily couple to preanalytical processors. Until that time, the challenge will be to create customized interfaces (both mechanical and electronic) for each instrument in each laboratory. Customers will be wary of adopting a labwide system from small companies because of their uncertain financial future. Maintaining customized interfaces and mechanics is generally not a profitable venture.

12.4.1. The IDS System

One preanalytical system is the IDS system (Fig. 12.7) [Coulter Corp., 11800 SW 147 Ave., Miami, FL, USA, tel. (305) 380-2652, fax (305) 380-2719]. One of the oldest and most respected names in laboratory diagnostics, Coulter Corporation (Miami, FL), has become the market leader in selling advanced laboratory automation in the United States and Europe. Benefitting from clear foresight, Coulter has formed an alliance with IDS (Kumamoto, Japan) to market their modular laboratory processor and sample distribution system. Specimens are placed into the system in racks in the input area. A cartesian robot removes each tube from the input carriers and places them onto the conveyor belt. The IDS device will transport specimens one at a time down the conveyor belt in individual holders that have a groove around the neck of the holder to retain them within a flange to improve their stability while moving down the conveyor belt.

The IDS system consists of modular conveyors that include mechanical traffic directors and holding areas. The conveyance system can be installed in many configurations to suit the geometry of most laboratories. Additional modules have been engineered to move specimens between floors in an individual specimen elevator. Smaller laboratories may decide to purchase only the centrifugation, aliquotting sections. After the system has placed the specimens in the individual carriers and read their bar codes, the tubes that require centrifugation are sorted from the remainder of the tubes.

Whole-blood tubes for which complete blood counts (CBCs) have been re-

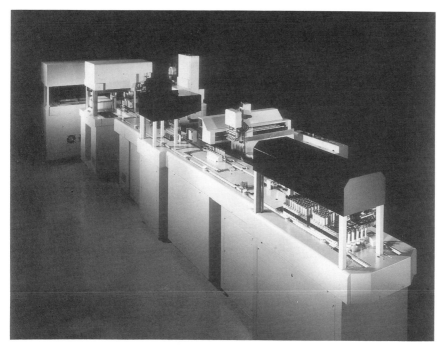

Figure 12.7. The Coulter automated sample preparation–aliquotting system is pictured. Specimens are loaded into the holding area in racks by the technologist. A cartesian robot, which is hidden by the black hood, picks up the tubes and places them into individual specimen carriers. Carriers proceed one at a time down the conveyor belt to the decapping, bar-code reading, serum-level detecting, centrifugation, and aliquotting stations. Technologists can remove the bar-code-labeled products at the other end. (Photo courtesy of Coulter Corp.)

quested are directed to the CBC analyzers. In the configuration currently available from Coulter, the tubes are lifted out of the specimen carriers by a dedicated device. The lifting device also rocks the tube to mix the contents and then inserts it into the *COULTER*®STKS analytical instrument. If the specimen is found to have abnormal results that require verification, it can be automatically shunted into a holding area after being returned to the conveyor mechanism. A manual differential then can be performed. Several automatic slide makers and stainers have already been interfaced to the system including the Omron Slide-maker/Stainer System.

Tubes that require centrifugation are directed to the centrifugation station. The centrifugation module will process up to 500 tubes per hour (see centrifugation above). After centrifugation a cartesian robot picks up five tubes at a time and places them into the laser scanner, which determines the red cell serum interface. In the case of insufficient sample volume, tests are then prioritized based on available serum so that most important tests are performed. The prioritization process takes place using a hierarchical matrix that the user has defined in the computer system. The next step on the conveyor belt is cap removal. The secondary tube labeler and aliquotting units produce bar-code labeled aliquots from the primary tube. The aliquotting module removes the caps and produces up to three labeled aliquots using a disposable tip. Aliquots are now placed into individual tube holders and sent along the conveyor belt for analysis.

Cartesian robots are employed at each analytical station to remove specimens from the carriers and place them directly into analytical instruments that have already been electronically and mechanically interfaced to the system. For instruments that are not linked to the system, a *pipetting station* employing disposable tips is used to load cups and tubes in rotors and racks that may be installed manually into an instrument.

The IDS device interacts in real time with the LIS to gather test request information and match it up with the appropriate tube. Primary tubes and secondary aliquots can be easily located within the system at any time. After the analytical process, the results can be reviewed by the host computer so that problem specimens are automatically sent back into the system for reanalysis or put aside for human intervention. After specimens have been analyzed, they are automatically placed into a refrigerated storage compartment for easy retrieval by robot. The storage capacity of one automated refrigerator is 3000 specimens.

More than 30 successful installations of the IDS system exist in Japan. These include Oita Prefecture Hospital and Tokyo University Hospital, as well as Metropolitan Reference Laboratories (contact David Hoover) in St. Louis, MO (USA).

12.4.2. The Hitachi Clinical Laboratory Integration System

Another preanalytical system is the Hitachi Clinical Laboratory Integration System (Fig. 12.8) [Boehringer Mannheim Corporation, 9115 Hague Road, P.O. Box 50446, Indianapolis, IN 46250-0446, tel. (800) 845-7355, fax (317) 576-4078]. Hitachi has developed a preanalytical processing system that has been used successfully in Japan for several years in over 40 sites. This product differs from the other systems described in this chapter because it is able to offer a full turnkey system to the entire analytical process, including preanalytical process automation devices, analyzers, and laboratory information system. Moreover, Hitachi recently announced the open architecture to hook up several vendors' instruments onto their system. Twelve types of instruments from eight different vendors have already been hooked directly to the systems in Japan. However, it is under a feasibility study to market the open architecture system in the United States. Hitachi instruments and systems will be distributed in the United States by Boehringer Mannheim Diagnostics.

The typical Hitachi system will be installed as a collection of devices connected by conveyor transportation devices. All systems will use the standard Hitachi specimen carrier, which is a five-position rack that accommodates 13 × 75, 13 × 100, 16 × 75, and 16 × 100 tubes. The process starts with up to 60 racks

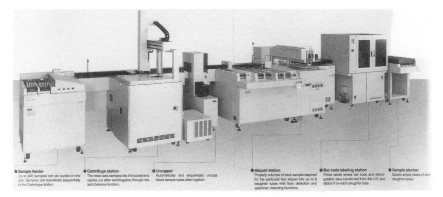

Figure 12.8. The Hitachi Clinical Laboratory Integration System consists of a sample feeder, centrifuge, uncapper, aliquot station, bar-code labeling station, and sample stocker. The aliquotter features the capability to produce eight daughter tubes with fibrin clot detection. (Photo courtesy of Boehringer Mannheim Diagnostics.)

(300 samples) being loaded into the sample feeder. Empty positions must be filled with blanks by the operator if the system includes an automatic centrifuge unit. Primary tubes may be sorted prior to any other specimen processing step. Specimens that require centrifugation will automatically be loaded into this device if necessary. The centrifuge has a 250-sample/h, 60-sample capacity and can be programmed to run when full, after an elapsed time, or stat. Standard spin time is 5 min at 2000g. Samples are then decapped at the rate of 300 tubes per hour. Aliquots in the form of cups, compatible with the online Hitachi analyzers, are prepared using disposable tips to eliminate carryover. Offline aliquots may also be produced in up to eight different forms (≤ 1 mL in volume). Larger volumes are easily accommodated by adding additional cycles. Fibrin clots and gels are automatically detected during the aliquotting process. Hitachi also owns the patents on the use of a spectrophotometer to examine the serum for icterus, hemolysis, or lipaemia. This technique is incorporated into their labwide automation system. Bar codes (code NW7, 39, 128, interleaved 2 of 5) are applied after aliquotting at the rate of 500 samples/h with automatic verification. Caps are then applied to the aliquots in the capper device. Sortation follows the capping step, allowing 500 tubes/h to be sorted into eight output streams. The primary tubes are passed into the specimen storage area or "stocker," which provides full trays for manual transportation to the refrigerator. In Japan they have included the use of specimen storage into an automated refrigerator. Specimen routing and temporary accumulation occurs in the turntable buffer.

System can be controlled by a workstation called "system controller" running under the UNIX environment. The System Controller graphically shows system status and alarms, as well as allowing setup of specimen volumes and sorting channels. Reports are printed at the workstation and electronic data is sent to the host LIS. All routing decisions are made by the system controller. Therefore, there is a single data interface between the integrated automated system and the host LIS that provides the test request and aliquot information and finally the test result. Hitachi can provide full turnkey system automation of the preanalytical processing area as well as whole clinical laboratory work area.

12.4.3. AutoLab Systems

Another group of preanalytical systems is AutoLab Systems [100 International Blvd. Etobicoke, Ontario, Canada, M9W 6J6, tel. (416) 675-4530, fax (416) 213-4086]). AutoLab has been created as the automation division of MDS Health Group Limited, in Etobicoke, Ontario, Canada. AutoLab products have been designed by a team of engineers, information handling specialists, and laboratory technologists to meet the needs of the MDS commercial laboratories, as well as laboratories all over the world. The AutoMed specimen-handling system is a series of modular devices (Fig. 12.9) designed and manufactured by Auto-Med Corporation [140-13120 Vanier Place, Richmond, British Columbia, Canada, V6V 2J2, tel. (604) 279-9293, fax (604) 279-9295] to automate the most labor-intensive tasks in specimen processing. These modules are integrated by Auto-Lab in their total laboratory automation solution. The AutoMed AutoSorter module takes input in the form of specimens placed in specimen transport carriers (STC) (See Section 12.1.1). Each STC is transported into the system, and the bar code is read from the tube. The sorter then moves each STC into a holding area destined for centrifugation or analytical process. The computer driving the system provides visual representation of the sorting process and keeps statistics on the numbers and identity of tubes that have been processed.

The AutoMed centrifuge can operate as a modular unit of receive STCs from the conveyance system. STCs are automatically loaded into the centrifuge. After spinning, the STCs are unloaded and placed in holding areas. The centrifuge has been rated at 64 STCs at one time and has a processing speed of 500 tubes/h. Multiple heads are used to accomplish this throughput.

Aliquotting is preformed automatically in the AutoQuot aliquotting module developed by William Godolphin and associates at AutoMed Corporation (Vancouver, British Columbia). The AutoQuot uses an individual disposable plastic device called a ThruQuot that is inserted through the rubber stopper on the test tube. Tubes are accepted from the conveyor system and placed into an indexing wheel. At the appropriate time, the test tube is inverted and a known quantity of air is injected through the ThruQuot device in the rubber stopper. Serum is then metered out into daughter aliquot tubes from the inverted primary tube. The primary tube must be inverted during this process, therefore, only serum separator tubes can be used. This unique method of dispensing from the primary tube should lend itself ideally to tests that cannot tolerate carryover such as polymerase chain reaction (PCR).

The test tube aliquotter can create as many aliquots as the laboratory demands provided there is enough serum. The AutoQuot is available as a single function unit or may be linked with an AutoSorter module that allows specimen aliquotting followed by sorting for selected analytical stations.

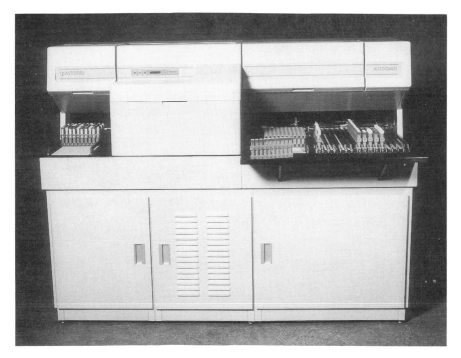

Figure 12.9. The AutoMed AutoQuot modular device will automatically aliquot, label, and sort medical specimens into analytical groups. Specimens can be transported individually in carriers that can be combined into any number of linear or matrix arrays. (Photo courtesy of AutoMed, a division of MDS Health Group.)

12.4.4. LAB-*InterLink*

LAB-InterLink (Fig. 12.10) [LAB-*InterLink*, Inc., 1011 South Saddle Creek Road, Omaha, NE 68106, USA, tel. (402) 449-0449, fax (402) 595-2951] has taken an approach to laboratory automation similar to that of IDS and Hitachi; however, they have some important differences. Each primary tube is placed into a patented individual carrier that carries a bar code that is linked electronically to the primary tube bar code. A series of conveyor rails, gates, elevators, and storage areas allow the carrier to be directed in a random-access manner to any analytical workstation within the laboratory. Positive specimen tracking is accomplished by bar-code readers in the specimen gates placed at periodic intervals along the rail. The system controller can then determine in real time the distribution of specimens in the system and avoid backup and congestion. An optional machine vision module can also determine cap color of each specimen to verify that the specimen was drawn into the correct tube.

The conveyor rails employed by LAB-*InterLink* are different from the conventional conveyor belt used frequently by industry. Each section (available in 10-, 5-, 3-, and 2-ft sections) contains a circular chain of wheels that ride on an internal member. As the chain is driven around this internal member, the wheels

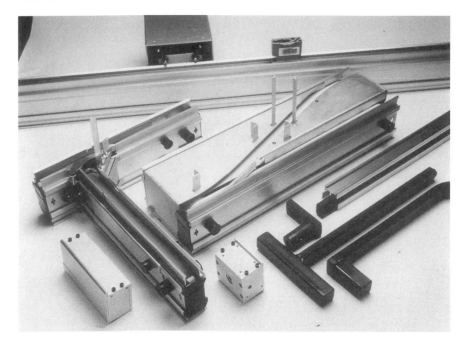

Figure 12.10. The LAB-*InterLink* conveyance system will transport specimens to any area of the laboratory using modular, user-installable conveyors. Conveyors will link to analytical instruments as well as commercially available automated centrifuges.

on the chain turn in the same direction but at a higher revolution. Specimens are effectively propelled along at a speed approximately 2.5 times the speed of the chain revolution. This system reduces friction and noise, however this system is noisier than the IDS, Hitachi, and AutoLab conveyor systems. Although specimen breakage in this system is highly unlikely, the specimen carrier is designed to contain spilled blood, as well as the conveyor and support I-beam. The main trunk of the LAB-*InterLink* conveyance system is suspended from the ceiling in a similar manner as that developed by Masahide Sasaki in Kochi, Japan.[3,4,13–16] LAB-*InterLink* has not yet released a product for integrating automatic specimen centrifugation into the conveyance system.

12.4.5. Rush Presbyterian St. Luke's Medical Center (Chicago, IL)

With over 3000 specimens per day, Kenneth Whisler, Ph.D., has taken a systems approach to laboratory automation. His group has taken a close look at the earliest phase of laboratory testing, namely, assuring proper specimen identification right at the patient bedside. Each patient carries a bar-coded wristband that is checked against the collection list before phlebotomy. The correctly labeled specimens are then loaded onto a conveyor system that dispatches into boxes which are then transported to the correct analytical area of the laboratory.

12.4.6. BDC

BDC [Biomedical Devices Corp., 40 West Howard Unit 404, Pontiac, MI 48058, tel. (810) 335-3535, fax (810) 335-3554] has produced an aliquotting device, the AAS, which has a midrange throughput of 300 primary tubes per hour if two aliquots are being made or 180 tubes per hour if five aliquots are made. The AAS was built for the Smith Kline Beecham Laboratories in Conshohocken, PA. Primary tubes are placed in six-position carriers that have an open architecture that allow bar-code reading. After reading the bar code on the primary tube, secondary tubes are automatically labeled with labels according to user specification (e.g., either identical to primary tube or different for each tube) after the system communicates with the LIS. After labeling the system again reads the bar code of the secondary tubes to verify correct label printing and placement. A special disposable cap piercing device is then automatically inserted through the rubber stopper in each primary vacutainer tube to allow closed primary tube sampling. The primary tube is then inverted automatically, and then positive pressure is applied to the contents of the primary tube to dispense a measured volume of serum into the secondary tubes. Since the primary tube must be inverted, only tubes containing serum separator may be used in this system.

The inserted device is similar in function to the ThruQuot developed by Andronics (see Section 12.4.3). Recent difficulty over potential patent infringement will have to be resolved. The BDC labeling technology, however, remains a proven reliable method to label specimen tubes.

12.4.7. Olympus

Olympus (Olympus America Inc., Clinical Instrument Division) has imported the Oasys (Fig. 12.11), a fully automated aliquotting system from Japan. This high-capacity system consists of an autoloader, sorter, and aliquotter. The autoloader will hold up to 300 primary tubes in 25 racks. Tubes are then transported by conveyor belt to an optical device that performs bar-code reading. The tube is then split into five or fewer bar-coded aliquot tubes. The system is one of the highest capacity systems on the market with a processing speed of 300 primary tubes split into 900 aliquots each hour. The system also has a sorter unit that can sort the aliquots into 50 user-defined bins.

Olympus America is also planning on importing a series of automated devices used currently in Japan. This line of products provides some of the highest capacity and throughput capabilities on the market today. Specific descriptions of these systems appear in Table 12.3.

12.4.8. EFL

EFL (Fig. 12.12) (EFL/Technidata, Entwicklung + Service fur Labortechnik GmbH Schillingsweg 15, 77633 Lahr/Schwarzwald, Germany) is a relatively new company that is becoming involved in clinical laboratory automation. They have

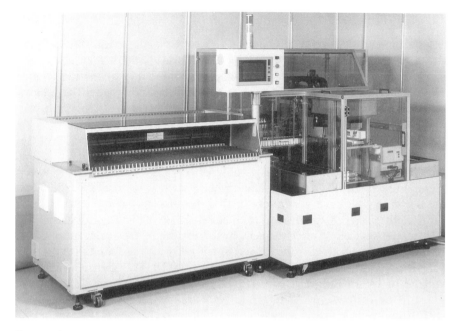

Figure 12.11. The Oasys offered by Olympus America will automatically aliquot primary specimen tubes into labeled secondary tubes at a rate of 300 tubes per hour. The finished tubes are available in a presorted format for easy transport to analytical instruments.

recently introduced the PV 3000, which is an automated sample splitting and distribution platform that employs a continuous conveyor belt in the form of a chain. The principal features of the system are a series of robotic devices that remove aliquots from specimens in the daisy chain and load them into rotors or racks, prefilled by technologists with labeled aliquots, for a wide variety of clinical analyzers. Inherent in the system is a high degree of flexibility in incorporating different clinical analyzer racks. Following centrifugation the tubes are manually placed into an open position on the conveyor chain. Optional modules will remove either Becton Dickinson Vacutainer caps or Sarstedt Monvette caps or provide clot detection and serum level detection. The PV 3000 uses a number of robotic arms for specimen splitting and loading into empty cups which have been pre-loaded into analyzer racks.

Throughput of the PV 3000 is in excess of 900 primary tubes per hour, but this figure can be doubled with double-armed manipulators. The system maintains continuous communication with the laboratory LIMS to provide distribution lists of racks, tubes, volumes, and error messages for each robotic workstation. Pipetting can be performed with either disposable tips or may use a washing unit to allow reuse of tips for less demanding analyses. Object-oriented software is used

TABLE 12.3. Preanalytical Processors

Company	Modules	Throughput and Features
A & T Clinlog	Stocker	1800/h
	Rackbuffer	3000/h
	Centrifuge	350/h
	Aliquotter	350/h
Autolab	Sorter	
	Centrifuge	500/h
	Aliquotter	
	Conveyance	Belt
	Carrier	Flexible single or group
Biomedical Devices	Robotic workcells	
Corporation (BDC)	Conveyance	"Silent chain"
	Aliquotter	
	Carrier	7-position rack
Daisen Sangyo Co.	Terume test-tube opener	4500/h
ELF Sample Distribution System	Conveyance	Chain
Hitachi	Uncapper	350/h
	Centrifuge	250/h
	Recapper	400/h
	Aliquotter	300/h
	Sorter	1000/h
	Stocker	600/h
	Refrigerator	300/h; cap 3000
	Conveyance	Belt
	Carrier	5-position rack
LAB-*InterLink*	Carrier	Individual
	Conveyance	Belt
	Robotic workcells	
Nagase	Aliquotter	340/h
	Centrifuge	550/h
	Stocker	300/h
	Robotic arm	150/h into Ektachem
	Conveyance	Belt
	Carrier	5-position rack
Nipro Co. Ltd.	Centrifuge	300/h
	Aliquotter	350/h
Olympus	Input device	940/h
	Decapper	940/h
	Centrifuge	480/h
	Aliquotter	9.80/h
	Conveyance	Belt
	Carrier	10-position rack
Shimadzo	Automated laboratory	120/h

(*continued*)

TABLE 12.3. *(Continued)*

Company	Modules	Throughput and Features
Sysmex	CBC/WBC differential system	120/h
	Reticulocyte System	80/h
	Slide film preparation	120/h
	Conveyance	Belt
Technomedica	Test-tube bar-code labeller	360/h

throughout the system running under the NeXTSTEP operating system. The system pictured in Figure 12.12 costs approximately $200,000.

12.4.9. Sysmex

At Sysmex (Fig. 12.13) [Sysmex Corp., Gilmer Road, 6699 RFD, Long Grove, IL 60047-9596, tel. (708) 726-3530, fax (708) 726-3505], major strides are being

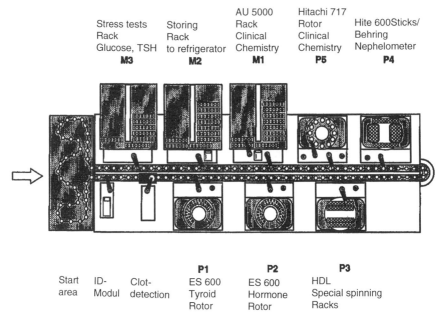

Figure 12.12. The EFL PV-3000 platform is an automated specimen distribution and splitting platform that employs a continuous conveyor belt in the form of a chain. Pictured is an overhead diagram of the system featuring an input area on the left and individual robotic devices that sample from the open tubes and transfer the aliquots to rotors and racks for analytical instruments.

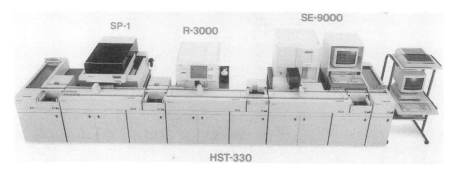

Figure 12.13. The Sysmex HST-330 is a completely automated hematology system capable of performing 120 CBC/WBC differentials per hour. In addition, it will perform 80 reticulocyte analyses, and 120 film preparations per hour. (Sp-1 = selective blood film preparation; R-3000 = reticulocyte analyzer; SE-9000 = CBC analyzer.)

made in the automation of the measurement of hematologic parameters such as erythrocyte, platelet, and white blood cell differentials in whole blood. The complete blood count (CBC) usually constitutes 30–50% of the average workload of a clinical laboratory. Since the CBC is performed on whole blood, there is little need for preanalytical processing of these specimens. Therefore, the efficiency of preanalytical processing can be dramatically improved by shunting these specimens as soon as possible to their own conveyance system after sortation.

The hematologic parameters measured in the CBC cannot be fully defined by cell counting hematology instruments. Therefore, the manual differential remains a necessary part of the hematologic profile for some patients. As a result of the need for manual differentials, additional instruments have become available that will create a blood film on a microscope slide ready for staining and viewing under the microscope.

Sysmex (a division of Toa Medical Electronics Co., LTD, Kobe, Japan) has developed the HST-series for complete automation of hematology including the CBC, white blood cell (WBC) differential, reticulocyte analysis, and blood film preparation. This modular unit consists of the SE-9000 CBC/WBCdiff instrument, R-3000 automated reticulocyte analyzer, and SP-1 slide preparer unit. Each of these instruments can be coupled in flexible configurations to an intelligent sample transportation system.

The automated process is started by generating a request for blood analyses on each specimen either manually by an operator or downloaded from the LIS. Specimens are placed into carriers that accommodate up to 10 specimens and can be accumulated in the preanalytical holding area (unlimited tube capacity). The computer that controls the system will then direct the rack to the appropriate analyzer on the basis of the tests requested. Bar-code readers are incorporated into the system to provide positive specimen identification. Current status of each specimen is available on the computer monitor, via a printed page, or directly transmitted to a laboratorywide process controller. The entire process can be interrupted at any time for emergency stat specimens. Once the automated hematology tests are completed, the positive specimens can be automatically directed to the SP-1, which prepares blood films prior to the manual differential performed by a technologist. The system depicted in Figure 12.13 has a throughput of 120 tubes per hour with the exception of the reticulocyte instrument, which has a throughput of 80 samples per hour. However, total system throughput is a factor of configuration.

The slide preparer can prepare a standard wedge smear by placing a drop of blood on the slide followed by dragging a coverslip across the drop to distribute it to create an increasing cell density wedge. The slide preparer can vary the amount of blood in the drop depending on the results of the CBC to provide optimal smear uniformity. A duplicate of the specimen identification number is then printed on each slide. Up to 300 slides can be made without the need for operator replenishment of slide cassettes. The finished slides are automatically placed in staining baskets that are removed by a human operator[17,18] and placed on commercially available automatic dip strainers to complete the staining process.

12.5. RELIABILITY AND MAINTENANCE

The systems described in this chapter have a high degree of complexity, which suggests that some of the labor savings accomplished by installing automation may be lost with increased maintenance costs. Stuart Wills, Manager of Coulter Worldwide Automation Systems, indicates that service will be required approximately every 10 months. Similar mean-time-between-failure (MTBF) data has been quoted by managers of the AutoMed 100 product. We will know how reliable these systems are only after significant experience has been gained from the different installation sites. It is expected that maintenance rates will differ from laboratory to laboratory based on the engineering expertise of the technologists. Furthermore, cultural differences are expected to influence maintenance rates since the United States and many developing countries do not have the technical expertise to support complex automation. Digital electronic and mechanical device troubleshooting are not currently components of the medical technology curriculum in the United States and Europe. In Japan, on the other hand, a greater number of medical technologists are trained to program computers and service these new devices.

LAB-*InterLink* has developed a training program that assists on site engineers and medical technologists in system repair using a step by step multimedia system. This novel approach may save LAB-*InterLink* thousands of dollars in supporting on site repair and save the clinical laboratory down time. Ideally, a combination of remote system monitoring by the vendor using modem links as well as multimedia training could virtually eliminate the need for repair staff.

12.6. FAULT TOLERANCE

Fault tolerant techniques are beginning to be understood and implemented into clinical laboratory automation. There are two basic objectives to fault tolerance: maintaining data integrity (assuring that data is not changed or destroyed) and data availability (assuring access to data despite failures). Fault tolerance can be achieved using protection, redundancy, and recovery methods. Data protection avoids predictable failures by creating systems with power protection and low-failure, high-quality engineering. Redundancy is provided by duplicate systems that will automatically activate on the failure of the primary system. If the protected redundant system fails, a recovery process is initiated to restore access to data.

Detecting errors is the foundation of fault-tolerant systems. Various methods are used to determine errors in data transmission including checksums and parity, timing checks, and self-checking logic (i.e., voting logic). Detecting power supply failures is another example of error detection. Uninterruptable power supplies have become affordable in recent years. These devices will automatically switch from line power to a battery backup should power failure occur. Disk mirroring, sending data to two disks at the same time, is used to protect data during hard-disk crashes. System failures that occur at the software level are caught and handled by special BIOS (basic input/output system) software that can intercept fatal errors and provide an orderly transition to a backup computer.

12.7. SUMMARY AND CONCLUSION

Laboratory robotics are one of many important solutions to healthcare cost containment. The added benefits, in addition to the cost savings, are improved precision, reduced turnaround, better worker morale, and improved laboratory safety. Although difficult to quantitate, improved analytical results will produce healthier patients at lower costs. This will result in further cost savings over those realized by the reduced requirement for labor and reagents. As more clinical laboratory scientists become familiar with advanced automation and robotics, the groundwork will be laid for the creation of flexible laboratories that will be adaptable to increasing future production as well as integrate into a larger networking production structure.

REFERENCES

1. Algeo LA: Financial pressure spurring move to introduce lab automation. *Adv News Mag* 5:8–9, 1993.
2. Felder RA, Boyd JC, Margrey KS, Holman W, Roberts J, Savory J: Robots in health care. *Anal Chem* 63:741A–747A, 1991.

3. Sasaki M: A fully automated clinical laboratory. *Lab Info Management* 21:159–168, 1993.

4. Sasaki M: An innovative conveyor belt system for a clinical laboratory. *IFCC* 3:31–33, 1991.

5. Standard specification for use of bar codes on specimen tubes in the clinical laboratory. ASTM Designation E1466-92.

6. Godolphin W, Bodtker K, Uyeno D, Goh L: Automated blood-sample handling in the clinical laboratory. *Clin Chem* 36:1551–1555, 1991.

7. Columbus RL, Palmer HJ: The integrated blood-collection system as a vehicle into complete clinical laboratory automation. *Clin Chem* 36:1548–1556, 1991.

8. Dudley AW, Lin JJ, Leu NC: Automatic balancing centrifuge (ABC). Poster presentation at the 1994 ASCP/CAP spring meeting.

9. Maclin E: Riding the next wave of laboratory automation: specimen handling. *Clin Chem News* 19:1–4, 1994.

10. Markin RS: Challenging the future clinical laboratory automation: a paradigm shift. *Clin Lab Management Rev*, Vol. 7, no. 3 /4 May–June:23–251, 1993.

11. Lob SW: Robotic transportation. *Clin Chem* 36:1544–1550, 1990.

12. Evans J, Krishnamurthy B, Pong W, et al: Creating smart robots for hospitals. Robots Conference (13th: 1989: Gaithersburg, Md.) Robots 13: conference proceedings, May 7–11, 1989, Gaithersburg, Maryland sponsored by *Society of Manufacturing Engineers,* Robotics International of SME. Dearborn, Mich.: Society of Manufacturing Engineers, c1989. UCI Sci Lib TJ210.3 .R65 1989 Bar.

13. Sasaki M: The belt line system; a complete automatic clinical laboratory using a sample transportation system. *Jpn J Clin Pathol* 32:119–126, 1984. (In Japanese.)

14. Sasaki M, Sonobe H, Koresawa S, Nishida M: An attempt at transporting laboratory samples. The establishment and further development of the belt line system. *Jpn J Clin Lab Auto* 10:82–90, 1985. (In Japanese.)

15. Sasaki M: The robotic system of the clinical laboratory. *Jpn J Clin Pathol* 35:1072–1078, 1987. (In Japanese.)

16. Sasaki M: How to make and manage clinical laboratory systems using robotic facilities. In Okuda K, ed: *Automation and New Technology in the Clinical Laboratory, Proc IUPAC 3rd Internatl Congress,* Kobe, Japan. (London: Blackwell Scientific Publications, 1988, pp 97–101.

17. Fernandes BJ, Abbott D, Pritzker KPH, Musclow E, Ray P, Atkinson J: Advanced laboratory systemization utilizing the HS-302. *Sysmex J Internatl* 3:154–159, 1993.

18. Kikuchi T, Okada K, Okayama N, et al: Evaluation of the NE-Alpha Integrated hematology system. *Sysmex J Internatl* 3:135–143, 1993.

13

Machine Vision in Laboratory Automation: Fundamentals and Applications

JOHN E. AGAPAKIS AND SARATH KRISHNASWAMY

CONTENTS

Handbook of Clinical Automation, Robotics, and Optimization, Edited by Gerald J. Kost with the collaboration of Judith Welsh.
ISBN 0-471-03179-8 © 1996 John Wiley & Sons, Inc.

13.1. INTRODUCTION

Over the past 10–15 years, machine vision—the extraction of useful symbolic descriptions from video images—has matured as a technology and is now considered an indispensable tool for manufacturing automation. Such manufacturing applications of machine vision include part presence/absence detection, part location and orientation determination, part recognition, quality inspection, precise two-dimensional (2D) or three-dimensional (3D) gauging, robot or other machine guidance, and process control. Machine vision applications are now common in industries that range from defense, aerospace, and electronics to automotive, pharmaceuticals, and consumer goods.

As the use of robotic automation in the laboratory becomes more widespread, the need for and application of machine vision technology has also expanded. Machine vision has been used in pharmaceutical research laboratories in automated compound screening applications for labware inspection, dissolution testing, procedure validation, and colony picking.[1,2] Most recently machine vision technology has also been used in DNA mapping & sequencing automation applications for colony picking, labware inspection, assay evaluation, and machine guidance.[3,4]

In recent years automated systems have been implemented in the clinical laboratory, driven by the increasing need to reduce costs, improve the quality and efficiency of laboratory tests, and protect human technicians from potentially hazardous clinical samples. Robotic sample handling systems have been used to increase the throughput of the clinical laboratory while minimizing exposure of personnel to samples.[5,6] As areas in the clinical laboratory become more automated, new applications for machine vision technology to facilitate automation have emerged. These applications range from sample identification and verification to evaluation of colorimetric information and feedback to automated sample-handling systems.

In this chapter we will present both the basics as well as examples of these emerging applications of machine vision in the automated laboratory. We will begin by giving an overview of a general-purpose machine vision system, describing how such a system is configured and some of the theory behind image processing and analysis—particularly those image processing/analysis algorithms relevant to laboratory applications. We will then describe applications of machine vision in the laboratory, examining how machine vision can be used for analytical purposes, quality control, and robot guidance.

13.2. MACHINE VISION FUNDAMENTALS

Machine vision systems are used to analyze images and produce useful symbolic descriptions of the scene or object being imaged. These descriptions are then used as sensory feedback necessary in carrying out some operation or task on the objects in the scene. For example, such symbolic descriptions could include a boolean (TRUE/FALSE) variable indicating the presence or absence of an object, a critical dimension of such an object that could be used to decide whether it is within tolerances, or its location and orientation that would allow a robot to grasp it.

13.2.1. Machine Vision System Architecture

The overall architecture of a machine vision system is schematically depicted in Figure 13.1. Such a system must perform the following four basic functions:

- Image acquisition
- Image processing
- Image analysis
- Interfacing to other equipment

Image acquisition is the process by which an image of the object or scene of interest is formed and converted to a digital representation that can be manipulated and interpreted by a computer. In general, light from the objects in the scene is first focused on the image sensor through the camera lens, and an electrical video signal is produced by the image sensor inside the camera; this video signal is digitized by the A/D (analog-to-digital) converter and turned into a 2D array of discrete intensity values in computer memory. This array of discrete intensity values forms the digital image, which may then be processed to produce other images and analyzed to produce useful symbolic descriptions from them.

Before the image in memory can be analyzed to generate any useful symbolic descriptions, it may be desirable to process the original image and generate new images in order to accentuate features of interest that must be extracted by the image analysis operations that follow (image preprocessing), improve the image quality by improving contrast or reducing noise (image enhancement), or eliminate the undesirable effects of image formation problems such as blurring, defocusing, or motion smear (image restoration). These operations produce a new image (output) from the original image (input) and are referred to as *image processing* operations. Image processing finds applications not only as a

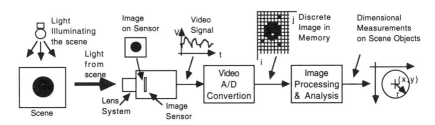

Figure 13.1. Idealized block diagram of a general-purpose machine vision system.

machine vision preprocessing step but also as a means to improve the ability of a person to interpret an image as, for example, in the case of enhancing x-ray images interpreted manually by a technician. It should be noted that in many machine vision applications, where the scene is constrained and lighting and image formation are carefully controlled, image preprocessing may not be always necessary.

The subsequent step of *image analysis* will extract the required useful symbolic descriptions from the original or preprocessed images. Such descriptions may be very simple (e.g., whether the part is present or absent) or very complex depending on the application. Often the ultimate result of image analysis is not only the extraction of features from the image but also the computation of real-world dimensional measurements. So, for example, it may not be sufficient to simply report back that the circular feature found in the image has a diameter equal to half the vertical size of the image but that the diameter of the circular object that was imaged is 5 mm or 7.5 m. This final step requires that sensor calibration information be available to allow mapping between the image and the real world.

Simple examples of image processing and analysis operations are shown schematically in Figure 13.2, where noise is first removed from the image, whereupon the boundaries of scene objects are then detected and used for the generation of the symbolic descriptions, which in this example are the real-world location and size of the circular feature.

It should be noted that the above mentioned image processing and analysis operations need not be applied to the entire image, but rather only one small region, which is typically referred to as a *region of interest* (ROI). Different processing or analysis operations can actually be applied to different regions of interest within the same image. The ROIs are typically rectangular but some machine vision systems allow the users to specify arbitrarily shaped ROIs using a graphical ROI drawing–editing tool. An example is shown in Figure 13.3.

Finally, a machine vision system typically allows *interfacing to other computers or equipment* that may be used to perform certain actions or tasks based on the vision feedback. Such interfacing may be as simple as a digital input line to trigger a vision inspection and one or more digital output lines set to high or low depending on the results of the inspection, or more complicated

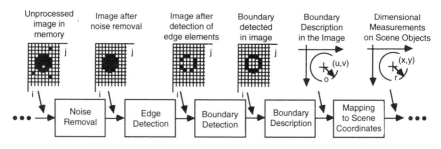

Figure 13.2. *Sample image processing and image analysis operations.*

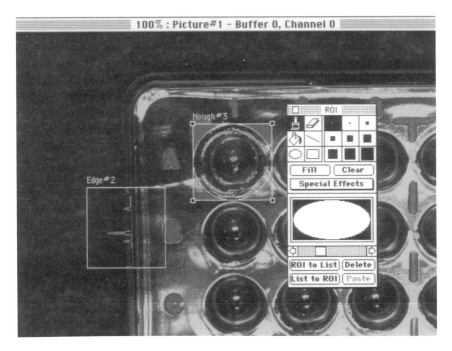

Figure 13.3. Microwell plate inspection. A rectangular ROI is used to find the edge of the plate, while an ROI with a circular mask is used for image analysis at the well. An ROI drawing tool is used to edit the mask.

involving, for example, communications to other computers over a serial line or a network connection.

Early machine vision systems were implemented on proprietary hardware and software platforms. Custom processing hardware was often incorporated to deal with the extensive image processing and analysis operations. This made such early systems expensive and difficult to use. More recently, the ever-increasing power and wide proliferation of personal computers have allowed the implementation of powerful and cost-effective machine vision solutions on such standard computer platforms. The price/performance ratios of such systems are continuously improving with every successive CPU generation. For example, the introduction of computers based on PowerPC RISC (reduced instruction set computer) CPUs in 1994 and their use in Acuity Imaging machine vision systems has resulted in a 3–12 times performance improvement in image processing and analysis operations as compared to the previous generation of CISC (complex instruction set computer)-CPU based systems. In addition, such open architecture systems also allow building powerful graphical user interfaces under industry-standard windowing environments and offer expandability through third-party hardware and software products.

The basics of image acquisition, image processing, and image analysis are discussed in some more detail in the following subsections.

13.2.2. Image Acquisition

This process typically involves the three basic steps of *image formation, image sensing,* and *image digitization.*

13.2.2.1. IMAGE FORMATION. Image formation refers to the process of capturing the light emitted from scene objects and focusing it on a sensing device where an image of the scene is formed. This is primarily the function of a lens in a camera. Understanding and modeling of the image formation process is important because extracting a symbolic description from an image can be thought of as the inverse process of image formation. Also, in applications where we can significantly constrain the environment, proper selection of the optics and/or the lighting approach can sometimes make a seemingly impossible machine vision task tractable. In general, models of the image formation process must provide answers to two questions:

- Where will the image of a known object be formed?
- How bright will such an image be?

Geometric optics are typically sufficient to provide an answer to the first question. Pinhole optics, the perspective transformation, and the simple paraxial formulas relating object distance, image distance, and focal length of the lens are the essential tools that most users of machine vision will need for this purpose. However, any further detailed exposition of optics fundamentals is outside the scope of this chapter. The reader is instead referred to the many excellent texts on optics[7,8] or review papers on optics[9,10] for machine vision. Another excellent source of information on optics is catalogs from vendors.[11]

The second question is the subject of photometry. For this treatment it is sufficient to mention that the brightness of the image is generally proportional to the brightness of the scene, and this, in turn, is related to both the illumination as well as the surface condition (diffuse or mirrorlike) of the object surface and its orientation with respect to the direction of incident illumination and direction of viewing. The image brightness is also proportional to the square of the lens *f*-number (the ratio of the lens opening and its focal length).

In practical terms, a user of machine vision will be faced with the selection of at least

- A lighting approach
- Light source(s)
- Optics (lenses and filters)

Some of the basic lighting schemes that may be employed include (shown in Fig. 13.4)

- Directional backlighting, which will produce a dark silhouette of the shape of the object—no surface detail will be visible.
- Directional frontlighting (dark or bright field produced with a camera at a low angle or in the same general orientation with the camera), and which will result in producing specular reflections or casting shadows that can be exploited in subsequent image analysis.
- Diffuse illumination using noncollimated lighting, which results in no shadows or specular reflections.

For light sources, some of the many options may include: conventional incandescent bulbs, fluorescent bulbs, xenon flash tubes, or LED (light-emitting diode) strobes, which freeze a moving object, lasers, infrared LEDs, x-ray tubes, and so on. Selections may depend on whether the object is stationary, whether it fluoresces, and other variables.

In terms of optics, decisions that must be made at a minimum include the type of lens (fixed-focal-length, zoom, macro, etc.), the lens focal length and f-number, the aperture (opening) of the lens, as well as the optics placement with respect to the part. These decisions will be determined by, and will thus affect, the magnification (the ratio of image to object size), the extent (width and height) of the field-of-view (the section of the scene visible by the sensor through the lens), the depth of field-of-view (the range around the distance of perfect focus within which objects are still in acceptable focus), and the brightness of the image. Again material found in some of the previously mentioned references coupled with a dose of trial-and-error can provide some of the required insight.

13.2.2.2. IMAGE SENSING. Most image sensors used in electronic imaging systems produce an electrical signal—a time-varying voltage level—whose instantaneous value corresponds to the image intensity under a point that is scanned across the image. This scanning—referred to as *raster scanning*—is what allows us to represent a 2D entity—the image intensity—in the form of a one-dimensional time-based signal. This signal is referred to as a video signal and commonly follows standards set by the television broadcasting industry. In conjunction to the intensity information, such a signal also typically contains timing pulses used to synchronize the beam scanning circuitry of a display device (composite video). A detailed description of such signals is beyond the scope of this chapter. However, references provide sufficient information on video signal concepts and standards.[12–14]

The video signal that is output from the sensor is produced by appropriately scanning in a rasterlike fashion some photosensitive surface where the distribu-

DIRECTIONAL
BACKLIGHT

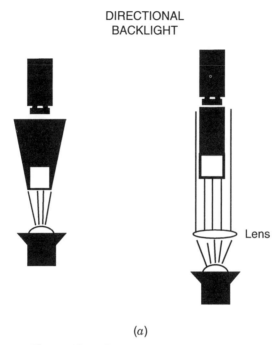

(a)

Figure 13.4. Common lighting approaches.

tion of electrical charges corresponds to the intensity distribution being sensed. Different image sensing devices employ different principles for the generation of such electrical charges. In general, mostly all image sensors depend on the generation of electron–hole pairs when photons strike a suitable material. Vacuum-tube based sensors (such as vidicon tubes found in low-cost surveillance cameras) employ electrons liberated from a heated cathode and scanned across the surface of a photosensitive target surface. There, differences in light intensity are translated to resistance changes. Thus a time-varying current flowing between the cathode and the target electrode is produced. In solid-state imaging devices (such as the most widely used CCDs, i.e., charge coupled devices), an array of discrete photosensitive elements isolated from each other and arranged in a grid forms the sensor surface. Electron–hole pairs are produced in each site in correspondence to the amount of light that has fallen at that particular location. Photoelectrons produced in each site move into an adjoining potential well and are shifted through charge coupling in a row-by-row fashion out of the sensor in the form of a conventional video signal. An alternative solid-state sensor configuration is in the form of a linear array. A 2D image is produced a line at a time by moving the part with respect to this line scan camera. More details can be found in the references.[8,12]

Solid-state sensors are preferable to tube-based sensors for machine vision applications because they (1) show little geometric distortion since the array of

DIRECTIONAL FRONT
LIGHTING

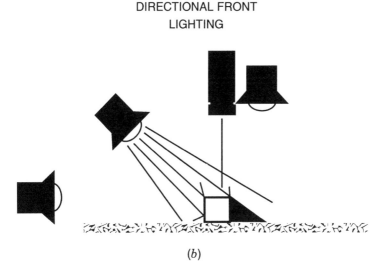

(b)

DIFFUSED TOP LIGHTING

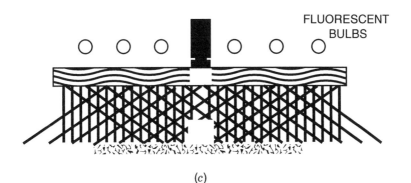

FLUORESCENT
BULBS

(c)

Figure 13.4. (*Continued*)

light-sensing elements is permanently built into the wafer and the location of the elements does not depend on beam scanning; (2) show immunity to mechanical vibration and shock; (3) are not affected by stray voltages and magnetic fields; (4) show rather low noise and high sensitivity; show low lag, burn, or sticking under bright illumination; (5) are more compact and more rugged than tube sensors; and (6) consume much less electrical power.

13.2.2.3. IMAGE DIGITIZATION. The video signal produced by the sensor must be *digitized* in order to be used in a computer. This is accomplished using a video A/D (analog-to-digital) converter that samples at a high speed the analog video signal and produces digital codes representing samples of the video signal

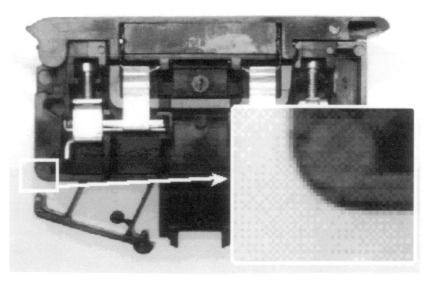

Figure 13.5. Digitized image is stored as a 2D array of discrete intensity values in computer memory.

value at discrete intervals along each raster scan line. The sampled signal is quantized in both time and value and thus produces a 2D array of discrete intensity levels (Fig. 13.5). These levels correspond to the distribution of intensities on the image sensor and thus the original scene which gave rise to the image.

The numbers of elements—also referred to as picture elements or *pixels*—in this discrete grid determines the *nominal spatial resolution* (see Fig. 13.6) of the digital imaging system or how well small details are reproduced. Since the intensity value for each pixel is the average intensity over the area covered by the pixel, details smaller than a pixel are not preserved in the digital image.* To increase resolution, we can either increase the number of pixels or reduce the field of view of the optics and thus use the same number of pixels over a smaller area of the object. This can be accomplished by bringing the lens closer to the object or by using a lens of a longer focal length.

The discrete levels of intensity that each pixel can take are referred to as *gray levels*. The number of gray levels determines the intensity or *gray-scale resolution* of the image and thus dictates how well the continuous variation of intensities of a natural scene is reproduced. The number of pixel elements and gray levels is determined by the available memory and the capabilities of the video A/D converter. Machine vision systems today commonly offer 640 × 480 spatial and 8-bit (256-level) gray-scale resolution.

*Actually, most image analysis schemes that are presented later in this chapter allow recovery of detail better than a pixel (subpixel resolution), often as low as 25% or 10% of a pixel.

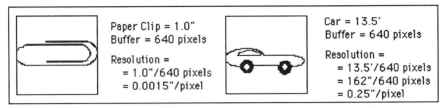

Figure 13.6. Two examples of computing nominal horizontal spatial resolution.

The gray-scale resolution as defined above is a characteristic of the vision system. The exact distribution of such values depends on the image. An *intensity histogram* provides a graphical representation of the distribution of gray-level intensities in the whole image or a localized region of interest. The histogram, which can be regarded as a discrete intensity probability distribution function, provides the number—or percentage—of pixels with intensities falling within each of a number of ranges of intensity values (the histogram bins). The distribution of pixels across different intensities in the histogram (see Fig. 13.7) provides important information about the image. For example, a histogram in which all image intensities are compressed in one cluster of low values signifies a dark image with a compressed dynamic range. As will be discussed in a later section, there are various techniques for expanding this range and thus making more image detail recognizable.

13.2.2.4. CAMERA CALIBRATION. Calibration of the camera is essential for relating image data to real-world dimensions, which is the final step of image analysis. The simplest way of performing this task is to specify the length of some given feature (a line, for example) in both the image and on the scene—such as, for example, imaging a ruler and noting the distance in pixels between inch

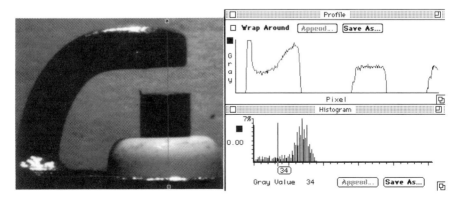

Figure 13.7. Intensity profile and histogram showing the intensity distribution along a vertical line and within a rectangular region of interest, respectively.

markings within the image. This simple calibration procedure essentially produces an average magnification factor for the entire image.

However, this method makes the assumption that the image plane and the plane of a 2D object that is being imaged are precisely parallel. Typically, this cannot be exactly the case. The camera may have some rotation relative to the scene, the sensor array within the camera may be offset or rotated, and other positioning errors may exist. A circle in the scene will be imaged as an ellipse and a square will appear as a trapezoid with the side furthest away from the camera appearing shorter, due to perspective.

The proper way of calibrating the system to account for perspective, rotation, and other such effects is to construct a 3×3 *calibration matrix* that serves as the overall transformation between world and pixel coordinates. The calibration matrix C relates the world plane (x,y) and the image (u,v) coordinate frames taking into account the world origin location $O = (O_x, O_y)$ and perspective P along the u and v axes. The matrix has the following form:

$$\begin{bmatrix} \dfrac{x}{u} & \dfrac{x}{v} & O_x \\[2mm] \dfrac{y}{u} & \dfrac{y}{v} & O_y \\[2mm] P_u & P_v & 1 \end{bmatrix}$$

Pixel points are represented as a three element vector $[u,v,1]^\mathrm{T}$, which, when multiplied by the calibration matrix, yields the corresponding world planar position $[x,y,1]^\mathrm{T}$ (multiplied by a scale factor). More generally, a 4×4 transformation matrix can be established to relate the 3D positions in the world to locations on the image plane. A detailed derivation can be found in the literature.[15]

In practice, the camera calibration matrix is calculated by providing the system with a sufficient number of corresponding pairs of world and image coordinates. Each pair of coordinates provides two simultaneous equations that are used to solve for the elements of matrix C. Generally, enough pairs of coordinates are used to create an overdetermined system of equations, whereupon a least-squared-error method is used to solve for C. The eight-dot calibration target shown in Figure 13.8, made in a wide range of sizes, can be used for this purpose; the vision system is provided with the world coordinates of the dot centroids, computes their image coordinates, and calculates C, along with a residual term indicating the precision of the fit.

13.2.3. Image Processing

Any operation that takes as an input an image and produces a new one as its output is typically referred to as an *image processing* or *filtering* operation. This encompasses both digital image processing operations that are performed in a computer on a digitized image as well as optical processing schemes that refer

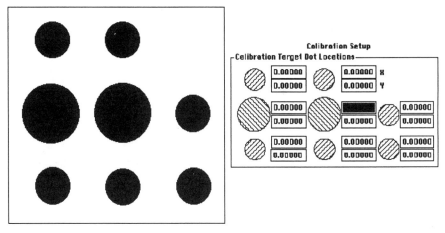

Figure 13.8. Eight-dot calibration target and user interface dialog used to enter the real-world coordinates of the dots.

to passing light rays (that form a continuous image) through an optical system (such as a lens element).

In this section we will briefly present some of the common image processing operations that are used in machine vision systems. These include

- Image intensity mapping operations
- Image arithmetic operations
- Linear filtering (convolution) operations
- Nonlinear filtering operations
- Morphological operations

13.2.3.1. INTENSITY MAPPING. These rather simple point-by-point image processing operations are used to map the intensity of each pixel in the input to another intensity in the output based on some user-defined mapping function. This mapping function is often referred to as an *input lookup table* (ILUT) and is implemented in hardware as an integral part of the frame grabber used to capture the images in memory. The mapping function can be defined either as a mathematical function (e.g., a linear, square root, cubic root, or logarithmic function), as an arbitrary set of input–output value pairs, or graphically as an arbitrarily shaped single-valued function.

Intensity mapping operations (see Fig. 13.9) may be used to improve the contrast of a dark image where most intensity values are concentrated in the low range of possible intensities. A simple linear mapping function expanding the narrow input dynamic range to a wider output range may be sufficient. Better results may be obtained by using a square or higher-order root function. The optimum such mapping function that will spread the image intensities in an as nearly as possible uniform fashion can be computed automatically through a

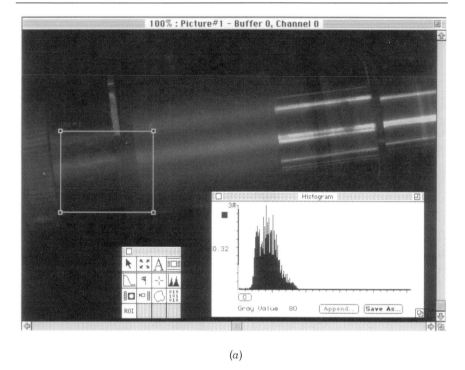

(a)

Figure 13.9. (a) Dark image of a syringe with image histogram; (b) same image with histogram equalization used to distribute pixel intensity mapping to a wider range.

process known as *histogram equalization.* It can be proved that this optimum mapping function is the cumulative histogram that graphically depicts the number of pixels with intensity values above—as opposed to at—a particular intensity level.

13.2.3.2. IMAGE ARITHMETIC. Image arithmetic and logic operations (add, subtract, multiply, divide, copy, OR, AND, XOR, NOT, etc.) operate on pixel values among multiple images or on different segments of a single image and are used to detect changes from image to image, deal with transient phenomena, compensate for the effects of nonuniform illumination, and perform complicated preprocessing operations by combining multiple simpler operations.

For example, motion in a scene might be detected by using a subtraction algorithm between two sequential images (see Fig. 13.10). Pixel values that are the same in the two images would produce a zero difference shown as black in the image, while changing pixel values would result in greater than zero differences and thus show up as lighter gray values. An example of such an application in the laboratory is the use of image subtraction to detect the presence of foreign or nonsoluble material in a vial filled with translucent liquid. By rotating the vial

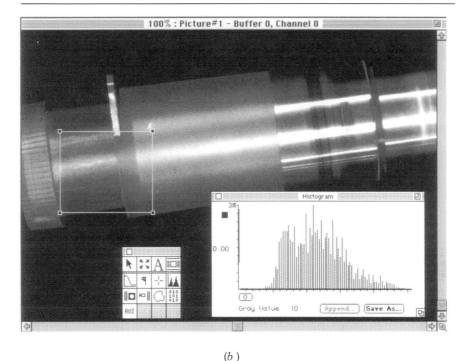

(*b*)

Figure 13.9. (*Continued*)

rapidly and stopping it suddenly, any material inside it will continue to move around. Taking multiple successive images and subtracting them from one another will detect any such moving particles but at the same time ignore any defects in the surface of the vial that will not move from image to image.

Similarly, such image subtraction can be used to detect missing parts or any other such changes in the objects of interest in the scene such as, for example, finding if the key in the images of Figure 13.11 has any missing teeth. After subtraction any differences between the model and the test image will show up as bright spots in a dark background and can be picked up during subsequent image analysis by simple counting the area of pixels with intensities above a certain value. Note that in order to compensate for any misregistration between the trained and test images the new image can also be offset and rotated as needed based on information extracted from the image itself.

Another use of image arithmetic operations is in compensating for inhomogenuities in the lighting used to illuminate the scene or in the transmissivity of optical media. The former situation may, for example, be caused by using a conventional light source over a relatively large surface area resulting in higher brightness directly below the source and decreasing intensities away from it. The latter may be caused by an unclean slide in a microscopy application or be due

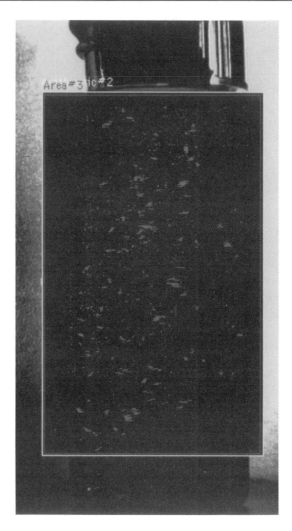

Figure 13.10. Use of image subtraction to detect foreign material in vial of clear liquid. Moving particulates show up as white flecks in the resultant image.

to vignetting effects in the lens, which would result in lower intensities around the edges of the field of view as compared with the values in the center of the image. To compensate in this last case we can subtract a blank image (e.g., taken with an empty microscope slide) from the actual image while adding a uniform offset to the result (equal to the average image intensity) to avoid negative intensity values. In the first case we can instead subtract a smoothed version of the image from itself, which could result in the removal of a nonuniform background. This allows straightforward image analysis techniques to be applied for counting of the dark cells.

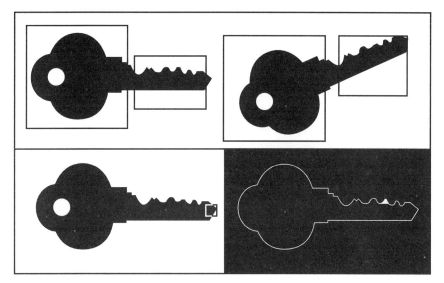

Figure 13.11. Use of image rotation followed by image subtraction to highlight a defect (missing tooth in key).

13.2.3.3. *LINEAR FILTERING (CONVOLUTION).* A filter or a general input/output system is characterized as being *linear* if linear combination of inputs results in the same linear combination of outputs and as *shift-invariant* if shifting the input image by a certain amount results in an equally shifted output. The behavior of such systems is amenable to mathematical description using *linear system* theory tools. Such mathematical machinery has originally been developed for continuous systems but can also be extended to operations on discrete images. A detailed coverage of these methods is given in the literature.[16–18]

An example of a linear image processing operation is spatial averaging (also referred to as *average* or *mean filtering*) (see Fig. 13.12). In the discrete case, each pixel in the output image is given an intensity value equal to the average of intensity values of its neighbors in the input image. A neighborhood can be specified as a 3×3, 5×5, or $n \times n$ square of pixels with the pixel under consideration in its center. Such a filtering scheme obviously results in a smoothed image where all sharp details (such as noise but also true intensity edges or peaks) are smoothed out.

Another way of describing this operation is then by considering a uniform mask of the form shown in Figure 13.13.

To compute the output image intensities, this mask is moved in a raster scan fashion on top of the pixel grid of the input image. At each location, the mask will lay over an image region of the same size. The corresponding output image intensity value at the center of this region will be equal to the average value of intensities in this region.

This value—equal to $[a + b + c + d + e + f + g + h + i]/9$—can also be

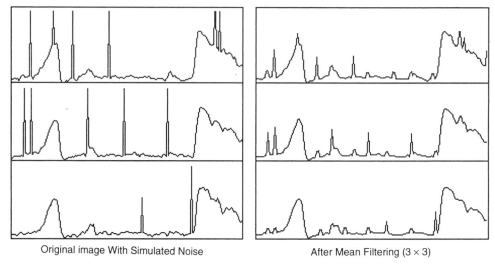

Original image With Simulated Noise   After Mean Filtering (3 × 3)

Figure 13.12. Horizontal intensity profiles across an image before and after mean filtering.

obtained by multiplying each element of the mask (here equal to $\frac{1}{9}$) with the underlying pixel intensity in the image and summing the individual products. This operation, which is called *convolution,* is schematically depicted in Figure 13.14. Of course, in the general case, the mask does not have to be uniform.

Linear filters can also be used for other purposes. The filter mask shown in Figure 13.15 is used to sharpen images. Since the sum of the terms in the mask is zero, when the filter is applied to uniform areas, the filter output is zero, while edge regions tend to be enhanced. This type of filter is also known as a *highpass* filter because it will pass areas of high spatial frequency (high rate of change of intensity values in the image) while limiting any uniform areas (low spatial frequency).

It should also be noted at this point that instead of using convolution to describe linear image processing operations in terms of their direct effect on image intensities, we can also describe them in terms of how they affect (accentuate or attenuate) fine or coarse image detail. So, the averaging filter described

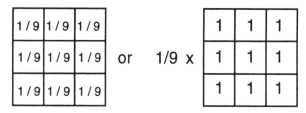

Figure 13.13. Uniform mask for average (mean) filtering of discrete images.

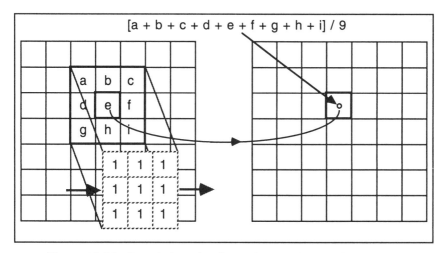

Figure 13.14. Convolution of a discrete image with a uniform mask.

in this section is a smoothing filter that attenuates fine image details such as edges or noise spikes, whereas the sharpening operations described above accentuate them.

This is analogous to describing the performance of a sound system in terms of how it affects the low or high frequencies (bass and treble response). In image processing, of course, frequency is defined with respect to space instead of time. So, for example, in the simple case of alternating black and white stripes in the image, spatial frequency is related to the number of lines per unit length (e.g., lines per millimeter). High spatial frequencies correspond to fine image detail, whereas low spatial frequencies are related to coarser features. Of course, since the image is a 2D entity, we must refer to spatial frequencies in both dimensions.

In addition to its intuitive appeal, describing a sequence of image processing operations in the *frequency domain* allows simplification of the computation of response by replacing convolutions with multiplications. The mathematical tool used in linear system theory to move back and forth between space and frequency domains is the *Fourier transform.* However, further discussion in this area is well outside the scope of this treatment. The interested reader is referred to the literature.[15,16]

13.2.3.4. NONLINEAR FILTERING. The linear mean filtering approach we discussed above is successful in smoothing the image, but it also has the disadvantage that the noise is not completely removed but simply reduced and spread out. Also, image details such as sharp edges are affected. Multiple solutions to this problem exist. For example, an alternative technique that would have better results than mere uniform averaging on such noisy images could involve comparing a pixel intensity with others in the neighborhood (vicinity) and changing it only when it is not within some tolerance of the average value. Obviously such a method is nonlinear.

-1	-1	-1
-1	8	-1
-1	-1	-1

(a)

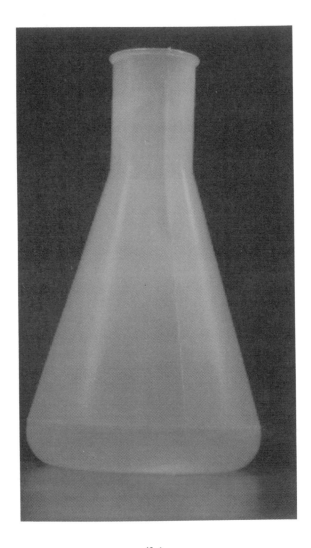

(b)

Figure 13.15. (a) Highpass sharpening filter kernel; (b,c) results of the operation on a flask image.

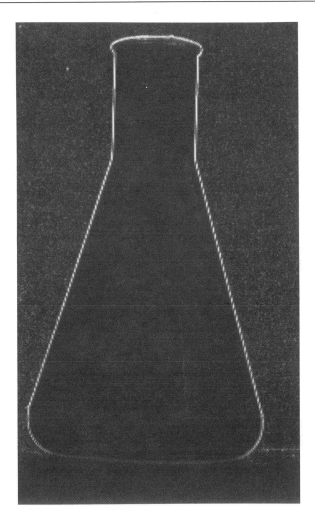

(c)

Figure 13.15. (Continued)

Another nonlinear alternative is to replace each pixel with the median value of intensities in its neighborhood. Such a median filter has the advantage that it chops off all noise spikes without affecting the sharp image detail found across an edge or line. A horizontal scan (the same as in the mean filtering example) across an input image and the median filtered output image is shown in Figure 13.16.

One disadvantage of median filtering is that the calculation of the median value of intensities requires sorting of all intensities in a window and thus is

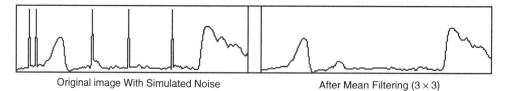

| Original image With Simulated Noise | After Mean Filtering (3 × 3) |

Figure 13.16. A horizontal scan across the image before and after median filtering.

more expensive than simple averaging. A solution proposed by Yang[19] computes the median from the histogram of intensity values in a window. This histogram is computed only once in the original position of a window. As the window slides across the image, the histogram is updated by removing all the pixels that were uncovered and adding all the ones that were now covered.

13.2.3.5. MORPHOLOGICAL PROCESSING. *Morphological operations* are used for noise suppression or feature enhancement, or to expose certain geometric relationships or structure in the image. These operators compute the intensity of a pixel in the output image based on the results of a logical (for binary morphology) or min–max (for gray-scale morphology) operation on the intensities of pixels within an arbitrarily shaped neighborhood around that pixel in the input image. Depending on the algorithm used and the size and shape of the neighborhood, different geometric features of an image can be enhanced or suppressed.

Morphological operations are classified as either binary or gray-scale. Common binary operations include erosion, dilation, opening, closing, skeletonization, convex hull, and so forth. Binary erosion performs a logical AND operation on the pixels of the neighborhood and assigns the result to the current pixel as shown in Figure 13.17. In this case, only when the entire neighborhood has the value zero (0) will the output value be one (1). That is, only a black pixel entirely surrounded by black will remain black. The end result is erosion of the boundary pixels of the regions in the image. Small regions or irregularities in the boundaries of the object are washed away, therefore removing noise in the original image while larger ones only lose perimeter pixels, in a pattern similar to peeling an onion. Such an operation would, for example, enable separation and accurate counting of objects that touch each other. Dilation is the opposite operation performing a logical OR operation on all pixels in the neighborhood and resulting in growing the object by a layer. Erosion as defined above should be more accurately referred to as "erosion of black" or as "dilation of white," whereas dilation should be referred to as "dilation of black" or "erosion of white." By changing the shape of the neighborhood over which the operations are performed one can erode or dilate the object along specific directions—for example, along the x or y axis.

Erosion followed by dilation is called "opening." It is called opening for topological reasons, but it has the effect of breaking small bridges between

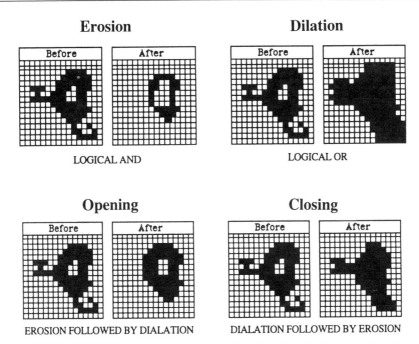

Figure 13.17. Simple binary morphology operations (erosion, dilation, opening, closing).

adjacent large regions. The macroscopic effect of the opening is to remove small regions or peninsulas. Dilation followed by erosion is called "closing" and has the opposite effect of opening. Closing eliminates small holes in objects. Opening followed by closing will therefore remove "salt-and-pepper noise" from an image. Other binary operations include *convex hull,* which will turn any blob into a convex object and *skeletonization,* which will turn an object into a thin skeleton.

Gray-scale morphology lowers or raises the gray-scale value of pixels in the ROI, depending on the result of neighborhood minimum–maximum operations. When applying these operators to light pixels, the preceding basic operators become

- *Erosion*—replaces each pixel with the darkest pixel (minimum intensity) in its neighborhood
- *Dilation*—replaces each pixel with the brightest pixel (maximum intensity) in its neighborhood
- *Opening*—erosion followed by dilation
- *Closing*—dilation followed by erosion

Other examples of more powerful gray-scale morphological operators include

- *TopHat*—original image minus opening (resulting in accentuating thin bright spots or lines of a given diameter or width and suppressing everything else)
- *Well*—closing minus original image (resulting in accentuating thin dark spots or lines of a given diameter or width and suppressing everything else)
- *Gradient*—dilated image minus eroded image (highlighting all edges)

Again, by appropriately selecting the size and shape of the structuring element, the lines of a particular orientation and thickness can be enhanced and all other detail can be rejected.

13.2.4. Image Analysis

To produce the symbolic descriptions necessary in any machine vision application, we need to be able to identify different entities in the image corresponding to separate and identifiable entities in the scene. These may be image regions corresponding to object surfaces or image contours corresponding to boundaries separating such regions. The main objectives of image analysis are to detect such features of interest (which may be regions of the image or boundaries between such regions), segment the image on the basis of such regions or contours (by picking, e.g., all bright objects in a dark background), and finally represent internally and generate descriptions of such features (e.g., by defining the perimeter and computing the area, centroid, or other geometric measures for every such region detected or by fitting a straight line through all collinear boundary points detected and returning the equation of such a line).

The following few sections present concepts and techniques used in such feature extraction, image segmentation, and image representation and description. All these techniques and methods are either region-based—when regions of contiguous pixels are detected and described—or contour based—when the boundaries of such regions are detected and described.

Specifically, the basic image analysis techniques covered in this chapter will include

- Binary image analysis: area counting and connectivity analysis
- Gray-scale analysis
- Edge detection
- Template matching by normalized correlation
- Detection of boundaries of known shapes by Hough transform methods

13.2.4.1. BINARY IMAGE ANALYSIS

Binary Images and Thresholding.   An image in which each pixel can take only one of two distinct values (0/1 or black/white) is referred to as a *binary image*. It can be produced from a gray-level image by selecting an intensity threshold and setting all pixels with intensities higher than the threshold value to 1 (white) and the rest to 0 (black). Analysis of binary images was the first vision processing technique widely used in manufacturing because binary images are easier to acquire, store, transmit, and process than are images with multiple gray levels. As we will see, both geometric and topological features—useful for recognition purposes —can be readily computed from binary images. Of course, such images do not contain any detail in the interior of a region. Instead, they provide information only on the outline of the object and are thus applicable only when the outline is sufficient to characterize the object.

A 2D discrete array $b(i,j)$ with values 0 or 1 on each pixel (i,j) can be used to describe a binary image. However, in most implementations, some form of encoding is actually used for the internal representation of the image. The most popular such technique is *run-length coding*.[16] This data compression scheme exploits the fact that along any particular scan line, long runs of ones and zeros are encountered. So instead of storing or transmitting pixels one-by-one, the lengths of each of these runs can be used. Algorithms have been developed and are widely used for the computation of geometric features of interest using these run lengths directly. Description of such algorithms is beyond the scope of this treatment but can be found in the references.[16]

The intensity histogram introduced in an earlier section is especially useful in the selection of an appropriate intensity level—threshold—which can be used to segment the image in two types of regions: regions with intensities above such a level and regions with intensities below. In an image of a dark object on a bright background or of an object with a hole where the dark and bright regions are approximately of the same size, the histogram shows two clear peaks (lobes). In such case, an appropriate threshold selection is a value in the valley between these two histogram lobes. This selection can be readily automated.

Thresholding a gray-level image to create a binary image is particularly straightforward when sufficiently high contrast exists between the object and the background in the original gray-level image. An example of such an image of industrial parts on a backlit surface is shown in Figure 13.18. As can be seen from a typical intensity profile along an arbitrary line, the intensities drop drastically from the maximum level in the background to the minimum intensity inside the objects. The histogram comprises primarily two sharp peaks at the object and background intensities and very little in between.

In most cases, the pixels on object boundaries have intensities in between those of the object and those of the background. The selected threshold value determines whether a pixel is classified as part of the object or the background and thus affects the size of the resulting blobs in the binary image. This effect is illustrated in Figure 13.19, which shows images of a dime on a nonuniform background. Depending on the threshold value selected the object found may also include part of the background, as shown in the first image.

Threshold selection becomes more difficult when the relative sizes of background and foreground objects are significantly different and have intensities

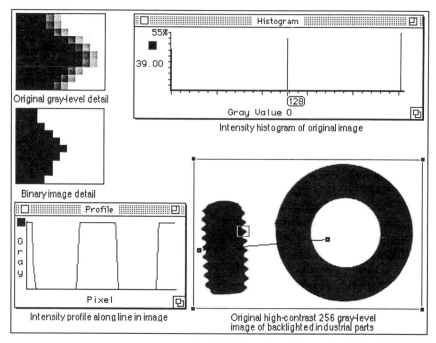

Figure 13.18. High-contrast image of backlit objects, histogram, intensity profile along a line, and thresholded image detail.

very close together. In such a case, the foreground corresponds to a small training tail of a large histogram lobe corresponding to the background. However, even in a case like this, there are approaches to automate the threshold selection by including in the histogram only pixels close to the boundaries between foreground and background. This will again make the histogram look nearly bimodal facilitating automatic threshold selection.

Area Counting. Area counting is the simplest binary image analysis scheme. This algorithm counts the total number of pixels within a region of interest that have intensities above or below a given threshold. This option can be used for very fast determination of presence or absence of a part, feature, or flaw in the image. An example of detecting defects in the printing of marks on disposable syringes is shown in Figure 13.20.

Blobs and Connectivity Analysis. *Connectivity analysis* is used to detect regions of connected pixels (also referred to as *blobs*) with intensities above or below a threshold and to compute many different geometric features for each blob (area, centroid, perimeter, major/minor axes, length, width, moments, roundness, bounding box dimensions, etc.) as well as topological features and statis-

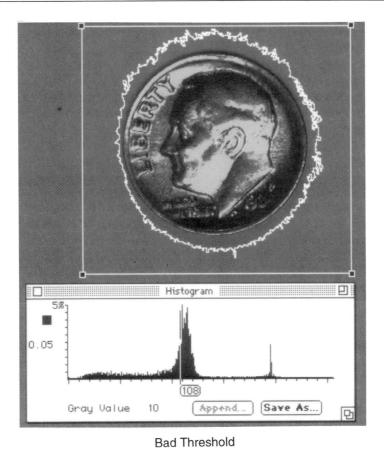

Bad Threshold

(a)

Figure 13.19. Effect of threshold selection.

tics across all blobs (number of parts, number of holes, etc.). These features can then be used for recognition purposes or as inputs to measurements computed from the image.

If multiple objects are visible in the image, several contiguous blobs of pixels with the same intensity will appear on a common background. Before any measurements can be computed for any specific blob, these blobs of connected pixels must be detected and labeled. This requires

- A criterion that determines whether a pixel is connected to another (connectedness)
- An algorithm for labeling different blobs and their topological relationships (as a blob within a hole within another blob, etc.)

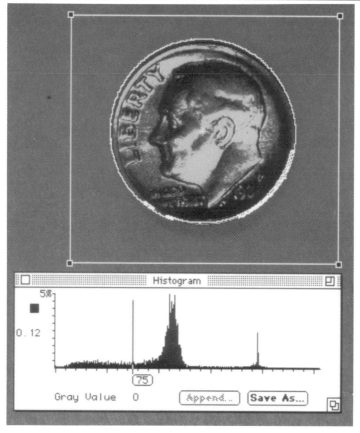

Good Threshold

(*b*)

Figure 13.19. (*Continued*)

In a rectangular pixel grid, three different possible connectedness criteria are possible, as shown in Figure 13.21. According to 4-connectedness, only the 4 pixels abutting a central pixel along a side are considered its neighbors. In 8-connectedness, all 8 pixels surrounding a central pixel are considered. It has been established that a 6-connectedness scheme is actually better than the other two, and this is what is used in most algorithms. Extensive work has gone into the development of robust and efficient algorithms that label the different blobs of connected pixels and also describe their topological relationships. The most widely used set of such connectivity algorithms was developed at SRI in the late 1970s.[16] One application of connectivity analysis is in cytometry (see Fig. 13.22).

Various geometric features can be computed for each blob. These can then be used as the basis for recognition or inspection. Averages and other statistics of these features may also be useful when we need to characterize images with

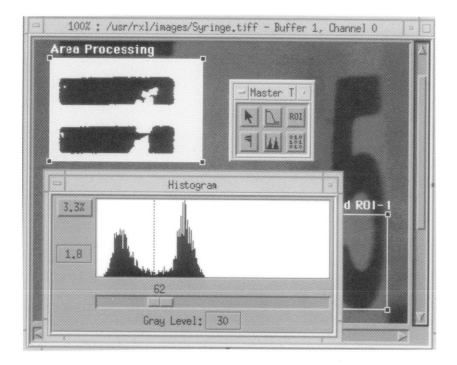

Figure 13.20. Area counting used to detect defects in printed marks on disposable syringes.

multiple similar blobs—such as porosity or other defects in an x-ray image or grains in a microphotograph. These geometric features, which can be computed from a binary image, include

- *Area* (*A*), which is equal to the sum of all blob pixels.
- *Perimeter* (*P*), which is the total number of pixels on the blob boundary. Because of the quantized nature of the boundary, this overestimates the actual blob perimeter[16] by a factor of $4/\pi$.

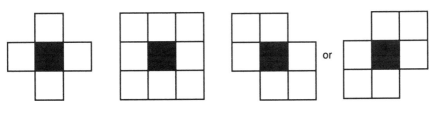

4-Connectedness   8-Connectedness   6-Connectedness

Figure 13.21. Connectedness criteria.

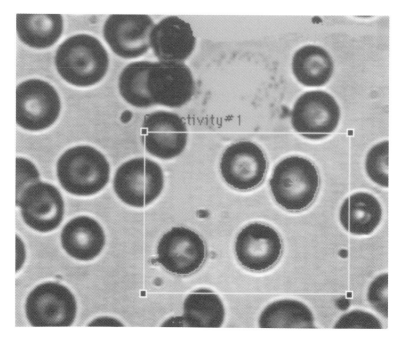

Figure 13.22. Connectivity analysis used to count blood cells.

- *First moments* around the x and y axes (M_x and M_y), which are found as the sum of all y or x coordinates of each pixel in the blob.
- x and y coordinates of the *centroid* (x_c, y_c) computed by dividing each first moment with area.
- *Second moments* (S_{xx}, S_{yy}, S_{xy}), which are the 2D equivalents of a 3D object's moments of inertia.
- *Minor and major axes* of the equivalent ellipse (one with the same moments of inertia). These are the axes of max and min second moment.
- *Roundness,* which is computed by dividing the minimum second moment by the maximum.
- *Width and length* along the x and y axes and along the major and minor axes.

See also Fig. 13.23.

Over 50 different geometric and topological features are typically made available by most image analysis packages.

13.2.4.2. Gray-Scale Analysis. Although binary image analysis is very powerful and sufficient for many applications, much more information can be extracted

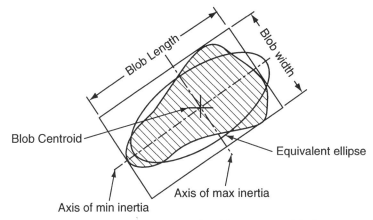

Figure 13.23. Simple measurements obtained from connectivity/blob analysis.

from the gray-scale images. All the algorithms highlighted in the remaining subsections of this section are operating on gray-scale images. The simplest, typically referred to as *gray scale analysis,* is often used to compute statistics such as min, max, mean, or standard deviation of pixel intensities within a region of interest. This computation can then be used to make judgments regarding the surface quality of an object and the presence or absence of surface features or defects.

13.2.4.3. Edge and Boundary Detection. *Edges* are boundary points separating regions of the image with pixels of different intensities. Such intensity changes may be due to a change in surface reflectivity or orientation on a real object surface, due to occlusion of one object by another, or due to shadowing. The transition between regions of different intensity is not abrupt because of blurring and limitations of the imaging device. An edge detection operator is an algorithm or filter which, when applied to the image, would result in some identifiable response along an edge (e.g., minimum, maximum, or zero).

As can be seen from the simple edge model of Figure 13.24, an edge can be modeled as a boundary between two regions of different intensities (B_1 and B_2). Along a direction normal to the edge, we have a step change in intensity. The first differences along such a step function can be readily computed and would show a maximum value at the location of the edge. The second differences can also be readily computed and would go through a zero crossing at the location of the edge. It can be further proved that both the edge strength and the edge direction of an arbitrarily oriented edge can be determined by appropriate combinations of the first differences along the x and y directions.

Thus, in order to detect edges one can compute the first differences along the x and y directions (also referred to as the x and y intensity gradients) and look for local maxima or the second differences and look for zero crossings. Alternatively such differencing operations can be viewed as convolutions with an

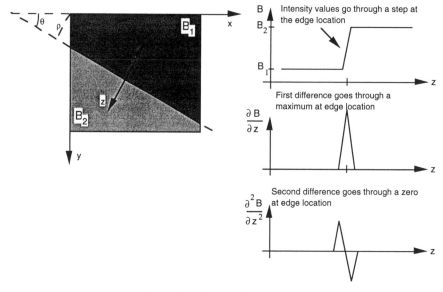

Figure 13.24. Simple edge model.

appropriate kernel. A variety of edge detection operators that are variants or appropriate combinations of the preceding direct discrete approximations of the x and y gradients have been proposed and are described in the image processing literature.[15,17] A particularly popular example is the Sobel operator (see Fig. 13.25). The image is convolved with the two x and y gradient kernels, and the absolute values of the resulting response are summed to produce an output image in which both the horizontal and the vertical edges will be enhanced.

Passing the entire image or a region of interest through an edge enhancement filter will accentuate edge points while suppressing uniform intensity pixels. To be useful in image analysis, all candidate edge points must then be linked and represented as boundaries (straight lines, circles, ellipses, or other

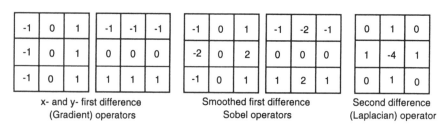

Figure 13.25. Common edge detection operators.

curves) corresponding to actual physical boundaries between objects in the scene.

When the general location and direction of an edge boundary is known, the edge detection process can be simplified by searching the image or region of interest along the horizontal, vertical, or user-specified directions looking directly for intensity transitions of the right size or for sufficiently high gradient values. This can be clearly seen in Figure 13.26, where searching for two horizontal edges is done along the vertical direction and searching for a circular boundary is done along the radial vector directions specified by the user.

After individual edge points on a boundary are detected, additional analysis is required in order to fit them into a representation and extract useful measures such as line equations or angles for straight boundaries, or circle centers and radii for circles, or other parameters for ellipses or more general boundary shapes. If no noise or spurious edge points are present, all detected edge points can be used in the line fit. Additional work is required to reject outliers. One

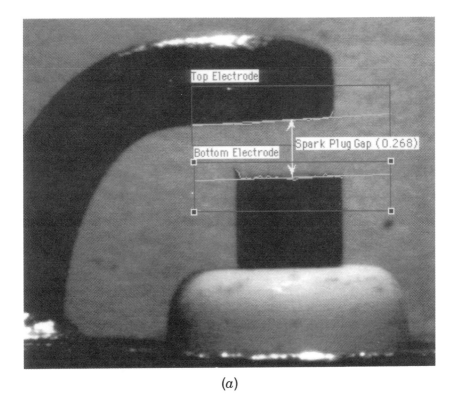

(a)

Figure 13.26. (a) Detection of nearly horizontal edges by searching along the vertical direction and (b) of edges on the perimeter of a circular hole by searching along user-specified radial directions.

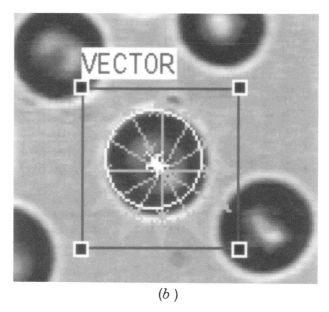

(*b*)

Figure 13.26. (*Continued*)

approach that is widely used in image analysis for rejecting such spurious points and keeping only points belonging to boundaries of known shape (straight lines, circles, or arbitrary shapes) is the Hough transform.

Although details about the approach are outside the scope of this treatment, it is important to note that this method can be used for detection of partially visible targets and can work on images with low contrast or varying intensities where other methods would not perform as well.

13.2.4.4. Template Matching by Normalized Correlation. *Normalized correlation* is used to locate a stored pattern of pixel intensities (template) in an image. This can be used for template matching and alignment operations. During training, a section of the image containing the object or pattern of interest is identified. This section, called a *template,* is subsequently used to locate the object in new images by searching for sections that are very similar to the template. The template is remembered by the system in full gray-scale detail, and the search is conducted in a way that is "normalized" or indifferent to variations in the level of illumination. During run time, the template image is stepped through a search window to find the best possible match between the template and the current image. When the best fit is found, the $x-y$ location of the best match and the correlation value are reported. The correlation value is a number between 0 and 1 that indicates the quality of the match (1 = perfect match, 0 = no correlation).

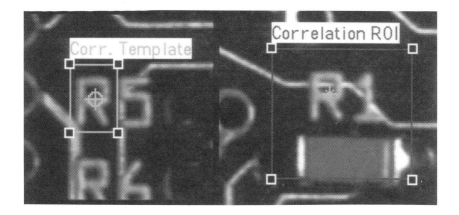

Figure 13.27. Detection of trained template using normalized correlation.

Normalizing the correlation value makes the algorithm less sensitive to variations in image intensity or noise and allows the algorithm to find the trained template even if intensity levels in the image vary or if part of the target is missing as in Figure 13.27. This approach can also be extended to deal with templates that may be rotated and/or scaled in the image by extending the search to these additional dimensions. Not only the template is found even if it is rotated or scaled but the angle of rotation and/or factor of magnification is also computed and returned. This is schematically depicted in Figure 13.28.

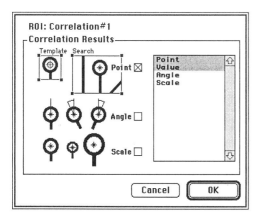
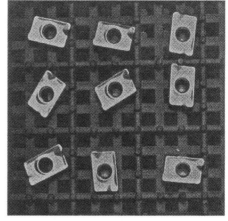

Figure 13.28. Selecting options for correlation search and typical image of randomly oriented parts where rotation-invariant search is necessary.

13.3. LABORATORY APPLICATIONS OF MACHINE VISION

Applications of machine vision can be generally classified under the following categories:

- Part presence/absence detection
- Part location and orientation detection
- Part identification
- Automated inspection
- Dimensional gauging
- Process monitoring and control
- Vision-guided robotics

These are also roughly the categories of applications in which machine vision can be applied in the automated laboratory. Frequently one vision system may be used in multiple combinations of these applications in a single automated laboratory procedure. For example, the vision system may be used to detect the presence of a sample, identify it through a bar code, determine its exact location and orientation, and feed that information to a robot system that will move it to another location. Further, given the power and flexibility of computer platforms today, a single system may act as the host for cell control, motion planning and control, and vision processing.

In this section we will present an overview of machine vision applications in the laboratory categorized along the general classes outlined above. Rather than attempting to completely categorize and document the many potential applications, we will provide only a brief "picture book" presentation of certain typical procedures and their basis in the machine vision fundamentals described in the previous section.

13.3.1. Part Presence/Absence Detection

Such uses of machine vision are very helpful in conjunction with a "blind" automated device, such as lab robots. One of the most common failure modes of a laboratory automation system occurs when apparatus such as laboratory consumables are missing or misplaced within the robot envelope. A frequently encountered example of this problem is in vial capping and uncapping stations. Many automated systems that perform this function today make use of special optical or touch sensors in order to verify the presence of the cap on the vial. Another example might be for test tubes or petri dishes in a dispenser. Most dispensers are loaded manually and in bulk by human technicians, then brought into the envelope of the lab robot for unattended use. In fact, dispensers are a preferred method of delivering these consumables as they make more efficient use of space within the envelope of the robot.[1] However, if the orientation of the consumable is not verified before handling—for example, if a petri dish is loaded in upside-down—potentially catastrophic errors can result. While some systems use touch sensing to make this sort of determination, this sensing modality brings up problems of contamination among samples and is preferably to be avoided.

As mentioned above, arrays of sensors can be built into automated workstations in order to avoid this type of problem. However, the same problem can be addressed more economically and robustly with machine vision in the case of a complete lab automation system, where many different locations exist where apparatus misalignment can create problems. This type of application is most commonly solved by looking for a specific feature—hence the "presence/absence" appellation. For example, determination of the orientation of petri dishes is made by using a gray-scale algorithm to look for a reflected gleam of light within the titled dish, indicating that the dish is right-side up (Fig. 13.29). The algorithm itself is relatively simple—most presence/absence applications are simply binary "yes/no" inspection tasks—however, considerable time is usually spent looking for a reliable feature on which to base the analysis. In the case of the optically clear petri dish principles of optics and reflected light were used to make the decision.

Most of the image analysis techniques discussed earlier can be applied in such part presence/absence detection applications. Even the simpler approaches will suffice in most cases. For example, a simple area count within an appropriately placed region of interest can be sufficient to detect the presence of a cap on a test tube or the presence of a correctly oriented flask (Fig. 13.30). Similarly, the detection of one or more unexpected edges along a user-specified vector direction may indicate that a foreign part is present on a surface that was supposed to be clear or that a pipette tip is in place.

13.3.2. Part Location and Orientation Detection

Location and orientation detection applications use machine vision to detect the exact location or orientation of a part that must be manipulated by a robot or other automated device. These applications frequently involve location of parts in coordinate systems that are moving relative to the fixed robot workspace, or sets of indexed positions. For example, a centrifuge rotor contains a set of fixed tube positions; however, the orientation of this set of positions changes as the rotor spins. A 96-well microwell plate also has fixed positions within the plate (the well locations), which can be moved as a set throughout the workspace. Machine vision can be used in both of these cases to identify specific positions or track the overall part translation and/or rotation.

In the example of a centrifugation procedure, the sample tubes are placed within the centrifuge, which spins them at high speed. After spinning, the tubes are removed and continue being processed. In order to remove the tubes from the centrifuge, the laboratory automation system must incorporate some means of ensuring that the position of the tubes postspin is known. There are two ways of making this possible. The centrifuge can be engineered either to stop at a

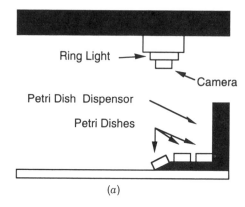

(a)

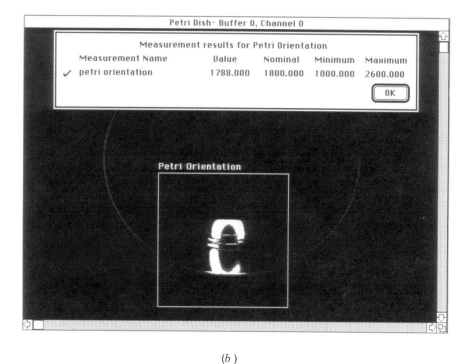

(b)

Figure 13.29. Verifying the correct orientation of petri dishes. The presence of reflections is detected as an indicator of whether or not the dish is upside-down.

predefined location or to provide position information through an encoder. The automation system then monitors the centrifuge position just as it would monitor any other robotic axis, and uses the position information at the end of a spin cycle to locate the tubes within the centrifuge. The alternative option—machine vision—eliminates the need for complex modification of the centrifuge and

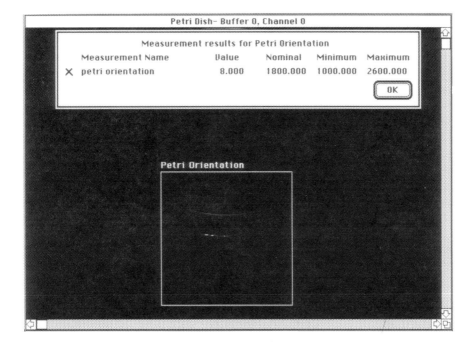

(c)

Figure 13.29. (Continued)

thus allows using in an automated setting conventional laboratory equipment.

The task of keeping track of the samples within the centrifuge can be solved by looking for fiducial reference marks placed on the centrifuge rotor, as shown in Figure 13.31. As the automated system loads tubes into the centrifuge, their (relative) positions are recorded. The vision system then uses the two fiducials to establish a reference frame within the centrifuge. After spinning, the fiducials are again located and the tube position transformed to the current ones.

If the positions of individual tubes within the centrifuge are not stored, machine vision can be used to search for tubes within the centrifuge wells (an example of a presence/absence type of application), as in Fig. 13.32a. The precise placement of regions of interest within the image can be accomplished using dynamic relocation of the ROIs based on vision feedback. Regions are initially created around individual centrifuge tube locations and set up to perform presence/absence tests (using an area counting algorithm or perhaps connectivity to look for a tube top). The same fiducial marks are used to orient the axes and establish an angle of rotation after the spin. The regions are then moved to the correct positions by recalculating the correct rotated position based on the new axis definition (Fig. 13.32b).

Similar techniques can be used to locate the wells in a microplate (see Fig.

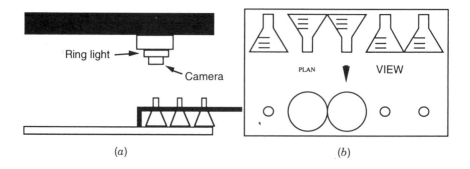

(a)   (b)

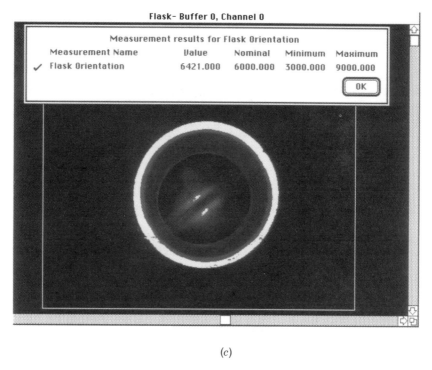

(c)

Figure 13.30. (a,b) Schematic of how machine vision may be used to verify correct flask orientation; (c,d) verification using area counting.

13.33). Edge/boundary detection schemes can be used to determine the locations of the edges of the microwell plate and thereby establish the local coordinate system. The wells themselves can then be found using offsets from the edges of the plate. This type of algorithm is particularly useful in systems where microplates are continually being transferred across the workspace or where results in individual wells (such as color changes) may be the basis of decision making about the remainder of the processing.

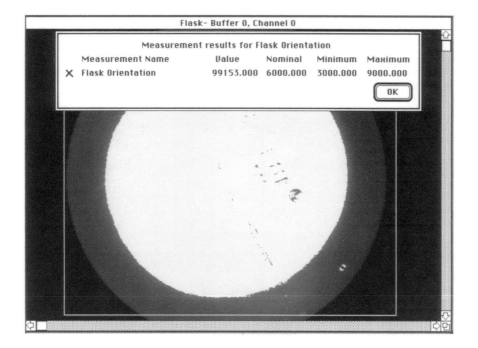

Flask- Buffer 0, Channel 0

Measurement results for Flask Orientation

	Measurement Name	Value	Nominal	Minimum	Maximum
X	Flask Orientation	99153.000	6000.000	3000.000	9000.000

OK

(d)

Figure 13.30. (Continued)

fiducial marks

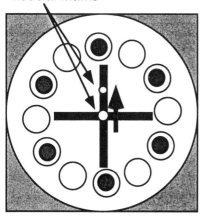
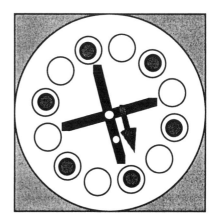

Figure 13.31. Schematic of how centrifuge angle is found using a fiducial mark placed on the centrifuge spokes.

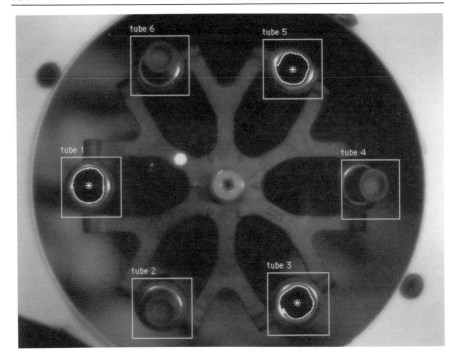

(*a*)

Figure 13.32. (*a*) Use of presence/absence methods to confirm tube presence in a centrifuge; (*b*) location of centrifuge tubes using fiducial reference mark and angle calculation.

13.3.3. Part Identification

One very common need in all laboratory environments is the accurate identification of specimen, compound, or reagent containers and/or the precise tracking of samples or specimens. Such identification can be done on the basis of some unique characteristic of a specimen container (such as, e.g., identifying the type of tests to be performed on a blood sample based on the color of color-coded sample caps; see Fig. 13.34).

The most common way to accurately identify and track samples is to use a label of some sort on the container. For example, bar code labels are now commonly used in laboratories to track samples as they are processed, either manually or by automation. These bar codes usually incorporate a code number that can be used as a "license plate" key to a database where information about the sample is stored. Bar codes are popular today because the time and effort required to read a code is relatively small; inexpensive bar-code readers can read the codes relatively quickly. Obviously, by adding bar-code reading capa-

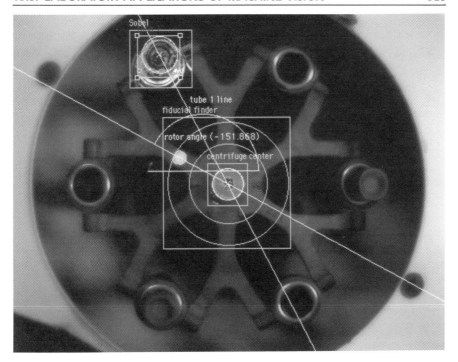

(b)

Figure 13.32. (Continued)

bilities to a machine vision system, additional savings can be realized. In addition, the user of a CCD array camera and image processing and analysis approaches instead of a laser based reader allows reading degraded bar codes in arbitrary orientations

However, bar codes have certain inherent limitations that have prevented their use in some classes of applications and limited their usefulness in others. These limitations (which include low information content, low data read/transfer reliability, need for precise and high-contrast printing, limited rotational tolerance, and lack of error-correction capabilities) have necessitated the development of alternative symbology approaches using two-dimensional (2D) codes that overcome linear symbology limitations and enable whole new classes of applications. On the basis of their characteristics and experience with their use in different applications and industries, these emerging 2D data codes seem to be uniquely suited for many novel identification applications in the laboratory and healthcare environments.

Such 2D codes are designed to be a small database within the symbol and can contain much more data than a regular bar code—up to 2000 characters in some cases at very high densities (60 characters of information can be readily carried

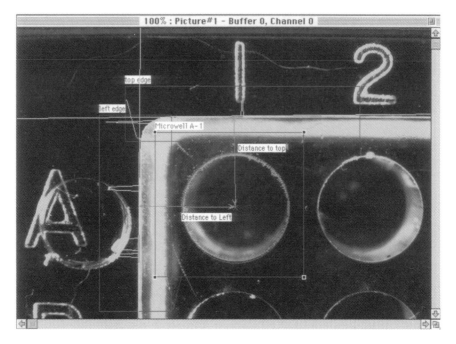

Figure 13.33. Location and orientation of wells on a 384-well microplate. Edge detection ROIs locate the top and left sides, while a Hough transform ROI confirms the well location.

in a 0.12 in.² matrix code). In addition, through built-in error correction, most 2D codes can deliver 100% of the data stored in the code even if the label is more than 50% damaged. Formulas embedded in the code reconstruct a missing portion of the symbol and recreate the original data. This allows the symbol to be stored in environments where damage is likely. Further, 2D codes require a contrast of only 20%, which means the code can be printed with chemical etch or photoengraving on surfaces such as semiconductor wafers or surgical instruments. It can even be printed using invisible ultraviolet inks. Matrix cell size can vary up to 50% within a single symbol and still be read with 100% accuracy. One common such code, the matrix code, is shown in Figure 13.35.

Problems encountered when reading such codes may include material surface defects such as scratches or dents, low-contrast printing or marking on certain materials or surfaces, faded code printing, or warping due to material stretching (which may turn a nominally rectangular code into a rhombus) or partial code occlusion by paint, marks, or other materials. Although some of these problems can be addressed through the built-in error-correction capabilities of the 2D codes, reading performance can be improved, or in some cases only

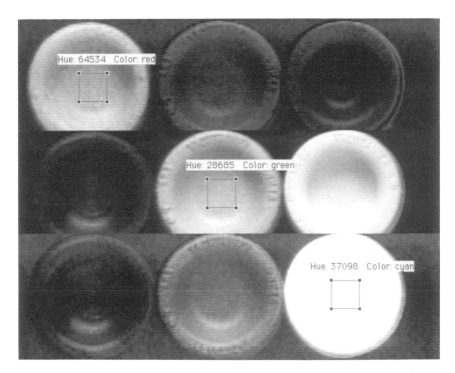

Figure 13.34. Use of color vision analysis (on red, green, and blue image planes) to determine type of tests to be performed on blood sample based on color-coded sample caps.

achieved, by applying sophisticated image processing and analysis capabilities available in a machine vision system.

Finally, other identification uses of machine vision are in optical character recognition (OCR) or optical character verification (OCV) where the vision system is used to read or verify human-readable characters. Since most accepted laboratory practices call for human-readable marking in addition to or instead of coded marking where possible, systems that are capable of interpreting human readable marks have significant potential in the laboratory.

13.3.4. Automated Inspection

The most prevalent application of machine vision in manufacturing is also useful in laboratory automation. *Automated inspection* tasks involve the execution of predefined vision sequences on samples in order to perform quality control. Generally such applications are used to weed out samples that are inappropriate

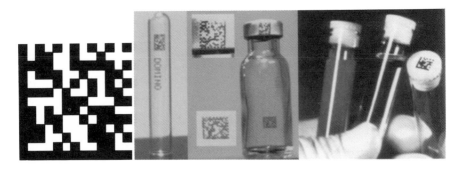

Figure 13.35. Matrix code close-up and its use on different lab consumables.

for automated processing, either because they are in some nonstandard form or because the sample requires specialized processing.

An example of this type of application is in the clinical laboratory for automated blood sample processing. Blood samples are frequently subject to quality problems that may hamper their analysis or require redirection to more specialized instrumentation. Among these sample problems are icterus (excessive bilirubin), hemolysis (evidence of damage to erythrocytes), and lipemia (excess lipids in serum). These sample quality problems can be characterized and classified visually: icteric serum samples tend to be yellow-orange, hemolyzed samples pink, and lipemic samples cloudy, as opposed to the normal straw color of serum. However, judgment of sample quality is not a binary decision; samples can show varying degrees of hemolysis, some of which may not require special processing. Laboratory technologists make use of special charts in order to compare the sample with standard archetypes and thus attempt to quantify the quality of the sample (Fig. 13.36a). Similarly, a machine vision system equipped to measure color changes can be used to quantify these slight changes in color gradient.

Another approach to inspecting serum samples would be to make use of a known background image, such as a line, to determine the opacity of the sample or to quantify the diffraction of light through the sample. As shown in Figure 13.36(b), as hemolysis increases, the clarity of the dark line in the background decreases. This reduction can be measured with a gray-scale algorithm.

Another example of an inspection application is the use of machine vision for

Figure 13.36. (a) Interference guides such as this one are used by laboratory technicians to gauge levels of hemolysis (top line), lipemia (center) or icterus (bottom) in serum samples; (b) gray-scale machine vision analysis on the image in (a) shows how a background line may be used to show increasing hemolysis. [Images courtesy of Eastman Kodak Company, Clinical Diagnostics Division, Rochester, NY.]

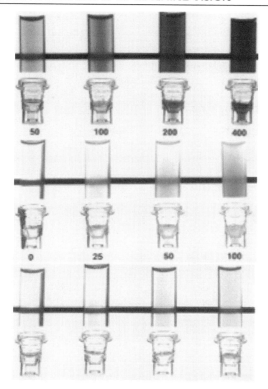

(a)

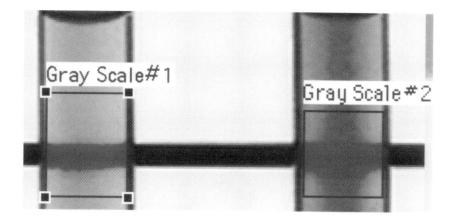

(b)

turbidity testing; that is, to determine whether a compound is soluble to a particular solvent. Simple area counting can usually be used for this purpose, as shown in Figure 13.37. However, special lighting may be required for an accurate test, depending on the color and clarity of the sample container and the morphology of the particulate inside. In addition, defects on the container such as scratches or labels can affect the accuracy of the area count. Image arithmetic methods might then be used to eliminate these static features, as explained in Section 13.2.3.2.

13.3.5. Dimensional Gauging

Dimensional gauging refers to using machine vision to compute precise measurements of parts. Although such applications are very common in manufacturing uses of machine vision, they are less common in laboratory automation applications. One example is the use of machine vision for quick volume or liquid level of fill measurements. Figure 13.38 shows a simple example where edge detection is used to detect the free surface of the liquid level as well as the liquid–liquid interface. The accuracy of the measurement depends on the resolution of the original image, as discussed in the first section. Once vision is used

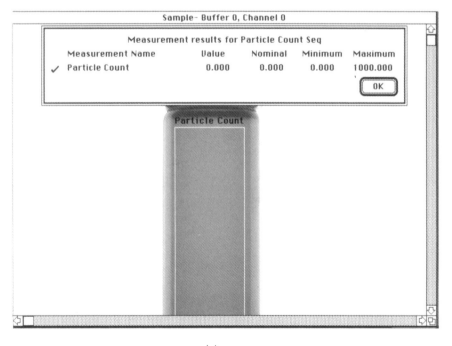

(a)

Figure 13.37. Use of machine vision to confirm sample dissolution in solvent.

to gauge the depth of the liquid interface, it is possible to forward this measurement to a robot controller or automated pipetting system and thus automate a liquid–liquid extraction task where the quantities of sample involved may not be known in advance.

Machine vision has also already been used for dimensional gauging purposes in gel electrophoresis,[20] where dedicated vision processing systems have been developed to quickly quantify markings on the gel.

13.3.6. Process Monitoring and Validation

A number of opportunities exist to use machine vision for automated process monitoring and validation. These may, for example, include

- Monitoring color changes that indicate the completion of a reaction
- Detecting precipitate formation in a clear solution
- Recording of selected video frames to record failed conditions or validate an automated laboratory procedure

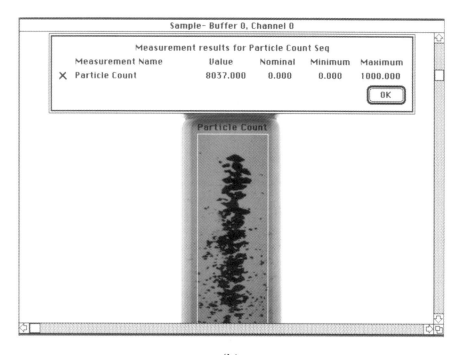

(b)

Figure 13.37. (Continued)

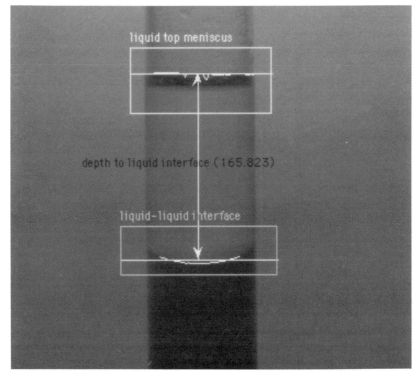

New ii Interface

Figure 13.38. Use of edge detection to perform simple level of fill and liquid–liquid interface measurements.

In this type of application the machine vision system is set up to execute a given image analysis sequence at periodic intervals and to trigger an output line when the sequence notes a change in a critical measurement. For example, in Section 13.3.1 we illustrated how a reflected light gleam could be used to determine whether a petri dish was properly oriented. In a laboratory automation system the vision workstation could monitor petri dishes as they are delivered from the dispenser and trigger an alarm whenever an inverted dish was found or, better still, modify the robotic procedure to account for the change in labware configuration (perhaps by directing the robot to turn over the dish).

Recording of video images of samples can also be effective for defending the accuracy of the sample preparation process, for example, in clinical sample analysis. An important consideration when storing images is their relatively large size; a full screen image may take up over 100 K (100 kilobytes) of storage space using current compression schemes. Depending upon the rate of sample processing and the time period over which images of samples must be maintained, very high capacity storage media may be required. Additionally, the time required to store the images should be taken into account when the rate of sample processing is very high.

Validation of the machine vision system itself can be relatively straightforward. The system can be provided with a number of known good/bad samples and the measurements recorded into a file for appropriate documentation. Repeated sequences should also be run to gauge the repeatability of system measurements and to estimate system sensitivity to noise conditions, variations in lighting, and the like.

13.3.7. Vision-Guided Robotics

Vision-guided robotics refers to applications of machine vision in laboratory automation that involve linking the vision system to a robotic device such as a robot or a motorized x–y positioning stage.[21-23] In these applications the feedback from the vision system must be transformed into coordinates that can be used by the robot. Quite often the same computer system that is performing the image analysis must also control the robot, calculate any coordinate transformations, and execute stored programs involving vision and motion.

Proper calibration of a vision-guided system is critical to obtaining accurate performance. The system is calibrated using a single-dot target, as opposed to the 8-dot target used to calibrate a stationary vision system (described in the previous section). The robot then moves the dot to eight planar positions underneath the camera (or the camera is moved to eight locations by the robot over the stationary dot). The image of the dot in these eight locations can then be used to calibrate the vision system to the motion system just as the standard 8-dot target is used, making the assumption that the motions made have been accurate (and hence that the motion system has already been calibrated). Location in the image plane determined by the vision system can then be transformed to locations in a particular plane of motion, given the current gross position of the camera or robot.

Once calibrated, the vision system can be used for three basic types of tasks in conjunction with a robot:

- Step-and-repeat operations (Fig. 13.39) where the same vision sequence is to be executed at an array of locations (such as for a microwell plate).
- Extended field-of-view measurements, where large measurements are made by a single camera at two locations instead of expanding the field of view to fit the entire object at a lower resolution. The information obtained by vision processing is combined with the length of movement to produce the actual measurement.
- Vision offsets where the results of vision processing are used to guide robot motion.

Vision offsetting typically is necessary in applications where some critical coordinate in the system remains unknown and hence cannot be preprogrammed into the robot program. An example of such an application is vision-guided

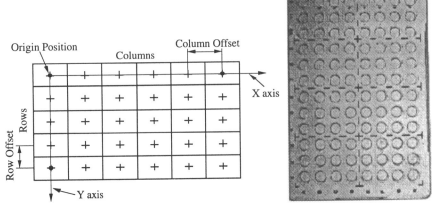

Figure 13.39. Grid configuration for common step-and-repeat operations and sample microwell plate where such approach would be necessary in order to perform the same inspection over each well of the plate.

colony picking.[22,24,25] In this application, a robot is used to transfer bacterial colonies from large plates filled with multiple colonies into individual containers, such as microwell plates or small petri dishes. All the source plates are different, since the colonies will grow at any location on the plate. In addition, certain colonies are inappropriate as samples either because they are too small, or because they have grown into another colony and are contaminated. Human technologists may also use other criteria, such as color, to make choices about which colonies to transfer.

Automation of this application requires a machine vision system to locate the colonies and to perform the classification required to select the appropriate colonies for transfer (Fig. 13.40). Furthermore, vision guidance is needed to direct a robot picking arm or a gantry device to the colonies selected. The steps involved in performing this vision-guided motion task include the following:

1. Calibrate the motion device and then calibrate the vision system to the motion device.
2. Acquire an image of the colonies.
3. Perform image processing to identify, locate, and sort the colonies.
4. Transform the colony locations into world locations.
5. Send the world locations to the robot in order to pick up colonies for transfer.

The first two steps were discussed in the previous section. The image processing steps required to locate and sort colonies are also relatively simple. First, some form of "anchor" position whose coordinates in world space are known must be located in the image. This may be a fiducial mark or other reference point that

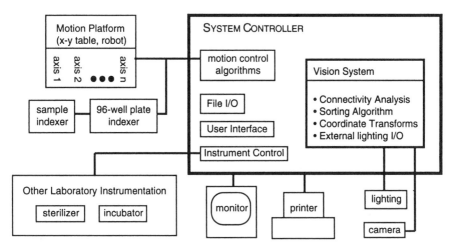

Figure 13.40. Schematic of a vision-guided colony picking system.

has been taught to the robot and that is also visible in the image of the colonies. Since both the world and image coordinates of the anchor are known, this point can serve as a link between points in the real world and points in the image plane. Within the vision sequence edge detection, circle finding, or other algorithms can be used to find the reference point coordinates in the image plane.

The colonies can then be located using a connectivity algorithm. Connectivity features such as blob area, gray value, or blob roundness are then recovered and used to classify colonies by size, color, and shape. A list of blob centroid locations is then created for those colonies that demonstrate sufficient size, appropriate color, and high roundness (since colonies that are touching other colonies will not show up as individual round blobs; see Fig. 13.41).

The system must then transform this list of coordinates from the image plane to real-world numbers. This task is accomplished by comparing distance measurements in the image plane between the colony centroid locations and the "anchor" reference point location. These distances are then converted to real-world distances using the calibration matrices established when the vision system was first calibrated, and these new real-world offsets are fed to the robot, which can now move to positions above the colonies and begin the picking and transferring operation.

A similar setup can be used to perform image analysis and robotic operations on microwell plates of varying sizes and formats. The edges of the plate are located with an Edge algorithm and individual well locations determined, as discussed above under Location and Orientation applications. In a vision-guided motion application the vision sequence can be used to determine specific wells of interest when the exact locations of the wells are not known with accuracy. Machine vision is particularly helpful with the smaller and more dense microwell formats such as the 384 (2 × 2)- and 864 (3 × 3)-well plates, and can be

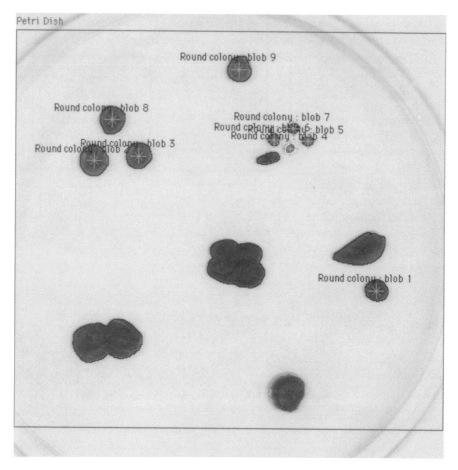

Figure 13.41. Connectivity processing is used to identify and sort simulated colonies on a petri dish. The centroid coordinates of colonies passing the sort are then transformed into world coordinates and forwarded to a robotic colony picking system.

easily modified to support arbitrary well configurations and formats as protocols and apparatus change. This flexibility gives the machine vision system a considerable advantage over fixed-format plate reading or micropipetting systems.

13.4. CONCLUSIONS

The applications described in Section 13.3 represent only a few examples of the many potential uses of machine vision in laboratory automation systems. Armed with an understanding of the basics of image processing and analysis, new users can build on the flexibility of the machine vision system to create unlimited applications. The rationale for use of a vision system in an automated laboratory closely follows that for laboratory automation itself: elimination of exposure of laboratory personnel to potential pathogens, reduction of the time needed for clinical sample preprocessing, increasing the accuracy of analysis, and lessening the costs associated with sample processing. Recent trends in lab automation are toward even greater throughputs, stricter tolerances on accuracy and repeatability of analysis, and significantly smaller scales, including nanovolumes of reagent and ultra-high-density microplate systems. The use of machine vision and vision-guided robotics to meet these demands on speed, quantity, and quality will sharply increase over the next few years until—as in the semiconductor and electronics industries—computer vision sensing and processing becomes an indispensable part of laboratory procedure as positioning and measurement tolerances fall beyond the limits of human capabilities.

ACKNOWLEDGMENT

Funding for applications described in this chapter was provided in part by a Small Business Innovation Research grant from the National Center for Research Resources, an institute of the National Institutes of Health, Bethesda, Maryland.

REFERENCES

1. Fouda HG: Robotics in biomedical chromatography and electrophoresis. *J Chromatogr* 492:85–108, 1989.
2. Ward KB, Perozzo MA, Zuk WM: Automated preparation of protein crystals using laboratory robotics and automated visual inspection. *J Crystal Growth* 90:325–339, 1988.
3. Watson A, Smaldon N, Lucke R., Hawkins T: The *Caenorhabditis elegans* genome sequencing project: first steps in automation. *Nature* 362:569–570, 1993.
4. Martin WJ, Walmsley RM: Vision assisted robotics and tape technology in the life-science laboratory: applications to genome analysis, *Bio/Technol* 8:1258–1262, 1990.
5. Boyd JC, Felder RA, Margrey KS, Martinez A, Savory J: Use of a robotic arm for specimen handling in a remote, unmanned clinical chemistry laboratory. *Clin Chem* 33:1560–1561, 1987.
6. Sasaki M: A fully automated robotics laboratory in Kochi Medical School. *Clin Chem* 35:1052, 1989.
7. Hecht E: *Optics.* Reading, MA: Addison-Wesley, 1987.
8. Fink DG, ed: *Television Engineering Handbook.* New York: McGraw-Hill, 1957.
9. VanDommelen, CH: Lighting for machine vision II: lighting techniques, design, and applications. *Electronic Imaging Conf,* 1992.
10. VanDommelen, CH: Fundamentals of camera selection for machine vision. *RIA/AIA Internatl Conf Robotics and Vision,* Oct, 1991.

11. Melles-Griot Inc: *Optics Guide 5* (catalog). Irvine, CA: Mellese Griot Inc., 1990.

12. Inoue S: *Video Microscopy.* New York: Plenum Press, 1986.

13. Jain AK: *Fundamentals of Digital Image Processing.* Englewood Cliffs, NJ: Prentice-Hall, 1989.

14. Ballard D, Brown C: *Computer Vision.* Englewood Cliffs, NJ: Prentice-Hall, 1982.

15. Gonzalez RC, Woods RE: *Digital Image Processing.* Reading, MA: Addison-Wesley, 1992.

16. Horn, BKP: *Robot Vision.* Cambridge, MA: MIT Press, 1985.

17. Haralick RM, Shapiro LG: *Computer and Robot Vision,* Vols. I, II. Reading, MA: Addison-Wesley, 1992.

18. Russ JC:*The Image Processing Handbook.* Boca Raton, FL: CRC Press, 1992.

19. Yang GJ, Huang TS: The effect of median filtering on edge location estimation. *Comput Graph Image Process* 15:224–245, 1981.

20. Redman T, Jacobs T: Electrophoretic gel image analysis software for the molecular biology laboratory. *BioTechniques* 10:790–794, 1991.

21. Agapakis JE, Cole WS, Krishnaswamy S, Lamoreaux PA: A vision-integrated robotic system for laboratory applications. Poster presentation. *3rd Annu Conf Automation, Robotics, and Artificial Intelligence Applied to Analytical Chemistry and Laboratory Medicine.* San Diego, CA: Jan 25, 1994.

22. Krishnaswamy S, Agapakis JE: Vision-guided motion applications in laboratory automation. Poster presentation. *Internatl Symp Laboratory Automation and Robotics,* Boston, MA, 1994.

23. Courtney P, Beck MS, Martin WJ: A vision guided life-science laboratory robot. *Meas Sci Technol* 2-2:97–101, 1991.

24. Meier-Ewert S, Maier E, Ahmadi A, Curtis J, Lehrach H: An automated approach to generating expressed sequence catalogues. *Nature* 361:375–376, 1993.

25. Parry RL, Chin TW, Donahoe PK: Computer-aided cell colony counting. *BioTechniques* 10:772–774, 1991.

CHAPTER

14

Image Analysis

WENDY A. WELLS AND VINCENT A. MEMOLI

CONTENTS

Handbook of Clinical Automation, Robotics, and Optimization, Edited by Gerald J. Kost with the collaboration of Judith Welsh.
ISBN 0-471-03179-8 © 1996 John Wiley & Sons, Inc.

14.1. INTRODUCTION

The major historical events shaping the subsequent development of quantitative pathology were the invention of the microscope by Antoni van Leeuwenhoek in the late seventeenth century and Lavoisier's studies in analytical organic chemistry in the 1770s.[1] Detailed descriptions of the cell nucleus and of human malignant cells, technical advances including an electric light source for the microscope and improved stains, fixatives and embedding media,[2] established the place of tissue morphology in the field of disease diagnosis by the early twentieth century.

Estimates of numerous cell parameters, such as size, shape, and texture, were first evaluated implementing the time-consuming disciplines of *karyometry*.[3] The *genetic* approach to karyometry, introduced in the beginning of the twentieth century by Hertwig,[4] Boveri,[5] and Erdmann,[6] postulated that the only cause of nuclear size variation was a change in the number or size of chromosomes. Functional changes of the cell were not considered. In spite of this rigid viewpoint, several important karyometric relationships were recognized, including the nuclear : cytoplasmic ratio.[4] Jacobj confirmed that this ratio remained the same after cell division but varied considerably during the process of cell division.[7] Work from the same scientist, and many others between 1925 and 1963, formed the basis of the principle of *chromosome constancy*, which stated that nuclear volume was directly dependent on the number and size of the chromosome population.

Favoring a *functional* approach to karyometry, other investigators observed an increase in nuclear volumes in ganglion cells after electrical stimulation;[8–10] the volume-reducing effect of starvation in cells of liver, pancreas, and kidney;[11] and the relationship between the age of an individual and the heart muscle fiber size.[12] Cell size changes were initially recorded empirically. Not until the 1950s was an adequate theory established to explain the dependence of nuclear size on the functional state of the cell and terms such as *functional edema, functional nuclear swelling and shrinking,* and *working hypertrophy,*[13,15] introduced.

The early planimetry methods of measurement utilized eyepiece micrometers, microplanimeters, and microprojection methods.[3] Later, the chemical identification of nucleic acids such as the Feulgen stain for DNA[16] and the methylgreen pyronin stain for RNA,[17] would be quantified using microspectrophotometric methods.

In the late 1940s, Papanicolou led the resurgence of interest in cell studies for the diagnosis of human disease.[18] An automatic scanning microscope for diagnostic purposes was first conceived, by Mellors, in the 1950s, who confirmed Caspersson's observations[19] that nuclear chromatin density could be used to distinguish normal, dysplastic and malignant exfoliated cervical squamous cells. The first semiautomated apparatus for the detection of cancer cells was developed between 1953 and 1956[2] although it did not include a computerized analytical system. Following the introduction of the computer,[20] Wied and his colleagues formed the basis of modern quantitative cytology.[21]

Today, the advent of inexpensive microprocessors, high-quality cameras and more affordable memory devices ensures that the many cost-effective and time-saving applications of image processing are amenable to operators with variable experience in applied computer sciences. The main techniques used in quantitative pathology today, and discussed in this chapter, are morphology, stereology, static and flow cytometry, digital image processing, and expert systems.

14.2. BASIC PRINCIPLES AND DEFINITIONS

Image processing is the manipulation of pictorial information to maximally enhance and evaluate the visual qualities of the original image. In this way, it is possible to exaggerate certain details in the digitized image not appreciated in the original form.

The steps in image processing and analysis are summarized in Figure 14.1. Applications for digital processing include the fields of astronomy, geology, particle physics, fluid mechanics, meterology, space exploration as well as medicine [MRI, CAT, U/S (magnetic resonance imaging, computerized axial tomography, ultrasound) scans and x-rays].

14.2.1. Image Types

The three image types are *optical, electronic,* and *digital.* The image field is usually defined with a microscope (optical manipulation), and the image information is transformed into an analog message via a videocamera tube and camera (electrical manipulation). At a set sampling frequency, the analog video signal is converted into a digital image forming a two-dimensional (2D) array of unit areas. Each unit area in a digitized image is called a *picture element* (pixel), sequentially arranged in rows and columns, left to right and top to bottom within the image file. The values of these pixels may be manipulated by an *intensity transformation function* (computer manipulation) and are then converted back to a pulse of voltages to be displayed on the computer monitor.

Although optical and electronic images can be processed more quickly, advantages of digital images are their increased flexibility and reproducibility (algorithmic format). Only part of the image needs to be utilized, and there is no information loss. Examples of image processing include image enhancement, geometric correction, image compression, identification of regions of interest (ROIs) in an image, and manipulation of image sequences, to be discussed in more detail later.

14.2.2. The Pixel

The pixel is defined by its location and intensity. The *image width* represents the number of pixels in a row within the image file. The *image height* represents the number of pixels in a column within the image file. Usually, pixels are *square* but they may be *rectangular* or *hexagonal.* The amount of information allocated to each pixel (gray value, color, direction) is measured in *byte* units, where 1 byte is equivalent to 8 bits. For an 8-bit image, each pixel has 1 byte (8 bits) of information such as 256 (2^8) gray values. This range of gray values (GVs) is known as the *gray scale,* where the pixel value of 255 is white and the pixel value of 0 is black. Pixel intensities between 0 and 255 are various shades of gray. For a 4-bit image, each pixel has 4 bits of information such as 16 (2^4) gray values. The minimum number of bits per pixel is 1, and an image that consists of single

Image analysis and Processing

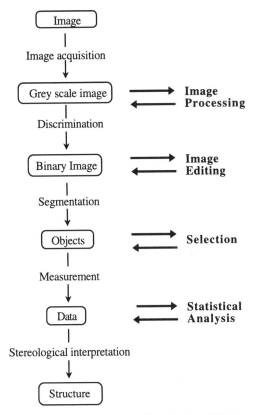

Figure 14.1. Image processing is the manipulation of pictorial information to maximally enhance and evaluate the visual qualities of the original image. (Reproduced, with permission of Plenum Press, from JC Russ, *Computer-Assisted Microscopy—the Measurement and Analysis of Images,* Plenum Press, New York, 199, Fig. 1-5.)

bit data is called a *binary image.* Such an image contains pixels that are either black (switched off) or white (switched on) and are represented by the pixel values 0 and 1, respectively.

14.2.3. The Histogram

The distribution of pixel number and value (e.g., GV/color) can be graphically represented in a *histogram,* which pictorially represents the number of pixels that appear in the image at each gray value[22] (Fig. 14.2). A tall, narrow histogram represents large numbers of pixels with equal or nearly equal gray values. In this *low-contrast* image, small points of detail are difficult to differentiate. A broad

Digitized image   Corresponding pixel values

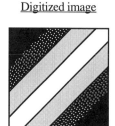

0	80	170	255
80	170	255	170
170	255	170	80
255	170	80	0

Frequency Histogram

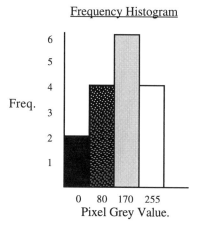

Figure 14.2. Each unit area in a digitized image is called a picture element (pixel), defined by its location and intensity within the image file. The pixel values can be represented in a frequency histogram.

histogram represents pixels of variable gray values. In this *high-contrast* image, the degree of image detail is markedly enhanced.

14.2.4. Resolution and Depth

Spatial resolution and image depth determine the *quality* of an image. Image resolution is defined by the number of pixels in the image and is a function of the application. Only the minimum resolution to perform a task is required. The resolution of most microscopic images is 512 × 512 pixels but in other cases, 30 × 50 pixels may be sufficient. Digital images are not always square.

Image depth is amplitude quantization or GV quantization, represented by the number of bits, m, used for each pixel. The number of possible GV's, G, is then given by

$$G = 2^m$$

The m index generally varies between 1 and 16, but may be as high as 64 for specialist applications. Eight-bit data is the most popular image depth currently used. Although the computer is capable of distinguishing between the 256 GVs (8-bit image), the human eye can distinguish only approximately 30 GVs (5-bit image). The more depth information required in an image, the greater the size of the image file.

Binary images, with pixel values of either 0 or 1 often result from operations performed on images of greater depth. As discussed later, 8-bit images can be segmented to produce a binary image to distinguish and delineate objects of interest.

14.2.5. Intensity, Transmittance, and Optical Density

The frequently used, and sometimes confusing, terms of intensity, transmittance, optical density, and gray value need to be defined and differentiated.

Intensity (I) of staining is expressed in terms of *average* gray levels but cannot be used to compare levels of staining in different regions. For example, immunohistochemical staining in a region with an average gray value of 100 is not stained twice as heavily as a region with an average gray value of 200.

Transmittance (T) is determined by the amount of regional staining, where T is the ratio of gray value in the region of interest to that of the incident or blank field light.

Optical density (OD) is a logarithmic function of transmittance. For the same object, at a fixed wavelength or temperature (etc.), the ratio of the intensity of incident light (I_t) to the intensity of transmitted light (I_i) is always the same; thus, if I_t is increased, then I_i will also be increased:

$$\therefore 0 \leq \frac{I_t}{I_i} \geq 1$$

As log (I_t/I_i) varies between $-\infty$ (opaque) and 0 (transparent), then:

$$OD = -\log\left(\frac{I_t}{I_i}\right)$$

An OD of 1 means that 0.1 of the incident light is transmitted.

An OD of 2 means that 0.01 of the incident light is transmitted.

An OD of 3 means that 0.001 of the incident light is transmitted.

The OD is an inherent property of the tissue. Gray values in a digitized image depend on camera calibration, microscope illumination, staining, and other variables. Neutral density filters of known ODs can be used to evaluate the equivalent GV for a given illumination, lens setting, or time. Using conversion tables, the OD for each GV can be found.

14.3. IMAGE ENHANCEMENT

14.3.1. The Human Visual System

Knowledge of the natural image enhancing characteristics of the human visual system may be helpful in understanding the computer manipulations required to reproduce similar qualities.[23] First, the relationship between illumination intensity on the rod and cone photoreceptors and perceived brightness is logarithmic rather than linear. Hence, for the same change in illumination intensity, there is a much greater change in the perceived brightness of darker regions in the image than brighter regions. By simply darkening an image, previously undetected details can be brought out (Fig. 14.3).

Second, the human eye displays a "simultaneous contrast effect" whereby the perceived brightness of an area is dependent on the intensity of the surrounding area. Given two identically sized images with the same gray-value intensity, the one with a black background will appear brighter than the one with a white background.

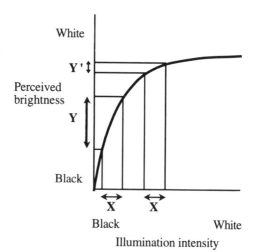

Figure 14.3. With a logarithmic response to perceived brightness, there is a much greater change in the perceived brightness of darker regions (*y*) than lighter regions (*y'*) for the same change in illumination intensity (*x*). [Reproduced with permission of the *American Journal of Clinical Pathology,* Volume 98, pages 493–501 (1992).]

Third, the human visual system is able to accentuate sharp intensity changes by employing the "Mach band effect." At the immediate interface of a dark region and a light region, the human eye perceives a more exaggerated change in the brightness transition than that which is actually present.

14.3.2. Intensity Transformation Functions

The two main techniques of image enhancement are defined in the *spatial* and *frequency* domains. *Spatial domain* enhancement describes the direct manipulation of the pixel values in the input image [Im1 (x,y)] and those in the output image [Im2 (x,y)] using a functional relationship, f. In *frequency-domain* enhancement, the processing techniques are based on modifying the Fourier transform of an image. The intensity transformation function (ITF) defines this variability in the shape of the histogram or contrast enhancement.[22] The ITF converts the raw image into a second image.

The *linear* function between the gray values (GVs) and the optical density is described as follows:

$$Im2 \ (x,y) = f[Im1 \ (x,y)]$$

where Im1 = pixel gray value at point (x,y) in the original image
Im2 = pixel gray value at point (x,y) in the modified image

Given that the *output* gray value of the ITF is solely dependent on the *input* gray value, and that the relative information between adjacent pixels remains the same, the specifications for individual pixels can be dropped:

$$GV2 = f(GV1)$$

where GV1 = the input gray value of image 1
GV2 = the output gray value of image 2

As a linear function:

$$GV2 = mGV1 + b$$

where m = slope of the line (a steep slope indicates better contrast)
b = intercept of the GV axis

A linear ITF with a fixed slope ($m = 1$) but variable-axis intercept (b value) is demonstrated in Figure 14.4. The overall relationship of the individual pixels in

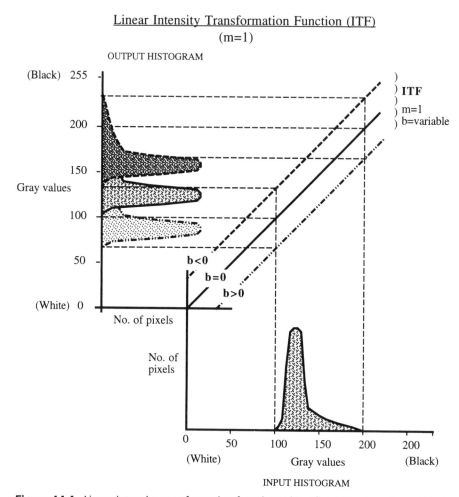

Figure 14.4. Linear intensity transformation function with a fixed line slope ($m = 1$) but variable axis intercept (*b* value). When $b > 0$, the transformed image appears universally paler. When $b < 0$, the transformed image appears universally darker. [Reproduced with permission of the *American Journal of Clinical Pathology*, Volume 98, pages 493–501 (1992).]

the image remain the same and so the shape of the input and output histograms are identical. But when $b > 0$, the gray value of every pixel is decreased by the same amount, and so the transformed image appears universally paler. When $b < 0$, the gray value of every pixel is increased by the same amount and so the transformed image appears universally darker. Figure 14.5 demonstrates a linear ITF with a fixed-axis intercept ($b = 0$) but increased line slope ($m > 1$). The

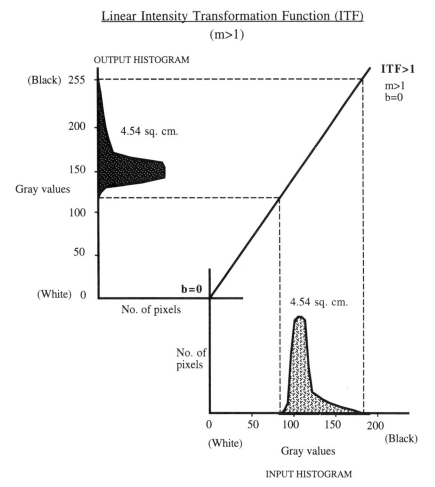

Figure 14.5. Linear intensity transformation function with a fixed axis intercept ($b = 0$) but an increased line slope ($m > 1$). The output histogram is broadened, representing a high-contrast output image. [Reproduced with permission of the *American Journal of Clinical Pathology*, Volume 98, pages 493–501 (1992).]

range of gray values displayed in the output histogram image is now increased. This broadens the output histogram and increases the contrast of the output image. In Figure 14.6, the axis intercept is fixed but the line slope is decreased ($m < 1$). The output histogram is narrowed, representing a low-contrast output image. *Nonlinear* ITFs enable contrast enhancement of one range of gray values in the image, leaving other regions of the image unaltered. Thus, certain features of an image can be accentuated above other areas.

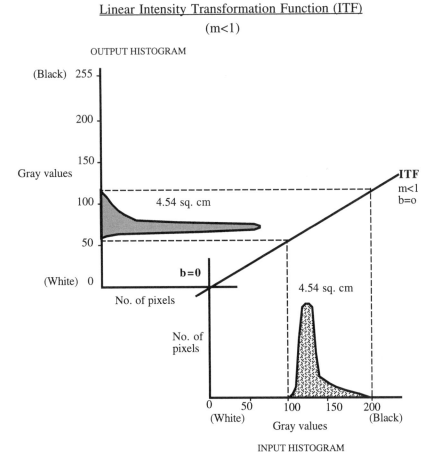

Figure 14.6. Linear intensity transformation function with a fixed-axis intercept ($b = 0$) but a decreased line slope ($m < 1$). The output histogram is narrowed, representing a low-contrast output image. [Reproduced with permission of the *American Journal of Clinical Pathology,* Volume 98, pages 493–501 (1992).]

14.3.3. Histogram Equalization

Histogram equalization is a functional operation whereby the distribution of gray values is spread as widely and evenly as possible to achieve near equal numbers of pixels per gray value.[22] In the ideal, well-represented image with good contrast, the relationship between the cumulative frequency of the GVs and the actual GVs approximates a straight line.

Consider an image with 10 possible GVs 0–9 with the relative frequencies given below:

GV	Frequency	Cumulative Frequency	
		Actual	Ideal
0	2	2	10
1	3	5	20
2	8	13	30
3	16	29	40
4	21	50	50
5	21	71	60
6	16	87	70
7	8	95	80
8	3	98	90
9	2	100	100

The original histogram, displaying GVs and their frequencies, is shown in Figure 14.7a. A transformed histogram, displaying GVs and their cumulative frequencies, is shown in Figure 14.7b. To improve this GV distribution, the *real* cumulative values can be grouped and mapped to the nearest *ideal* cumulative value. With similar grouping, each real pixel gray value can be mapped to the closest ideal pixel GV in order to construct an equalized histogram with near equal numbers of pixels per GV (Fig. 14.7c).

14.3.4. Lookup Tables

Lookup tables (LUTs), indexed by the values of the original image, enhance the image output display. No information is lost. Each value from the input image is converted to the relevant entry in the LUT and then displayed in the output image as the new value. A gray-value input image can be represented as a pseudocolor output image using a separate LUT for each of the primary colors red, blue, and green. If an input image point is mapped to LUT values set at a maximum intensity for red, blue, and green, then the output image point will be white. If an input image point is mapped to LUT values set at a maximum intensity for red, but zero intensity for blue and green, then the output image point will be red. The human eye may not be able to distinguish between pixels with gray values of 100 and 101, but if all input GVs of 100 are mapped to an LUT with maximum intensity for red and all input GVs of 101 are mapped to an LUT with maximum intensity for blue, then the output image will exhibit clearly defined pseudored and pseudoblue colors.

14.3.5. Image Smoothing

Smoothing algorithms may be used to correct defects present in the image commonly referred to as "noise." Noise may be either *random* (stochastic) or

Histogram Equalization

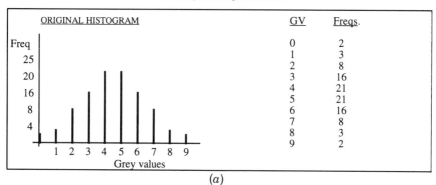

GV	Freqs.
0	2
1	3
2	8
3	16
4	21
5	21
6	16
7	8
8	3
9	2

(a)

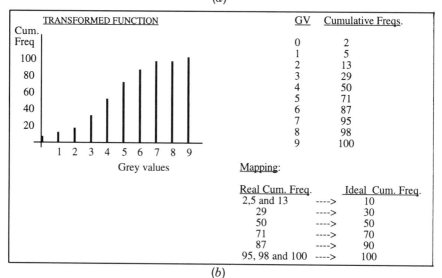

GV	Cumulative Freqs.
0	2
1	5
2	13
3	29
4	50
5	71
6	87
7	95
8	98
9	100

Mapping:

Real Cum. Freq.		Ideal Cum. Freq.
2,5 and 13	---->	10
29	---->	30
50	---->	50
71	---->	70
87	---->	90
95, 98 and 100	---->	100

(b)

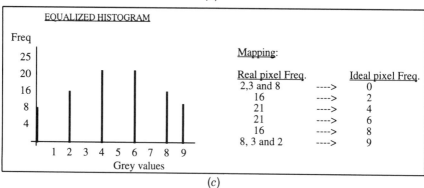

Mapping:

Real pixel Freq.		Ideal pixel Freq.
2,3 and 8	---->	0
16	---->	2
21	---->	4
21	---->	6
16	---->	8
8, 3 and 2	---->	9

(c)

Figure 14.7. (a) Original histogram displaying GVs and their frequencies; (b) transformed histogram displaying GVs and their cumulative frequencies; (c) equalized histogram with near equal numbers of pixels per GV.

periodic. Most of the random noise can be eliminated simply by *averaging* together many captured images. The problem pixels, which are randomly present at different locations in each image, are averaged out and removed. Another method is *background subtraction.* A blank area is captured and subtracted pixel by pixel from the image to be smoothed.

If the random noise still persists in the image after averaging or background subtraction, *templates or convolutions* can be used. A template comprises an array of fixed values that is systematically placed over each pixel point in the image to be enhanced. Most commonly, the template value (T) is multiplied by the corresponding pixel in the image (P). The ($P \times T$) values are then added together and the central pixel in the smoothed image acquires this new value. This convolution is repeated throughout the image for every pixel. Templates can be any size although they are commonly (3×3) or (4×4).

If the template (T) equals

$$\begin{array}{ccc} T_1 & T_2 & T_3 \\ T_4 & T_5 & T_6 \\ T_7 & T_8 & T_9 \end{array} = \begin{array}{ccc} 1 & 2 & 3 \\ 4 & 5 & 6 \\ 7 & 8 & 9 \end{array}$$

and the area in the image over which the template is laid (P) is equal to

$$\begin{array}{ccc} P_1 & P_2 & P_3 \\ P_4 & P_5 & P_6 \\ P_7 & P_8 & P_9 \end{array} = \begin{array}{ccc} 2 & 2 & 3 \\ 5 & 6 & 6 \\ 4 & 4 & 4 \end{array}$$

then, the new central pixel value will be equal to

$$(P_1 * T_1) + (P_2 * T_2) + (P_3 * T_3) \cdots (P_9 * T_9)$$
$$= (1 * 2) + (2 * 2) + (3 * 3) + (4 * 5) \cdots (9 * 4)$$

Gaussian smoothing replaces the brightness value of each pixel in the image with a value representing the average of the central pixel and its surrounding eight neighbors. The disadvantage of a center weighted smoothing kernel method is degradation of edge sharpness and the image as a whole.

The *median filter* is the best method for removal of *random* noise. Using the *one-dimensional (1D) median filter,* an image line is scanned and the median value for every three neighboring pixel GVs replaces the original central pixel.

Consider the image scan line of GVs where GV 6 represents a noise point and the change in GVs to 4, 3, 4 represents an edge in the image.

$$1 \quad 0 \quad 1 \quad 1 \quad 1 \quad 6 \quad 1 \quad 1 \quad 4 \quad 3 \quad 4 \quad 4$$

Using the 1D filter, the noise is removed but edge distinction is maintained and the scan line of GVs becomes

$$1 \quad 1 \quad 1 \quad 1 \quad 1 \quad 1 \quad 1 \quad 1 \quad 3 \quad 4 \quad 4$$

Using the *2D median filter,* the brightness value of each pixel in the image and its eight neighbors are ranked in order, and the median value (the fifth brightest) is used to replace the original central pixel. The disadvantage of the median filter is that it can be very time-consuming.

The gaussian kernel and the median filter operate in the *spatial domain.* They deal with each individual pixel and its neighbors based on the physical or spatial relationship to each other. This class of operations is generally ineffective in removing periodic noise. In order to delete this type of noise, one must rely on processing operations that take place in the *frequency domain.* The most familiar example is the application of the *Fourier transformation,* details of which are beyond the scope of this chapter.[24] In brief, the convolutions are carried out on the transformed image rather than the original image. The latter can be recovered by applying the inverse of the original transform function. Noise contributes heavily to the high-frequency content of the Fourier transform. Noise reduction can be achieved by attenuating a specific range of high-frequency components in the transform of a given image, using *lowpass filtering.*

14.3.5. Image Sharpening or Focusing

The *laplacian kernel* is a nondirectional second derivative that will not alter the pixel values in uniform or smoothly varying regions, but will extenuate regions of change such as edges and lines. For example:

$$\begin{array}{ccc} -1 & -1 & -1 \\ -1 & 8 & -1 \\ -1 & -1 & -1 \end{array} \qquad \text{(the template values sum to 1)}$$

or

$$\begin{array}{ccc} 0 & -1 & 0 \\ -1 & 4 & -1 \\ 0 & -1 & 0 \end{array} \qquad \text{(the template values sum to 1)}$$

Areas of change are highlighted, while the areas of uniformity are suppressed. This convolution kernel mimics the inhibition used by the human visual system and responds strongly to discontinuities in an image irrespective of their orientation. If a laplacian image is added back to the original image, the edges will be enhanced but the overall contrast is markedly reduced.

Thus, the use of sharpening operators should be used only to improve the visual appearances of images and not as a precursor to improved processing. Since the laplacian filter is a highpass filter, it is most sensitive to points and least sensitive to edges. Thus it may increase the amount of noise present in an image due to isolated points.

14.3.7. Color Schemes and Filters

Color images (RGB, CMY, HSI) are more informative than their monochrome counterparts, especially when processing and analyzing images obtained from histologically stained tissues. Light is electromagnetic radiation with a wavelength in the approximate range 400–700 nm. As seen by human eyes, the light appears as *violet* at the bottom of the range and as *red* at the top of the range. A broad band of all visible wavelengths appear *white*. A broad band with a greater *intensity* of one wavelength will give a *pastel* shade. If there is a red bias, the result will be a pink shade.

The *additive or primary colors* (RGB system) are red, green, and blue. By mixing these colors other colors are produced (Fig. 14.8*a*). The *subtractive or secondary colors* (CMY system) are cyan, magenta, and yellow. When pigments or filters are used to subtract a portion of the light spectrum, the effect is the opposite to the RGB system (Fig. 14.8*b*).

Color is produced by absorption of light. An object appears blue-green to the human eye because all the yellow, red and orange light has been absorbed. Yellow, magenta, and cyan absorb the blue, green, and red thirds of the spectrum, respectively, but each passes the other two colors.[25]

Yellow	*absorbs*	blue	and	*reflects*	red and green
Cyan	"	red	"	"	green and blue
Magenta	"	green	"	"	red and blue

There are many methods available for describing color spaces. In biology, the most useful is the *Hue saturation intensity scheme* (HSI system). Hue is the attribute of *pure* color: pure red, pure cyan, pure magenta. Saturation is the *shade* of a color: how much *white* is added to the pure color. A fully saturated color has a *low* white component. Intensity is the overall *brightness* of the color.

With the RGB system, it is necessary to examine *all* three color components in the image. With the HSI system, the examination of any one component, such as intensity, may be adequate. As a result, image processing times can be reduced using the HSI rather than the RGB system. In applications that perform gray scale operations, only the *intensity* component of the HSI system need be employed. A similar system, also used, is the *Hue lightness saturation scheme* (HLS system).

Because the human eye routinely assimilates image information from color sources, its scope of pictorial analysis is reduced when viewing an image with just gray values. This is well demonstrated by observing, via image analysis, low-intensity immunoreactivity staining with the visualizing substrate diaminobenzidine (DAB). When the brown substrate is converted into gray values, the immunostaining may be barely distinguishable from surrounding areas. Some of this lost detail can be recovered, and the thresholding sensitivity increased, using color filters (additive and subtractive).

Many commercial image analysis systems advocate the use of immunohistochemical counterstains other than standard haematoxylin.[26] The reason for

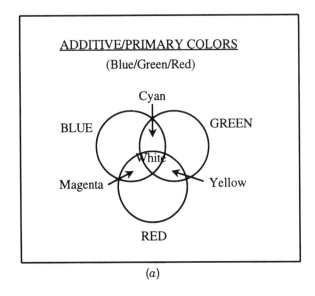

(a)

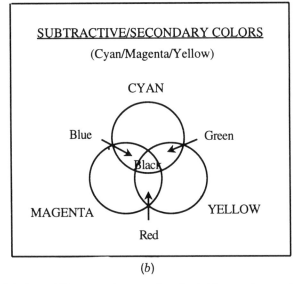

(b)

Figure 14.8. (a) The additive or primary colors (red, blue, and green) together give white. [Reproduced with permission of the *American Journal of Clinical Pathology,* Volume 99, pages 48–56 (1993.]; (b) the subtractive or secondary colors (cyan, magenta, and yellow) together give black. [Reproduced with permission of the *American Journal of Clinical Pathology,* Volume 99, pages 48–56 (1993).]

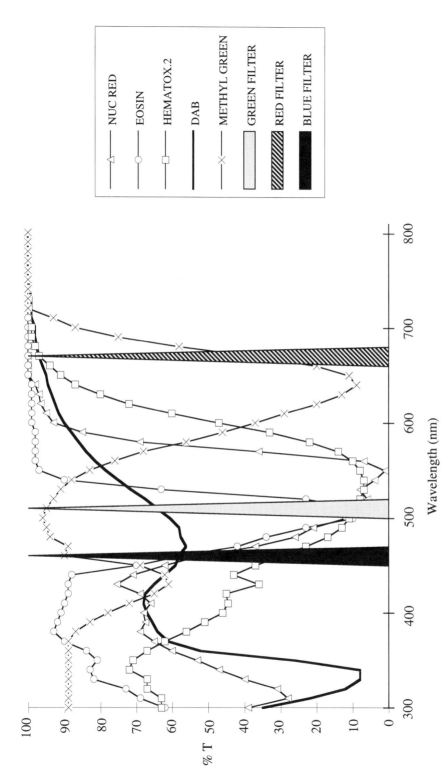

Figure 14.9. Graphic representation comparing the light transmission (T) of commonly used laboratory reagents to diaminobenzidine (DAB). [Reproduced with permission of the *American Journal of Clinical Pathology*, Volume 99, pages 48–56 (1993).]

this relates to the specificity of staining by the chosen counterstain (whether nuclear, cytoplasmic, or both) and the percent transmission of the counterstain color is compared to that of the visualizing substrate in the immunohistochemical technique used.

Many combinations of filters and counterstains can be used. Spectral studies of commonly used reagents and counterstains in our laboratory (eosin, hematoxylin, methylgreen, neutral red, and DAB) demonstrated variable degrees of light transmission for each (Fig. 14.9). Bandpass filters only allow transmittance of light of a certain wavelength and can be inserted anywhere between the light source and the camera. Using certain combinations of reagents, counterstains, and filters, the areas of immunohistochemical staining identified by the DAB in the captured image appear better contrasted and can be thesholded and analyzed more sensitively. For example, with DAB specific immunostaining limited to the nuclei, then the counterstain to use is nuclear specific methylgreen. The reason is that at two distinct wavelengths, separated by bandpass filters, methylgreen shows the best spectral separation from DAB (Fig. 14.10). With a red bandpass filter in place at a wavelength of 650 nm, the brown-red light of the DAB is maximally transmitted and that of methylgreen is mainly absorbed. Now, all the nuclei in the digitized image will show a darker gray-level value than the background. These can then be thresholded to obtain the total nuclear area. With a green bandpass filter in place at a wavelength of 500 nm, the green light of methylgreen is maximally transmitted and that of the DAB is mainly absorbed. Now, the nuclear immunostaining in the digitized image is represented in a darker gray-level value than the unstained nuclei and can be separately thresholded to obtain a value for the percentage of nuclear immunostaining.

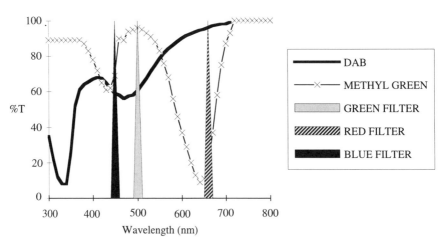

Figure 14.10. Differences between light transmission of methylgreen counterstain and DAB are maximum at the wavelength defined by the green bandpass filter. [Reproduced with permission of the *American Journal of Clinical Pathology,* Volume 99, pages 48–56 (1993).]

14.4. INSTRUMENTATION

Equipment for quantitative microscopy may be nonautomatic, semiautomatic, or automatic.[27] Nonautomatic methods for stereological point counting require a projection microscope and eyepiece graticules. Semiautomatic methods, to collect planimetric data, require digitizing graphic tablet systems consisting of a microcomputer, a cursor-coupled electromagnetic sensitive digitizing tablet, and a video overlay. Automatic methods utilize the digital image processor, detailed below, and the flow cytometers.

The four main components of an image processing system are the image capture device, image storage, an image display device, and the image processing unit.

14.4.1. Image Capture

As powerful as computer analysis can be, its abilities will always be secondary to the natural processing skills of the human brain. If the human eye cannot perceive a certain feature in the digitized image, then no amount of computer manipulation will be able to create information that is fundamentally missing from the captured image. Hence the importance of optimal image capture.

An image capturing device converts the image into a voltage signal that is then digitized for computer input. *Videocameras* are of two basic types: those using a *picture tube* (photoconductive), such as the vidicons, plumbicons, and saticons; and those with a *solid-state sensor* (silicon detectors), such as the charge-coupled devices (CCDs) and the charge-injection devices (CIDs).[28]

In image processing today, the CCDs are the most commonly used cameras. There are three main groups of CCD cameras: the monochrome CCD, the single-chip CCD, and the three-chip CCD. The *monochrome cameras* are of low cost and possess a standard "c" mount. This provides direct attachment of the camera, without any lenses, such that the optics of the microscope become the lens and the image is focused directly onto the sensing element of the camera. The gamma value, representing the slope of the curve relating output voltage to input light intensity on a log–log scale, is one (1). A positive gamma will compress the histogram at the bright end while expanding the dark end. Negative gamma values will have the opposite effect on an image. Any enhancing filters can also be used.

The *single-chip CCDs* are economical with red-blue-green output, a standard "c" mount, good sensitivity, and acceptable performance at both ends of the optical spectrum. They are easy to use, with minimal adjustments required and straightforward measurement calibration. Disadvantages are low-to-medium spatial resolution, "aliasing," and a signal-to-noise ratio (SNR) unequal for different colors. The gain, black level, and gamma value must also be controlled.

The *three-chip CCDs* are excellent performance, simple-to-use color cameras, with good color stability and a low SNR ratio. Their disadvantages relate mainly to the internal prism structure spitting the light beam into three pickup tubes representing each color. This may result in some decrease in sensitivity or poor image alignment. They are also expensive cameras without a built-in "c" mount.

14.4.2. Storage Devices

A digital image, consisting of 512 × 512 pixels, each of which is quantized into 8 bits, would occupy *0.25 Mbytes* of storage space. The 16-bit equivalent image would require *512 kbytes of storage* space. Thus, providing adequate bulk storage facilities is an important aspect in the design of an image processing system.[24]

Digitized images are best processed while stored in the random-access memory (RAM or video memory buffer). It is very time-consuming to write to and from the disk. The principal disk storage media available are threefold: (1) *magnetic disks* with a capacity of 700 Mbytes, holding 2800 images (512 × 512), (2) *magnetic tapes* (high density, 6400 bytes/in.) storing a 512 × 512 image in four foot of tape, and (3) *optical disks* with a capacity of 4 Gbytes holding approximately 16,000 images per disk.

14.4.3. Display and Recording Devices

The principal display devices are monochrome and color TV monitors, cathode-ray tubes (CRTs), and printing image display devices. Details of these devices are beyond the scope of this chapter.[29]

14.4.4. Commercially and Personally Compiled Systems

Image analysis systems may be commercially tested and purchased or personally compiled. It is evident that the expensive component in any system is the image processing software. The hardware is almost identical in most instances. Obvious advantages of a commercial system include their internal quality assurance using provided calibration slides, "user conferences" for improvement and educational sessions, as well as regular, backup servicing by the company concerned. Advantages of a personally compiled system are a more reasonable cost, the ability to interact as a workstation in the computer environment of choice, and increased flexibility of the required applications.

Many commercial image analysis systems are available on the market and have been summarized elsewhere.[30] However, in spite of the manufacturers promises, it is rare to purchase an image processing system that is suitable for every application. It is invariably necessary to make minor modifications to both hardware and software. Certainly, it is recommended that a larger storage disk than seems necessary at the time is purchased.

In today's economic climate, many medical institutions do not have, readily available, the $150,000 required to purchase a commercially developed image analysis system. As in our institution, the alternative is to compile a personal system by individually purchasing the hardware systems as well as a software packet with adequate operational processing capabilities. Goals for the first image analysis system in our laboratory were that the system should be practically affordable, maximally standardized, and not require extensive changes in technical procedures, reagents, or histotechnologist training. It also had to be a MacIntosh compatible computer system so that it could be integrated into the MacIntosh environment of our institution. The cost of our system was $8300. Details of the hardware have already been described in detail.[30] The software we use is an image processing and analysis program, "*IMAGE,*" developed by Wayne Rasband at the National Institute of Health (Research Services Branch, NIMH). The cost of any image processing system is directly proportional to the complexity of the analytical software. To our good fortune, this software is available, free, on the public-domain computer system. Our results are transported to the Microsoft "*EXCEL*" program (Microsoft Corp., Redmond, WA) and statistical analyzed is facilitated using the *DATA DESK* program (Data Description, Inc., Ithaca, NY).

14.4.5. File Formats

A digital image is a graphical representation of an array of values stored sequentially left to right within the image file. These values, which are usually integers between the range of 0 and 255, represent the intensities of pixels or describe the color components of the pixels within the image. Theoretically, the image size may be any size, although the display is obviously restricted by the characteristics of the output device.

The image file structure comprises an image *header,* the image *body* or data, and the image *trailer.* The file header incorporates information relating to image size and type, the pixel size and the scaling parameters. A *signature* introduces the file type. If it is not present, the process may abort if the encoder cannot find it. The file body records the position of individual pixel values within the image. This critical positional information ensures that the correct pixel values are placed at the appropriate location within the reconstructed image, written sequentially from left to right for each row and from top to bottom. The file trailer contains information, defined by the user, recording the factors required to reconstruct the image, such as the filter type or the zoom factor.

Currently available graphical file formats are numerous, sometimes complicated and remain to be standardized.[31] Commonly used file formats include the *Tag Image File Format* (TIFF™—Aldus Corp. and Microsoft Corp., Redmond, WA);[32] the *Graphics Interchange Format* (GIF™—CompuServe Inc., Columbus, OH); the *MRC Image Format* (Medical Research Council, UK) for the Bio-Rad Confocal Image System); the *Targa Image Format* (Truevision, Inc., Indianapolis, IN), a popular format for personal computers; the *Visualization File Format* (VFF), developed by Sun Microsystems Inc. and utilizing an ASCII header; and the *Sun Rasterfiles,* a workstation file format with provisions for GV and color images.

An *image converter* can be used to transfer images between common formats. However, for conversion between proprietary formats, the existing image must first be converted to a *raw* image file and the required header then created. The new file comprises the combined information of the header and the raw image file.

14.4.6. Image Compression

The disadvantage of storing high-resolution images is that the image files can be extremely large and occupy excessive amounts of disk space. A three-color image (1024 × 1024 pixels) will occupy 3-Mbyte memory. A confocal data set will occupy approximately 30MB of the disk storage space. The transfer speed of large files is also greatly reduced.

Image compression involves data coding in such a way that a sequence of image bits is replaced with an encoded version that occupies less storage space. The regions of interest in the image must be saved and the remainder of the image discarded. Only the bits that are required to convey the correct image information need be stored. All noise must be removed from the image before it is compressed. *Lossless* compression (image-preserving) algorithms maintain 100% of the image information; hence, the precompressed and postcompressed images are identical. *Lossy* compression algorithms permit some degree of image degradation and the postcompressed image is not the same as the precompressed image. The degree of compression is expressed as the ratio of storage space for the image before and after compression. A compression ratio of 20 : 1 indicates that the compressed image occupies only 20% of the space of the original image.

Simple, commonly used compression methods include run-length encoding and difference mapping:

1. Using *run-length encoding* (RLE), the pixel intensities are examined along a scan line and mapped to a sequence of number pairs. Each number pair consists of a pixel intensity and a frequency. Take the following scan line of GVs:

    80   80   80   85   90   90   90   93   93   93   93   91   91

Number pairs: (80   80   80)   85   (90   90   90)   (93   93   93   93)   (91   91)
                         3   1   3   4   2

                  RLE = 80   3   85   1   90   3   93   4   91   2

The disadvantage of this method is seen if all of the neighboring pixel GVs occur only once. This may result in the encoded scan length actually doubling.

2. Using *difference mapping,* only the difference between the neighboring pixels is recorded. With the same GV scan line:

 80   80   80   85   90   90   90   93   93   93   93   91   91

Difference = 0   0   +5   +5   0   0   +3   0   0   0   −2   0

Difference
mapping   = 80   0   0   +5   +5   0   0   +3   0   0   0   −2   0

Particularly in a noisy image, such as this, the difference mapping method is more efficient than the RLE method.

Other commonly used encoding methods include *Huffman coding,*[33] *LZW coding,*[34] and *2D coding* (contouring, quadtree representation, and Hilburt space-filling curves).[29]

14.5. IMAGE PROCESSING TOOLS

14.5.1. Thresholding (Global and Local)

Segmentation of the image into meaningful data by a computer is performed using two general principles. In one, the object of interest can be found by discovering areas where pixel values are homogenous and thresholding these regions. In another, when objects do not differ appreciably from their surroundings, one must rely on edge detection.[35]

Thresholding refers to the segmentation of a single or known range of gray values within the image and will discriminate objects of interest based on their brightness relative to each other. This powerful tool is easily applied in many instances such as identifying numbers of mitoses or assessing the distribution of immunohistochemical staining. However, in many biological specimens, the inherent contrast is low and the structures present exhibit a similar tendency to absorb and scatter light. In these cases, discussed in more detail later, varying counterstains and complementary color filters are used to enhance the image for analysis.[36]

Unlike edge detection algorithms that perform multiple operations on each pixel, methods that segment an image based on pixel values are much quicker since they work on the entire image at once. The threshold range can be selected by the observer using *manual* pointing but within- and between-operator consistency is often poor. Even so, this may be the best method of thresholding at the present time and with the available technology.

Automatic thresholding techniques for setting threshold limits are also useful, but they are far from perfect. They can be classified as either *global* or *local*. Using global methods, all the areas of interest have the *same* threshold. Global techniques may be either *point-dependent* (depend solely on the individual pixel gray values) or *region-dependent* (where information of neighboring pixels is taken into consideration). Using local methods, the thresholding values *vary* throughout the image.

Commonly used *global, point-dependent* thresholding methods include the Standard histogram or Mode method, the P-Tile method (percentile), and Otsu's method although many other methods exist.[36]

14.5.1.1. STANDARD HISTOGRAM OR MODE METHOD. Bimodal distributions are commonly used to separate out two objects within an image.[37] A threshold at the minimum gray value between the two histogram peaks can be used to separate such objects. However, this simple method cannot be applied to images with many unequal peaks or broad, flat valleys in the histogram. Smoothing methods may need to be implemented to average out the histogram values.

14.5.1.2. P-TILE METHOD (PERCENTILE). To use this method, it is assumed that the image comprises dark objects in a light background.[38] The percentage of the total image that represents the object of interest is known. For example

Let 5% of the image represent the object of interest
Let 95% of the image represent the background

The histogram of pixel gray values is constructed. The histogram is then scanned until the cumulative value of pixel numbers represents the required percentage of the total. The threshold selected will distinguish the 5% of pixel gray values within the object of interest and the 95% of pixel gray values in the background.

14.5.1.3. OTSU'S METHOD. The histogram of the pixel gray values in a certain image may show two distinct peaks of varying height and width representing two areas of interest in that image. A threshold gray value is selected between these two peaks, dividing the histogram into two areas, A_1 and A_2. The variance of the gray values within each area A_1 and A_2 is then computed. This is repeated for varying threshold values throughout the histogram.[39]

The optimum threshold to best separate the two regions of interest in the image can be represented by a maximization of the between-group variance (i.e., a maximum difference in gray value variance between A_1 and A_2) with respect to the within group variance (i.e., minimum variance variability within A_1 and within A_2).

14.5.1.4. LAPLACIAN HISTOGRAM. An example of a global, region-dependent thresholding method is the *high-gradient pixel histogram method (laplacian histogram)*. Within an image, an edge can be represented, using pixel gray values, as

5 5 5 6 7 8 9 9 9

Using a laplacian convolution $(-1 \quad -2 \quad -1)$:

5 5 5	becomes	$-5 \quad -10 \quad -5 = 0$
5 5 6	becomes	$-5 \quad -10 \quad -6 = -1$
5 6 7	becomes	$-5 \quad -12 \quad -7 = 0$ etc.

Thus, the preceding edge is represented as

$$0 \quad -1 \quad 0 \quad 0 \quad 0 \quad +1 \quad 0 \quad 0$$

(the value -1 represents where the slope starts, and $+1$ where the slope stops).

In an image, the shoulder points edging an object of interest can be identified using the laplacian convolution, distinguishing it from the background gray values that have no edges (and are therefore unaffected by the convolution). A smoother, more regular histogram can then be constructed and the threshold distinguishing the object and the background better identified.

14.5.1.5. QUADTREE SPLIT/MERGE TECHNIQUES. An example of a local thresholding method is the *split-and-merge techniques using quadtrees.* The image is subdivided into a set of arbitrary, disjointed regions. Assuming that the image is square, it is split into four quadrants. A certain property, P (based on gray value, texture, color, etc.), is applied to all the pixels in the quadrants. If this property is present in the entire area, then the quadrant is considered complete. If not, the quadrant is further subdivided into four subquadrants and the property P is reapplied. Any pair of adjacent regions can be merged if the property P is still satisfied. All the pixels in one region are set to a constant value, or alternatively the pixels at the edge of each region are highlighted to distinguish the boundary.

14.5.2. Point and Line Detection

Methods for the detection of points, lines, and edges are based on the use of 3×3 spatial "masks," laid over 9 pixels in the image. The values in these masks are often weighted to accentuate certain features. This is applied to the nearest neighbors of an image pixel to give new pixel value. The mask weights must be *zero-summed* and should display some sort of *symmetry.*

14.5.2.1. POINT DETECTION. The basic masks for point detection (*point symmetrical*) are

-1	-1	-1		0	-1	0
-1	8	-1	or	-1	4	-1
-1	-1	-1		0	-1	0

14.5.2.2. LINE DETECTION. The basic masks for line detection are

(A)			(B)			(C)		
−1	−1	−1	−1	2	−1	−1	−1	2
2	2	2	−1	2	−1	−1	2	−1
−1	−1	−1	−1	2	−1	2	−1	−1
	horizontal			vertical			diagonal	

Consider a region in an image:

$$
\begin{matrix}
10 & 15 & 10 \\
80 & 97 & 103 \\
25 & 17 & 31
\end{matrix}
$$

Mask *A* will accentuate the horizontal, central values:

(10 × −1)	(15 × −1)	(10 × −1)		−10	−15	−10
(80 × 2)	(97 × 2)	(103 × 2)	⟶	160	194	206
(25 × −1)	(17 × −1)	(31 × −1)		−25	−17	−31

For the same image region, mask *B* will "cancel out" the weighting system:

(10 × −1)	(15 × 2)	(10 × −1)		−10	30	−10
(80 × −1)	(97 × 2)	(103 × −1)	⟶	−80	194	−103
(25 × −1)	(17 × 2)	(31 × −1)		−25	34	−31

To *outline* certain parts of an image, these horizontal, vertical, and diagonal masks can be combined.

14.5.3. Edge Detection

An *edge* can be defined as an area that corresponds to a sudden shift from one pixel value to another.

The *Robert's cross edge* operator is an algorithm that delineates edges but does not change the original image.[40] Two brightness derivatives, obtained at right angles to each other and each orientated at 45° to the pixel grid, are used to determine the magnitude of the slope change. This method has the added benefit of providing information regarding the direction of the edge but may be sensitive to any noise that is present.

The *Sorbel and Kirsh* operators are also used as edge detectors.[41] These algorithms use kernels similar to the laplacian filter, but they are more sensitive to edges than points. The operator derivatives comprise 3 × 3 grids, representing a total of 9 pixels. For each operator grid, the brightness value of the central pixel is the sum of the surrounding eight pixel values. By rotating this operator grid on pixels throughout the image, the number of edges found in a given direction can be graphed.

14.5.4. Logical Operators

Despite all of the previously mentioned image processing tools, with few exceptions, the image is still not fully segmented for obtaining measurements. Because objects may still overlap, many measurements are benefited if performed on a *binary image*. A binary image converts all the pixels present in the threshold range to the maximum pixel value ("on"), and all the pixels outside this threshold range, to the minimum pixel value ("off"). Binary image manipulation, unlike the previous image processing tools, works directly on the image itself.

14.5.4.1. BOOLEAN-TYPE-OPERATORS. The simplest image processing technique used on binary images is to logically combine them into a single image. *Boolean-type operators*[28] are AND, OR, EX-OR (exclusive OR), and NOT. The NOT statement simply inverts the previous operation. All the pixels previously turned on are turned off. The AND statement combines two images, emphasizing features that are shared by both images. The OR statement is used when combining two images acquired by implementing different procedures such as differing threshold ranges. The EX-OR operation of two images gives a result in which pixels are turned on when they are "on" in either original image but not both (Fig. 14.11*a*).

14.5.4.2. NEIGHBOR OPERATORS. These operators respond to the feature in or the shape of the object in question. *Erosion* is an example of a neighboring operator. Each binary pixel is examined, and if any of its neighbors are "off," the pixel itself is turned "off." The net effect is to reduce the features around the periphery of an object. Complementary to this process is *dilatation* where the periphery of an object will be added. These two simple operators are very useful when used in combination. *Closing* represents the dilatation operation followed by the erosion operation. As a result, surface indentations in the image are smoothed out and any central holes are filled. *Opening* represents the erosion operation followed by the dilatation operation (Fig. 14.11*b*).

14.5.5. Counting and Labeling

An object is a connected component. If all the pixels within one object are given the same label, when connected, then each object can be separately identified and labeled. Counting techniques include propagation labeling, tracking, and boundary/border following.[29] Stereological methods can also be employed, as will be discussed later.

Logical Operators

Boolean operators

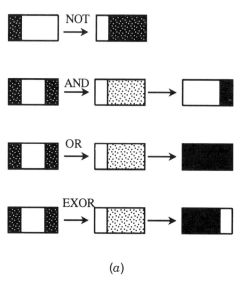

(a)

Neighborhood operators

OPENING (erosion then dilatation)

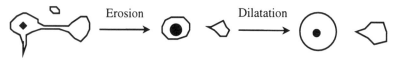

CLOSING (dilatation then erosion)

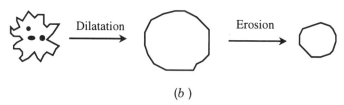

(b)

Figure 14.11. (a) Boolean operators are simple image processing techniques used to logically combine binary images into a single image; (b) the neighborhood operators respond to the feature in or the shape of the object to be analyzed.

14.5.6. Skeletonization and Thinning

Skeletonization is the characterization of an object as a sticklike figure (Fig. 14.12). Theoretically, the process should be reversible. Skeletonization reduces objects within the image to medial lines of unit width. It enables objects to be represented as simplified data-structures and helps structural analysis. It also reduces storage requirements for object characterization. The main disadvantage of skeletonization is that it involves massive computation. For this reason, simplified *thinning* methods are often used as a substitute.[28]

14.5.7. Texture Analysis

Texture refers to the pattern of pixel regularity. The regular pixel values of a chessboard pattern have one texture. An area of exactly similar pixel GV may exhibit another texture. By identifying repeating patterns, the range of applications for texture analysis varies from image segmentation to the evaluation of picture interference, bacterial colonies, or landscape surfaces.[29]

There is no formal definition for textural analysis; hence, there is more than one approach to analyzing this property, often used in combination. The main methods used are *statistical, structural* and *spectral*. In brief, the statistical methods use the frequency distribution of image gray values, described by histogram moments. Co-occurrence matrices identify the texture properties in local areas of an image, between neighboring pixels, rather than over the entire image.

Structural approaches are based on an attempt to match a small window of an image with one or more areas in the main image. The more often there is a direct match between the two, the more likely that texture periodicity is present. The best match is obtained when the differences in pixel values between the window and main image regions are minimized (the square of the differences = 0). With increased variability, the square of the differences increases accordingly.

SKELETONIZATION

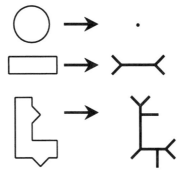

Figure 14.12. Skeletonization reduces objects within the image to medial lines of unit width and enables them to be represented as simplified data structures.

The Fourier spectral method is ideally suited for describing the directional periodicity of near-periodic 2D patterns in an image.[24] Features in the image are converted to a waveform that can be analyzed for periodicity. This waveform represents a discontinuous function, approximated by a series of *sinusoidal* functions (sine or cosine) of different amplitudes and frequencies with Fourier coefficients, *a* and *b* and an *i*th harmonic:

$$\Sigma \ [a(i) * \cos(i * x) + b(i) * \sin(i * x)]$$

The *square of the coefficients* $\{a(i)^2 + b(i)^2\}$ is called the energy or *power* spectrum. The Fourier spectrum transforms first along the rows and then along the columns. A power spectrum (power vs. GV frequencies), generated from the image, can be used to describe texture. Prominent peaks in the spectrum give the principal direction of the texture patterns. The locations of these peaks indicate the fundamental spatial period(s) of any texture patterns. Eliminating periodic components and inverting leaves nonperiodic image elements that are amenable to statistical techniques such as *lowpass, median bandpass,* and *highpass* filtering.

14.6. FLOW AND STATIC CYTOMETRY

Flow and static cytometry are now widely used to quantify DNA analysis for many diagnostic and prognostic applications.[42,43] In the early 1960s, the scientific basis of *flow cytometry* and cell sorting was established.[44] Cell nuclei, in suspension, are labeled with fluorescence dyes such as DAPI, propidium iodide or ethidium bromide, which bind proportionally to the amount of nuclear DNA. The cell nuclei are hydrodynamically focused within the flow chamber where light from a laser source exits the fluorescent dye. A photomultiplier system correlates the fluorescent staining with the amount of DNA for each nucleus.

The technique of *static cytometry* measures properties of tissues or cells, on slides rather than in cell suspensions, using digitized images. The tissues are stained with a dye, the Feulgen stain,[16] which binds to nuclear DNA. Its absorption, and its optical density in the digitized image, is proportional to the amount of DNA. Unlike immunohistochemical staining, Feulgen staining is stoichiometric. The greater the Feulgen staining intensity, the greater the loss in transmitted and measured light (Beer–Lambert absorption law).[43]

The objective interpretation of the DNA histograms for both techniques includes details of the DNA index, cell cycle analysis (G_0/G_1, S, and G_2/M) and the coefficient of variation. DNA quantification by image analysis from Feulgen-stained correlates well with the results from flow cytometry in fresh and frozen touch preparations,[45,46] tissue sections,[47–49] and cytology effusions.[50]

Although both methods of cell analysis are complementary, advantages of static cytometry over flow cytometry include (1) better sampling by histological correlation; (2) a wider range of tissue processing techniques, including cytospins and touch imprints as well as tissue sections; (3) the ability to use limited material such as fine-needle aspirates or hypocellular effusion fluids; (4) visual control of cells, particularly rare events; and (5) the supplementary information of prognostic indicators, such as Ki-67, BrdU, and PCNA, assessed on comparable paraffin blocks. However, static cytometry requires strict adherence to standardization protocols for tissue fixation, preparation, and staining to maintain a low coefficient of variation.

The flow cytometer offers (1) higher resolution, (2) faster processing speeds, (3) reproducible staining, (4) cell sorting facilities, and (5) lower coefficients of variation in the histogram.

14.7. STEREOLOGY

14.7.1. Definitions

Stereology, a word coined by Hans Elias in 1963,[51] is a set of simple and efficient rules, used in the quantification of 3D microscopic structures.[52] The necessity for stereology stems from the nature of conventional microscopy where thin tissue sections are a prerequisite for microscope analysis. With only small amounts of raw data, estimates of many structural parameters can be made.

Interpretation of 2D sections to obtain information about the spatial distribution of elements within 3D can be misleading. Consider randomly cutting a sphere with a cutting plane. There is only a small probability of cutting the sphere through the exact center, and hence the diameter of the profile is likely to be smaller than the diameter of the sphere. From a *single* random cut, it is impossible to deduce any feature of the original sphere. However, if *many* random cuts are taken, it becomes possible to obtain spatial information representative of the sphere.

Traditional stereology formulas were based on *random* sectioning of the tissue in question. Isotropic uniform random (IUR) sections were obtained by cutting the usual block of tissue and randomizing the orientation before embedding. Histopathological entities like lymphomas can still be considered isotropic if the objects of interest are homogeneously and randomly distributed throughout a tissue. But many biological tissues, such as skeletal muscle or skin, exhibit a degree of layered organization and orientation (anisotropy), making unbiased stereological sampling difficult. Some of the many isotropic sampling methods now used in pathological research and diagnosis are outlined below.[53–55]

Dimensional information lost during tissue sectioning can be recovered statistically. Sectioning causes geometrical features of dimension D to appear with D-1 dimensions; for example,

Geometric Feature			Geometric Feature after Sectioning	
(Volume)	L^3	$\longrightarrow$	L^2	(area)
(Area)	L^2	$\longrightarrow$	L^1	(line)
(Line)	L^1	$\longrightarrow$	L^0	(point)

Geometric probes of different dimensions are used to estimate certain features in 3D objects. If points are randomly thrown into a space, the number of points appearing in any 3D feature will be proportional to the volume of the feature. This may be achieved by taking a random section through an object and *randomly* placing a 2D raster of points (grid probe) on the resulting plane. As derived later, a 2D raster of lines is used to estimate surface area, and a 2D raster of plane profiles provides an estimate of object length. For instance,

	Probe		Features Estimated	
(Points)	L^0	$\longrightarrow$	L^3	(volume)
(Lines)	L^1	$\longrightarrow$	L^2	(area)
(Planes)	L^2	$\longrightarrow$	L^1	(length)
(Volumes)	L^3	$\longrightarrow$	L^0	(number)

Stereological estimates are derived as ratios and hence usually relate measurement parameters of an object to the volume of tissue containing that object.

Volume density $= Vv = V/V =$ volume of interest/reference volume
Surface density $= Sv = S/V =$ surface area of interest/reference volume
Length density $= Lv = L/V =$ length of interest/reference volume
Numerical density $= Nv = N/V =$ number of objects of interest/reference volume

14.7.2. Volume Density Estimation and Cavalieri's Principle

To obtain a density measurement, it is imperative that the reference volume be known. *Cavalieri's principle* is used for measuring the *reference volume* of an object. The object is systematically sliced into section(s). The sections needed to be of equal *thickness* (t) but the starting position of the first slice must be random. The projected *surface area* (a) of each slice is estimated using the point-counting method or computerized pixel counting. The *volume* (V) of the object may be estimated by multiplying the distance between the sections by the sum of the projected surface area. If the distance between the slices is not uniform, the average slice thickness may be used.

$$V = t * \Sigma(a * s)$$

The *volume density* [V/V_{ref}) may be obtained by counting the *number of points* that fall within the objects of interest (P)] and dividing it by the number of points that fall within the *reference space* (P_{ref}). Therefore

$$\frac{P}{P_{ref}} = \frac{V}{V_{ref}}$$

14.7.3. Numerical Density Estimation

Stereology utilizes an array of basic tools to estimate numerical density, detailed elsewhere.[54,55] These include the *unbiased counting frame,* the *physical dissector,* and the *double dissector.*

14.7.3.1. THE UNBIASED COUNTING FRAME. This is designed for counting profiles in a *two-dimensional* tissue slice in order to estimate the number of profiles per area of the counting frame (numerical density). Object profiles that fall within the randomly placed frame are counted, provided they do not touch the exclusion edge (solid line) of the frame or its extensions (solid line with arrows).[56] In Figure 14.13*a*, one profile (checkered) lies within the counting frame and another (spotted) lies on an edge of the frame. Two other profiles (hatched) lie on the exclusion edges of the frame. The number of profiles that can be counted in this case are *two* (the checkered and the spotted). Using this method of counting, different techniques and observers can be compared. Cellularity can be defined as the number of cells per unit area rather than cells (or mitoses) per field of unknown size and magnification.

14.7.3.2. THE PHYSICAL DISSECTOR. This is a probe that samples isolated objects, with uniform probability, in *three-dimensional* space.[57] Two serial histological sections, a distance (b) apart, are compared. If the particles of interest appear within one section (the *reference* section) and not the other section (the *lookup* section), these particles are counted. The number of particles (Q) are counted as they disappear when moving through the specimen. In Figure 14.13*b*, three profiles are identified in the lookup slice and four profiles are identified in the reference slice. Thus, Q is *five*. Knowing the object magnification, the distance (b) between sections and the area (a) of the dissector, the volume (V_{dis}) of the dissector probe can be calculated:

$$V_{dis} = a * b$$

Particles are counted between many randomly selected consecutive tissue sections using the same dissector of constant volume (V_{dis}).

An estimate of the *number of particles* (N) in the entire specimen, of volume V_{ref}, is

$$N = \frac{\Sigma Q * V_{ref}}{\Sigma V_{dis}}$$

Thus

$$\text{Numerical density} \left(\frac{N}{V_{ref}} \right) = \frac{\Sigma Q}{\Sigma V_{dis}}$$

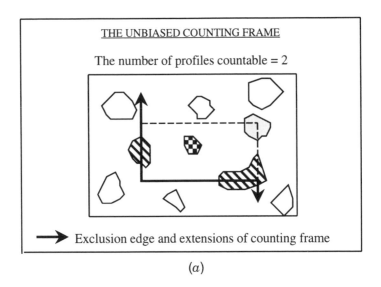

(a)

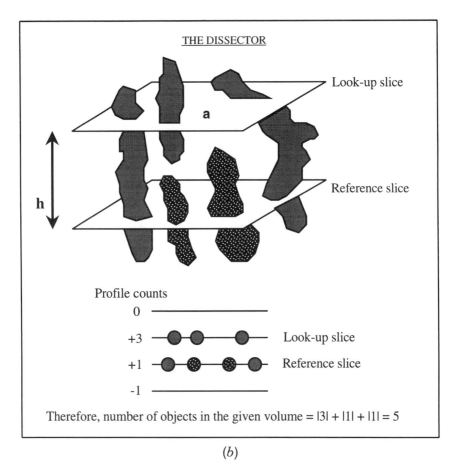

(b)

Figure 14.13. (a) The unbiased counting frame used to obtain numerical estimations; (b) the physical dissector used to obtain numerical estimations.

14.7.3.3. THE DOUBLE DISSECTOR. This is used to estimate the density of different-sized cell populations in the same thin section. Consider estimating the numerical densities of synapses and neurons in brain tissue. The granule cells are confined to the granular layer and the synapses are located in the molecular layer. The volume of the two reference spaces need to be deduced separately. By applying two different-sized dissectors to each tissue compartment, the two densities are then estimated from uniform samples of the granular and molecular references spaces.

14.7.4. Surface Density Estimation

Consider calculating the surface density of all Golgi apparatus membranes in a standard unit of organ volume. Surface area estimation may be obtained using the *mean linear intercept method*. The probe comprises grid lines intercepting at grid points. The probe is placed over an IUR tissue section containing Golgi apparatus. The grid lines will pierce the Golgi apparatus in proportion to the amount of their surface area and the total length of the grid lines. The number of intersections between the grid lines and the boundaries of the Golgi apparatus is then calculated.[58]

The stereological equations for surface density estimation (S/V) as defined by Tomkeieff[59] is

$$\frac{S}{V} = \frac{2I}{L}$$

where S = total surface area of the objects of interest (e.g., Golgi apparatus)
V = the volume of the container space containing the object of interest
I = the number of intersections between the test lines and the objects
L = the total length of line used in the test grid

Since the length associated with one grid point = 2 * 1, the total length (L) of line associated with all the grid points = (2 * 1) * N (where N = number of grid points).

14.7.5. Length Density Estimation

The probability that a given structure is hit by a randomly positioned cutting plane is proportional to its length or height. The probe used for length density estimation in IUR sections comprises an unbiased 2D counting frame containing a regular lattice of planes. This is laid over the tissue sections and the number of profiles crossing the object of interest (Q) is noted.

If the total area associated with each 2D counting frame is known (A), the following equation can be applied to estimate length density:

$$\frac{L}{V} = \frac{2Q}{A}$$

where L = total length of the objects of interest
V = the volume of the container space containing the object of interest
Q = the number of profiles counted
A = the area within which profiles are counted

14.7.6. Particle Sizing

Direct methods of estimation include selecting particles according to the dissector rule and measuring the volume of each particle using the *Cavalieri* principle. *Point-sampled* intercept measurements use point-counting systems to sample the particles and measure only the volume of the particles that are selected by the points.[60,55] Indirect methods estimate the mean volume of particles as Vv/Nv and the mean surface area of particles as $Sv/Nv.$

14.7.7. Future Directions of Stereology

New software packages are available today which can be applied to images of histological sections captured with a standard light microscope and attached videocamera. These integral systems for stereological data processing can now display each histological section on the computer screen, superimpose the geometric probe of choice over the image, compute the stereological parameters required from the digitized images, and tabulate and store the data, as well as carry out any statistical analysis required. However, disadvantages of stereological techniques are that the random sectioning required throughout a tissue block results in the destruction of that block. Also, stereological techniques are not applicable to tissue samples, such as cytospin preparations, which cannot be sectioned unless embedded in media such as agar or Araldite. Training in stereological principles, technical transfer of new methodology to the user community and information organization are three important future directions for biological stereology.[58]

14.8. CONFOCAL LASER SCANNING MICROSCOPY

A patent application in 1957 by Marvin Minsky (U.S. Patent 3,013,467) provides the earliest published account of a confocal microscope.[61] In spite of the desire for scientists, at this time, to observe living processes in three dimensions, several factors were instrumental in the slow progress of confocal technology. These were the eclipsing developments of the electron microscope, the lack of laser, light-source technology, and the embryonic computer capabilities at that time, which were unable to handle vast amounts of image data.

Using standard epiillumination fluorescence microscopy, fluorescent molecules (fluorochromes) emit light of a given wavelength when excited by incident light of a different (shorter) wavelength.[62] Detection sensitivity and specificity of the chosen fluorochrome can be obtained with the insertion of filters that block all light wavelengths other than those being emitted by the fluorochrome. For example, fluorescein isothiocyanate (FITC) and tetramethyl B rhodamine isothiocyanate (TRITC) are excited by blue (488-nm) and green (514-nm) light, respectively and emit green (514-nm) and red (540-nm) light, respectively. The three filters used in a standard fluorescence microscope are described in Figure 14.14.

The confocal microscope can be used as a standard epifluorescence microscope, but it also has the ability to filter out interfering light that does not originate from the plane of focus. It offers improved optical resolution and contrast as well as high photometric precision. Before the light reaches a detector, such as a photomultiplier tube, it passes through a small confocal aperture placed at optically the same point as the focus plane of the scanned beam of light. Hence, only exactly focused light returning from the specimen will reach the photomultiplier through the confocal aperture (Fig. 14.15). By scanning across the surface of the specimen, the photomultiplier tube electronics convert

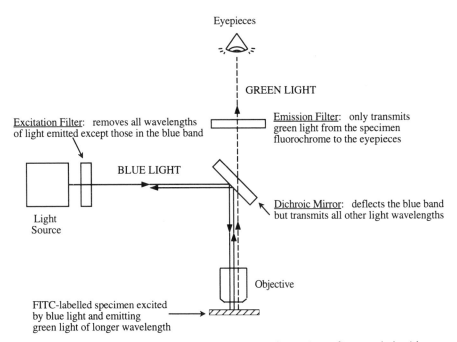

Eyepieces

GREEN LIGHT

Excitation Filter: removes all wavelengths of light emitted except those in the blue band

Emission Filter: only transmits green light from the specimen fluorochrome to the eyepieces

BLUE LIGHT

Dichroic Mirror: deflects the blue band but transmits all other light wavelengths

Light Source

Objective

FITC-labelled specimen excited by blue light and emitting green light of longer wavelength

Figure 14.14. An epifluorescence microscope with a fluorochrom fluorescein isothiocyanate (FITC)-labeled specimen. (Adapted from DJ Rawlins, *Light Microscopy*, 1992, with permission from BIOS Scientific Publishers Ltd.)

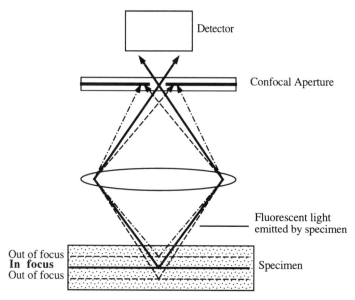

Figure 14.15. In the confocal microscope, only exactly focused light returning from the specimen will reach the detector through the confocal aperture. (Adapted from DJ Rawlins, *Light Microscopy,* 1992, with permission from BIOS Scientific Publishers Ltd.)

the emitted light into an electrical voltage that is digitized and then viewed on the computer screen. Output data is stored on hard disk and then transferred to optical disk devices or mainframe computers. To facilitate accurate optical sectioning and reconstruction, the focus is driven, in precise increments of 1/1000 multiples, by a z-axis controller or stepping motor. Multiple sections through the tissue can be analyzed rapidly, using dedicated rendering software, to build up a 3D image of the specimen and to obtain direct measurements, such as volume.

In the same way that Köhler illumination, optimal magnification, resolution, and mounting media influence the quality of a captured image, the confocal microscope also requires certain calibrations. In a confocal image, the light intensity distribution of a luminous point object is known as its *point spread function* (PSF). In an aberration-free optical system, virtually the entire intensity of the PSF is concentrated in the central spot. A light intensity distribution can also be displayed as an *airy disk.* This comprises a central, bright spot surrounded by alternating bright and dark rings, representing reinforced and canceled wavelengths, respectively, emitted from the periphery of the luminous point object. This is detailed elsewhere.[63]

The diameter of the PSF central spot will represent the smallest resolvable image element. In other words, the limit of resolution for the microscope is reached if the principal maximum of one diffraction disk coincides with the first dark ring of another disk. Abbe[64] described the relationship of this resolving power as

$$d = \frac{1.221}{NA_{obj} + NA_{cond}} \qquad (14.1)$$

where d = the minimum distance that the diffraction images of two points in the specimen can approach one another laterally before they converge and can no longer be separately resolved

l = wavelength of light used for observation

NA_{obj} = numerical aperture of the objective lens

NA_{cond} = numerical aperture of the condenser lens

The numerical aperture (NA) of any lens describes the relationship between the refractive index (n) of the medium between the lens and the specimen and the angle (ϕ) at which the light passes through the lens. Hence

$$NA = n(\sin\phi)$$

Substituting Eq. (14.2) into Eq. (14.1), we obtain

$$d = \frac{1.221}{2[n(\sin\phi)]}$$

Another term for distance d is the full-width half-maximum (FWHM) spread function, which refers to the overlap of two PSFs such that at the point where both PSFs are full width, they are both half the maximum height (Fig. 14.16). If the two specimen points are too far apart, then intermediate information will not

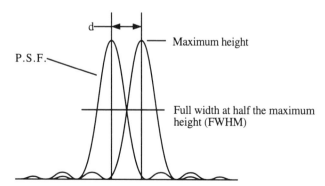

Figure 14.16. The point spread function used to evaluate the minimum thickness of optical sections.

be represented in either PSF and it will be lost. If the two specimen points overlap by too much, then the information in one PSF will be almost exactly the same as the information in the other PSF. By using the FWHM spread function, then one can calculate optimal thickness of the optical sections. The value of the FWHM dictates the thickness (and hence the number) of sections in the z direction through the tissue section. Obviously, the chosen optical section size cannot exceed the FWHM, or else valuable information will not be represented.

14.9. 3D RECONSTRUCTION AND TOPOLOGY TECHNIQUES

Three-dimensional (3D) reconstruction is the construction of 3D images from 2D images. Prior to the advent of modern microscopes and computer systems, various modeling procedures such as hand-drawn graphic plates or wax plates were laboriously stacked and aligned to build up a 3D image. In 1972, computer 3D reconstruction was introduced[65] and became an important method for visualizing the connectivity of biological structures.[66]

As previously described, the confocal laser scanning microscope (CLSM) produces datasets of optical slices through the tissue of interest, which can then be reconstructed and analyzed using dedicated rendering software. But such an expensive microscope is not absolutely necessary. Access to a personal computer, a 3D reconstruction program, a digitizing graphic tablet with photographs or projection facilities, and a stack of 2D images ensures that 3D reconstruction techniques can be utilized by most pathologists.

Practical difficulties in 3D reconstruction have been outlined elsewhere and include image registration and the choice of data to input.[67] Registration is the alignment of the tissue sections in the stack of 2D images. Artificial reference registration points must be positioned in relation to each tissue section to ensure correct alignment. These may be external marks in the tissue or wax block such as drilled holes or inserted nerve fibers.[68] Cactus spines (genus *Mammillaria*) have also been introduced into the tissue block before embedding.[69] As an alternative to external registration points, a stage micrometer may be laid over the boundary contours of each section. The number of data or registration points included in each tissue section depends on the complexity of the tissue structure. An estimation of the number of slices required for adequate reconstruction can also be performed.[70] Tissue distortion in the three dimensional reconstruction of consecutive tissue sections may relate to variations in tissue fixation or processing and be exaggerated by using suboptimal numbers of tissue sections in the stack. Large numbers of variable serial sections will reconstruct with a serrated outline, whereas too few sections may result in a serious misrepresentation of the true shape.[71]

For data entry, consecutive photographs of each tissue section can be sequentially projected onto a digitizer tablet, the registration points having been recorded. Software programs are now available for the actual reconstruction[72] and can be completed in minutes rather than days. Details of the various methods used are described elsewhere.[42]

Three-dimensional reconstruction and topology techniques are continuously being developed, but are not, as yet, considered as routine tools for the pathologist. Collaboration with a computer scientist is recommended until the software becomes more affordable and user-friendly.

14.10. CLINICAL APPLICATIONS OF IMAGE ANALYSIS

Clinical applications of image analysis are listed in Table 14.1.

14.10.1. Introduction

In the field of diagnostic pathology, it is generally considered that experienced pathologists make reliable and reproducible diagnostic decisions.[73] The theoret-

TABLE 14.1. Clinical Applications of Image Analysis

Counting (cell numbers, mitotic rate, nucleoli, pyknotic nuclear debris)	
Mitotic–karyorrhexis index	Prognostic factor in childhood neuroblastomas
Numbers of AgNors	Prognostic indicators in skin, breast, prostate
Basic morphometry (area, perimeter, diameter, shape factors, contour ratios)	
Breslow levels	Skin malignant melanomas
Microinvasion depths	Cervical squamous-cell carcinomas
Electron microscopy	Sizes of neurosecretory granules
Nerve myelination	Peripheral and central demyelinating diseases
Osteoid: mineralization ratios	Metabolice bone disease, chemotherapy responses
Nuclear characteristics	Prognostic prediction and diagnostic adjunct
Immunohistochemistry	
High sensitivity	Proliferative activity/BrdU
	Ileal IgA in antibody-secreting cells
Low sensitivity	Estrogen/progesterone receptors
	Oncogene expression (*c-erb*-B2)
	Proliferative antigen detection (PCNA)
Flow and static cytometry	DNA and proliferative (*S*)-phase analysis
Stereology	Particle number, volume, and area densities
Confocal microscopy	Tissue organisation, volume/area evaluation
3D reconstruction	Anatomical connectivity, tissue organisation
Cytogenetics	Metaphase location, segmentation, shape recognition
Autoradiography	Receptor localization, physiological quantitation
Department workstations	Image and data storage/archiving
	Text and image pathology reporting
	Conference presentations
Telepathology	Robotic control of microscopic slide stages
	Remote frozen-section diagnosis service
	Image compression, transmission, and storage

ical analysis of this ability suggests a tendency to disregard unimportant details, and to simplify the observed images into models with structural interrelations specific for the pathological diagnosis being considered. In order to apply the appropriate criteria for a given diagnosis, the experienced pathologist is able to select the relevant areas and regions in the tissue to study, at the macroscopic, microscopic, and ultrastructural levels.[74] Diagnosis making may be a fast-acting template recognition procedure or an analytical process, both often subconscious.

Whatever the hierarchical organization employed to reach the correct diagnosis, analytical morphometry requires a conscious, rather than subconscious, construction of the model leading to the correct diagnosis. The knowledge of a pathologist who is unable to specify or articulate the criteria used to make a particular pathological diagnosis cannot be transferred or reproduced by others.

The two types of lesions available for morphometric measurements in the field of pathology are described as discrete and continuous.[75] Discrete lesions require very specific criteria for their correct diagnosis; an example is the non-caseating granuloma of sarcoidosis. Interobserver and intraobserver agreement is high. Continuous lesions can range from complete benignity to highly reactive to malignant. The interobserver and intraobserver agreement is often very poor, and it is for these cases that morphometric analysis can be most useful.

The criteria required to apply morphometric measurements as a clinical tool can be divided into four levels.[76,77] *Level I* studies define single or combined quantitative measurements that can distinguish different groups, diagnostically or prognostically, with set sensitivity, specificity, and efficiency thresholds. *Level II* studies confirm level I findings using a different patient group, but within the same laboratory. Level II studies reduce the effects of tissue processing and measurement variables. *Level III* studies confirm level I findings using a different patient group in an independent laboratory, thereby excluding interlaboratory and interobserver variations. *Level IV* studies confirm level I–III findings when routinely applied in the same laboratory. Level IV confirmation should be achieved before the morphometric measurements can be used as a clinically diagnostic tool. Continued quality control of the measuring system is required with regular equipment calibration and measurement repeatability tests.

The applications of image analysis and processing in biology and pathology can be broadly divided into two groups, namely tumor diagnosis or prognosis and nontumor interests.

14.10.2. Counting

Simply counting elements such as numbers of cells, mitoses, nucleoli, or pyknotic nuclei is greatly facilitated by automated or manual identification of the elements, thresholding of their gray value, and subsequent analysis. Examples include the counting of Alcian-blue stained metaplastic cells in the stomach;[78] silver-stained nucleolar organizer regions (AgNORs) in skin,[79,80] breast,[81,82] prostate,[83] liver,[84] bladder,[85] and thyroid;[86] and pyknotic or karyorrhectic nuclear debris as another prognostic indicator in childhood neuroblastoma.[87,88]

14.10.3. Basic Morphometry

Routine uses for the surgical pathologist include Breslow measurements for malignant melanomas of skin and microinvasive depths in cervical squamous cell carcinomas. The microscopic image can be captured in seconds, and a traced calibrated ruler marker can be automatically measured from the computer screen. In the same way, the number and size of neurosecretory granules or viral inclusions in digitized electron microscopy images can be routinely evaluated.

Morphometric methods in bone pathology, such as the measurement of trabecular bone volume, relative osteoid volume, and the osteoid index, can be used in the evaluation of metabolic bone disease.[89] Many semiautomatic programs are now available for measuring bone surfaces, although colored, rather than gray-value images, are usually required.[90] Image processing is also used for the evaluation of bone tumor necrosis after chemotherapy[91] and the differential counts of hematopoietic cells in bone marrow trephines.[92]

Using digitized electron microscopic images of nerve, the quantification of myelination in nerve biopsies is useful in the diagnosis of neuropathies as well as in the assessment of nerve regeneration after reconstructive surgery.[93]

All software packages vary in their ability to deal with the evaluation of nuclear characteristics. Fourier's analysis applied to 2D profiles and including such parameters as area, perimeter, mean diameter, and coefficience of variation of each contour, has been used to differentiate normal lymphocytes from a chronic lymphocytic lymphoma.[94] A combination of nuclear shape indices, such as indentation, convolution, cleaving, and ellipsing, provide a good method of quantitative assessment in non-Hodgkin's lymphoma.[95] Nuclear profiles have also helped to differentiate reactive and malignant mesothelial cells from adenocarcinomas in cytological effusion specimens[96] and the morphometric characteristics of prostatic intraepithelial neoplasia.[97] In tissue biopsies, mean nuclear areas have helped distinguish between reactive and malignant pleural mesothelial cells, between endometrial hyperplasias and endometrial adenocarcinomas, and between borderline and frankly malignant ovarian tumors. Interobserver and intraobserver agreement of malignancy grading has also been improved, using similar parameters, in diagnosing and differentiating grades of malignancy in endometrial, ovarian, and urothelial tumors.[76]

Nuclear chromatin pattern quantitation is considered a more sensitive reflection of the functional state of the nucleus than the DNA content. Performed on Feulgen-stained specimens, geometric, densitometric, textural, and topographic features can be extracted.[42] Mean nuclear area, size, and textural features such as chromatin distribution and optical density have been used as prognostic predictors in carcinomas of bladder,[98] ovary,[99] endometrium[100,101] breast,[48,102,103] and stomach.[103] Varying chromatin patterns have been utilized in the differentiation of polyomavirus-infected and malignant urothelial cells.[104]

14.10.4. Immunohistochemistry

With the advent of monoclonal antibodies against estrogen receptors, both semi-quantitative[105,106] and quantitative[107] methods of immunohistochemical localization have been shown to give acceptable sensitivities and specificities as compared with biochemical methods. Rather than reporting a biochemically evaluated estrogen receptor level expressed in femtomoles per milligram of tumor protein, a value for the percentage of nuclear staining is given.[26,108] This becomes increasingly important as the size of biopsied tissue diminishes and the need for a battery of diagnostic and prognostic indicators increases. Instead of dividing up fresh tissue for distribution amongst the biochemistry, flow cytometry, electron microscopy, and histochemistry laboratories, the development of more universal fixatives and quantitative image analysis methods, ensures that much of the required information can be obtained from a single paraffin-embedded tissue block.

Examples of discrete, *high*-sensitivity immunohistochemical staining include the assessment of cellular proliferative activity using the nuclear stain bromodeoxyuridine (BrdU) and highly specific immunostaining such as ileal IgA in antibody secreting cells. In these cases, the immunoreactivity is limited, in relatively dense quantities, to the nucleus. Thus, gray-value differentiation by thresholding, between stained nuclei, unstained nuclei, cytoplasm, and background is possible.

However, as is seen commonly with numerous antibodies, the immunostaining may be of *low* sensitivity. Examples of such antibodies include oestrogen and progesterone antibodies, oncogene expression such as *c-erb*-B2[109,110] and proliferative antigen expression such as PCNA[111,112] and Ki-67.[113] In these cases, the reactivity may range from focal to marked and be complicated by varying degrees of both cytoplasmic and nuclear staining, as well as background staining. Variable counterstains and color filters can be implemented to enhance the immunostaining maximally, as described previously.

The intensity of oncogene expression (*c-myc* and *H-ras*), labeled by *in situ* hybridization using biotinylated complimentary DNA probes, has been quantified with computerized color-image analysis in dysplastic Barrett's esophageal mucosa.[114]

14.10.5. Flow and Static Cytometry

The evaluation of ploidy status and the proliferative *S*-phase fraction of tumor cell suspensions or tissue blocks (fresh-frozen or paraffin-embedded), is now carried out routinely in many laboratories.

In breast cancer, abnormal ploidy correlates with histologically poorly differentiated tumors,[115,116] positive nodal status,[117,118] clinical relapse independent of stage,[118,116] and shortened survival.[119,120] Although not always true,[121] a high S-phase fraction in breast tumors usually correlates with a less favorable prognosis.[122–125] Tumors with DNA aneuploidy and a high proliferative index are also more likely to be estrogen and progesterone receptor negative.[126,120,127,128]

In lymphomas, a moderate or high proliferative activity (>10–12% S phase) has been correlated with intermediate or high-grade lymphomas (NCI Working Formulation).[129–131] In Hodgkin's disease, a proliferative activity of >10%, together with the histological subtype and an older age at diagnosis, correlates with poor disease prognosis.[132]

Reduced survival times and poor prognosis are associated with abnormal DNA or aneuploidy in colonic cancer,[133] ovarian cancer,[134] non-small-cell[135] and small-cell[136] pulmonary carcinoma, renal-cell carcinoma,[137,138] prostatic carcinoma,[139,140] hepatocellular carcinoma,[141] and melanocytic lesions.[142] Diploid or normal DNA content has been reported to be found more commonly in partial moles and suggests a lower premalignant potential.[143]

Static cytometry provides densitometric not only variables for cell cycle analysis but also morphometric features and chromatin analysis as previously described.

14.10.6. Stereology

Stereological techniques have been employed for the morphometric analysis of numerous tissues. In hepatology, correlations have been made between a morphometric study of liver cell structure and a stereological and biochemical analysis of subcellular fractions.[144] The same investigator used stereological methods, with micrographs, to characterize pancreatic exocrine cell membranes so that changes in individual membrane compartments, or movements of a membrane between compartments, could be detected.[145] In the adrenal gland cellular changes within mitochondria and smooth endoplasmic reticulum, associated with certain stresses, stimulations or inhibiting steroid synthesizing enzymes have been characterized and compared with extensive biochemical data.[52] Structural differentiation in normal and pathological states has been studied in oral mucous membrane epithelium.[146]

In prognostic studies, stereological estimates of nuclear volume in tissue sections have been shown to provide an independent prognostic variable in squamous cell carcinomas of the uterine cervix[147] and prostate.[148] In malignant melanoma, although 2D nuclear profile areas did not provide significant prognostic information, nuclear volume measurements were found to be a highly sensitive parameter for malignancy grading.[149] Stereological estimates of mean nuclear volume have also been shown to correlate with histopathological grading of bladder transitional carcinoma and have been used to predict those tumors most likely to recur.[150,151] However, other investigators have found marked intratumor variation and poor correlation between nuclear volume and both cytological and architectural grades in endometrial adenocarcinomas.[152]

In diagnostic pathology, the value of stereological volume estimates seems limited. One study, carried out retrospectively on archival breast tissue sections and cytology smears using a point–line intercept method, identified a distinct nuclear volume range in benign cytology and histology specimens, respectively, as compared to a larger nuclear volume range in malignant cytology and histology specimens, respectively.[153]

14.10.7. Confocal Microscopy

The confocal laser scanning microscope (CLSM) has provided new insights into 3D cell and tissue organization by accurately imaging, and aligning, multiple, noninvasive optical sections through labeled biological specimens. Examples include the development of single neurons over time,[154] the spatial distribution and quantitation of megakaryocytes in human bone marrow tissue,[155] the quantification of immunolabeled axon terminals,[156] the activity of single cells within intact and functioning brain (or a tissue slice preparation) using voltage-sensitive fluorescent dyes,[157] the 3D analysis of chromosomes,[158] and the three-dimensional distribution of chromatin in neuroblastoma.[159]

The value of direct measurements in prognostic and diagnostic pathology, obtained using the CLSM, has only just started to be assessed. The confocal microscope has been used to differentiate otherwise undiagnosable cell clusters in thick, cytobrush cervical smears by highlighting chromatin patterns, mitotic figures and glandular architecture.[160] The technology has been used to evaluate the volume of epidermal nuclei in thick skin sections.[161] One of the authors (WAW) recently devised a method to establish the reliability and accuracy required to obtain a range for the nuclear : cytoplasmic ratio of normal, human mesothelial cells, using a confocal microscope and dedicated rendering software. The volume measurements obtained were compared and contrasted with those estimates acquired using point-counting stereological methods.

14.10.8. 3D Computer Reconstruction

As well as making measurements, such as surface areas and volumes, 3D computer reconstruction has greatly enhanced our understanding of organ and tissue connectivity. Reconstruction of the fetal notochord has provided clues to the pathogenesis of the chordoma.[162] Connections between neuronal synapses have been evaluated.[163] The distribution of chemical components, such as dopamine in midbrain neurons, has been mapped and the reconstruction of anatomical structures, such as colonic crypts, undertaken.[164]

14.10.9. Cytogenetics

In the field of cytogenetics, with or without a fluorescent microscope, image analysis provides a rapid and efficient means of determining and quantifying metaphase location, segmentation, and shape recognition.

14.10.10. Autoradiography and Cellular Fluorescence

Autoradiography involves image visualization with light- or dark-field illumination followed by photographic documentation onto a graphics tablet attached to a microcomputer. Applications include localization of a receptor population (neurotransmitters, drugs, enzymes, ion channels); steroid receptor assays, physiological quantitation (blood flow, pH, protein synthesis, glucose utilization rate), and immunocytochemistry.[165] Applications for the microscopy of fluorescent probes include the assessment of image membrane potential probes, fluorescein-labeled antisperm, and calcium sensitive probes.

14.10.11. Departmental Workstations

The rapidly expanding computer science concepts of hypermedia, image and data storage, laboratory databases, decision analysis, and artificial intelligence are now being embodied into the concept of a workstation whereby pathologists can organize information acquisition, processing, and subsequent storage.[166] Such a microcomputer based workstation may be able to (1) apply mathematical and graph analysis to patient-related data; (2) possess tools for image processing and analysis; (3) incorporate gross, microscopic, and electron-microscopic images into a final surgical pathology report; (4) store image data for conferences; and (5) utilize educational programs with medically oriented software. Other workstations, utilizing computer-assisted microscopes, have shown that reproducible quality control is now feasible in routine cytological screening.[167]

14.10.12. Telepathology

Telemedicine is the practice of medicine at long distance using telecommunications and has been utilized for over 30 years.[168,169] With rapidly advancing and cost-effective technologies, not only can the pathologist organize information in departmental workstations, but it is feasible to (1) robotically control light-microscope slide stages so that digitized images of tissue sections, blood smears, and cytology smears can be diagnosed by consultant experts in different medical institutions;[170,171] (2) provide a remote frozen-section diagnosis service in outreach institutions;[173] (3) integrate both static and real-time dynamic imaging so that diagnostic fields can be actively selected and the focus or illumination adjusted; and (4) optimize image compression, transmission, and storage facilities.[173]

14.11. SOURCES OF ERROR AND STANDARDIZATION

In 1990, the Committee for Diagnostic Quantitative Pathology Working Group of the European Society of Pathology called for the widespread standardization of preparatory techniques, interpretational criteria and internal quality assurance in the field of image analysis.[174,175] The main sources of error in quantitative image analysis relate to tissue preparation, image quality, and measurement reproducibility.

14.11.1. Tissue Preparation

Standardized specimen sampling, denoting the optimal number of sections that should be taken from a solid tumor, varies depending on the tumor size and type. The influence of variations in fixation[176] and instrumentational features have been well studied.[177] Only small differences in histological preparatory techniques, such as varying exposure for acetone and formalin fixation, or conditions for dehydration, paraffin-embedding, section thickness, water-bath temperature, deparaffinization, and staining, can drastically alter the optical density of cells and tissue. Stretching of sections on water baths after cutting affects cytoplasm and intercellular tissues but not nuclei.[71] Cytoplasmic measurements are more sensitive to fixation and processing variations than are nuclear measurements. Some investigators embed in water-soluble methacrylate in order to avoid carrying out additional dehydration steps and prevent tissue shrinkage.

In general, as few staining reagents and counterstains should be used as possible with the actual staining time strictly controlled.[178,179] The advent of automated immunohistochemical staining machines may play an increasingly important role in the field of image analysis where standardization of staining is paramount.[180] The fading effect, over time, of repeated measurements on methylgreen counterstain and immunohistochemical reagents can result in a linear change in the gray-valued threshold range required to identify the progressively less darkened immunostained regions.[30]

14.11.2. Image Capture

Camera calibration can be carried out using neutral density filters of known optical density. An optimal image sampling rate can be obtained using the discrete Fourier transformation of an image, which states that sampling should be done at twice the frequency of the highest frequency present in the image.[24] Glare, from the object of interest, can be corrected by ensuring optimal settings of the microscope according to Köhler's illumination rules[181] as well as correcting with neutral density filters. Irregular surges in the light source can be controlled with a standardized light source. Uneven background shadowing can be eliminated by subtracting a blank background gray-scale image from the captured image of interest. The gain or contrast adjustment on a camera describes the relationship between the input illumination and the output voltage.[165] For image processing, the gain setting must be fixed if a comparison of illumination levels from different regions in the same specimen is to be made. The black level adjustment on a camera represents the lowest level of illumination capable of producing a voltage from that camera. For image processing, this black level must be preset since the darkest regions of each captured image are not usually constant.

14.11.3. Measurement Reproducibility

Reproducibility describes how well repeated measurement assessments of the same objects, from one population, agree. A number of factors determine reproducibility. Variations in the spatial, densitometric and spectral characteristics of objects will influence their ease of segmentation.[182] The variation in coefficient of variance for segmentation of high-sensitivity Feulgen nuclear staining is small compared to the variability in segmentation of low-sensitivity immunohistochemical staining for estrogen receptor antigens.[183] The operator's experience has a great impact on inter- and intraobserver variation of measurements; the more experienced the operator, the better the reproducibility.[184]

In diagnostic studies, an established and ongoing quality-control program is vital to ensure reliable and meaningful morphometric measurements. New methods for quantitation must be compared against established techniques measuring the same parameter or alternatively, the mean values of experienced operators may be used as reference values.[42] Multivariate analysis of more than one morphometric parameter may provide better distinctions in areas of diagnostic overlap.[185,186]

14.12. ANALYSIS OF QUANTITATIVE RESULTS

All medical research should follow a study design. Image processing is no exception.[187] If the experimental design is wrong, the results will be meaningless. The study protocol should include a full description of the aims, methods, and subjects, with the inclusion and exclusion criteria clearly defined. The information supplied must be sufficiently detailed to be easily interpreted by new investigators or advising statisticians. The expected findings must be defined and the need for financial support or evaluation by an ethical committee considered. Important general concepts include experiment simplicity, types of study (observational, experimental, prospective, retrospective), sample size calculations, control of bias, randomization, control groups, blinding, method comparison (accuracy), and repeatability.

14.13. SUMMARY

With the advent of highly sophisticated and affordable microprocessors, cameras, and microcomputers, the analysis of enhanced, digitized microscopic images in the medical field provides a means of quantifying, in a small way, the complex, natural image processing capabilities of the human brain. Image processing is now considered cost-effective, accurate, labor-saving, and reproducible. It will be improved still further with the routine use of color cameras. Particularly in the field of three-dimensional imaging, the new software techniques for image processing, analysis, and feature discrimination are continuously developing. This software can be used by operators with only limited knowledge of the background theories involved. But, in order to appreciate and usefully implement the numerous applications of image processing, it helps to understand its distinct vocabulary, its basic algorithmic tools and its limitations.

Today, the pathologist is required to make more and more sophisticated and complete diagnoses on less and less tissue. With image cytometry, a morphological diagnosis, quantitative histochemical analysis of receptor, oncogene and proliferative antigen expression, DNA ploidy analysis, and proliferative index determination, can be made on the same paraffin-embedded histological sections. Similar studies can be carried out on fine-needle aspirate samples and cytologic smears. The image analyzer can be part of a pathologists workstation for data measurements, presentation, and storage. Whether the system is commercial or personally compiled, standardization procedures and quality assurance issues must be adhered to conscientiously. Quantitation and image processing in medicine is most successful when there is a full collaboration between biomedical, microscopi, statistical, and computer experts.

REFERENCES

1. Swift H: Analytical microscopy of biological materials. In Wied G, ed: *Introduction to Quantitative Cytochemistry.* New York: Academic Press, 1966.

2. Koss L: *Anal Quant Cytol* 4:251–256, 1982.

3. Palkovits M, Fischer J: *Karyometric Investigations.* Budapest: Akadémiai Kiadó, 1968.

4. Hertwig R: *Biol Zbl* 23:49–62, 1903.

5. Boveri T: *Jen Z Naturwiss* 39:445–524, 1905.

6. Erdmann, R: *Arch Zellforsch* 2:76–136, 1909.

7. Jacobj W: *Arch Entw Mech* 106:124–192, 1925.

8. Hodge C: *Am J Psychol* 1:479–486, 1888.

9. Vas F: *Arch Mikr Anat* 40:375–389, 1892.

10. Mann G: *J Anat Physiol* 29:100ff, 1894.

11. Morpurgo B: *Virchows Arch Pathol Anat* 152:550–552, 1898.

12. Schiefferdecker P: *Arch Physiol* 165:499–564, 1916.

13. Benninghoff A: *Mon Zool Ital* 61(Suppl):84–89, 1953.

14. Puff A: *Med Diss* (Marburg), 1950.

15. Eichner D: *Z Zellforsch* 37:406–414, 1952.

16. Feulgen R, Rossenbeck H: *Symposium Soc Exper Biol no. 1* 135:203–248, 1924.

17. Brachet J: *Nucleic acids in the cell and the embryo*, Conference 1947 Symposium of the So Biol Nucleic Acid 1:207–224, 1947.

18. Koss L: *Acta Cytol* 21:639–642, 1977.

19. Caspersson T, Santesson L: *Acta Radiol* (Suppl) 46:1–105, 1942.

20. Prewit J, Mendelsohn M: *Ann NY Acad Sci* 128:1035–1043, 1966.

21. Bahr G, Bartels P, Wied G, Koss L: In Automated Cytology, Koss L, ed: *Diagnostic Cytology and Its Histopathologic Bases.* Philadelphia: Lippincott, 1979, pp. 1123–1186.

22. Inoue S: *Video Microscopy.* New York: Plenum Press, 1986.

23. Baxes G: *Digital Image Processing: A Practical Primer.* Englewood Cliffs, NJ: Prentice-Hall, 1988.

24. Gonzales R, Wintz P: *Digital Image Processing.* Reading, MA: Addison-Wesley, 1987.

25. Benzschawel T: *Human factors influence effective use of color in information displays.* 1:16–21, 34, 1985.

26. Bacus S, Flowers J, Press M, Bacus J, McCarty K: *Am J Clin Pathol* 90:233–239, 1988.

27. Baak J: *Pathol Res Pract,* 1987.

28. Russ J: *Computer-Assisted Microscopy: The Measurement and Analysis of Images.* New York: Plenum Press, 1990.

29. Low A: *Introductory Computer Vision and Image Processing.* London: McGraw-Hill, 1991.

30. Wells W, Rainer R, Memoli V: *Am J Clin Pathol* 99:48–56, 1993.

31. Kay D, Levine J: *Graphics File Formats.* New York: Windcrest/McGraw-Hill, 1992.

32. Webster G: *EXE Mag* 7:33–40, 1992.

33. Huffman D: *Proc Inst Electr Radio Eng* 40:1098–1101, 1952.

34. Welch T: *IEEE Comput* 17:8–19, 1984.

35. Haralick R, Shapiro L: Image Segmentation Techniques, *Computer Graph Image Process* 29:100–132, 1985.

36. Sahoo P, Soltani S, Wong A: *Comput Vis Graph Image Process* 41:233–260, 1988.

37. Prewitt J, Mendelsohn M: *Ann NY Acad Sci* 128:1035–1053, 1966.

38. Doyle, W: *J Assoc Comput Mach* 9:259–267, 1962.

39. Otsu N: *IEEE Trans Syst Man Cybernet* SMC-8:62–66, 1978.

40. Pratt W: *Digital Image Processing.* New York: Wiley, 1978.

41. Sobel I: *Camera Models and Machine Perception.* Palo Alto, CA: Thesis (Ph.D.) Dept. of Electrical Engineering, Stanford University, 1970.

42. Baak J: *Manual of Quantitative Pathology in Cancer Diagnosis and Prognosis.* Berlin: Springer-Verlag, 1991.

43. Coon J, Weinstein R: *Diagnostic Flow Cytometry.* Baltimore: Williams & Wilkins, 1991, pp. 1–17.

44. Kamentsky L, Melamed M, Derman H: *Science* 150:630–631, 1965.

45. Suit P, Bauer T: *Am J Clin Pathol* 94:49–53, 1990.

46. Bauer TW, Tubbs RR, Edinger MG, et al: A Prospective Comparison of DNA Quantitation by Image and Flow Cytometry, *Am J Clin Pathol* 93:322–326, 1990.

47. McFadden P, Clowry L, Daehnert K, Hause L, Koethe S: *Am J Clin Pathol* 93:637–642, 1990.

48. Dawson A, Norton J, Weinberg D: *Am J Pathol* 136:1115–1124, 1990.

49. Sapi Z, Hendricks J, Pharis P, Wilkinson, E: *Am J Clin Pathol* 99:714–720, 1993.

50. Rijken A, Dekker A, Taylor S, Hoffman P: *Am J Clin Pathol* 95:6–12, 1991.

51. Elias H: Address of the president. In *Proc 1st Internatl Congress Stereology*, Congressprint, Wein, Feldberg, Germany, 1963, pp. 1–2.

52. Weibel E: *Stereological Methods: Practical Methods for Biological Morphometry.* London: Academic Press, 1979.

53. Baddeley A, Gundersen H, Cruz-Olive L: *J Microsc* 142:259–276, 1986.

54. Gundersen H, et al: *APMIS: acta pathologica, microbiologica et immunologica Scandinavica* 96:379–394, 1988.

55. Gundersen H, et al: *APMIS: acta pathologica, microbiologica et immunologica Scandinavica* 96:857–881, 1988.

56. Gundersen H: *J Microsc* 111:219–223, 1977.

57. Sterio D: *J Microsc* 134:127–136, 1984.

58. Bolender R: *Microsc Res Tech* 2:255–261, 1992.

59. Tomkeieff, S: *Nature* 155:24, 1945.

60. Gundersen H, Jensen E: *J Microsc* 131:291–310, 1983.

61. Hall A, Browne M, Howard V: *Proc RMS* 26:63–70, 1991.

62. Ploem J, Tanke H: *Introduction to Fluorescence Microscopy.* Oxford, UK: Oxford University Press and Royal Microscopical Society, 1987.

63. Muchel F: *Zeiss Inform* 30:20–27, 1988.

64. Abbe, E: *Anatomy* 9:413–468, 1873.

65. Levinthal C, Ware R: *Nature* 236:207–210, 1972.

66. Whimster W: *Pathol Res Pract* 185:594–597, 1989.

67. Salisbury J, Whimster W: *J Pathol* 170:223–227, 1993.

68. Burston W, Thurley K: *J Anat* 91:409–412, 1976.

69. Deverell M, Whimster W: *Pathol Res Pract* 185:620–605, 1989.

70. Deverell M, et al: *Analyt Cell Pathol* 5:253–263, 1993.

71. Deverell M, Bailey N, Whimster W: *Pathol Res Pract* 185:598–601, 1989.

72. Holman J, Cookson M, Dykes E: *Med Info* 14:173–184, 1989.

73. Bartels P, Bibbo M, Wied G: *Acta Cytol* 20:62–67, 1976.

74. Oort J: *Analyt Quant Cytol Histol* 7:164–166, 1985.

75. Langley F, Baak J, Oort J: In Baak J, Oort J, eds: *A Manual of Morphometry in Diagnostic Pathology.* Berlin: Springer-Verlag, 1983, pp. 6–14.

76. Baak J: *Analyt Quant Cytol Histol* 9:89–95, 1987.

77. Baak J: *Acta Stereol* 2:307–311, 1983.

78. Rubio C, Uribe A, Svensson A, May I: *Analyt Quant Cytol Histol* 10:115–119, 1988.

79. Crocker J, Skilbeck N: *J Clin Pathol* 40:885–889, 1987.

80. Fallowfield M, Cook MG: *Histopathology* 14:299–304, 1989.

81. Dervan P, Gilmartin L, Loftus B, Carney D: *Am J Clin Pathol* 92:401–407, 1989.

82. Smith R, Crocker J: *Histopathology* 12:113–125, 1988.

83. Helpap B: *Histopathology* 13:201–211, 1988.

84. Crocker J, McGovern J: *J Clin Pathol* 41:1044–1048, 1988.

85. Cairns P, Suarez V, Newman J, Crocker J: *Arch Pathol Lab Med* 113:1250–1252, 1989.

86. Montironi RAB, Scarpelli M, Matera G, Albrti R: *J Clin Pathol* 44:509–514, 1991.

87. Shimada H, et al: *JNCI* (*J Natl Cancer Inst*) 73:405–416, 1984.

88. Wells W, Rainer R, Memoli V: *Determination of the Mitosis-Karyorrhexis Index, a Prognostic Indicator in Neuroblastoma, by Macintosh-Based Image Analysis* (abstract), Atlanta, GA, 1992.

89. Byers P: In Avioli L, Krane S, eds: *Metabolic Bone Disease.* London: Academic Press, 1977.

90. Salisbury J, Deverell M, King S: *Histomorphometric Analysis of Bone Biopsies from Normal Subjects: Comparison of Quantitation Using Eye-Piece Graticules and IBAS 2000,* Basel, Switzerland, Aug 29–Sept 1.

91. Picci P, Bacci G, Campanacci M: *Cancer* 56:1515–1521, 1985.

92. Wilkins B, O'Brien, C: *J Clin Pathol* 41:558–561, 1988.

93. Usson Y, Torch S, Saxod R: *Analyt Cell Pathol* 3:91–102, 1991.

94. Strojny P, Traczyk Z, Rozycka M, Bem W, Sawicki W: *Analyt Quant Cytol Histol* 9:475–479, 1987.

95. Stevens M, Fazzalari N, Crisp D: *Analyt Quant Cytol Histol* 9:459–468, 1987.

96. Oberholzer M, et al: *Analyt Cell Pathol* 31:25–42, 1991.

97. Petein M, et al: *Am J Clin Pathol* 96:628–634, 1991.

98. Sowter C, Slaven G, Sowter G, Rosen D, Hendry W: *Analyt Cell Pathol* 3:1–9, 1991.

99. Miller B, Lavia L, Horbelt D: *Cancer* 67:1318–1321, 1991.

100. Fu Y, Ferenczy A, Huang I, Gelfand M: *Analyt Quant Cytol Histol* 10:139–149, 1988.

101. Bocking A, Chatelain R: *Analyt Quant Cytol Histol* 11:177–186, 1989.

102. Dawson A, Austin R, Weinberg D: *Am J Clin Pathol* 95:S29–S37, 1991.

103. Haroske G, Kunzel KD, Theissig F: *Analyt Cell Pathol* 3:11–24, 1991.

104. Koss L, Sherman A, Eppich E: *Anal Quant Cytol* 6:89–94, 1984.

105. McCarty K Jr, Miller L, Cox E, Konrath J, McCarty K Sr: *Arch Pathol Lab Med* 109:716–721, 1985.

106. Hanna W, Mobbs B: *Am J Clin Pathol* 91:182–186, 1989.

107. Esteban J, Battifora H, Warsi Z, Bailey A, Bacus S: *Mod Pathol* 4:53–57, 1991.

108. Baddoura F, Cohen C, Unger E, DeRose P, Chenggis M: *Mod Pathol* 4:91–95, 1991.

109. van Diest P, Baak J, Chin D, Theeuwes J, Bacus S: *Analyt Cell Pathol* 3:195–202, 1991.

110. Bacus S, Bacus J, Slamon D, Press M: *Arch Pathol Lab Med* 114:164–169, 1990.

111. Sebo T, Roche P, Witzig T, Kurtin P: *Am J Clin Pathol* 99:668–672, 1993.

112. Siitonen S, Isola J, Rantala I, Helin H: *Am J Clin Pathol* 99:226–231, 1993.

113. Jordan P, et al: *Am J Clin Pathol* 99:736–740, 1993.

114. Abdelatif O, et al: *Arch Pathol Lab Med* 115:880–885, 1991.

115. Feichter G, Mueller A, Kaufmann M: *Internal J Cancer* 41:823–828, 1988.

116. Fallenius A, Franzen S, Auer G: *Cancer* 62:521–530, 1988.

117. Harvey J, de Klerk N, Berryman I: *Breast Cancer Res Treat* 9:101–109, 1987.

118. Hedley D, Rugg C, Ng A, Taylor I: *Cancer Res* 44:5395–5398, 1984.

119. Auer G, Ericksson F, Azavedo E: *Cancer Res* 44:394–396, 1984.

120. Moran R, Black M, Alpert L, Straus M: *Cancer* 54:1586–1590, 1984.

121. Muss H, Kute T, Case D: *Cancer* 64:1894–1900, 1989.

122. Hedley D, Rugg C, Gelber R: *Cancer Res* 47:4729–4735, 1987.

123. Kallioniemi O-P, et al: *Eur J Cancer Clin Oncol* 23:277–282, 1987.

124. Clark G, et al: *N Engl J Med* 320:627–633, 1989.

125. Kallioniemi O, Blanco G, Alavaikko M: *Cancer* 62:2183–2190, 1988.

126. Raber M, et al: *Cytometry* 3:36–41, 1982.

127. Olszewski W, Darzynkiewicz, ZPPR, Schwartz M, Melamed M: *Cancer* 48:985–988, 1981.

128. Olszewski W, Darzynkiewicz, ZPPR, Schwartz M, Melamed M: *Cancer* 48:985–988, 1981.

129. Braylan R, Benson N, Nourse V: *Cancer Res* 44:5010–5016, 1984.

130. Juneja S, et al: *J Clin Pathol* 39:987–992, 1986.

131. Cowan R, Harris M, Jones M, Crowther D: *Br J Cancer* 60:904–910, 1989.

132. Joensuu H, Klemi P, Korkeila E: *Am J Clin Pathol* 90:670–673, 1988.

133. Giaretti W, et al: *Cancer* 67:1921–1927, 1991.

134. Iversen O-E, Skaarland E: *Cancer* 60:82–87, 1987.

135. Zimmerman P, Hawson G, Bint M, Parsons P: *Lancet* 530–533, 1987.

136. Jackson-York G, Davis B, Warren W, Gould V, Memoli V: *Cancer* 68:374–379, 1991.

137. de Kernion J, et al: *Cancer* 64:1669–1673, 1989.

138. Grignon D, et al: *Cancer* 64:2133–2140, 1989.

139. Winkler H, et al: *Mayo Clinic Proc* 63:103–112, 1988.

140. Nativ O, et al: *Mayo Clin Proc* 64:911–919, 1989.

141. Fujimoto J, Okamoto E, Yamanaka N, Toyosaka A, Mitsunobu M: *Cancer* 67:939–944, 1991.

142. Slater S, Cook M, Fisher C, Wright N, Foster C: *Histopathology* 19:337–344, 1991.

143. Hemming J, Quirke P, Womack C, Wells M, Elston C: *J Clin Pathol* 40:615–620, 1987.

144. Bolender R: *Internatl Rev Cytol* 55:247–289, 1978.

145. Bolender R: *J Cell Biol* 61:269, 1974.

146. Schroeder H, Münzel-Pedrazzoli S: *J. Microsc* 92:179, 1970.

147. Sørenson F, Bichel P, Jakobsen A: *Cancer* 69:187–199, 1992.

148. Nielsen K, Berild G, Jørgensen P, Wies N: *J Microsc* 154:63–69, 1989.

149. Sørenson F: *Cancer* 63:1784–1798, 1989.

150. Nielsen K, Colstrup H, Nilsson T, Gunderson H: *Virch Arch* (*Cell Pathol*) 52:41–54, 1986.

151. Nielsen K, Ørntoft T, Wolf H: *Cancer* 64:2269–2274, 1989.

152. Nielsen A, Nyholm H: *Histopathology* 22:17–24, 1993.

153. Neal H, Hurst P: *Diagn Cytopathol* 8:293–298, 1992.

154. Bacon J, Gonzalez C, Hutchison C: *Trends Cell Biol* 1:172–175, 1991.

155. Zhang Y: *Cytometry* 12:308–315, 1991.

156. Mossberg K, Arvidsson U, Ulfhake B: *J Histochem Cytochem* 38:179–190, 1990.

157. Fine A, Amos W, Durbin R, McNaughton P: *Trends in neurosciences* 11:346–351, 1988.

158. Houtsmuller, A.B., Oud J.L., van der Wort, H.T.M., Baarslag, M.W., Krol, J.J., Masterd, B., Mans, A., Brakemhoff, G.J. and Nanninga, N: *J Microscopy*, 158, 235–248, 1990.

159. Brakenhoff G, van der Voort H, van Spronsen E, Linnemans W, Nanninga N: *Nature* 317:748–749, 1985.

160. Boon M, Kok L, Sutedja G, Dutrieux R: *Acta Cytol* 37:40–48, 1993.

161. Zhu Q, Tekola P, Baak J, Beliën J: *Analyt Quant Cytol Histol* 16:145–547, 1994.

162. Salisbury J, Deverell M, Cookson M, Whimster W: *Reconstructed Three-Dimensional Images of Fetal Notochords: Clues to the Pathogenesis of Chordoma* (abstract), Heraklion, Crete, 1992.

163. Rydmark M, Jansson T, Berthold C-H, Gustavsson T: *J Microsc* 165:29–47, 1992.

164. Campbell F, Garrahan N, Deverell M, Whimster W, Williams G: *Application of a Computer Aided Design System to the Dimensional Reconstruction of Colonic Crypts* (abstract), Manchester, UK, 1992.

165. Conn P: *Quantitative and Qualitative Microscopy.* San Diego: Academic Press, 1990.

166. Shultz E, Brown R: *Am J Clin Pathol* 95 (Suppl 1):S50–S57, 1991.

167. von Hagen V, Morens A, Krief B: *Analyt Cell Pathol* 3(4):249–256, July 1991.

168. Riggs R, Purtillo D, Connor D: *JAMA* 228:600–602, 1974.

169. Jutra J: *AJR. American Journal of Roentgenology* 82:1099–1102, 1959.

170. Weinstein R: *Clin Lab Management Rev* 6:182–184, 1992.

171. Wold L, Weiland L: *Clin Lab Management Rev* 1:174–175, 1992.

172. Nordrum I, Engum B, ER: *Hum Pathol* 22:514–518, 1991.

173. Krupinski E, Weinstein R, Bloom K, Rosek L: *Adv Pathol Lab Med* 6:63–87, 1993.

174. Montironi R, Whimster W: *Pathol Res Pract* 186:817–820, 1990.

175. Esteban J, et al: *Am J Clin Pathol* 95:460–466, 1991.

176. Baak J, Noteboom E, Koevoets, J: *Analyt Quant Cytol Histol* 11:219–224, 1989.

177. Bacus J, Grace L: *Appl Optics* 26:3280–3293, 1987.

178. Jordan S, Brayer J, Bartels P, Anderson R: *Analyt Quant Cytol Histol* 10:37–46, 1988.

179. Deverell M, Whimster W, Salisbury J: *Pathol Res Pract* 185:555–557, 1989.

180. Tubbs R, Bauer T: *Arch Pathol Lab Med* 113:653–657, 1989.

181. Rawlins D: *Light Microscopy.* Bios Scientific Publishers, in association with the Biomedical Society, 1992.

182. Smeulders A, Dorst L: *Analyt Quant Cytol Histol* 7:242–249, 1985.

183. Kosma V, et al: *Analyt Quant Cytol Histol* 7:271–274, 1985.

184. Gamel J, Gleason J, Williams H, Greenberg R: *Analyt Quant Cytol Histol* 7:174–177, 1985.

185. Bartels P: (1979–1983). *Analyt Quant Cytol* 1:20–28, 1979 - 5:229–235, 1983.

186. Baak J, Langley F, Hermans J: In Baak J, Oort J, eds: *A Manual of Morphometry in Diagnostic Pathology.* Berlin: Springer-Verlag, 1983, pp. 32–34.

187. Altman D: *Practical Statistics for Medical Research.* London: Chapman & Hall, 1991.

15

Automation of Molecular Genetics and Diagnostics

EMILY S. WINN-DEEN

CONTENTS

15.1. DNA PURIFICATION

The key to good molecular assay performance is beginning with properly isolated and purified DNA or RNA. These nucleic acids may be isolated from a

Handbook of Clinical Automation, Robotics, and Optimization, Edited by Gerald J. Kost with the collaboration of Judith Welsh.
ISBN 0-471-03179-8 © 1996 John Wiley & Sons, Inc.

number of clinical sources, including blood, amniocytes, buccal cells, sputum, vaginal or urethral swabs, and stool. The source of the sample and the assay in which it will be used determines how the nucleic acid should be isolated. For example the heme in red blood cells can interfere with DNA polymerase so that care must be taken in preparation of blood samples for polymerase chain reaction (PCR). Highly purified DNA is needed if the samples will be digested with restriction enzymes for Southern blotting. Some infectious organisms such as *Mycobacterium tuberculosis* are particularly difficult to lyse and require especially stringent conditions.

All nucleic acid purification methods begin with cell lysis.[1] Mammalian cells can be lysed by boiling or treatment with detergent. Other cells require a lysis methods tailored to the characteristics of that cell. After lysis, many purification methods remove detrimental proteins such as nucleases through treatment with proteinase K in the presence of EDTA and extraction with phenol. Other methods pass the cell lysate through a resin to trap proteins. After removal of the protein, the nucleic acid is generally alcohol-precipitated to yield high-molecular-weight DNA. Many of these purification methods are relatively straightforward to do manually, but some involve several separation, centrifugation, and precipitation steps where errors can occur. Samples can be mislabeled, dropped or cross-contaminated, and pipetting errors can be made at any of the many steps. Some samples such as human blood and tissue may contain infectious agents and therefore require special precautions for handling. Additionally, the chemicals used in the classic phenol/chloroform extraction procedure are hazardous. For these reasons automation of DNA preparation is highly desirable.

There are several approaches to automation on the market today. In the AutoGen (Integrated Separation Systems, Natick, MA) system classic manual procedures are mimicked by a robotic instrument. The operator loads 1 mL of cultured cells or blood into a microcentrifuge tube and places it into the centrifuge module. Empty tubes and pipette tips are also loaded into the unit, and the cycle begins. Microprocessor control allows all subsequent reagent deliveries, aspirations, and centrifugations to be handled by the instrument. These steps include cell concentration, lysis, neutralization, deproteination, precipitation, DNA washing, and resuspension. The Model 540 can process up to 12 samples to purified DNA in 40 min. Protocols are available for isolation of DNA or RNA from blood, plasmids, cosmids, phages, plant cells, tissue suspensions, and bacterial cultures.

The Beckman (Palo Alto, CA) Biomek® 1000 workstation, a generic x, y, z pipetting robot, has also been adapted to isolation of genomic DNA.[2] The method involves automation of DNA isolation by anion-exchange chromatography on Qiagen-100 columns (Chatsworth, CA). The robot handles all the liquid manipulations, including loading cells onto the column, washing the column, and eluting the DNA. Using this method, DNA from 8–12 samples of $\sim 10^6$ cells each can be isolated in less than one hour. DNA prepared in this way is suitable for PCR or for allele-specific hybridization applications.

The GENEPURE™ 341 nucleic acid purification system from Perkin Elmer

Corporation, Applied Biosystems Division (Foster City, CA) features on-line chemistry reagents and a unique reaction vessel available in three volumes (7, 14, and 30 mL) that can be heated and rotated. In a typical protocol, samples from blood, tissue, cell culture, plants, plasmids, bacteria, or viruses are added to the reaction vessel. Hot lysis buffer containing proteinase K is added and gentle agitation is used to open the cells. After lysis is complete, phenol/chloroform is added, and the sample is extracted using gentle agitation. The reaction vessel returns to a horizontal position and phase separation is encouraged by the addition of heat. The lower layer (organic) is transferred to waste until the in-line conductivity meter senses the aqueous layer. Phenol extraction can be repeated if desired. The DNA is then precipitated by the addition of ethanol/sodium acetate and collected onto a special filter cartridge. After additional ethanol washing, the filter cartridge is removed and the DNA is redissolved in the appropriate buffer. DNA purified in this manner is suitable for most molecular biology applications, including sequencing, PCR, and restriction digestion. Alternate protocols for RNA purification are also available. Not all end uses require complete DNA purification; for them, a fast, nonorganic cycle can be used. This instrument can process eight samples to purified DNA in 2–4 h, depending on the cycle chosen.

Another approach to automation of DNA isolation is the Pharmacia Biotech (Piscataway, NJ) EasyPrep™ system. This system can process either 12 or 24 samples simultaneously using positive pressure to force the purification reagents through an assortment of filtration devices. It can be used to purify synthetic oligonucleotides, PCR products from gel slices, and DNA from bacteria or plasmids. PCR products can be purified in 30 min with a recovery of 95%, while preparation of DNA from plasmids takes about one hour and yields 15–20 μg of DNA from 1 mL of cultured cells. Each of these methods automate some of the steps where human errors inevitably take place.

15.2. DNA SEQUENCING

DNA sequencing, which has traditionally been a research tool, is the gold standard reference method for molecular diagnostics. Sequencing of a number of affected individuals is also used to gather the epidemiological data needed to characterize the mutation spectrum in inherited diseases. These data are then used as a basis for development of diagnostic reagents to screen for the mutations most commonly associated with any given disease. In cases where this mutation spectrum is large, sequencing is now used for routine diagnostic work as well. Diagnostic sequencing has already been applied to a variety of problems, including HLA (human leukocyte antigen) typing,[3,4] diagnosis of inherited diseases caused by point mutations in the hypoxanthine phosphoribosyltransferase[5,6] and apolipoprotein B[7] genes, p53 tumor suppresser gene mutations,[8] and epidemiology of infectious diseases such as cholera[9] and HIV.[10,11]

15.2.1. DNA Sequencing Using Radioactive Labels

DNA sequence analysis is based on either chemical degradation of DNA[12] or random chain termination of DNA polymerase extension products with dideoxynucleotides.[13] Originally all DNA sequence analysis was done using radioactive markers such as ^{32}P or ^{35}S. The Sanger sequencing method is depicted in Figure 15.1. In this method, a reaction mix containing a primer, DNA polymerase, and the four deoxynucleotide triphosphates (at least one of which is radioactively labeled) is prepared and then divided into four aliquots. A limiting amount of either A, T, C, or G dideoxynucleotide triphosphate is added to each of the four aliquots so that the dideoxy-A tube ends up containing all of the fragments which contain terminal A, the dideoxy-T tube ends up containing all the fragments that contain terminal T, and so on. After the sequencing reactions are completed, the A, T, C, and G aliquots are each loaded onto a separate lane of a denaturing acrylamide gel and separated by high-voltage electrophoresis. The gel is then transferred to a solid support and subjected to autoradiography. The sequence is read by following the bands between the A, T, C, and G lanes. This method offers a relatively simple means of analyzing DNA sequences and was quickly adopted by the research community. However, the pipetting and transfer required are quite tedious, and accurate interpretation of base sequence from the autoradiograms requires skill and careful attention to detail.

Creation and analysis of the autoradiogram is one part of the radioactive sequencing process that has been chosen for automation. In order to eliminate the need to transfer after electrophoresis, two instruments are now available that combine electrophoresis and transfer into a single operation (Intelligenetics/Betagen AutoTrans System, Mountain View, CA; Hoefer TE 2000 TwoStep™, San Francisco, CA). Both electrophorese a sample down a vertical gel and, as the DNA elutes off the bottom of the gel, it is deposited onto a constantly moving membrane web. With the AutoTrans system a computer controls web speed, electrophoresis voltage, temperature, and buffer recirculation, while the Two-Step™ controls only web speed and temperature.

Several companies have written highly sophisticated software that interacts with a densitometric film scanner to find lanes, detect bands, correct for smiling, and read out the sequence. Scanner–software packages are available from Millipore Corporation, Bedford, MA (Bio Image® 60S), Molecular Dynamics, Sunnyvale, CA (DNAscan™ software for use with the ImageQuant™ workstation or 325 Computing Densitometer), and United States Biochemical, Cleveland, OH (SciScan™ 5000 with BioAnalysis™ software). These systems can significantly improve on the eyestrain associated with manual interpretation of sequencing autoradiograms. Variation in band mobility between lanes, and lanes that do not run straight down the gel make radioactive sequencing difficult to interpret electronically. Chemistry anomalies such as compressions and stops also make instrument interpretation difficult.

Automation of the actual radiation measurement can replace traditional auto-

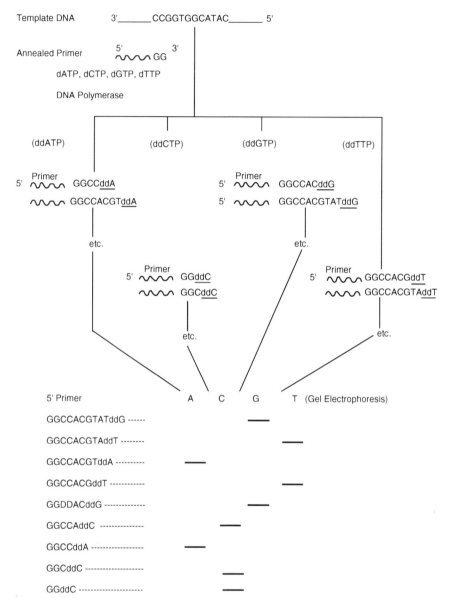

Figure 15.1. Schematic of the Sanger dideoxy sequencing method. (Artwork courtesy of Ellson Chen, Perkin Elmer Corporation, Applied Biosystems Division.)

radiography with direct reading of the radioactive blot. The Intelligenetics/ Betagen Betascope 603 Blot Analyzer™ images patterns of radioactivity from [32]P- or ^{35}S-labeled blots by tracing the path of high-energy beta emission through two measurement planes, each consisting of three frames of tightly spaced wires, within a gas-filled chamber. The instrument provides real-time visualization of the radioactive areas of the blot and computer analysis of the counts coming from each area. This system is simple and easy to use. Its one drawback is that for samples that are weakly labeled the instrument may be tied up for many hours counting a single blot. Conversely, in the Molecular Dynamics PhosphorImager, the gel transfer is placed in a cassette that contains a $BaFBr:Eu^{+2}$ medium to capture all the energy released by beta particles.[14] The beta particles excite an electron of the Eu^{+2} ion. This electron is then trapped in the $BaFBr^-$ complex and results in the oxidation of Eu^{+2} to Eu^{+3}. Only after exposure is complete, are the phosphor screens placed in the PhosphorImager. The 633 nm light from a helium–neon laser converts the Eu^{+3} to an excited state, Eu^{+2*} which, in turn, emits a photon at 390 nm as it returns to the ground state. These photons are counted by the PhosphorImager and their locations determined. This medium has a greater dynamic range than conventional x-ray film and requires much shorter exposure times. Since the instrument is used only for reading the medium, multiple gels can be exposing the phosphor plates at the same time in a manner analogous to autoradiography.

15.2.2. DNA Sequencing Using Fluorescent Labels

Several years after the first description of the Sanger enzymatic sequencing chemistry a group of researchers at California Institute of Technology (Pasadena, CA) and Applied Biosystems developed fluorescent DNA sequencing.[15,16] Fluorescence-based DNA sequencing utilizes Sanger sequencing reactions run exactly as they are for radioactive sequencing except that a fluorescently labeled primer is substituted for the radioactive label. In single-color systems (Pharmacia A.L.F., Licor Model 4000, and Amersham VISTRA) the products from the fluorescent primers are each run in separate gel lanes in a manner analogous to radioactive sequencing. In the A.L.F. system the excitation laser is stationary and its' light enters through the side of the gel.[17] The 40 lanes of the gel are each equipped with a separate fixed detector to collect the emitted light.

In addition to the absence of moving optical parts, the system's laser light passes directly into the gel, thus minimizing problems with fluorescence of the glass plates. This system can determine about 350 bases for 10 sequences simultaneously (3500 bases per gel). However, it still suffers from the main problems that plague conventional radioactive sequencing, variation in electrophoretic mobility between lanes, and its effects on accurate base calling. Some of this is addressed by software that analyzes four lanes at once to assure that only one peak is found for any given base position. However, fixed detectors make it difficult to compensate for lanes that do run straight down the gel.

The Licor Model 4000 sequencer (Lincoln, NE) uses an infrared fluorescent dye-labeled primer and an inexpensive helium–neon laser similar to those used to read compact disks.[18] The 10-mW solid-state laser diode used for excitation at 785 nm and the confocal microscope objective/avalanche photodiode detector at 820 nm used for emission detection have allowed miniaturization of the instrument optics. This, in turn, has allowed the complete optics package to be mounted onto the scanning platform, giving flexibility in scan speed and scan width. Like the A.L.F., this instrument uses a single dye, and A, C, G, and T reactions must be run in separate lanes. Up to 11 samples can be run simultaneously (44 lanes). Data is analyzed using the system's Base ImageIR™ software with typical performance of 450 bases per sample with 99% accuracy. The Amersham VISTRA DNA sequencer also uses a long-wavelength fluorescent dye, Texas Red, and an inexpensive helium-neon laser. Similar to the A.L.F., the laser is focused via fixed lenses through the entire width of the gel. It can run up to eight samples (32 lanes) and read 500 bases of data per lane with an accuracy of $\geq 98.5\%$ in a 6-h electrophoresis run. Another single-color approach reported recently involves using rhodamine X-labeled fluorescent primers to run the sequencing reactions.[19] After running the samples out on a gel, the gel and plates are placed into a fluorescent image scanner and excited with a 15-mW green laser at 532 nm. The emitted light is monitored at 605 nm and an image is created. This hybrid technique allows the user to review the sequence data quality quickly and return the gel to the electrophoresis chamber for further separation if initial resolution is not sufficient.

In the four-color fluorescent DNA sequencing system (Model 377, Perkin Elmer, Applied Biosystems Division), the A reactions contain a primer labeled with one dye, while the T, C, and G reactions use the same primer sequence, but are each labeled with a different rhodamine or fluorescein dye. The dyes are chosen such that they are all excited by the argon ion laser used in the instrument, but emit at wavelengths that are approximately 20 nm apart (535, 555, 580, and 605 nm). The overlap in the fluorescence emission spectra of the dyes requires software that is capable of doing multicomponent analysis to separate the four different-colored signals. By using these special software algorithms the different colored bands are clearly resolved. The variation in electrophoretic mobility caused by the differing dye structures is controlled by insertion of a variable length spacer arm between the dye and the 5' end of the primer, decreasing relative mobility shifts to approximately one quarter of a base.[20]

After the sequencing reactions are complete, the A, T, C, and G tubes are pooled together and the DNA is ethanol processed. The DNA is then resuspended in loading buffer and then loaded onto an acrylamide gel. Because of the unique emission spectra of each of the four dyes, the A, T, C, and G samples can be coelectrophoresed in a single lane. Each fragment's fluorescence is excited by directing the argon laser through a small area in the glass plates near the bottom of the gel. Light emitted from the dye-labeled DNA fragments passing through this area is focused by a collection lens through a four-wavelength-selectable filter (540, 560, 580, 610 nm) into a photomultiplier tube (PMT) and digitized signals from the PMT are then transferred to the computer for interpretation. Software is also used to analyze emission wavelength, peak height, shape, and interval to provide automatic base calling. This approach allows up to 36 A, T, C, and G sets to be run simultaneously on the instrument, giving a fourfold increase in the throughput per gel. Currently 700 bases of sequence information can be obtained per lane with 98% accuracy, corresponding to 25,200 bases of sequence information per gel. An additional advantage of this multicolor approach to sequencing is the elimination of the lane-to-lane drift, which can cause difficulty in interpretation of data in single color and radioactive sequencing systems.

Further simplification of the fluorescent sequencing chemistry was achieved by placing the fluorescent label on the dideoxyterminator instead of on the primer.[21] Four modified fluorescein dyes were chosen to minimize shifts in relative mobility between the four bases, while still allowing differentiation of the four dyes from their emission spectra. This approach has several advantages. First, it eliminates the need to synthesize fluorescently labeled primers for each sequence one wishes to analyze. Use of dye terminators also allows the A, T, C, and G reactions to take place in a single tube, thus cutting the chemistry required reagents by a factor of 4. By placing the dye on the terminator, signals from false terminations do not interfere with reading the sequence.

15.2.3. Robotic Preparation of Sequencing Reactions

With the advent of automated, high-throughput fluorescent sequencers came the need to automate the sequencing chemistries run prior to gel electrophoresis. Accurate, repetitive pipetting of small volumes in multiple reaction tubes is tedious and provides numerous opportunities for operator error. Several companies have provided a solution to this problem. The Beckman Biomek® workstations (Models 1000 and 2000) can be adapted through the purchase of specific modules to perform DNA sequencing.[22,23] Applied Biosystems' Catalyst™ is a dedicated robotic workstation designed specifically for molecular biology and sequencing applications.[24] The Amersham VISTRA DNA Labstation also has the ability to perform all the pipetting and heating steps required for a variety of sequencing applications and is user-programmable. The Beckman and Applied Biosystems units process 96 reactions at once in a microtitre well format starting from purified DNA, while the Amersham unit can handle up to 72 samples a day. The Beckman unit has interchangeable pipetting heads and uses disposable tips, with a minimum pipetting volume of 2.0 μL. The Applied Biosystems unit has a single, fixed pipetting probe designed to achieve the greater pipetting accuracy required for the submicroliter volumes used in microsequencing applications. All three units provide for hands-off running of standard sequencing chemistries.

Researchers at the Institute of Physical and Chemical Research in Japan have automated the sequencing process on a production scale for the Human Genome Project.[25] This project was initiated by Akiyoshi Wada at the University of Tokyo in 1981 and funded by the Japanese Science and Technology Agency and several private companies. The Human Genome Analyzer (HUGA) consists of a production line of machines that carry out the different steps of DNA analysis from DNA isolation to input of the final sequence data into a computer database. Computer-controlled robots transfer microtitreplates and gel casting cassettes between various stations on the analyzer, which can run unattended and generate up to 108,000 bp (basepairs) of sequence per day. This production-style sequencing is probably not suitable for the average lab's needs, but will provide a mechanism for large-scale sequencing such as the current Human Genome Project.

15.2.4. Sequencing by Hybridization

Since its first description[26] the concept of sequencing by hybridization has captured the imagination of many scientists. This method differs from both Sanger[13] and Maxam–Gilbert[12] sequencing in several ways. It does not require the creation of DNA fragments and subsequent electrophoretic separation of those fragments. Instead it depends on differentiation of the binding of perfectly matched probes from probes containing one or more base mismatches. In the early design of this method by scientists in Yugoslavia, cloned DNA fragments to be sequenced were immobilized on filters and then probed with a large number of probes. Using 8-mer probes, this method requires probing with 65,536 probes to cover all possible 8-mer sequences. This is clearly a daunting task, so early feasibility work was done with a smaller number of probes covering only short target sequences.[27,28] In these studies 2.9% of the probes gave similar signals when there was either a perfect match or only one base mismatch. The remaining probes showed significantly higher signal with perfect matches compared to mismatches, as is required for this method to work. Differentiating perfect matches from single-base mismatches is a fundamental problem with any system based on probe hybridization. In order to better understand and solve the differentiation of perfectly matched probes from those containing mismatches, a group in Oxford began systematic investigations into the factors affecting perfect match/mismatch hybridization.[29–31] In the process of these studies they also changed the format of the assay system, developing chemistry to synthesize immobilized probe arrays directly on a glass slide using standard DNA synthesis chemistry.[32–36] These probe arrays could then be interrogated with a variety of radioactively labeled DNAs, the hybridization pattern seen with phosphor imaging,[14] and used to determine sequence. An improvement on the solid phase synthesis of probe arrays was made when scientists from Affymax (Palo Alto, CA) applied technology developed originally for synthesis of peptide arrays to synthesis of oligonucleotide arrays.[37,38] Their approach makes use of the photolithography techniques used in the manufacture of silicon chips for the electronics industry and applies them to the production of oligonucleotide arrays on silicon chips. Using light-sensitive blocking groups and photolithography masks, they are able to specifically activate any spot on the chip for base addition. Using this technique 256 tetramers were synthesized on a 1.28 × 1.28-cm array using 16 chemical reaction steps in only 4 h.[38] Epifluorescence microscopy was then used to assess hybridization of fluorescently labeled DNA target to the various probe positions. Using these glass or silicon supports, oligonucleotide arrays have been designed for sequence analysis and mutation screening in the β-globin,[39] cystic fibrosis transmembrane regulator,[40] Fragile X,[41] and p53[42] genes. Recently the use of an ultrasensitive charge-coupled device (CCD) has also been reported for analysis of hybridization of radioactively or fluorescently labeled DNA to oligonucleotide arrays.[43] The technique of sequencing by hybridization offers the possibility to create a "universal" sequencing chip that could in theory be reused many times to determine the sequence of many DNA fragments. The first practical application of this technology will probably be arrays dedicated to resequencing known genes, many of which are clinically important. However, the required instrumentation and software for detection of hybridization events and reconstruction of sequence from complex hybridization patterns still requires much further development before it is ready for routine clinical laboratory use.

15.3. SOUTHERN BLOTTING

Restriction fragment-length polymorphism (RFLP) analysis by Southern blotting was one of the earliest techniques developed for analysis of sequence variation.[44] Two of the most common uses for Southern blotting in the clinical laboratory today are for assessing B- and T-cell rearrangements in malignant leukemia and lymphoma[45] and in the molecular diagnosis of Fragile X mental retardation.[46] In this technique highly purified DNA is digested with a restriction enzyme to form small pieces that are then subjected to agarose gel electrophoresis. Sequence changes within the recognition site for the restriction enzyme cause the appearance or disappearance of an enzyme cutting site and thus a change in fragment size. These changes in fragment size, or RFLPs, are detected by blotting the separated fragments onto a membrane and then hybridizing the membrane with ^{32}P-labeled probes to "light up" specific parts of the DNA. The areas where the probes have hybridized are then detected by placing the membrane against a piece of x-ray film and performing autoradiography.

There have been various approaches to automating different segments of this intensely manual and time consuming process.[47] Analysis of the autoradiogram can be done with computing densitometers used to measure the intensity of the bands from the exposed x-ray film and are available from several manufacturers (Personal Densitometer™, Molecular Dynamics, Sunnyvale, CA; Bio Image™ Gel Scanner, Millipore, Bedford, MA; Optical Imaging System, Ambis, San Diego, CA). Traditional autoradiography can also be replaced by direct reading of the radioactive blot (Betascope™, Intelligenetics/Betagen; Matrix™, Packard Instruments, Meriden, CT; Ambis 1000/4000). If a radioactively labeled molecular weight standard has been included in a lane of the gel, the computer can also construct a standard curve, and then determine the size of any unknown bands. Higher throughput can be obtained by using phosphor imagers (Phosphor-Imager, Molecular Dynamics; Molecular Imager™, Bio-Rad, Hercules, CA). With these instruments, each blot is placed in a cassette that contains a medium to capture the energy released by beta particles releasing photons. These photons are counted and their locations determined. These media have a greater dynamic range and require much shorter exposure times than does conventional x-ray film. Since the instrument is used only for reading the medium, multiple blots can expose multiple phosphor plates simultaneously in a manner analogous to the autoradiographic part of the Southern blotting process. These systems are still a relatively expensive replacement for x-ray film. Recently chemiluminescence has been used to replace radioactivity as a detection system.[48] Probes are labeled with biotin during synthesis. After hybridization, the probes are exposed to alkaline phosphatase conjugated to avidin. A chemiluminescent substrate for alkaline phosphatase, disodium 3-(4-methoxyspiro[1,2-dioxetane-3-2'-tricyclodecan]-4-yl) phenyl phosphate (AMPPD), is then added and the light produced on dephosphorylation of the AMPPD is captured by exposure of the blot to Polaroid or x-ray film.

One of the most commonly used Southern blotting systems found in clinical laboratories today is the Oncor (Gaithersburg, MD) Probe Tech™ instrument line, which facilitates the electrophoresis and blotting portion of the process. These instruments have a gel chamber and controls to select which reagents pass through that chamber. The chamber looks like a normal agarose gel electrophoresis chamber, except that the support beneath the gel is made of a porous plastic, allowing vacuum to be placed under the gel. Using this system, gels are poured in the usual way, and samples are loaded and electrophoresed. Following electrophoresis a piece of membrane is placed underneath the gel, and, using vacuum transfer, the DNA fragments are completely transferred from the gel onto the membrane within 90 min. The Probe Tech minimizes the handling of the gel, and takes about 6 h off the time required to complete the blotting process. This system offers convenience for the first part of the Southern blotting process; however, the final step of hybridization to a labeled probe must still be done in the traditional manual manner. Another approach to automation of this step in the Southern blotting process is via the direct transfer provided by the Autotrans 7000 (Intelligenetics/Betagen) and the TE 2000 Two Step™ (Hoefer) systems described in Section 15.2.1. The samples electrophorese down a vertical gel, and as the DNA elutes off the bottom of the gel, it is deposited onto a constantly moving membrane web. This approach is potentially simpler than the Oncor approach, and eliminates the need to handle the gel at all, but requires very precise tolerances on the moving parts. These are two different approaches to automation of the same part of the Southern blotting process.

15.4. NUCLEIC ACID AMPLIFICATION METHODS

15.4.1. Polymerase Chain Reaction

Over the past few years several methods have been described to amplify a specific target nucleic acid sequence.[49] The polymerase chain reaction (PCR) was the first of the target amplification procedures.[50] Two primers, one for each strand, are used to direct selective chain replication by DNA polymerase. As each chain is replicated, it creates a copy of the original template. Thermal denaturation of these copies from the original template results in four strands, which can be replicated in the next cycle. By employing successive cycles of high-temperature thermal denaturation and lower-temperature primer annealing and chain extension, exponential amplification of the target sequence bracketed by the two primers is achieved. A thermal stable DNA polymerase permits this amplification procedure to be carried out in a programmable thermal cycler without the need to add more polymerase after each denaturation cycle.[51]

Over the past 10 years this amplification method has been extensively developed. Diagnostic applications abound. The extreme sensitivity of this method (single copies of a target sequence can be detected) has led to its application in the detection of numerous infectious organisms, such as HTLV-1,[52] which have been difficult to culture. Applications in genetics include detection of point mutations with either competitive oligo priming (COP)[53] or amplification refractory mutation systems (ARMS)[54] where mismatches between the primer and the mutant template result in loss of PCR product. Deletions and insertions are handled by bracketing the suspect area with PCR primers and observing the size of the PCR product formed. Translocation mutations, common in cancer, can be detected by choosing primers from the two different chromosomes involved in the translocation and observing whether any PCR product is formed.

Automation of PCR began with automation of the thermal cycling required for the alternation between high-temperature denaturation of the double-stranded template and lower-temperature primer annealing and extension. The first commercial thermal cycler, developed by Perkin-Elmer Corporation (Norwalk, CT), was a programmable heating block. Improvements on this method over the past few years include special thin-walled amplification tubes to facilitate thermal exchange between the block and the reagents, introduction of a heated lid that eliminates the need to cover the reaction with oil in order to prevent evaporation during thermal cycling, and a new heating block designed to handle the microscope slides used for *in situ* PCR applications. The capacity of these block-style cyclers is generally 20–50 tubes, one 96-well microtiterplate or 10 slides. Most brands are manufactured with a built-in cooling source, although some lower-priced brands require an external source. Other companies have taken slightly different approaches to automating thermal cycling. Stratagene (San Diego, CA) markets a robotic cycler that moves the tubes between blocks held at various temperatures in imitation of the original manual method. Others such as BIOS (New Haven, CT) and Enprotech (Natick, MA) use forced-air ovens to cycle. Although this cycling method is considerably slower than the heating block approach, since cooling is achieved passively, the capacity is greater and 4 micro-titerplates or 200 tubes can be cycled simultaneously. Extremely rapid thermal cycling can now be done in capillary thermal cyclers such as those from Idaho Technology (Idaho Falls, ID) or A.B. Technology (Pullman, WA). By cycling in small thin-walled glass capillaries, cycle times of less than a minute are possible, greatly reducing total PCR time.

After completion of the PCR reaction the products must be detected. In most early work, products from amplification reactions were evaluated by simple gel electrophoresis using gels stained with an intercalating dye such as ethidium bromide. Later they were quantitated by gel electrophoresis on a fluorescent DNA sequencer. Some sequencer manufacturers provide specialized software for fragment analysis (Genescan 672, Applied Biosystems; Fragment Analyzer™, Pharmacia). Very small quantities of DNA (100 attomoles) are required for analysis. Use of a multicolor DNA sequencer allows the inclusion of a dye-labeled molecular-weight standard as an internal reference in each lane, and automatic size calling of each band.[55,56] This is especially important in identity testing where variations in electrophoretic mobility between lanes, or between gels run on different days or in different labs, can raise doubts as to whether an individual should be included or excluded as a result of the analysis. The single-color Pharmacia system handles this same problem by allowing the computer to overlay bands from a molecular-weight marker lane with a data lane, providing size calling of the fragments in the data lane.

Quantitative fluorescent gel electrophoresis has been successfully applied to the analysis of multiplex PCR reactions for Duchenne muscular dystrophy (DMD).[57] The multicolor detection capability of the fluorescent DNA sequencer allows the nine DMD PCR reactions[58,59] labeled in blue to be run in the same lane with a tandem repeat marker (pYNZ22)[60] for sample identification labeled in green, and a molecular-weight marker labeled in red (GENESCAN-1000 ROX, Applied Biosystems). Analysis of DMD families using this approach has also shown that automated fluorescent gel electrophoresis can be used for gene dosage studies of carriers as well as affected individuals who have deletions or duplications of specific portions of the DMD gene. Recently, gene dosage studies for aneuploidy analysis by automated fluorescent gel electrophoresis have also been reported.[61] The combination of size determination, quantitation, and internal standardization makes automated fluorescent gel electrophoresis a powerful tool for analysis of amplification products.

Automated gel electrophoresis has also been used in the detection of point mutations using single-strand conformational polymorphism (SSCP) analysis of PCR products.[62] PCR product is denatured and allowed to assume a single-stranded conformation that depends highly on the specific nucleic acid sequence and this conformation confers a specific electrophoretic mobility under nondenaturing conditions. Single-base changes (mutations or polymorphisms) can cause visible shifts in this electrophoretic mobility. The Pharmacia PhastSystem™ allows the user to electrophorese the PCR products on a precast gel at different carefully controlled run temperatures. Typically two different temperatures, one cool ($< 10°C$) and one nearer ambient, are run to maximize the chance of detecting conformational polymorphisms. The gel is then silver-stained by the system (45 min at 30–50°C) and the bands visualized. Electrophoresis is rapid (< 1 h), and the sharp bands simplify SSCP interpretation. This technique has been applied successfully to point mutation detection in the *ras* and p53 oncogenes and phenylketonuria.[62–64]

Although the most common detection method for PCR products is gel electrophoresis, dot blot,[65,66] HPLC,[67-69] and microtiterplate detection[70] methods have also been developed. The Amplicor™ system marketed today by Roche Diagnostic Systems (Nutley, NJ) use a microtiterplate capture method to detect the PCR products. DNA is prepared from the clinical sample, and the PCR is run using a biotinylated primer. The PCR product is denatured and then removed from the amplification tube, added to microtiterplate wells coated with a capture probe, and allowed to be hybridized to the wells. Unbound PCR products are removed with a standard microtiterplate washer and a horseradish peroxidase–avidin conjugate added. The avidin binds to any biotinylated PCR product present and can then be detected with tetramethylbenzidine (TMB) by absorbance measurement at 450 nm on a microtiterplate reader. Assays based on this chemistry are available for *Chlamydia trachomatis, M. tuberculosis,* HCV, HTLV-1, HTLV-2, and HIV. The next-generation tests from Roche will run on a modified Cobas clinical analyzer, the Cobas Amplicor™. After off-line sample preparation is completed using a kit specially tailored for each analyte, the prepared samples are loaded into the thermal cycler rack. Twelve samples can be cycled simultaneously, and the two on-board cyclers give an overall amplification capacity of 24 samples. After amplification the instrument's pipette pierces the top of the PCR tube and transfers the PCR product to the detection station. There the PCR products are captured on magnetic beads coated with up to six different probes and hybridization is detected colorimetrically in a manner similar to the microtiterplate assay. This new format provides multiplex detection capability, which will be used in panel tests for chlamydia/gonorrhea, mycobacteria genus/species, and cystic fibrosis mutations.

Scientists at Kodak (Rochester, NY) have been busy developing another approach to PCR automation.[71] Their assay also requires off-line sample preparation. The prepared samples are then combined with the PCR reagent containing biotinylated primers and loaded into a unitized reagent pouch. The pouch is heat-sealed, and the rest of the assay, including detection, occurs within the pouch. The first chamber of the pouch is used for thermal cycling. Heater/cooler units clamp onto each side of the pouch, sandwiching the reagent bubble. Hot start PCR within the pouch is made possible through the use of a proprietary monoclonal antibody-bound Taq polymerase. During the first high-temperature denaturation step the antibody is denatured, releasing active polymerase. Rapid cycling (1 min/cycle) is possible due to extremely efficient thermal transfer. After cycling, the PCR product is squeegeed into the detection area, which contains seven spots of immobilized latex particles coated with capture probes. Two of the detection areas are dedicated to positive and negative controls, and the remaining five spots are used for analyte detection. As in the Roche system, the biotinylated PCR product bound to the capture probe is detected colorimetrically using horseradish peroxidase conjugated to streptavidin to oxidize a leuko dye. After completion of the assay, the pouch is simply thrown away, eliminating any of the issues surrounding contamination control for PCR.

PCR of the future may well be done in a similar self-contained manner, but miniaturized to fit onto a silicon chip. Wilding and coworkers[72] have already demonstrated feasibility of this concept by creating a PCR chip through photo-lithographic etching of small (15 × 17-mm) silicon chips. Small-volume PCR (5–10 µL) was carried out in these chips using a computer-controlled Peltier heater/cooler. In the future microminiaturization of both PCR and amplification product detection may result in cheap unitized PCR devices capable of multiplex analyte detection.

15.4.2. Ligase Chain Reaction

The ligase chain reaction (LCR) is probably the most well-developed amplification system after PCR.[73,74] It relies on a pair of probes that hybridize immediately adjacent to one another in a DNA target and are then joined together with a DNA ligase. When this process is carried out on both strands of the DNA target, and the reaction is thermal-cycled with a thermal stable ligase between a denaturation temperature and an anneal/ligate temperature, exponential amplification results. Millionfold amplification can be achieved in ~2 h. This method has been applied to the detection of numerous infectious organisms, including HIV-1, HPV, *C. trachomatis,*[75] *Neisseria gonorrhea,*[76] *M. tuberculosis*[77] and *Listeria monocytogenes.*[78] It has also been used to look for point mutations or small deletions such as those found in important genetic diseases such as sickle cell anemia[74,79] and cystic fibrosis.[80]

As with PCR, the first part of the LCR process that can be automated is the thermal cycling. LCR can be run in any of the thermal cyclers used for PCR. Detection of the ligation products can be done by simple gel electrophoretic separation of the ligated product from the starting probes.[73,74] Fluorescent electrophoresis has also been applied to the detection of LCR products in an assay for *M. tuberculosis*[77] and analysis of β-globin[79] and cystic fibrosis[80] mutations. Alternatively, if one of each probe pair is labeled at its 5' end and its partner labeled at its 3' end, a doubly labeled ligation product is produced. This product can then be captured and analyzed in a microtiter plate using standard ELISA reagents.[70,81] Abbott (North Chicago, IL) has developed their own approach to LCR automation. Sample preparation is done manually, and then the LCR reactions are run in specialized unit dose reagent tubes in a conventional thermal cycler. The tubes are designed with thin, pierceable lids for detection of LCR products on the Abbott LCx clinical analyzer. Using the approach described above for microtiterplate detection, a bifunctionally labeled LCR product is captured on antibody-coated microparticles in the LCx and detected with a second antibody conjugated to alkaline phosphatase and a fluorogenic substrate, 4-methylumbelliferyl phosphate. The doubly labeled LCR product is thus distinguished from the singly labeled LCR probes. Using the Abbott system, LCR products from 24 samples can be analyzed simultaneously in about 30 min. Abbott is developing LCR-based assays for HIV, HPV, *C. trachomatis,*[75] *N. gonorrhea,*[76] and *M. tuberculosis.*

15.4.3. Q-Beta Replicase Amplification

The Q-beta replicase amplification scheme is based on RNA replication.[82–86] Starting with an RNA target and a sequence-specific primer that also contains the T7 promoter sequence, reverse transcriptase is used to synthesize a DNA strand. This DNA strand, which now contains the T7 promoter sequence on the 5′ end, is then annealed to MDV-1 RNA (a natural template for Q-beta replicase) containing as part of its sequence an area that is also a target-specific probe. T7 RNA polymerase is then used to create an RNA template that contains both the T7 promoter and the MDV-1 sequence. This RNA template can then be rapidly replicated by Q-beta replicase, an RNA-directed tRNA polymerase from bacteriophage Q-beta. A billionfold amplification can be achieved in 30 min at 37°C.[87,88]

GENE-TRAK (Framingham, MA) has automated this process on their Galileo™ instrument. This instrument uses unitized test packs that contain all required reagents divided into reagent, reaction, waste, and read areas. Sample is prepared off-line and then added to the test pack with a syringe. All further steps of the assay are carried out in the test pack by the Galileo™, which directs the reagents through the test pack and also contains the detection optics. It can run up to 10 samples at a time, with the result for the first sample available in ~3 h. Because of the extremely high level of amplification possible with this method, it was necessary to develop a method to clean up the target prior to amplification with Q-beta replicase. A target-specific probe is used to capture the target molecules on magnetic beads. The beads are washed, and then the target is released from the beads by denaturation. The released target is then moved to a second area of the cartridge and captured with a second probe bound to magnetic beads. After a second washing, the target is again released from the magnetic beads and is annealed to the replicatable probe, and amplification is initiated. Finally products from the amplification reaction are mixed with an intercalating dye and detected in the read area of the test pack by measuring the increase in fluorescence as amplification product accumulates. Test packs for *M. tuberculosis* and other respiratory and sexually transmitted infectious diseases are planned for this system.

15.4.4. Nucleic Acid Sequence–Based Amplification

The nucleic acid sequence–based amplification system (NASBA) depends on RNA polymerase rather than DNA polymerase.[89,90] Starting with an RNA target and a DNA primer containing an RNA polymerase promoter sequence on the 5′ end and a target-specific sequence on the 3′ end, a cDNA is produced using reverse transcriptase. Instead of thermal denaturation, NASBA uses RNase H to digest the RNA strand of the DNA:RNA duplex and create single-stranded DNA. The single-stranded DNA is copied with reverse transcriptase and a second primer to yield DNA:DNA duplex. In the presence of T7 RNA polymerase, the

DNA:DNA duplex now serves as a template for generation of multiple copies of RNA transcript. Millionfold amplification in one hour is possible with an initial amplification rate of tenfold every 2.5 min. This technique has been applied to the detection of human papilloma virus[91] and HIV-1.[92–95]

As an isothermal process, a simple heating block serves to "automate" the amplification process. In the instrument system being developed at Organon Technika (Durham, NC), the NASBA® QR system, detection of products from NASBA amplification is done using electrochemiluminescence.[96–99] After amplification is completed, the RNA product is hybridized with a target-specific probe labeled with biotin and with a second target-specific probe labeled with tris(2,2'-bipyridine) ruthenium(II) (TBR). The biotinylated complex is captured with streptavidin-coated magnetic beads and placed into the autosampler. Once in the NASBA® QR system, the sample is aspirated into the detection cell and the bead-bound NASBA products are concentrated by the magnetic arm. Assay buffer containing tripropylamine (TPA) flows through the cell to wash the beads. When the flow stops and voltage is applied, the TPA and TBR^{2+} are both oxidized to produce TPA^+ and TBR^{3+}. The TPA then deprotonates to yield a TPA free radical, which, in turn, reacts with TBR^{3+} to produce an excited-state TBR^{2+*}. The TBR^{2+*} decays to ground state, emitting light at 620 nm that is detected with a photomultiplier. After light measurement is complete, cell cleaner flows through the detection cell into a waste container, and analysis of the next sample is begun. Analysis time in the NASBA® QR system is ~1 min per sample. This system has been applied to quantitation of HIV-1 RNA.

Today automated molecular genetic methods are a reality. Instrument/reagent systems are being commercialized specifically for the clinical laboratory. The resemblance to the more familiar clinical analyzers has made the technology more transparent to the user. Bar codes and automated data analysis will allow these analyzers to mate up with laboratory information systems and provide for direct downloading of patient results into the central laboratory computer. These "high tech" assays are rapidly becoming routine clinical techniques as automation makes them more user-friendly.

REFERENCES

1. Sambrook J, Fritsch EF, Maniatis T: *Molecular Cloning: A Laboratory Manual.* New York: Cold Spring Harbor Laboratory Press, 1989.
2. Mischiati C, Fiorentino D, Feriotto G, Gambari R: Use of an automated laboratory workstation for isolation of genomic DNA suitable for PCR and allele-specific hybridization. *BioTechniques* 15:146–151, 1993.
3. Kaneoka H, Lee DR, Hsu K-C, Sharp GC, Hoffman RW: Solid-phase direct DNA sequencing of allele-specific polymerase chain reaction-amplified HLA-DR genes. *BioTechniques* 10:30–34, 1991.
4. Santamaria P, Boyce-Jacino MT, Lindstrom AL, Barbosa JJ, Faras AJ, Rich SS: HLA class II

"typing": direct sequencing of DRB, DQB, and DQA genes. *Hum Immunol* 33:69–81, 1992.

5. Gibbs RA, Nguyen P-N, McBride LJ, Koepf SM, Caskey CT: Identification of mutations leading to the Lesch-Nyhan syndrome by automated direct DNA sequencing of *in vitro* amplified cDNA. *Proc Natl Acad Sci* (USA) 86:1919–1923, 1989.

6. Gibbs RA, Nguyen P-N, Edwards A, Civitello AB, Caskey CT: Multiplex DNA deletion detection and exon sequencing of the hypoxanthine phosphoribosyltransferase gene in Lesch-Nyhan families. *Genomics* 7:235–244, 1990.

7. Leren TP, Rodningen OK, Rosby O, Solberg K, Berg K: Screening for point mutations by semi-automated DNA sequencing using Sequenase and magnetic beads. *Bio-Techniques* 14:618–623, 1993.

8. Kovach JS, McGovern RM, Cassady JD, et al: Direct sequencing from touch preparations of human carcinomas: analysis of p53 mutations in breast carcinomas. *J Natl Cancer Inst* 83:1004–1009, 1991.

9. Olsvik O, Wahlberg J, Petterson B, et al: Use of automated sequencing of polymerase chain reaction-generated amplicons to identify three types of cholera toxin subunit B in *Vibrio cholerae* O1 strains. *J Clin Micro* 31:22–25, 1993.

10. Wike CM, Korber BTM, Daniels MR, et al: HIV-1 sequence variation between isolates from mother-infant transmission pairs. *AIDS Res Hum Retroviruses* 8:1297–1300, 1992.

11. Wolinsky SM, Wike CM, Korber BTM, et al: Selective transmission of human immunodeficiency virus type-1 variants from mothers to infants. *Science* 255:1134–1137, 1992.

12. Maxam AM, Gilbert W: A new method for sequencing DNA. *Proc Natl Acad Sci* (USA) 74:560–564, 1977.

13. Sanger F, Niklen S, Coulsen AR: DNA sequencing with chain terminating inhibitors. *Proc Natl Acad Sci* (USA) 74:5463–5467, 1977.

14. Johnston RF, Pickett SC, Barker DL: Autoradiography using storage phosphor technology. *Electrophoresis* 11:355–360, 1990.

15. Smith LM, Fung S, Hunkapiller MW, Hunkapiller TJ, Hood LE: The synthesis of oligonucleotides containing an aliphatic amino group at the 5' terminus: synthesis of fluorescent DNA primers for use in DNA sequence analysis. *Nucl Acids Res* 13:2399–2412, 1985.

16. Smith LM, Sanders, JZ, Kaiser RJ, et al: Fluorescence detection in automated DNA sequence analysis. *Nature* 321:674–679, 1986.

17. Ansorge W, Sproat B, Stegeman J, Schwager C, Zenke M: Automated DNA sequencing: ultrasensitive detection of fluorescent bands during electrophoresis. *Nucl Acids Res* 15:4593–4602, 1987.

18. Middendorf LR, Bruce JC, Bruce RC, et al: Continuous, on-line DNA sequencing using a versatile infrared laser scanner/electrophoresis system. *Electrophoresis* 13:487–494, 1992.

19. Ishino Y, Mineno J, Inoue T, et al: Practical applications in molecular biology of sensitive fluorescence detection by a laser-excited fluorescence image analyzer. *Bio-Techniques* 13:936–943, 1992.

20. Connell C, Fung S, Heiner C, et al: Automated DNA sequence analysis. *BioTechniques* 5:342–348, 1987.

21. Prober JM, Trainor GL, Dam RJ, et al: A system for rapid DNA sequencing with fluorescent chain-terminating dideoxynucleotides. *Science* 238:336–341, 1987.

22. Wilson RK, Yuen AS, Clark SM, Spence C, Arakelian P, Hood LE: Automation of dideoxynucleotide DNA sequencing reactions using a robotic workstation. *BioTechniques* 6:776–787, 1988.

23. Civitello AB, Richards S, Gibbs RA: A simple protocol for the automation of DNA cycle sequencing reactions and polymerase chain reactions. *DNA Sequence* 3:178–223, 1992.

24. Cathcart R: Advances in automating DNA sequencing. *Nature* 347:310, 1990.

25. Swinbanks D: Japan's human genome project takes shape. *Nature* 351:593, 1991.

26. Drmanac R, Labat I, Brukner I, Crkvenjakov R: Sequencing of megabase plus DNA by hybridization: theory of the method. *Genomics* 4:114–128, 1989.

27. Stezoska Z, Pauneska T, Radosavljevic D, Labat I, Drmanac R, Crkvenjakov R: DNA sequencing by hybridization: 100 bases read by a non-gel based method. *Proc Natl Acad Sci* (USA) 88:10089–10093, 1991.

28. Drmanac R, Drmanac S, Stezoska Z, et al: DNA sequence determination by hybridization: a strategy for efficient large scale sequencing. *Science* 260:1649–1652, 1993.

29. Maskos U, Southern E: Parallel analysis of oligodeoxyribonucleotide (oligonucleotide) interactions. I. Analysis of factors influencing oligonucleotide duplex formation. *Nucl Acids Res* 20:1675–1678, 1992.

30. Southern E, Maskos U, Elder JK: Analyzing and comparing nucleic acid sequences by hybridization to arrays of oligonucleotides: evaluation using experimental models. *Genomics* 13:1008–1017, 1992.

31. Maskos U, Southern E: A novel method for the analysis of multiple sequence variants by hybridization to oligonucleotides. *Nucl Acids Res* 21:2267–2268, 1993.

32. Maskos U, Southern E: Oligonucleotide hybridizations on glass supports: a novel linker for oligonucleotide synthesis and hybridization properties of oligonucleotides synthesized *in situ*. *Nucl Acids Res* 20:1679–1684, 1992.

33. Maskos U, Southern E: A study of oligonucleotide reassociation using large arrays of oligonucleotides synthesized on a glass support. *Nucl Acids Res* 21:4663–4669, 1993.

34. Beaucage SL, Caruthers MH: Deoxynucleoside phosphoramidites—a new class of key intermediates for deoxypolynucleotide synthesis. *Tetrahedron Lett* 22:1859–1862, 1981.

35. Matteucci MD, Caruthers MH: Synthesis of deoxyoligonucleotides on a polymer support. *J Am Chem Soc* 103:3185–3191, 1981.

36. Vu H, McCollum C, Jacobson K, et al: Fast oligonucleotide deprotection phosphoramidite chemistry for DNA synthesis. *Tetrahedron Lett* 31:7269–7272, 1990.

37. Fodor SPA, Read JL, Pirrung MC, Stryer L, Lu AT, Solas D: Light-directed, spatially addressable parallel chemical synthesis. *Science* 251:767–773, 1991.

38. Pease AC, Solas D, Sullivan EJ, Cronin MT, Holmes CP, Fodor SPA: Light generated oligonucleotide arrays for rapid DNA sequence analysis. *Proc Natl Acad Sci* (USA) 91:5022–5026, 1994.

39. Maskos U, Southern E: A novel method for the parallel analysis of multiple mutations in multiple samples. *Nucl Acids Res* 21:2269–2270, 1993.

40. Cronin MY, Barniv Z, Morris MS, et al: Detection of cystic fibrosis gene mutations by hybridization to GeneChip™ probe arrays. *Clin Chem* 40:656, 1994.

41. Wehnert MS, Matson RS, Rampal JB, Coassin PJ, Caskey CT: A rapid scanning strip for tri- and dinucleotide short tandem repeats. *Nucl Acids Res* 22:1701, 1994.

42. Sheldon EL, Shah NA, Barone D, et al: Probe chips for the analysis of gene sequences. *Clin Chem* 40:662, 1994.

43. Eggers M, Hogan M, Reich RK, et al: A microchip for quantitative detection of molecules utilizing luminescent and radioisotope reporter groups. *BioTechniques* 17:516–524, 1994.

44. Southern EM: Detection of specific sequences among DNA fragments by gel electrophoresis. *J Mol Biol* 98:503–517, 1975.

45. Cossman J, Uppenkamp M, Sundeen J, Coupland R, Raffeld M: Molecular genetics and the diagnosis of lymphoma. *Arch Pathol Lab Med* 112:117–127, 1988.

46. Caskey CT, Pizzuti A, Fu Y-H, Fenwick RG, Nelson DL: Triplet repeat mutations in human disease. *Science* 256:784–789, 1992.

47. Winn-Deen ES: Automation of electrophoretic techniques for DNA analysis— evolution of the Southern blot. *Lab Robot Auto* 4:337–342, 1992.

48. Bronstein I, Voyta JC, Lazzari K, Murphy O, Edwards B, Kricka LJ: Rapid and Sensitive detection of DNA in Southern blots with chemiluminescence. *BioTechniques* 8:310–314, 1990.

49. Persing D: *In vitro* nucleic amplification techniques. In: Persing DH, Smith TF, Tenover FC, White TJ, eds: *Diagnostic Molecular Microbiology: Principles and Applications.* Washington, DC: American Society for Microbiology, 1993, pp. 51–121.

50. Saiki RK, Scharf S, Faloona F, Mullis KB, Horn GT, Erlich HA, Arnheim N: Enzymatic amplification of β-globin genomic sequences and restriction site analysis for diagnosis of sickle cell anemia. *Science* 230:1350–1354, 1985.

51. Lawyer FC, Stoffel S, Saiki RK, Myambo KB, Drummond R, Gelfand DH: Isolation, characterization, and expression in *Escherichia coli* of the DNA polymerase gene from *Thermus aquaticus. J Biol Chem* 264:6427–6437, 1989.

52. Kwok S, Ehrlich G, Poiiesz B, Kalish R, Sninsky JJ: Enzymatic amplification of HTLV-I viral sequences from periferal blood mononuclear cells and infected tissues. *Blood* 72:1117–1123, 1988.

53. Gibbs RA, Nguyen P-N, Caskey CT: Detection of single base differences by competitive oligonucleotide priming. *Nucl Acids Res* 17:2437–2448, 1989.

54. Newton CR, Graham A, Hepinstall LE, et al: Analysis of any point mutation in DNA. The amplification refractory mutation system (ARMS). *Nucl Acids Res* 17:2503–2516, 1989.

55. Mayrand PE, Hoff LB, McBride LJ, et al: Automation of specific gene detection. *Clin Chem* 36:2063–2071, 1990.

56. Mayrand PE, Corcoran KP, Zeigle JS, Robertson JM, Hoff LB, Kronick ME: The use of fluorescence detection and internal lane standards to size PCR products automatically. *Appl Theor Electroph* 3:1–11, 1992.

57. Kronick M, Ziegle J, Robertson J, Fenwick R: Simultaneous detection of PCR products informative of human disease and human identity: a novel method for internal sample identification. *Am J Hum Genet* 47:A225, 1990.

58. Chamberlain JS, Gibbs RA, Rainer JE, Nguyen PN, Caskey CT: Deletion screening of the Duchenne muscular dystrophy locus via multiplex DNA amplification. *Nucl Acids Res* 16:11141–11156, 1988.

59. Chamberlain JS, Gibbs RA, Rainer JE, Caskey CT: Multiplex PCR for the diagnosis of

Duchenne muscular dystrophy. In Innis MA, Gelfand DH, Sninsky JJ, White TJ, eds: *PCR Protocols: A Guide to Methods and Applications.* San Diego, CA, Academic Press, 1990, pp. 272–281.

60. Nakamura Y, Ballard L, Leppert M, et al: Isolation and mapping of a polymorphic DNA sequence (pYNZ22) on chromosome 17p. *Nucl Acids Res* 16:5707, 1988.

61. Mansfield ES: Diagnosis of Down syndrome and other aneuploidies using quantitative polymerase chain reaction and small tandem repeat polymorphisms. *Hum Mol Genet* 2:43–50, 1993.

62. Orita M, Suzuki Y, Sekiya T, Hayashi K: Rapid and sensitive detection of point mutations and DNA polymorphisms using the polymerase chain reaction. *Genomics* 5:874–879, 1989.

63. Dockhorn-Dworniczak B, Dworniczak B, Brommelkamp L, Bulles J, Horst J, Bocker WW: Non-isotopic detection of single strand conformation polymorphism (PCR-SSCP): A rapid and sensitive technique in diagnosis of phenylketonuria. *Nucl Acids Res* 19:2500, 1991.

64. Mohabeer AJ, Hiti AL, Martin WJ: Non-radioactive single strand conformation polymorphism (SSCP) using the Pharmacia PhastSystem. *Nucl Acids Res* 19:3154, 1991.

65. Bugawan D, Saiki RK, Levenson CH, Watson RM, Erlich HA: The use of nonradioactive oligonucleotide probes to analyze enzymatically amplified DNA for prenatal diagnosis and forensic HLA typing. *Bio/Technology* 6:943–947, 1988.

66. Saiki RK, Walsh DS, Erlich HA: Genetic analysis of amplified DNA with immobilized sequence-specific oligonucleotide probes. *Proc Natl Acad Sci* (USA) 86:6230–6234, 1989.

67. Katz ED: Quantitation and purification of polymerase chain reaction products by liquid chromatography. *J Chrom* 512:433–444, 1990.

68. Katz ED, Dong MW: Rapid analysis and purification of products of polymerase chain reaction by high-performance liquid chromatography. *BioTechniques* 8:546–555, 1990.

69. Katz ED, Haff LA, Eksteen R: Rapid separation, quantitation and purification of products of polymerase chain reaction by high-performance liquid chromatography. In White BA, ed: *Methods in Molecular Biology,* Vol. 15: *PCR Protocols: Current Methods and Applications.* Totowa, NJ: Humana Press, 1993, pp. 63–74.

70. Nickerson DA, Kaiser R, Lappin S, Stewart J, Hood L, Landegren U: Automated DNA diagnosis using an ELISA-based oligonucleotide ligation assay. *Proc Natl Acad Sci* (USA) 87:8923–8929, 1990.

71. Findlay JB, Atwood SM, Bergmeyer L, et al: Automated closed vessel system for *in vitro* diagnostics based on polymerase chain reaction. *Clin Chem* 39:1927–1933, 1993.

72. Wilding P, Shoffner MA, Kricka LJ: PCR in silicon microstructure. *Clin Chem* 40:1815–1818, 1994.

73. Wu DY, Wallace RB: The ligation amplification reaction (LAR)—amplification of specific DNA sequences using sequential rounds of template-dependent ligation. *Genomics* 4:560–569, 1989.

74. Barany B: Genetic disease detection and DNA amplification using cloned thermostable ligase. *Proc Natl Acad Sci* (USA) 88:189–193, 1991.

75. Dille BJ, Butzen CC, Birkenmeyer LG: Amplification of *Chlamydia trachomatis* DNA by ligase chain reaction. *J Clin Micro* 31:729–731, 1993.

76. Birkenmeyer L, Armstrong AS: Preliminary evaluation of the ligase chain reaction for specific detection of *Neisseria gonorrhoeae, J Clin Micro* 30:3089–3094, 1992.

77. Iovannisci DM, Winn-Deen ES: Ligation amplification and fluorescence detection of *Mycobacterium tuberculosis* DNA. *Mol Cell Probes* 7:35–43, 1993.

78. Wiedmann M, Czajka J, Barany F, Batt CA: Discrimination of *Listeria monocytogenes* from other *Listeria* species by ligase chain reaction. *Appl Environ Micro* 58:3443–3447, 1992.

79. Winn-Deen ES, Iovannisci DM: Sensitive fluorescence method for detection DNA ligation amplification products. *Clin Chem* 37:1522–1523, 1991.

80. Winn-Deen ES, Iovannisci DM, Brinson E, Eggerding F: Application of DNA probe ligation to genetic disease analysis. *Clin Chem* 39:727–728, 1993.

81. Winn-Deen ES, Batt CA, Wiedmann M: Non-radioactive detection of *Mycobacterium tuberculosis* LCR products in a microtiter plate format. *Mol Cell Probes* 7:179–186, 1993.

82. Levison R, Spiegelman S: The cloning of a self-replicating molecule. *Proc Natl Acad Sci* (USA) 69:3038–3042, 1968.

83. Meile EA, Mills DR, Kramer FR: Autocatalytic replication of a recombinant RNA. *J Mol Biol* 171:281–295, 1983.

84. Chu BC, Kramer FR, Orgel LE: Synthesis of an amplifiable reporter for bioassays. *Nucl Acids Res* 14:5591–5603, 1986.

85. Lizardi PM, Guerra CE, Lomeli H, Tussie-Luna I, Kramer FR: Exponential amplification of recombinant-RNA hybridization probes. *Biotechnology* 6:1197–1202, 1988.

86. Lomeli H, Tyagi S, Prichard CG, Lizardi PM, Kramer FR: Quantitative assays based on the use of replicatable hybridization probes. *Clin Chem* 35:1826–1831, 1989.

87. Prichard CG, Stefano JE: Detection of viral nucleic acids by Qβ replicase amplification. *Med Virol* 10:67–80, 1991.

88. Cahil P, Foster K, Mahan DE: Polymerase chain reaction and Qβ replicase amplification. *Clin Chem* 37:1482–1485, 1991.

89. Guatelli JC, Whitfield KM, Kwoh DY, et al: Isothermal, *in vitro* amplification of nucleic acids by a multienzyme reaction modeled after retroviral replication. *Proc Natl Acad Sci* (USA) 87:1874–1878, 1990.

90. Compton J: Nucleic acid sequence-based amplification. *Nature* 350:91–92, 1991.

91. Haycock PV, Radany EW: Detection of HPV sequences in cultured cells by *in situ* amplification and hybridization with enzyme-linked oligonucleotides. *FASEB J* 5:1661a, 1991.

92. Bush CE, Donovan RM, Peterson WR, et al: Detection of human immunodeficiency virus type 1 RNA in plasma from high-risk pediatric patients by using the self-sustained sequence replication reaction. *J Clin Micro* 30:281–286, 1992.

93. van Geman B, Kieevits T, Schukkink R, et al: Quantification of HIV-1 RNA in plasma using NASBA™ during HIV-1 primary infection. *J Virol Meth* 43:177–188, 1993.

94. van Geman B, Kieevits T, Nara P, et al: Qualitative and quantitative detection of HIV-1 RNA by nucleic acid sequence-based amplification. *AIDS* 7 (Suppl. 2):S107–S110, 1993.

95. Bruisten S, van Geman B, Koppelman M, et al: Detection of HIV-1 distribution in different blood fractions by two nucleic acid amplification assays. *AIDS Res Hum Retroviruses* 9:259–265, 1993.

96. Kenten JH, Casadei J, Link J, et al: Rapid electrochemiluminescence assays of polymerase chain reaction products. *Clin Chem* 37:1626–1632, 1991.

97. Kenten JH, Gudibande S, Link J, et al: Improved electrochemiluminescent label for DNA probe assays: rapid quantitative assays of HIV-1 polymerase chain reaction products. *Clin Chem* 38:873–879, 1992.

98. Anderson MS, Di Cesare JL, Katz ED: An electrochemiluminescence-based detection system for quantitative PCR. *Am Biotech Lab* vol. 11 no. 8:10, July 1993.

99. DiCesare J, Grossman B, Katz E, Picozza E, Ragussa R, Woudenberg T: A highly sensitive electrochemiluminescence-based detection system for automated PCR product quantitation. *BioTechniques* 15:152–157, 1993.

CHAPTER

16

Immunoassay Automation: From Concept to System Performance

DANIEL W. CHAN

CONTENTS

Handbook of Clinical Automation, Robotics, and Optimization, Edited by Gerald J. Kost with the collaboration of Judith Welsh.
ISBN 0-471-03179-8 © 1996 John Wiley & Sons, Inc.

419

16.1. INTRODUCTION

16.1.1. Meeting the Challenges of Today's Clinical Laboratory

The clinical laboratory is faced with increasing challenges (Table 16.1). These include the chronic shortage of qualified technologists, limited laboratory space and shrinking resources, and external challenges such as healthcare reform, managed care competition, cost compression, and increased regulation of the testing laboratory. The Clinical Laboratory Improvement Amendment of 1988 (CLIA '88) is currently being implemented. This legislation has placed additional burden on the laboratory in quality assurance, proficiency testing, and reaffirmation of skill. Despite these challenges, the users have higher expectations for laboratory services.

In order to meet these challenges, the clinical laboratory has to become more efficient by incorporating creative solutions and adapting to changes. One such solution is to increase automation of laboratory procedures and integrate these automated systems. Since most clinical laboratory procedures are labor-intensive, automation will reduce the dependence of the labor requirement. Furthermore, smaller clinical laboratories could perform a larger menu of tests "in house" rather than sending them to outside laboratories. This not only reduces expenses but also increases revenue and improves turnaround time of testing. With the availability of automated devices designed for point-of-care testing, laboratory tests may be relocated to "near patient."

16.1.2. History of Immunoassay Automation

During the last 20 years, major advances have been achieved in automating routine clinical chemistry procedures. Discrete and random-access analyzers provided a wide spectrum of chemistry tests around the clock to meet the clinical demands of rapid testing. Recently, more attention has been focused on automating the sample handling and processing steps, especially with the concern of infectious specimens from patients with hepatitis and AIDS.

Automating specialized procedures, such as immunoassay, have lagged behind, especially for heterogeneous immunoassay (i.e., an assay requiring a physical separation of the bound from unbound antigens). The homogeneous

TABLE 16.1. Challenges of Today's Clinical Laboratory

Shortage of technologists
Limited laboratory space
Limited available resources
Healthcare reform
Cost compression
Increased laboratory regulations

immunoassay (i.e., an assay requiring no physical separation of bound and unbound antigens) can be adapted to general chemistry analyzers; however, the heterogeneous immunoassay requires a dedicated analyzer.

The first attempt was to automate radioimmunoassay (RIA). Several systems were introduced in the late 1970s. These systems included the Centria (Union Carbide), Concept 4 (Micromedic), ARIA II (BD), and Gammaflow (Squibb). These systems, with limited throughput and testing menu, were not as reliable and cost-effective as the users expected. Automation of immunoassay would not be successful until nonisotopic systems became available.

This chapter is based on another recent publication entitled *Immunoassay Automation: A Practical Guide.*[1] The focus is on the concept, principles, issues, and performance of automated immunoassay systems. The detailed description of specific automated systems are cited in the references. For the latest model of a particular system, literature should be requested from the manufacturer of the system. In the ever-changing world of the automated immunoassay system, this approach will have longer lasting value.

16.2. AUTOMATION OF IMMUNOASSAY

16.2.1. The Changing Concept of Automation

The total laboratory testing process starts with the ordering of laboratory tests. A complete test menu should be provided together with instructions for blood collection device and with bar-code label for positive identification. The sample should be centrifuged in a closed system and transferred onto the automated system for direct sampling. The actual testing procedure may include a separation step of the bound from unbound antigen if it is a heterogenous immunoassay. No physical separation step is needed if it is a homogenous immunoassay. The detection system could be multiapproach, such as spectrophotometry and fluorimetry. Finally, electronic data processing and quality control should facilitate result verification and reporting. A computer terminal located at the user's site will shorten the turnaround time of testing.

The traditional idea of automation is to adapt the reagent on the automated instrument for the central clinical laboratory. Such instrumentation mechanized all the necessary steps in an immunoassay procedure, including pipetting, incubation, washing, and detecting the signal. The automated system performs a large variety of test mixes at the same time with fairly high throughput. The ability to access the sample and test selection continuously is a key feature of this type of automation.

A different approach is a smaller batch or selective instrument. These systems tend to have lower throughput. They are designed for smaller laboratories or decentralized locations. For larger laboratories, multiple systems are required. Examples are the IMX by Abbott Labs, the Stratus by Baxter Diagnostics.

In a broader sense, the concept of automation could include disposable devices designed for quick, mostly qualitative tests, such as ICON (Hybritech, Inc.) and test packs (Abbott Labs) for pregnancy testing. These devices use membrane technology with monoclonal antibodies immobilized on them. A qualitative result will be obtained in a few minutes by the presence of color development. Quantitative results could be obtained by reading on a photometer. These devices are self-contained "automation in a box" without instrumentation. Most of these devices are intended for use in the point-of-care setting.

In reality, all three types of automation may be applicable in a clinical laboratory, whether large or small. A large clinical laboratory may perform all tests on the day shift. During the evening shift, its testing may resemble a medium-size clinical laboratory. While on the night shift, it is more like a small clinical laboratory. The need to perform tests off site from the central laboratory is increasing, such as in the emergency room, outpatient clinic, and remote medical-care locations as well as the patient's home. Automated systems could be located at those sites and connect with the central laboratory by computer link for monitoring quality control, result reporting, and test interpretation.

16.2.2. The Components of Automation

An automated system consists of three major components: instrument, reagent, and computer. A system will not be successful unless all three components are functioning well as a unit. These three components are interdependent. The format of the reagent will determine the design of the instrument. The limits of the instrument design may require modification of the reagent and the immunoassay procedure. The computer program could optimize the reaction condition, the sequence of reagent addition, and the order of sample testing. It will expedite data processing and management as well as result reporting. Therefore, we should consider the issues of automation as an integrated system.

16.2.3. The Issues of Automation

Immunoassay is an analytical procedure involving antigen–antibody binding reaction. After the binding takes place, separation of bound antigen–antibody complex from unbound antigen is needed before the unknown antigen can be quantified. The following are some key issues to be considered.

16.2.3.1. COMPETITIVE OR IMMUNOMETRIC ASSAY. Traditional RIA is based on the principle of competitive protein binding. The radioactive-labeled antigen competes with the unlabeled antigen for a *limited* amount of binding sites on the antibody. "Sensitivity" as defined by the minimum detectable amount is affected by the affinity constant of the antibody, the nonspecific binding, the specific activity of the labeled antigen, and the experimental error in the measurement of bound and unbound antigen. In the development of an immunoassay, the competitive approach conserves the use of antibody in the assay since the antibody concentration is limited.

Immunometric assay could be optimized for better sensitivity than the competitive immunoassay. The maximal sensitivity can be achieved with a large concentration of labeled antibody with high specific activity, low amount of nonspecific binding by the labeled antibody, high-affinity constant of the labeled antibody, and small experimental errors in measuring the bound labeled antibody.

The decision on whether to choose a competitive or immunometric assay will depend on the size of the analyte. The choice for small analytes is the competitive immunoassay; for large analytes, the immunometric assay. Immunometric assay provides both sensitivity and specificity needed for peptide hormones, for example, parathyroid hormone (PTH) and adrenocorticotropic hormone (ACTH). The specificity of measuring the intact molecule of PTH could exclude the PTH C-terminal fragments that accumulate in renal disease.

16.2.3.2. SAMPLE MANAGEMENT. The sample management system is becoming increasingly important as the concern of infectious specimens rises. A random-access device is preferred since test requests vary with each individual patient. Furthermore, random access will allow the laboratory to perform testing continuously and eliminate the batching and scheduling of tests.

A sample management system could include sample processing and introduction to the instrument. Positive identification, including bar-code labeling, should be applied at the blood collection step. The primary blood drawing tube could be centrifuged and transferred to the testing step. The concept of centrifugation along the axis of the tube will allow direct sampling through the top of the tube. Another approach is the use of an automating cap removal device. Either approach will allow the sample management system to be fully automated.

The sample introduction system should be designed to minimize carryover. Carryover is not a major problem for general chemistries since the physiological ranges of most analytes are rather limited. However, carryover could be a significant problem for hormones and tumor markers. It is not uncommon to have a 10^5-fold difference in the values of tumor markers. An ideal target for carryover is less than one part per million (< 1 ppm). To minimize carryover, the design of the sampler such as the shape, size, and materials is important. Adding a washing step in between each sampling may help reduce carryover.

16.2.3.3. SIGNAL DETECTION. The type of signal detection system is determined by the signal or the label of the reagent. The choice should be based on the technical performance and economic considerations. A system should be able to achieve the sensitivity of most clinically important analytes, with acceptable precision, and be easy to build, relatively inexpensive, common, and easy to troubleshoot. Three types of detection systems that fit these criteria have been used in most automated systems.

Spectrophotometry is probably the most popular detector. Enzyme immunoassay (EIA) could be homogenous or heterogenous. In the heterogenous assay, the two most frequently used enzymes are alkaline phosphatase and peroxidase.

Fluorimetry is widely used for both homogenous and heterogenous immunoassay. Some systems use enzymes to convert a substrate to a fluorescent product, while others use both spectrophotometry and fluorimetry in the same system. In theory, fluorimetry is capable of detecting as little as 10^{-14} mol of a compound, while spectrophotometry can detect only 10^{-8} mol. In practice, the sensitivity is significantly reduced because of the background noise from the endogenous fluorophore (e.g., bilirubin, protein, and lipids). Time resolved fluorescence technique such as the DELFIA system by Wallac may somewhat reduce this problem.

Luminometry is gaining popularity rather quickly. Luminescence immunoassay (LIA) has the potential of achieving the highest sensitivity. Most LIAs are heterogenous assay. Taking advantage of the inherent sensitivity, Nichols Diagnostics developed an ultrasensitive thyrotropin (TSH) assay that is capable of measuring TSH down to 0.005 mIU/L (milli–international unit per liter).

16.2.3.4. DATA MANAGEMENT. The data management system is the commanding center. Table 16.2 lists the desirable characteristics of a data management system.

In order to manage the automation effectively, the data management system should control as many steps in the total testing process as defined earlier. The system should be designed to be user-friendly and allow a technologist to perform the crucial daily functions efficiently.

Diagnostics of instrument malfunction are important for troubleshooting purposes. Troubleshooting can be performed by the operator or with remote diagnostics through modem or satellite connection to the manufacturer. Modern instruments should contain built-in sensors for the proper operation of the system. Examples are "detector of short sample" by the pipettor. Continuous monitoring and self-adjusting may be necessary for a truly "walkaway" automation.

A real-time, on-line quality-control (QC) system allows the technologist to make a quick decision on the acceptability of the laboratory result. In this

---

TABLE 16.2. Desirable Characteristics of a Data Management System

Ability to manage as many steps as in the total testing process
User-friendliness with easy access to the routine daily function
On-line quality control
Diagnoses of instrument malfunctions for troubleshooting purposes
Sample and patient identification—bar-code label
Data reduction and management
Lab management functions—workload recording, turnaround time, and quality assurance (QA) productivity
Bidirectional interface with host computer

verification step, an "exception" list of results could be generated for further investigation. Results not in the exception list will be allowed to pass through to the reporting step. The rules for the exception list should be user-defined.

Sample and patient identification should be done by a bar-code device with a unique identifying label generated as early as possible in the history of the sample. This label will provide positive identification throughout the entire testing process. It should contain all the testing information and provide a link to the patient identification. An automated system should be able to communicate with the host computer with a bidirectional interface. A buffer to store laboratory data will be important in the event that the host computer is down.

Other management functions will be useful for a laboratory to evaluate the testing data, workload recording, turnaround time, productivity, quality assurance, and the efficiency of the operation. However, these management functions are less critical and should not interfere with the daily operating routines.

16.2.3.5. LIMITATIONS OF AUTOMATION. One limitation of automation is the need for capital equipment acquisition. Most fully automated systems use dedicated reagents. The closed system "locks in" the laboratory to use all the reagents from the same manufacturer, even though they may not have the same quality. The choice of tests is also limited by that particular system. The commitment for an automated system is usually 3–5 years. The quality of reagent may change; however, the instrument will also be obsolete.

The throughput of most automated systems using heterogeneous format is 30–120 tests per hour. All instruments require maintenance and service. The total dependence of an automated system means that the entire immunoassay system may be shut down. The limited throughput as well as the reliability issue cause many laboratories to acquire more than one system. Finally, one should not overlook the human factor. Most instruments are advertised as "walkaway." However, as technologists walk away from the instrument, they are concerned about the outcome of the testing: What if the instrument malfunctions and none of the results are acceptable?

16.3. AUTOMATED IMMUNOASSAY SYSTEMS

16.3.1. Homogeneous Immunoassay Systems

Homogeneous immunoassay requires no physical separation of bound and unbound antigen. The major advantage is the ability to adapt reagent to the existing clinical chemistry analyzer. For example, the enzyme-multiplied immunoassay technique (EMIT) by Syva Company could be used on the BMC-Hitachi analyzer. The automated homogeneous immunoassay systems use small sample size and low reagent volume, and provide fast turnaround time. The calibration curve is stable for at least several days to weeks. This allows the laboratory to perform tests at any time without having to recalibrate the system. The efficiency is enhanced by saving technical time, quality control, and reagent expenses.

Most homogeneous immunoassay takes advantage of the size difference between unbound antigen (small) and antigen-bound antibody complex (large). The differences in the sizes may limit the changes in signal detection. This will, in turn, limit the dynamic ranges of the assay and, to a certain extent, the sensitivity as well. Since there is no separation of the patient sample from the final signal detection, the specificity may be compromised. Interference from patient's sample may cause high background signal or compete with the binding site. Some tests require sample pretreatment to eliminate interference. For example, digoxin assay requires an acid precipitation (TDx analyzer by Abbott Labs) before analysis. In general, small analytes such as drug, thyroid, and steroid hormone that are present in relatively high concentration could use the homogenous format. On the other hand, large molecules such as protein antigens would be difficult to measure by the homogeneous immunoassay because of poor sensitivity and unacceptable imprecision.

16.3.1.1. OPEN SYSTEM. An "open system" consists of a general-purpose instrument designed to perform chemistry tests. Immunoassay reagent could be adapted to the instrument if it shares the same sample delivery and the detection device, and requires no physical separation of unbound from bound antigen (homogeneous). For example, the BMC-Hitachi analyzers 747 and 911 are designed to perform routine chemistry tests such as glucose, cholesterol, and alkaline phosphatase. The EMIT reagent could be adapted to this instrument because it uses the same pipetting device and the spectrophotometric detection step.

Because immunoassay may require more than one reagent or reaction step than the simpler chemistry test, not every general chemistry instrument could be used for homogeneous immunoassay. For example, the "cloned enzyme-donor immunoassay" (CEDIA) reagent for vitamin B_{12} and folate uses reagent components that require four reagent addition steps. The Hitachi 704 analyzer is not designed to handle these many steps, whereas the Hitachi 911 analyzer is. The open systems do have the advantage of the user's choice of reagent and potential competitive edge of more than one reagent. With the introduction of CLIA '88 and the U.S. Food & Drug Administration (FDA) approval process, open systems will have to specify the reagent and the instrument combination in the FDA approval process. Examples of these systems are listed in Table 16.3.*

16.3.1.2. CLOSED SYSTEM. A "closed system" is one that uses specific reagent designed for a particular instrument. Generally, the same company produces

*The following abbreviations are used in Tables 16.3–16.7. *Reagent:* CEDIA—cloned enzyme donor immunoassay, EIA—enzyme immunoassay, EMIT—enzyme multiplied immunoassay technique, FIA—fluorescent immunoassay, FPIA—fluorescent polarization immunoassay, LIA—luminescent immunoassay, PETINIA—particle enhanced turbidimetric inhibition immunoassay. *Format:* CB—coated bead, CT—coated tube, CW—coated well, CF—coated filter paper, MF—multilayer film, PF—particle filter, MP—magnetic particle, TB—turbidimetric. *Test:* A—all, D—drug, H—hormone, T—tumor marker, ID—infectious disease.

TABLE 16.3. Open Homogeneous Immunoassay System

Instrument	Reagent
Hitachi 747, 911	CEDIA, EMIT
Olympus AU5000	EMIT
Miles Chem 1	EMIT
Roche cobas/Mira	EMIT
Beckman Array	Nephelometric

both the instrument and reagent, although there are a few exceptions. For example, the popular TDx analyzer by Abbott Diagnostics uses fluorescent polarization immunoassay (FPIA) reagents made by Abbott. Because there are so many TDx analyzers for the testing of therapeutic drugs, FPIA made by other companies became available. The DuPont ACA analyzer uses the particle-enhanced turbidimetric inhibition immunoassay (PETINIA). The advantage of a closed system is that the overall quality of the performance can be better controlled by the company. The disadvantage is usually higher price of the reagent. Examples of these systems are shown in Table 16.4.

16.3.1.3. COMBINED HOMOGENEOUS IMMUNOASSAY SYSTEM. The "combined" homogeneous immunoassay system (Table 16.5) uses either open or closed reagents and has the ability to measure both small and large molecules. Most of these systems are available for research use only. They incorporate a unique approach so that both large and small molecules can be measured in a homogeneous format. In addition to immunoassay, the electrochemiluminescence (ECL) technology has been applied to the detection of nuclear acid, for example, the IGEN system. The Copalis system, which uses flow cytometry could be used to detect markers on the cell surface in addition to the coupled particles for immunoassay. The real-time immunodiagnostics employing optical immunobiosensor (OIB) developed by BMC uses conventional competitive or immunometric assay with fluorescent conjugate. The fluorescence produced by the evanescent wave generated by the molded polystyrene optical fiber is detected by an immunosensor. This allows a short reaction time of < 5 min while achieving similar sensitivity as conventional immunoassay.

TABLE 16.4. Closed Homogeneous Immunoassay Systems

Instrument	Reagent	Reference
Abbott TD, AD	FPIA	2
Dupont ACA	PETINIA	3
Roche Cobas	FPIA	4

TABLE 16.5. Combined Homogeneous Immunoassay System

Instrument	Reagent	Detection	Reference
Sienna Biotech	Copalis	Flow cytometry	5
BMC	FIA	OIB	6
IGEN	LIA	ECL	7

16.3.2. Heterogeneous Immunoassay Systems

Heterogenous immunoassay is more versatile. It can measure both small and large analytes. With a physical separation step, it eliminates most interfering substances present in the patient's sample prior to quantification. The separation step, together with the potential of using larger sample size, will improve the sensitivity. The immunometric assay tends to have a broader dynamic range of the standard curve. The peptide hormone and tumor marker are ideally measured by immunometric assay, for example, human chorionic gonadotropin (hCG) and prostate-specific antigen (PSA). The disadvantages of heterogenous immunoassay are that it is more labor-intensive and time-consuming, and requires a dedicated immunoassay analyzer.

16.3.2.1. SEMIAUTOMATED IMMUNOASSAY SYSTEM. An automated instrument could be built on multiple blocks. These building blocks may be linked by computer program or mechanically attached together. In most semiautomated systems, these blocks function separately, for example, the pipetting of reagent, the incubation of the reaction mixture, the bound/free separation by washing the solid phase, the signal detection, and the data management steps. These systems operate according to the batch concept, with testing of all samples for the same analyte. Most fully automated heterogenous immunoassay systems are relatively slow, with throughput of 30–120 tests per hour. Therefore, a high-volume testing laboratory may benefit from using a semiautomated system that performs the most labor-intensive steps, leaving the less time-consuming steps for the technologist. Examples are shown in Table 16.6.

16.3.2.2. FULLY AUTOMATED IMMUNOASSAY SYSTEM. Fully automated immunoassay systems link all the separate components of the semiautomated system and allow the testing to be completed from the sample addition to result reporting. Depending on the ability of the system to select sample for analysis on demand, the fully automated system can be further subdivided into batch, selective, and continuous access systems. The batch immunoassay systems have been the primary working systems in the clinical laboratory (Table 16.7a). These systems are small in size and relatively slow in throughput and are being replaced by the random-access systems. The selective system is similar to the batch system; however, the selective system can perform more than one test for a given specimen. Once the reaction starts for a particular batch of specimen, no more

TABLE 16.6. Semiautomated Immunoassay System

Company	Instrument	Reagent	Format	Test	Reference
Kodak	Amerlite	LIA	CW	H	8
Hybritech	Photon QA	EIA	CB	T	9
DuPont	ACA Plus	EIA	MP	A	10
Nichols	CLS	LIA	CB	H	*
Abbott	Commander	EIA	CB	ID	*

specimen can be added until the testing is complete. It is useful for laboratories with a relatively large test volume (Table 16.7b). Because of their inability to test continuously, selective systems are also being replaced with the truly continuous, random-access systems. These systems allow continuous access of the testing process by adding additional specimen and reagent. The throughput varies from 30 to 150 tests per hour (Table 16.7c). Examples of two automated systems are shown in Figures 16.1 and 16.2.

TABLE 16.7. Automated Immunoassay Systems

Company	Instrument	Reagent	Format	Test	Reference
a. Batch Automated Immunoassay System					
Abbott	IMX	FIA	PF	A	11
Baxter	Stratus II	FIA	CF	H,D	12
b. Selective Automated Immunoassay System					
BMD	ES-300	EIA	CT	A	13
BioRad	Radius	EIA	CW	H	14
BioMerieux	VIDAS	FIA	CW	A	15
Syva	Vista	FIA	MP	A	16
c. Continuous Access Immunoassay System					
Abbott	AxSym	FIA & FPIA	PF	A	17
BD	Affinity	EIA	CT	H	18
Behring	Opus	FIA	CF/MF	A	19
Biotrol	System 7000	EIA	MP	A	20,21
Ciba	ACS-180	LIA	MP	A	22,23
DPC	Immunlite	LIA	CB	H	24
Miles	Immuno 1	EIA	MP/TB	A	25
Roche	Cobas Core	EIA	CB	A	26
Sanofi	Access	FIA	MP	A	27
Serono	SR-1	EIA	MP	H	28
Tosoh	AIA-1200	FIA	MP	A	29
Wallac	AutoDELFIA	tFIA	CW	A	30

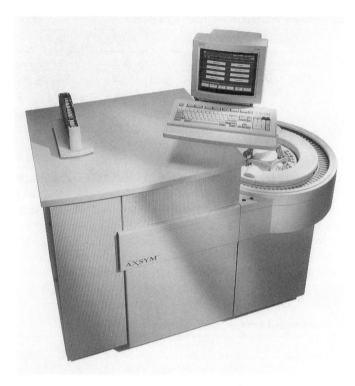

Figure 16.1. The Abbott AxSym automated immunoassay system.

16.4. PERFORMANCE OF IMMUNOASSAY SYSTEM

16.4.1. Defining Goals and Objectives

The first step in the evaluation of an automated immunoassay system is to define the goals and objectives of automation. There should be significant improvements in both system performance and laboratory operation.

Automation is the solution for consolidating workstations and thereby reducing the labor requirements, in terms of both number and skill level of the technologist. Most automated systems are able to achieve 2–4-week calibration stability, allowing more frequent testing without the increased cost of daily calibration. The random-access feature of the automation should eliminate the "batch" concept; there will be no need to schedule tests. This will enhance the turnaround time.

Automation should improve the technical performance of the assay such as precision and sensitivity. Most assays could be performed in a single tube rather than in duplicate. This reduces not only the total assay time but also the cost of reagent. The total cost of the testing should be reduced as the savings in labor

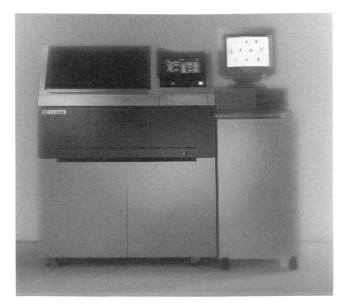

Figure 16.2. The Tosoh AIA-1200DX automated immunoassay system.

and the reagent could offset the cost of the instrument. The overall goal of automation is to improve the efficiency and the outcome of the testing.

16.4.2. Technical Performance

Technical performance is the first step in the evaluation of an automated immunoassay system. The system should be tested in the order of precision, sensitivity, accuracy, patient comparison with another method, and lot-to-lot variation.

16.4.2.1. PRECISION. Precision—or more appropriately, imprecision—is probably the most important technical aspect of the system. Automation should improve precision to the point that single testing is acceptable. Both within-run and between-run precision should be evaluated. The acceptable level of precision is about 5–10% CV (coefficient of variation) in the useful concentration ranges. For random-access systems, the precision should be determined in both random-access and batch modes to see if there are any differences.

Since precision is the most important aspect of the technical performance, identifying and controlling the source of imprecision is quite important. The reagent components of a system predetermine the extent of imprecision, both the affinity constant and the concentration of the antibodies used in the reagent. For immunometric assay, the antibody conjugate will determine the amount of signal generated. The stability and the consistency of the substrate will affect the enzyme reaction and the final color production. The accurate assignment of the calibrator value and the stability of the calibrator is important. Other components that affect the precision are diluent, wash solution, quench solution, and quality-control samples. The matrices, pH, ionic strength, and lyophilization process will also influence the overall precision.

Interference can cause imprecision. Nonspecific interference such as hemolysis, lipemia, and icterus as well as specific interference such as heterophilic antibodies will affect both the accuracy and precision. Samples with extremely high concentrations of analyte will affect precision in either of two ways: (1) the high concentration of this sample could carry over into the next sample or (2) it may cause a high-dose hook effect. The apparent low value will be rather imprecise.

16.4.2.2. SENSITIVITY. *Sensitivity* in the immunoassay automation context is usually defined as the detection limit of an assay. Several approaches to the determination of sensitivity do not yield the same result.

The minimum detectable dose (MDD) is calculated from the mean $+2$ SD (standard deviation) of 20 replicates of the zero calibrator performed within a run. It is usually calculated based on the response (absorbance) and read off the calibration curve to obtain the MDD. This approach usually gives the best (lowest) MDD possible and is the accepted industry standard. However, the MDD calculated in this manner is unrealistic and is seldom reproducible from day to day. The value of between-run MDD (on different days) is usually higher than the within-run MDD.

Another approach is to use patient samples with zero analyte concentration in determining sensitivity since calibrator does not always resemble patient material. A patient's serum is diluted with the assay diluent to below the detection limit of the assay. The sensitivity is determined at the dilution where the percent recovery found is no longer close to 100% of the expected value.

16.4.2.3. ACCURACY. The analytical accuracy is the ability of a system to determine the true value of the analyte. Methods for assessing accuracy include recovery, linearity, parallelism, interference, carryover, and calibration stability.

Recovery is an indirect assessment of accuracy. It tests the system's ability to measure a known amount of analyte. The experiment is done by adding a known amount of analyte (A) to a base (B) and measuring the concentration (C). The percentage of recovery can be calculated by $100\% \times (C - B)/A$.

The dilution experiment is an assessment of the relative recovery of the system. The diluent is usually the assay buffer or the zero calibrator. In addition, saline or another patient sample could also be used to assess the matrix effect. Linearity indicates that the responses are proportional and the final concentration calculated from the curve is linear. Good parallelism indicates that the assay fulfills one of the fundamental principles of immunoassay; that is, the unknown antigen gives the same response as the standard antigen.

16.4.2.4. INTERFERENCE. Dilution beyond the calibrator curve may indicate assay problems like "high-dose hook effect" in an immunometric assay or the presence of interference. At extremely high analyte concentrations, the antibody binding sites may be saturated with antigens, making the antibodies unavailable to form a sandwich, that is, antibody–antigen complexes. The end result is the severe underestimation of the analyte concentration. This is a particular problem with analytes that could be present in wide concentration ranges.

Heterophilic antibodies have been reported to cause false positive results in immunometric assay.[31] Since most monoclonal antibodies are developed from a hybridoma using the mouse system, the presence of antimouse antibodies in a patient's serum will lead to false-positive results. To minimize this problem, mouse serum has been added to the reaction medium to absorb mouse antibodies. Some assays use other scavenger antibodies or *Fab* fragments rather than the whole immunoglobulin in the assay. Genetically engineered chimeric antibody with a combined mouse and human immunoglobulin molecule has also been used. In addition to the problem of endogenous antibodies, immunotherapy of cancer patients with toxin-labeled antibody in the blood circulation as well as human antimouse antibodies (HAMA) will cause interference.[32] High titers of rheumatoid factors will also cause false-positive results in immunometric assay.

Other nonspecific interferences, such as lipemia, hemolysis, and icterus, may affect the separation and detection using the spectrophotometric or fluorometric measurement. Substances may be present in the serum that cross-react with the antigen for the antibody. In the digoxin assay, digoxin-like immunoreactive substance (DLIS) have been identified to cause false positives in neonates, pregnant women, and patients with renal or liver diseases.[33]

16.4.2.5. CARRYOVER. Carryover is a potential problem for the automated immunoassay system. For most analytes of immunoassay, the physiological ranges are quite broad. It is particularly troublesome for tumor markers. One would require a carryover rate of less than one part per million.

16.4.2.6. CALIBRATION STABILITY. The stability-of-calibration curve can be determined by the daily QC results over a period of weeks or months. Trend analysis and other statistical analysis may be helpful. Some assays require running one calibrator with each run. The absorbance of this calibrator is compared to the stored curve, and the ratio is calculated. The variation of this factor may be a useful indicator of the extent of shift in the calibration curve. If the QC values show a declining trend, calibration may be in order; however, the bias introduced during the recalibration may be a significant component of the overall imprecision of the system.

16.4.2.7. METHOD COMPARISON. Despite the potential shortcomings of method comparison, it is still useful if one realizes the limitations for such comparison. If the reference method is a definitive method, the results of method comparison could be used to establish the analytical accuracy of the new method. When the clinically defined patient samples are used in method comparison, the clinical accuracy of the new method can be established. The comparison to the reference method can be used to identify outliers if the reference method has good precision. When the current method is the reference method, one can decide whether the reference ranges need to be changed. With a good correlation coefficient but slope not equal to one, one can adjust the reference ranges by the slope factor. If the correlation coefficient is poor (i.e., significantly less than 1.0), it will be difficult to assess the reference ranges.

16.4.2.8. LOT-TO-LOT VARIATION. Whenever possible, the technical performance of multiple lots of reagents should be evaluated. A recommended protocol is shown in Table 16.8.

To check in a new lot of reagent, one should record the lot number of all components. In the event of inconsistent performance, the component information will facilitate troubleshooting of the causes. The most frequent lot change is the tracer in the RIA and the conjugate in the EIA. This may produce rather dramatic changes in the absolute absorbance or the amount of radioactivity. When the calibrator lot changes, shifts in QC and patient results may occur. The tolerance limit of the manufacturers vary from 5 to 10% or 1 to 2 SD of the difference between lots.

The absorbance of the calibrator is a good indicator of lot-to-lot variation of the conjugate. The slope of the calibration curve changes significantly according to its absorbance. This may affect the sensitivity, linearity, and precision of the assay. For qualitative assay, the positive or negative result will greatly depend on the differences in the absorbance of the zero and the positive cutoff calibrator. Minimum acceptable absorbance values should be set for such assays, such as the EMIT assay for abuse drugs, to avoid false-positive results.

The parameters generated from the data reduction of the calibration curve could be evaluated. These parameters include the slope, intercept, coefficient of correlation, and standard error estimate. Such parameters could be recorded for quality control and troubleshooting purposes. If there is any indication of nonlinearity—for example, a patient with high analyte value by the old lot and lower value by the new lot of reagent—a linearity study should be performed. If both primary and secondary wavelengths are used, one should compare patient results obtained by both wavelengths.

TABLE 16.8. Protocol for Lot Checkin

1. Record lot numbers of all components.
2. Evaluate the absolute and the differences of the signal response of the high and low calibrators.
3. Evaluate the characteristics of the calibration curve.
4. Evaluate the replicate CV.
5. Evaluate QC shifts.
6. Compare patient results between the old and new lots.
7. Check linearity, if necessary.

16.4.2.9. BETWEEN-INSTRUMENT VARIATION. The performance of an individual instrument may not be the same as another instrument, even if both instruments are the same model of the same manufacturer. The alignment and the adjustment of the optical system may be slightly different, which could produce different results. The accuracy of the pipetting system may vary. The temperature of the incubator could be different. Although each and every component of the system has its own specification, any two particular instruments may perform at opposite ends of the tolerance limit. The same reagent used in different instruments could also produce different results. If more than one automated system is to be used, it is important that the performance of each automated system be evaluated and the test results compared to the other system.

16.4.3. Clinical Performance

The goal of a clinical evaluation is to assess the ability of a system to provide accurate test results in a timely fashion for clinical use. The need could be for disease screening, diagnosis, or management.

16.4.3.1. PREDICTIVE VALUE OF THE DIAGNOSTIC TEST. The determination of reference values is rather time-consuming and requires a large healthy population ($n \geq 120$). Statistical analysis using the mean $\pm$ 2 SD for a population with gaussian (normal) distribution is the most frequently used method. For non-gaussian distribution, percentile method is probably the simplest approach. For tests with relatively specific applications, for example, creatine kinase isoenzyme MB (CK-MB) in the diagnosis of acute myocardial infarction (AMI), or tumor markers in the diagnosis and management of cancer, a decision level is more appropriate than the upper limit of the normal population. The decision level can be determined using a predictive value model.

The predictive value model includes sensitivity, specificity, and efficiency of a test. By varying the decision level, sensitivity and specificity will change in opposite directions. A higher decision level will reduce the sensitivity but increase the specificity. An optimal decision level can be selected on the basis of the highest possible efficiency.

A useful approach to evaluate multiple tests for the same analyte is the receiver operating characteristic (ROC) curve. The ROC curve can be constructed by plotting sensitivity versus 1− specificity, or true-positive rate versus false-positive rate. The advantage of ROC curve is the display of the performance over the entire decision levels. One can pinpoint the decision level where the optimal sensitivity and specificity can be achieved. By superimposing the ROC curves of more than one test method, one can select the best methodology. A better test is one that displays higher true-positive rate and lower false-positive rate. An example is the comparison of prostate-specific antigen (PSA) to prostatic acid phosphatase (PAP) in the diagnosis of prostatic cancer.[34] The preparation of a ROC curve has been discussed in detail by Zweig and Robertson.[35]

16.4.3.2. DISTRIBUTION OF PATIENT VALUES. The predictive value model is difficult to use for analytes that are not diagnostic for a single disease. Most, if not all, tumor markers are elevated in more than one disease condition. Carcinoembryonic antigen (CEA) has been shown to be elevated in colorectal, lung, breast , and pancreatic carcinoma as well as in benign conditions. The reference values for CEA in the healthy population are higher for smokers than non-smokers. Using the predictive value model, it is necessary to select a population which includes disease and nondisease groups. The clinical question asked should be used to define the disease group. The outcome of the sensitivity and specificity will greatly depend on the inclusion of the number and groups of patients. In this situation, the actual distribution of patient values may be more informative. The distribution of tumor marker values is usually shown as the percentage of patients with elevated values using various cutoff values in as many groups of healthy, benign, and cancerous patients. These groups are selected from past experiences of other similar markers. An example is CA 549.[36]

16.4.3.3. DISEASE MANAGEMENT. Disease management is applied mainly for analytes such as tumor markers that are used in the monitoring of treatment and progression of cancer. To determine the success of surgery, one would expect that an elevated marker prior to surgery should fall after a successful operation. The extent of the decrease in the marker value will depend on the pretreatment tumor involvement. To detect the recurrence of cancer after a successful initial treatment, one would expect that the marker value will be steady, possibly within the reference values of healthy individuals. When the marker value starts to trend upward, it may indicate the recurrence of cancer. To monitor the effectiveness of cancer therapy, one would expect that the marker value should increase with progression of cancer. With the regression of cancer, the marker value should decrease. For stable patients, the marker value should not change.

16.4.4. Operational Performance

An important benefit of automation is enhancing the efficiency of the laboratory operation. Two major issues are the improvement of system operation and the impact of automation on laboratory operation.

An automated system should require minimum servicing, both scheduled and unscheduled. Reliability of an automated system is critical since automation usually means consolidation of procedures into a system. Therefore, malfunction of the system could shut down the entire immunoassay laboratory.

It is difficult to compare throughput of various systems. Most available systems are 30–180 tests per hour. One should also evaluate the throughput in terms of patient samples per hour and samples per working day. It is more realistic to evaluate the throughput on the basis of your own workload and the physician's ordering pattern. The throughput based on patient samples will depend on the calibration and quality-control frequencies as well as the batch size. The less frequent the calibration and quality control of a system, the closer the real throughput of patient samples will be to the theoretical throughput.

The impact of automation on the laboratory operation is mainly on the mechanization of the testing procedure and the consolidation of workstations. The random-access feature of the automation will facilitate the workflow and shorten the turnaround time.

To evaluate an automated system, one should examine the steps of testing that are mechanized. A totally automated system, including all the steps of the total testing process, is possible by combining computer technology for order entry and results reporting with a robotic device for sample application and analysis. Automation will change the job function of a technologist from a technician to a data manager and quality-control officer. Through workstation consolidation, it will reduce the labor requirement in terms of both skill level and number.

The major benefit of automation is in the consolidation of workstations. The reduction in bench space and personnel should be evaluated. The disadvantage of consolidation is the total dependence on the system. In the event of malfunction, the entire immunoassay testing will be shut down. One should consider backup options and redundant systems to ensure continuous testing. The extent of such consolidation will depend on the degree of random accessibility. A selective system capable of analyzing multiple tests in a batch format will achieve intermediate consolidation, such as the ES-300 analyzer by BMD. A truly random-access system with a broad menu and high throughput should allow maximum consolidation into one workstation for immunoassay testing, as, for example the AIA-1200 analyzer by Tosoh Medics. This type of system should eliminate scheduling of analytical runs. Tests will be performed as the sample arrives in the laboratory, and the turnaround time should be improved.

16.4.5. Economic and Human Issues

With the changing healthcare delivery system, the laboratory is under considerable pressure to reduce costs. Four aspects of the cost improvement will be examined in the economic performance of an automated immunoassay system: productivity, labor requirement, system cost, and total cost.

Productivity is defined as the output of product per full-time equivalent (FTE) of laboratory personnel. The product could be measured by the number of tests or work units. The work unit per FTE is a better indicator than the number of tests per FTE, since tests vary in their complexity. In the process of arriving at the final productivity, one should examine other testing support activities. These include calibration, quality control, duplicate testing, dilution of sample with values in excess of the highest calibration, and repeat testing due to system malfunction. A system that requires frequent calibration, quality control, and repeat testing will result in lower productivity of patient results.

The labor component represents the greatest potential in cost improvement. Both the skill level and the number of FTEs needed to operate the system will be affected by automation. Automation demands different skills and training, but not necessarily less skill. The number of technologists should be reduced because of the consolidation of workstations. Any reduction in the labor requirement is not beneficial unless this saving can be turned into additional productivity.

The cost of acquiring and operating a system includes instrument, reagent, disposables, maintenance, service contract, and quality control. Most laboratories often negotiate the price for the instrument and reagent while other operating costs are not appreciated. Examples include the service contract, maintenance, disposables, and quality control. The annual service contract is often priced at about 10% of the instrument cost. Unscheduled downtime could be costly for both the laboratory and the hospital.

Disposable items can be costly on a daily basis if a system uses disposable curvettes, pipettes, tips, and other disposable instruments. Quality control (QC) is essential but does not generate revenue. The cost of QC is determined by the frequency of QC and the QC material. The cost of reagent should be analyzed not only per test but also per patient. A number of factors will affect reagent usage and hence reagent cost. Examples are single versus duplicate testing, frequency of calibration, QC, retesting of samples with values greater than the assay dynamic range, and malfunction of the system. The other factor is waste; it is usually between 5 and 20%.

In addition to the cost items discussed earlier, some other hidden costs are seldom appreciated. One should examine the total cost to include quality assurance and impact on the healthcare provider. Quality assurance has become increasingly important. The impact of turnaround time and the level of laboratory service on the hospital is difficult to measure. One indicator is the length of stay of patients in the hospital. Any avenue to reduce the length of stay will save hospital money. An automated system could provide more frequent testing and better turnaround time. This may lead to faster diagnosis and workup of the patient and expedite discharge of the patient from the hospital.

Finally, one should not forget about human issues in automation. The first issue is safety. A system should be designed to ensure safety of the operator. Safety issues relate to injury due to mechanical moving parts, infections from biological hazards (e.g., AIDS, hepatitis virus), and potential fire hazards. Computer programs for the operation of the system should be user-friendly. Psychological factors should be considered for a walkaway instrument. For example, error messages should be indicated as soon as a problem occurs. An audible alarm should be used to alert the operator of such an occurrence.

16.5. FUTURE TRENDS

The design of the future automated immunoassay system will depend on the need of the testing site, quality expectation, and technological advances.

Where will the testing of patients be done in the future—central clinical laboratory, decentralized locations, physician's office, or patient's home? It is possible that a trained technologist could perform laboratory tests in the patient's home using a portable testing device. Alternatively, a sample can be collected by the patient and transported to a testing center. Reports could be transmitted by fax.

Outpatient testing could be performed at a testing center in a convenient location away from the patient's home. It depends on the need of turnaround time, the complexity of the test, and the cost. I believe that the turnaround time issue will be less critical in the future as more automation will include pre-analytical variables such as order entry, sample collection, transportation, processing, and result reporting. At the present time, such preanalytical variables often cause significant delay in the testing process.

For inpatients, a hospital laboratory needs a system with a large menu and continuous access to different samples and tests. A commercial laboratory needs an automated system with higher throughput since most of the testing is routine in nature. The continuous-access feature is less critical. I believe more centralization of laboratory testing will occur to improve efficiency. Therefore, the need for such high-throughput instrumentation will be in demand.

System integration will be the next level of automation. Since an individual system may not fulfill all the needs of a particular laboratory, multiple systems of the same or different types could be linked together with a common sample processor. The data generated by the different instruments could be reported by a common data management system. Furthermore, a totally integrated immunoassay system would be able to perform all the steps in the total testing process.

Technological advances in immunoassay automation will result in miniaturized systems with better sensitivity, less interference, more consistency, and faster testing time. Designer antibodies with higher affinity and specificity could be used to improve sensitivity and analyte selectivity. Labels could be chosen to have higher signal for quantitation. Homogeneous immunoassay will facilitate sample handling and shorten reaction time, as for example, in the BMC system using optical fiber evanescent-wave fluoroimmunosensor. Multiple analytes could also be performed simultaneously using different labels, as for example, in the time-resolve fluorescent system (DELFIA). The other approach is the use of different sizes of particles, as in the Copalis system. The laser detector of the flow cytometer could produce signals at different positions according to the size of the particle.

Finally, automated immunoassay systems should be designed to meet the clinical need and expectation of the user. It should include as many steps as possible in the total testing process. A system composed of individual modules may be the best approach. The module may be able to perform a group of tests suitable for a unique clinical setting, such as an emergency room, critical-care unit, and outpatient clinic for a specific medical discipline. Clinical settings would be the determining factor of the test menu on a particular system rather than the traditional laboratory disciplines of chemistry, microbiology, and hematology. Such modular systems would be most suitable for the changing needs of the clinical laboratory testing in the 1990s and beyond.

REFERENCES

1. Chan DW: In Chan DW, ed: *Immunoassay Automation: A Practical Guide.* San Diego, CA: Academic Press, 1992, pp. 1–367.

2. Wong SH: TDx systems. In Chan DW, ed: *Immunoassay Automation: A Practical Guide.* San Diego, CA: Academic Press, 1992, pp. 317–341.

3. Litchfield W, Craig AR, Frey WA, Leflar CC, Looney CE, Luddy M: Novel shell/core particle for automated turbidimetric immunoassays. *Clin Chem* 30:1489–1493, 1984.

4. Goldsmith BM: Cobas-Fara II analyzer. In Chan DW, ed: *Immunoassay Automation: A Practical Guide.* San Diego, CA: Academic Press, 1992, pp. 129–135.

5. Bodner AJ, Britz J: Copalis technology. In Chan W, ed: *Immunoassay Automation: An Updated Guide to Systems.* San Diego, CA: Academic Press, in press.

6. Mahoney W, Lin JN, Brier RA, Luderer AA: Real-time immunodiagnostics employing optical immunobiosensor. In Chan DW, ed: *Immunoassay Automation: An Updated Guide to Systems.* San Diego, CA: Academic Press, in press.

7. Blackburn GF, Shah HP, Kenten JH, et al: Electrochemiluminescence detection for development of immunoassays and DNA probe assays for clinical diagnostics. *Clin Chem* 37:1534–1539, 1991.

8. Faix JD: Amerlite immunoassay system. In Chan DW, ed: *Immunoassay Automation: A Practical Guide.* San Diego, CA: Academic Press, 1992, pp. 117–127.

9. Frye RF: The Photon-ERA immunoassay analyzer. In Chan DW, ed: *Immunoassay Automation: A Practical Guide.* San Diego, CA: Academic Press, 1992, pp. 269–292.

10. Vaidya HC, Zuk PJ, Ballas RA: ACA plus accessory for the ACA discrete clinical analyzer. In Chan DW, ed: *Immunoassay Automation: An Updated Guide to Systems.* San Diego, CA: Academic Press, in press.

11. Chou PP: IMx system. In Chan DW, ed: *Immunoassay Automation: A Practical Guide.* San Diego, CA: Academic Press, 1992, pp. 203–219.

12. Kahn SE, Bermes EW: Stratus II immunoassay system. In Chan DW, ed: *Immunoassay Automation: A Practical Guide.* San Diego, CA: Academic Press, 1992, pp. 293–316.

13. Sagona MA, Collinsworth WE, Gadsden RH: ES-300 immunoassay system. In Chan DW, ed: *Immunoassay Automation: A Practical Guide.* San Diego, CA: Academic Press, 1992, pp. 191–202.

14. Bussel J, Edwards R: Radius immunoassay system. In Chan DW, ed: *Immunoassay Automation: An Updated Guide to Systems.* San Diego, CA: Academic Press, in press.

15. Ng R: VIDAS system. In Chan DW, ed: *Immunoassay Automation: An Updated Guide to Systems.* San Diego, CA: Academic Press, in press.

16. Li TM: The Vista immunoassay system. In Chan DW, ed: *Immunoassay Automation: A Practical Guide.* San Diego, CA: Academic Press, 1992, pp. 343–349.

17. Painter P: The AxSym system. In Chan DW, ed: *Immunoassay Automation: An Updated Guide to Systems.* San Diego, CA: Academic Press, in press.

18. Chan DW, Kelley C: Affinity immunoassay system. In Chan DW, ed: *Immunoassay Automation: A Practical Guide.* San Diego, CA: Academic Press, 1992, pp. 83–94.

19. Lehrer M, Miller L, Natale J: The OPUS system. In Chan DW, ed: *Immunoassay Automation: A Practical Guide.* San Diego, CA: Academic Press, 1992, pp. 245–268.

20. Frier C, Kan B, Cicquel T: Biotrol system 7000: automated immunoassay analyzer. *J Clin Immunoassay* 14:111–114, 1991.

21. Dellamonica C, Frier C: Routine use of a Biotrol System 7000 in a private laboratory. *J Clin Immunoassay* 15:242–245, 1992.

22. Dudley RF: The Ciba Corning ACS 180 automated immunoassay system. *J Clin Immunoassay* 14:77–82, 1991.

23. Smart JB: The Ciba Corning ACS 180—a user's perspective. *J Clin Immunoassay* 15:246–251, 1992.

24. Babson AL: The Cirrus IMMULITE automated immunoassay system. *J Clin Immunoassay* 14:83–88, 1991.

25. Ehresman DJ, McQueeney L: Immuno 1 automated immunoassay system. In Chan DW, ed: *Immunoassay Automation: An Updated Guide to Systems.* San Diego, CA: Academic Press, in press.

26. Huber PR: Cobas Core immunochemistry analyzer. In Chan DW, ed: *Immunoassay Automation: An Updated Guide to Systems.* San Diego, CA: Academic Press, in press.

27. Guitard M: The access immunoassay system. In Chan DW, ed: *Immunoassay Automation: An Updated Guide to Systems.* San Diego, CA: Academic Press, in press.

28. Demers LM: SR1 immunoassay system. In Chan DW, ed: *Immunoassay Automation: A Practical Guide.* San Diego, CA: Academic Press, 1992, pp. 277–292.

29. Chan DW: AIA-1200 immunoassay system. In Chan DW, ed: *Immunoassay Automation: A Practical Guide.* San Diego, CA: Academic Press, 1992, pp. 95–115.

30. Gudmundsson TV, Olafsdottir E: AutoDELFIA system. In Chan DW, ed: *Immunoassay Automation: An Updated Guide to Systems.* San Diego, CA: Academic Press, in press.

31. Boscato LM, Stuart MC: Heterophilic antibodies: a problem for all immunoassays. *Clin. Chem* 34:27–33, 1988.

32. Kricka LJ, Schmerfeld-Pruss D, Senior M, Goodman DB, Kaladas P: Interference by human anti-mouse antibody in two-site immunoassays. *Clin Chem* 36:892–894, 1990.

33. Soldin SJ: Digoxin—issues and controversies. *Clin Chem* 32:2–12, 1986.

34. Rock RC, Chan DW, Bruzek DJ, Waldron C, Oesterling J, Walsh P: Evaluation of a monoclonal immunoradiometric assay for prostate-specific antigen. *Clin Chem* 33:2257–2261, 1987.

35. Zweig MH, Robertson EA: Clinical validation of immunoassay: a well-designed approach to a clinical study. In Chan DW, ed: *Immunoassay Automation: A Practical Guide.* San Diego, CA: Academic Press, 1987, pp. 97–128.

36. Chan DW, Beveridge RA, Bruzek DJ, et al: Monitoring breast cancer with CA 549. *Clin Chem* 34:2000–2004, 1988.

CHAPTER

17

Automated Clinical Laboratory Systems

MASAHIDE SASAKI, KATSUMI OGURA, HIROMI KATAOKA, AND JUN IMAMURA

CONTENTS

17.1. INTRODUCTION

Clinical laboratory tests, especially tests using blood and urine specimens, have traditionally consisted of a series of time-consuming procedures including obtaining and preparing the samples, performing the tests, and reporting the results. Recent technological developments, however, have permitted the automation of many of these procedures. In particular, new developments in microcomputerization and microchemistry have resulted in major improvements in analyzing technology. For example, equipment for performing clinical labora-

Handbook of Clinical Automation, Robotics, and Optimization, Edited by Gerald J. Kost with the collaboration of Judith Welsh.
ISBN 0-471-03179-8 © 1996 John Wiley & Sons, Inc.

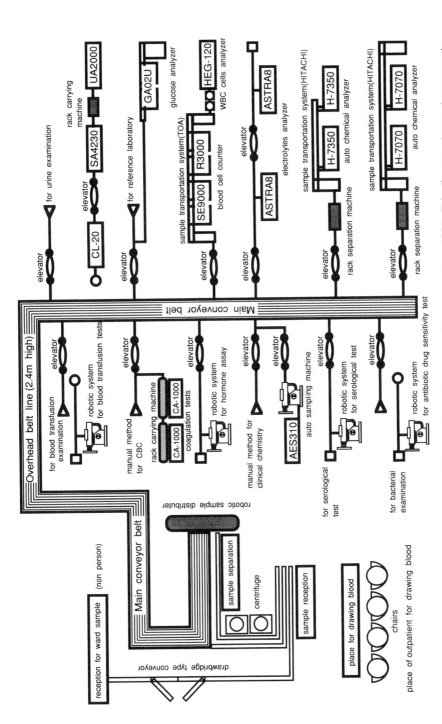

Figure 17.1. Outline of the belt line system. We have been developing this system since 1981. This diagram shows the system in September 1994. Samples are positioned on the main conveyor belt by the robotic sample distributor, then carried and distributed to each analyzing section via the conveyor belt, elevators, and other transferring machines. Automated analyzing systems in each section then perform the diagnostic tests.

443

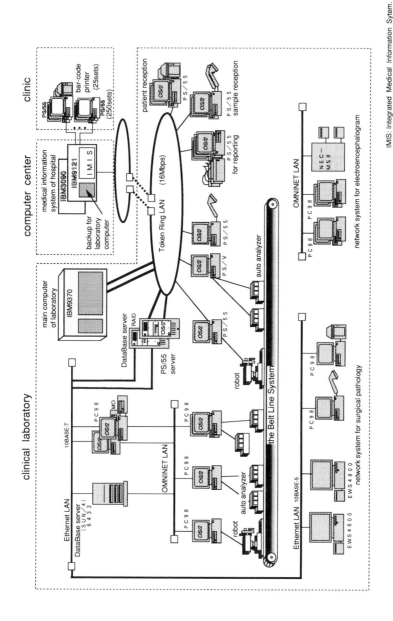

clinical laboratory

computer center

clinic

Figure 17.2. Outline of the computer system. This diagram shows the network system in April 1994. We installed and connected local-area networks (LANs) to control the Belt Line System and to transfer data to and from the host computers via the Token Ring LAN. We also developed software used in the system. This system contributes substantially to realizing our goal of rapid and accurate laboratory testing.

IMIS: Integrated Medical Information Sytem.

tory tests has been developed that permits dozens of tests to be performed simultaneously using small sample amounts.

The clinical laboratory of today requires an efficiently designed analysis system. In order to design an efficient system for processing clinical laboratory tests, one of the most important tasks is the construction of a logical sample-carrying system. In this regard, we developed the Belt Line System[1-3] (Fig. 17.1), which consists of several automated analyzers connected to a series of conveyer belts. The Belt Line System functions within the Integrated Medical Information System (Fig. 17.2). Test-tube racks containing samples are distributed to analyzing equipment throughout the laboratory via the conveyer belts. After the tests are performed, the results are automatically printed or transmitted to the host computer. The robotic systems for blood transfusion tests and antibiotic sensitivity tests are not currently connected to the Belt Line System.

Since automated analyzing machines were not commercially available, we designed and constructed a robot-aided analyzing system. In the following pages, we describe applications of the robotic analyzing system to serum hormone analysis, serological agglutination tests, blood transfusion tests, antibiotic sensitivity tests, and serum electrophoresis.

17.2. APPLICATION OF ROBOTICS TO SERUM HORMONE ANALYSIS

Objectives. We designed and constructed a fully automated robotic diagnostic testing facility using the DELFIA system (Pharmacia Co., Sweden) developed by Soini, et al.[4,5] and an industrial robot (model RT-3000, Seiko Electronics Co., Japan). The DELFIA system is a time-resolving fluoroimmunoassay system using the fluorescent substance europium (EU). This system has better reproducibility, and sensitivity equal to or greater than the radioisotope assay (RIA) system. The DELFIA system analyzing procedure is not complicated but requires a time-consuming 1.5–5.0 h for each diagnostic test. In order to reduce the staff time required to perform the tests manually, we designed and constructed a fully automated analyzing system using the model RT-3000 robot and the DELFIA system connected to the Belt Line System[6] (Fig. 17.3).

Diagnostic Tests. We perform the following clinical laboratory tests using the DELFIA system test strips: Thyrotropin (TSH), Triiodothyronine (T3), Thyroxin (T4), Prolactin, Lutropin (LH), Follitropin (FSH), Choriogonadotropin (hCG), and Cortisol.

System Design. This system consists of a basic robot surrounded by other equipment (Fig. 17.4).

Basic robot. The robot, model D-TRAN RT-3000 (Seiko Electronics Co., Japan) employs quadraaxial robotics in cylindrical coordinates. Its movements are characterized by extreme accuracy and precise positional reproducibility. The robotic microcomputer is programmed with a controller supplied by the manufacturer.

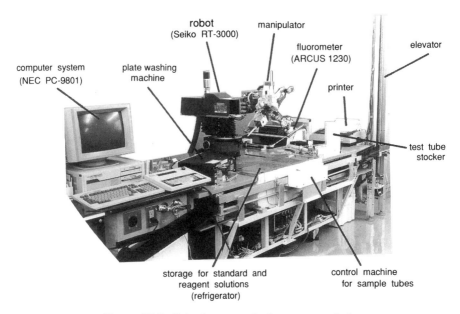

Figure 17.3. Robotic system for hormone analysis.

Robotic manipulator. The manipulator is a windmill-shaped device attached to the arm of the RT-3000 robot to which two electronic digital pipettes, EDP-250 and EDP-2500X (Rainin Instrument Co., USA), have been attached. Handgrips have also been attached for handling the 12-well plate, also called the strip, and the reagent tubes.

Storage system for standard solution and other reagents. The storage system consists of a 4–8°C humidified incubator that holds 32 strips. It also includes a cabinet for storing reagents and control sera that is shaken at intervals. The inside of the cabinet is humidified to avoid drying of the reagents.

Test-tube stocker. This cabinet stocks plastic test tubes (14 × 100 mm, Greiner Co., Sweden). It is designed to serve the test tubes one by one to the robotic manipulator for making tracer solution (europium dissolved buffer).

Control machine for sample tubes. Sample tube racks are carried on the conveyor belt to the control machine. A pipette attached to the manipulator then withdraws a measured amount of the sample from the first tube and transfers it to a well on the strip. After the sampling procedure, the sample rack is sent forward and the sampling sequence is repeated on the next tube.

DELFIA system instruments. The DELFIA system includes plate shakers (fast and slow), a plate washer for the strip, and a fluorometer—ARCUS-1230—and its printer.

Control unit. We installed a 32-bit personal computer, PC-9801 (NEC Co., Japan) for receiving test orders and for controlling the analyzing system. We also developed software that is designed to graphically display steps in process on the CRT screen.

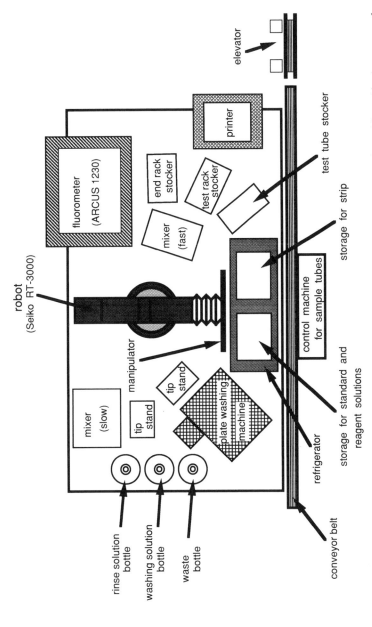

Figure 17.4. Arrangement of the robotic system for serum hormone analysis. The robot is positioned in the center of the system to facilitate interactions with surrounding equipment.

447

Testing Procedures. When a sample rack reaches the control machine, the robot scans the barcode identification number on the rack to confirm the tests to be performed. If the sample is the first sample of the day, the robot prepares aliquots of control solutions and performs the sampling procedures. According to information shown on the test order, an aliquot of the sample is transferred to one of the wells in the strip with control sera in wells 11 and 12. The sample rack is then sent forward, and sampling of the next sample tube is performed. The robot advances to the analyzing step after 10 tubes are sampled. Steps in the analyzing procedure are shown in Table 17.1.

We programmed the robot to perform similar procedures simultaneously in order to streamline the complicated process of analyzing multiple samples and to reduce the processing time necessary to complete the tests.

Effectiveness

Accuracy. Accuracy of each assay and correlation with the conventional RIA method are shown in Table 17.2. Reproducibility was satisfactory for all assays except the Cortisol test. Therefore, we utilize this system for analyzing hormone levels other than Cortisol.

Stability. In automating the DELFIA system, it is important to assure that the reagents in the strip wells remain stable within the incubator. After conditioning studies, we added a procedure in which a small volume of buffer solution is transferred to the wells in the strip. With the addition of this procedure, reagents remain stable for more than 48 h.

Processing speed. Since this system can perform multiple tests simultaneously, the processing speed is 70 samples per 90 min.

Safety. The control system monitors the movement of the robot and the strip using 29 fiber-photoelectric cells (reflecting sensors) during the testing process. In the case of robot malfunction, the computer stops the local system and alerts laboratory staff by displaying a warning on the computer screen and by sounding an alarm.

17.3. APPLICATION OF ROBOTICS TO SEROLOGICAL AGGLUTINATION TESTS

Objectives. The robotic system for agglutination tests performs the red blood cell (RBC) agglutination test or its alternative, the gelatin beads aggregation test (Fig. 17.5). To increase efficiency, this system is connected to the Belt Line System. When samples are transported to the serological testing room, the system automatically determines the tests to be performed according to the barcode identification. The robot withdraws sera and formulates a stepping dilution on a 96-well microplate. Red blood cells or gelatin beads are added to the plate wells, and the plate is shaken. Following the completion of these procedures and an appropriate reaction period, the robot transports the plate to the technicians who judge the test results.[7,8]

TABLE 17.1. Examinations and Their Procedual Steps for DELFIA System by the Robotic System

Step	Procedures	Assay							
		TSH	T3	T4	Prolactin	LH	FSH	hCG	Cortisol
1	Prewashing (times)	1	1	1	1	1	1	1	1
2	Sample or standard solution (µL)	50	50	25	25	25	25	25	25
3	Buffer (µL)	200	100	200	200	200	200	200	100
	Tracer solution (µL)		100						
	Antibody solution (µL)								
	Mixing, fast/slow (min)	2/240	0/90	0/90	0/90	0/45	0/180	2/60	0/120
4	Strip washing (times)					1	2	3	
	Tracer solution (µL)					200	200	200	
	Mixing, fast/slow (min)					0/15	2/0	2/30	
	Standing (min)						30		
5	Strip washing (times)	6	4	4	6	6	6	6	6
	Enhancement solution (µL)	200	200	200	200	200	200	200	200
	Slow mixing (min)	5	5	5	5	5	5	5	5
6	Standing (min)	10–15			10–15			10–15	
7	Measure by ARCUS 1230	O	O	O	O	O	O	O	O

449

TABLE 17.2. Accuracy of Measurement of Each Hormone Assay and Correlation with RIA Method

Unit	TSH (mIU/L)	T3 (ng/L)	T4 (µg/L)	Prolactin (µg/L)	LH (IU/L)	FSH (IU/L)	hCG (IU/L)	Cortisol (µg/L)
Accuracy								
Test 1 n	12	12	12	12	12	12	10	12
Mean	1.474	769.03	80.92	2.341	2.522	3.884	1.500	30.73
SD	0.049	16.77	3.07	0.127	0.117	0.104	0.158	5.10
CV (%)	3.355	2.181	3.793	5.430	4.621	2.682	10.44	16.60
Test 2 n	12	12	12	12	12	12	10	12
Mean	352.18	6873.5	207.24	253.04	256.83	242.35	5138.6	292.80
SD	5.117	125.45	6.56	13.551	7.121	9.099	247.27	25.66
CV (%)	1.453	1.825	3.166	5.355	2.773	3.754	4.812	8.763
Correlation with RIA								
n	50	50	50	50	50	50	—	50
Slope	0.958	0.919	0.992	0.846	1.089	1.011	—	0.902
Intercept	0.843	−79.59	5.00	−2.644	−1.542	0.019	—	2.00
r	0.9979	0.9956	0.9937	0.9945	0.9982	0.9961	—	0.9729

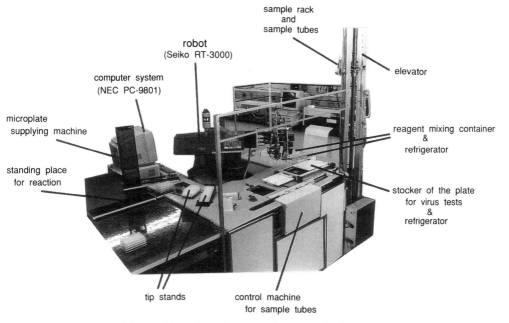

Figure 17.5. Robotic system for serological tests.

Diagnostic Tests. We perform the following agglutination tests using the robotic system: Thyroid test, microsome test, TPHA for syphilis, ASK test, RA test, mycoplasma test, anti-DNA test, and HIV test. This system can be used for any test performed by RBC agglutinating reaction or gelatin aggregating reaction.

System Design. This system consists of a basic robot surrounded by other equipment (Fig. 17.6).

Basic robot. The robot, model D-TRAN RT-3000 (Seiko Electronics Co.) has four axes driven by DC-servo motors, with ± 0.025 mm positional reproducibility, and covering bellows on every cylinder.

Robotic manipulator. An aluminum disk plate (300 mm in diameter) is connected to the manipulator. Attached to the disk plate is a digital multichannel pipette (Titertek Co., USA) for reagents, a multistepping pipette (Model 25/50, Titertek Co., USA) for stepwise dilution, and an electronic digital pipette (Model EDP-250x, Rainin Instrument Co., USA) for sera sampling. A vacuum table for transporting microplates is also attached to the disk plate. This equipment is driven by compressed air.

Automatic reagent mixing container. Reagents used for serum agglutination tests contain red blood cells or beads with specific antigens or antibodies conjugated on the surface. In order to assure accurate and uniform reaction conditions, it is important that these reagents be mixed continuously. However, vigorous mixing may result in antigen or antibody particles being removed from

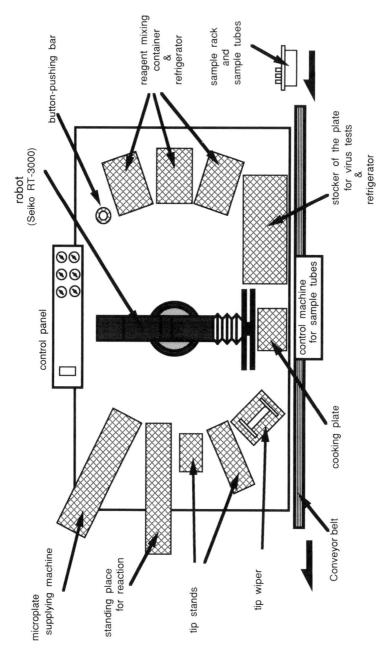

Figure 17.6. Arrangement of the robotic system for serological tests. The button-pushing bar is used to change the settings of the electronic digital pipette. The robot presses the pipette head against the bar which depresses the buttons on the pipette head.

these surfaces. To mix the reagents without damaging the antigens or antibodies, we developed a special reagent mixing container. The container consists of two tanks differing in size and depth. When the container is inclined upward 30° reagent moves from the larger to the smaller tank, thereby mixing the reagent solution and minimizing reagent waste (Fig. 17.7).

Hot plate. We use a hot plate to prepare and mix the reaction mixture. It is designed to hold the microplate and automatically mix the reaction mixture.

Microplate supplying machine. This equipment serves microplates one by one from stock. The robot grasps the microplate with its handgrip and transfers it to the hot plate.

Pipette tip selector. Pipette tips are exchanged for each procedure to avoid contamination. The pipette tip selector serves tips selectively for wells in use. Use of this server reduces reagent waste.

Control unit. We have developed software for the robot's computer using D-TRAN assembly robot language. We have connected this computer to a personal computer PC-9801 (NEC Co., Japan) to permit the transmission of test orders from the host computer directly to the robotic system.

Testing Procedures. The procedures used in this system are the same as those used in conventional manual testing. The robot is so accurate that it can reproduce precise movements of the pipette tip, such as positioning the tip on the wall of the well after ejecting the reagent.

Sample-handling steps are shown in Fig. 17.8. Laboratory technicians deposit samples in the rack at the starting point of the conveyer belt. The sample rack is transported via the conveyer belt to the robot in the serological testing room. The robot removes a reaction microplate from the microplate supplying machine and positions it on the hot plate. Using the pipette EDP-250X, the robot transfers a specific volume of sera to the microplate wells. After each tube has been sampled, the sample rack is removed from the robotic system. The robot prepares the necessary dilution and performs the testing procedure on each sample. In the final step, laboratory technicians examine the microplate and judge the results.

Effectiveness. Robotic testing is generally more accurate than conventional manual methods due to the precise movements of the robotic system. Each plate (eight tests) is completed in 6 min; processing time is therefore 10 samples (80 tests) per hour. Important advantages of this system include a reduction in specimen handling errors and a decrease in the risk of infection to laboratory technicians.

17.4. APPLICATION OF ROBOTICS TO BLOOD TRANSFUSION TESTS

Objectives. The robotic system for blood transfusion tests performs blood typing and cross-matching tests[7,8] (Fig. 17.9). This system is basically the same as the application for agglutination tests.

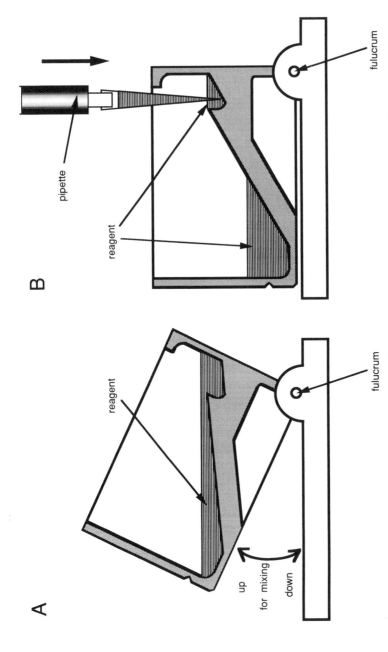

Figure 17.7. Automatic reagent mixing container. This container consists of two reagent tanks differing in size and depth; (A) When the container is tilted up and down, the reagent mixes as it moves from one tank to another; (B) reagent waste is avoided by withdrawing reagent from the smaller tank.

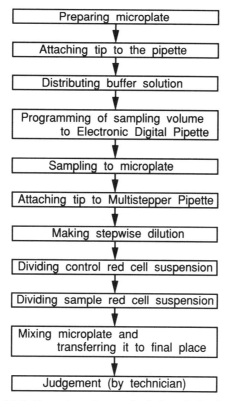

Figure 17.8. Procedures for serological agglutination tests.

The robotic system rapidly performs tests on donor blood, including testing for syphilis, spirochetes, hepatitis viruses, human T-cell leukemia viruses (HTLVs), and human immunodeficiency viruses (HIVs). Blood typing and cross-matching tests are performed using the agglutination test. Because of the importance of these tests, laboratory technicians judge the test results. On the other hand, procedures for performing the liver function tests also necessary for selecting appropriate blood donors are totally automated. The system performs all procedures from sampling to the reaction using robotic manipulation, followed by automated judgment by spectrometry using a microplate reader (Toyosoda Co., Japan).

Diagnostic Tests. We perform blood typing [ABO, Rh(D)] and cross-matching (major and minor). We also test for HB antigen, HB antibody, TPHA for syphilis, HTLV-I antibody, HIV antibody, serum total protein, albumin, and GPT (ALT) for blood donor compatibility.

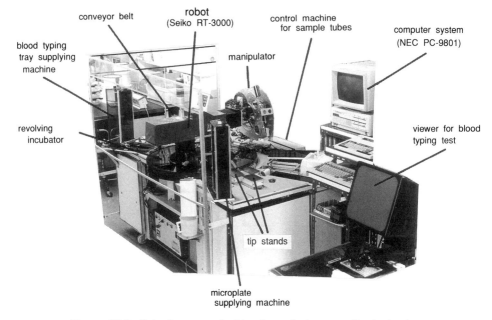

Figure 17.9. Robotic system for blood transfusion tests (back view).

System Design. This system consists of a basic robot surrounded by other equipment (Fig. 17.10).

Basic robot. The application of the robotic system for blood transfusion tests is similar to the one for serological agglutination tests. The robot has been modified for this purpose by the installation of a special handgrip for grasping the microplates and blood typing trays.

Special equipment. We have developed the following special equipment for blood transfusion tests:

Blood Typing Tray. We have designed a special tray with two 20 (5 × 4) well CEA testing plates (Ono Medicine Co., Japan) connected with cloth tape for use during the centrifugation procedure. The cloth tape functions as a hinge. The two sides of the tray remain flat when positioned on the hot plate during the reaction process, and angle at approximately 120° during centrifugation to avoid spilling samples during rotation (Fig. 17.11).

Blood Typing Tray Supplying Machine. This equipment serves the blood typing trays one by one to the robot. The robot grasps the trays with its handgrip. The blood typing tray supplying machine has almost the same mechanism as the microplate supplying machine described in Section 17.3.

Revolving Incubator. Cross-matching tests require an incubation period of 15 min at 37°C after the bromelin solution has been added. To provide for this incubation period, we built a revolving incubator around the robot

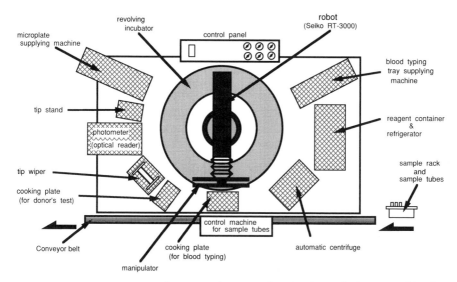

Figure 17.10. Arrangement of the robotic system for blood transfusion tests. After incubation, the blood typing tray is transported from the revolving incubator to the automatic centrifuge. In the centrifuge, the tray is held at an angle of 120° during rotation.

using a turntable. The blood typing tray is positioned on the turntable after the reaction mixture has been prepared. The tray is removed after the 15 min incubation period. The robot performs other procedures during this period.

Centrifuge for the Blood Typing Tray. This centrifuge is specially designed to accommodate the hinged blood typing tray. Its funnel-shaped rotor avoids spilling the samples during rotation. The rotor stops in a position that allows the robot to insert and remove the blood typing tray.

Multiple Test Modes and Sample Preparation

Multiple test modes. In order to perform the many complicated blood transfusion tests reliably and rapidly, sample racks are affixed with a test identification barcode on the front surface. The robotic system automatically scans the barcode to select one of the following test modes:

Mode 1: ABO group and Rh(D) blood typing

Mode 2: ABO group, Rh(D) and cross-matching test (Bromelin method)

Mode 3: Eight blood transfusion tests

Mode 4: ABO group and the blood transfusion tests including Rh (D)

Sample preparation. Since blood transfusion tests require blood plasma (or serum) and red blood cells, manual sample preparation is necessary. Sample

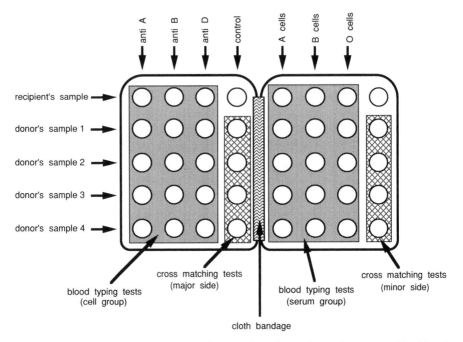

Figure 17.11. Blood typing tray and the location of samples and reagents. The blood typing tray consists of two 20-well plates connected with cloth tape. The cloth tape functions as a hinge allowing the tray to be positioned at an angle within the centrifuge.

serum and RBC suspensions are supplied separately in different tubes. The serum and RBCs of the recipient and donor are carried on a sample rack. Thus, one sample rack can hold samples for four donors per recipient. The sample number is checked just before the rack enters the robotic system by a reflecting infrared sensor, and an appropriate volume of reagent is drawn into the pipette tip. This procedure reduces wasted reagent solution.

Testing Procedures

Blood typing and cross-matching. The laboratory technician separates sample blood into serum and blood cells, places these samples on the sample rack with barcode identification, and positions the rack on the conveyor belt. Subsequent procedures are performed by the robotic system (Fig. 17.12). When the sample rack reaches the system, the handgrip on the manipulator transfers a blood typing tray from the supplying machine to the hot plate. If the sample is from a blood donor, a cross-matching plate is also transferred to the hot plate. Using a pipette on the manipulator, the robot divides the blood testing reagents into the appropriate wells on the blood typing tray. Red blood cells are suspended in normal saline to a concentration of 5%, and the suspension is also divided into the wells. For the cross-matching test, a measured amount of bromelin solution is added after the serum and 5% red blood cell suspension have been transferred to the tray. The tray containing the reaction mixtures is then shaken to mix the reagents and placed on the turntable to be incubated for 15 min at 37°C. After the reaction is completed, the tray is centrifuged for one min and transferred to the judging table. Sample and reagent positions on the blood typing tray are shown on Fig. 17.11.

Blood donor identification. During the blood typing and cross-matching tests described above, other compatibility tests are simultaneously performed on the donor blood samples. Donor sera is transferred to a 98 well, flat bottom microplate and a stepwise dilution is prepared. Then reagents are added to the reacting wells. After the reagents have been mixed, the microplate is incubated until the reaction is complete. Then the robot transports the microplate to the microplate reader for measurement. Results of the serological tests are judged by technicians. A flowchart of the blood transfusion test is shown in Fig. 17.12.

Effectiveness. The robotic system has reduced the staff time necessary to perform these tests as well as provided the additional advantages discussed below.

Accuracy. The accuracy of the system is dependent mainly on the accuracy of

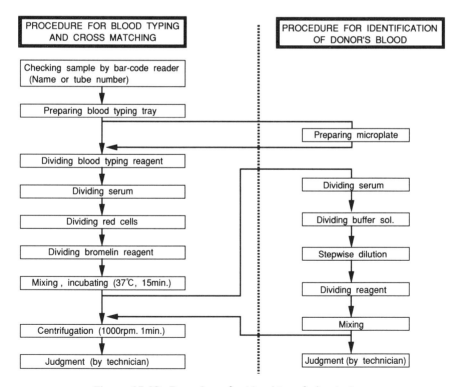

Figure 17.12. Procedures for blood transfusion tests.

the pipettes. The coefficient of variation (CV) is generally less than 1.5%, which is superior to the manual method using the same pipettes.

Reproducibility. Reproducibility is excellent due to the precise manipulation capabilities and procedural accuracy of the robotic system.

Processing speed. Processing speed for the four test modes is as follows:

Mode 1: 60 samples per hour

Mode 2: 4 donors for 4 recipients per hour

Mode 3: 12 samples per hour

Mode 4: 4 donors for 2 recipients per hour

Safety. This system reduces the possibility of disease transmission to laboratory technicians from physical contact with the samples. However, there is a risk of physical injury due to robotic movement. To reduce this risk, we have installed a fence surrounding the robotic system.

17.5. APPLICATION OF ROBOTICS TO ANTIBIOTIC SENSITIVITY TESTS

Objectives. The minimum inhibitory concentration (MIC) in antibiotic sensitivity tests is measured by two methods: plate dilution and solution dilution. In the case of solution dilution, the macrodilution method uses test tubes for stepwise dilution of antibiotic drugs, and the microdilution method uses microplates. Due to the complicated nature of these protocols, however, many clinical laboratories do not perform these procedures during routine testing. We have therefore sought to apply robotics to the microdilution method.[9] After the culturing chambers have been manually inoculated with bacteria, the robot automatically cultures the bacteria, prepares the dilution of ordered antibiotic drugs, and monitors growth of the bacteria. Thus, the MIC can be calculated automatically (Fig. 17.13).

Diagnostic Tests. We now test the MIC for 16 types of antibiotic drugs of the 24 commercially available.

System Design. This system is composed of two robots surrounded by other equipment (Fig. 17.14).

Basic robots. We employ two robots, model RT-3200 and model RT-2000 (Seiko Electronics Co., Japan). The RT-3200 is an improved version of model RT-3000 with enhanced speed and a wider moving area. The RT-2000 is similar in function but slightly smaller than the RT-3000.

Syringe culture chambers. We utilize 10 mL disposable syringes with 18 gauge needles (1.20 mm ϕ × 38 mm) as bacterial culture chambers (Fig. 17.15).

Transportation unit for the culture chambers. This equipment transfers the syringe culture chambers to the robotic system. The transportation unit includes

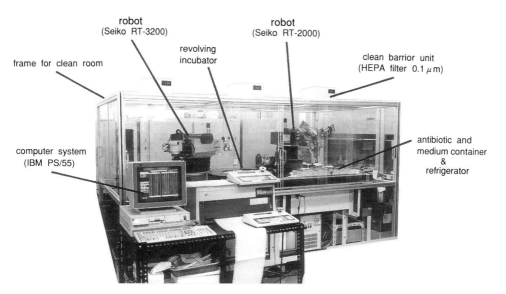

Figure 17.13. Robotic system for antibiotic drug sensitivity tests.

a refrigerator to prevent bacterial growth when a large number of samples precludes immediate processing.

Windmill incubator. This 37°C incubator holds 40 culture chambers. The incubator is designed to rotate vertically in a windmill pattern thereby mixing the culture medium within the syringe culture chambers. Gas is expelled from the syringes when the needles are pointed upward (Fig. 17.15). A photometer monitors bacterial growth during each rotation.

Antibiotic drug panel unit. The antibiotic drug panel unit prepares a stepwise dilution of 16 types of antibiotic drugs as ordered by the clinicians. The model RT-2000 robot uses 8 channel pipettes for dividing reagents and for preparing the stepwise dilution. The robot is surrounded by a pipette tip selector, a refrigerated stirrer for drugs and reagents, and a medium container (Fig. 17.14).

Culturing unit. The culturing unit controls the transfer of culture chambers and microplates between units as well as dividing the culture medium. This unit consists of a robot, model RT-32000, surrounded by other equipment. The robot uses its handgrip to manipulate the culture chamber, microplates, and 8 channel pipette.

Turntable unit. The turntable unit incubates microplates for 40 samples (a total of 80 microplates) at 37°C with continuous shaking. It stops the rotation at a position that allows the robot to remove the microplate to monitor bacterial growth.

Result judging unit. This unit consists of two microplate readers (Toya-soda Co., Japan) which periodically monitor bacterial growth in the culture chambers.

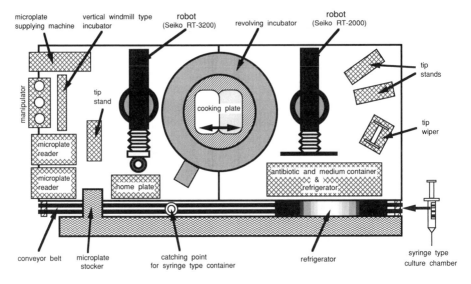

Figure 17.14. Arrangement of the robotic system for antibiotic drug sensitivity tests. Samples are supplied to this system in disposable syringe culture chambers. The culture chambers are incubated in a windmill incubator before the sensitivity tests are performed.

Control unit. We installed a 32-bit IBM 5550-T0A personal computer system to control the overall system of antibiotic sensitivity testing.

Testing Procedures

Preparation by technicians. After culturing for 10–12 h on an agar plate, a sample of the bacterial colony is drawn into the needle of a syringe culture chamber. The bacteria is inoculated into the culture medium and the inoculated medium is drawn into the syringe. The syringe is then transferred to the robot via the transportation unit.

Robotic manipulation. The RT-3200 robot inserts the culture chambers into the windmill incubator with its handgrip. The robot removes two microplates from the microplate supplying machine and positions them on the hot plate. Then the RT-2000 robot prepares a stepwise dilution of antibiotics as ordered using 16 types of antibiotic drugs and the diluting medium.

After bacterial growth has reached an appropriate concentration, the RT-3200 robot removes the culture chamber from the windmill incubator and divides the bacterial suspension into the antibiotic dilution. The robot then carries the plates to the turntable unit for an incubation period of 2 h at 37°C. After incubation, the robot transports the plates to the microplate reader to check the sensitivity. The robot then returns the plates to the turntable and continues the incubation process. The bacterial growth is monitored every two hours for up to 12 h. After 12 h, the technician prints the results and reports them to the clinicians.

Effectiveness

Accuracy. In order to calculate the accuracy of the robotic system, we programmed the microdilution method according to the National Committee for Clinical Laboratory Standards (NCCLS).[10] We used *Escherichia coli* (ATCC® 25922), *Pseudomonas aeruginosa* (ATCC® 27853), and *Enterococcus faecalis* (ATCC® 29212) as control strains of bacteria. We used carbenicillin (CBPC), piperacillin (PIPC), ticarcillin (TIPC), cefoperazone (CPZ), cefotaxime (CTX), amikacin (AMK), gentamicin (GM), and tobramycin (TOB) as control antibiotics. We have achieved results within the same dilution with the exception of tests with *E. coli* and CBPC, *E. coli* and PIPC, and *E. faecalis* and CBPC in which results differed by one well.

Reproducibility. We have conducted 20 trial studies using three bacterial strains and eight types of antibiotics. After a 6-h culture, *E. coli* and *E. faecalis* demonstrated 100% reproducibility (160/160 tests); *P. aeruginosa* showed one well difference in 4 of 160 tests.

Efficiency. Installation of the windmill incubator has improved efficiency and accuracy in measuring the MIC. After inoculation in the culture chamber, bacterial growth reaches an appropriate concentration within a 60–80 min incubation period. We have conducted several trial studies using short-term 4-, 6-, 8-, and 10-h cultures and an overnight 16-h culture. These studies revealed a high correlation between the two methods; 82% of intestinal bacteria in 6 h, 90% of glu-

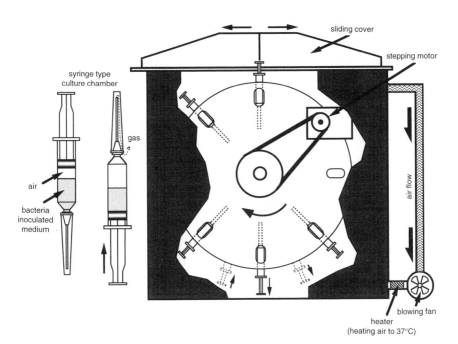

Figure 17.15. Vertical windmill incubator. A syringe culture chamber is shown on the left. The culture chambers, containing bacteria inoculated medium, are placed in the vertical windmill incubator for preliminary culturing.

cose nonfermentation bacteria in 8 h, and 82% of Gram-positive bacteria in 10 h showed MICs within one well of the result of the overnight culture. These results suggest that preliminary sensitivity test results can be reported to clinicians after a 6–8-h period.

Sterility. We have covered the entire robotic system with acrylic panels and installed three air-filtrating blowers (Clean Barrier Unit®, Kondo Kogyo Co., Japan) with 0.1 mm high-efficiency particulate air filters (HEPA filter). Each blower filters 0.5–1.0 m³ of airflow per minute. With the installation of this equipment, bacterial contamination has been reduced to 0.3 per microplate well.

17.6. APPLICATION OF ROBOTICS TO SERUM ELECTROPHORESIS

Objectives. The AES310 electrophoresis system (Olympus Co., Japan) is fully automated. After the technician transfers sample sera to a special tray, AES310 blots the samples on a Separax® or Sartorius® membrane, completes the electrophoresis process, and charts the results. We connected this automated apparatus and the robotic sampling system to the Belt Line System to create a fully automated electrophoresis system. Samples transported on the conveyer belt are processed with appropriate control serum, as ordered on the sample tube barcode.[11,12]

Diagnostic Tests. This system performs electrophoreses for serum albumin, α_1-, α_2-, β- and γ-globulin.

System Design. This system consists of a robot surrounded by other equipment (see Fig. 17.16 and Fig. 17.17).

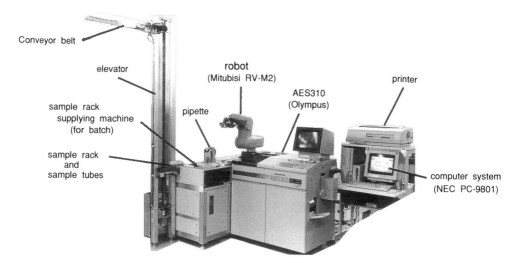

Figure 17.16. Fully robotic sampling system for serum electrophoresis.

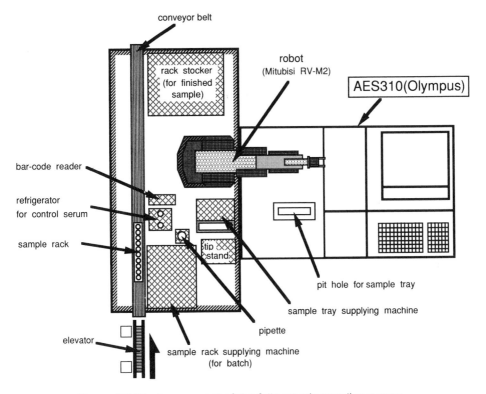

Figure 17.17. Arrangement of the fully robotic sampling system.

Basic robot. The basic robot in this system is a Move Master® model RV-M2 (Mitsubishi Electric Co., Japan). This vertical multiple joint robot is small, quiet, and accurate. Its long arm includes a special handgrip and extends 570 mm to cover a wide area.

Sample rack carrying unit. This equipment consists of a conveyer belt, sample rack supplying machine, and a sample rack stocker. It is directly connected to the Belt Line System but also designed to accept manual insertion of a sample rack.

Serum tray supplying machine. To increase efficiency, AES310 is designed to blot ten samples simultaneously. For this purpose, we use a 25 × 130 × 8 mm plastic tray with ten engraved 3.5 × 10 × 1.5 mm grooves. The serum tray supplying machine holds five of these trays and serves them one by one to the robotic handgrip.

Sampling unit. The sampling unit consists of a sampling pipette, tips, and tip remover. This unit facilitates the robot's handling of the pipette during sampling.

Refrigerator for control serum. The refrigerator for control serum maintains a temperature of 8–10°C.

Control unit. A personal computer controls AES310 and the surrounding equipment. We used a personal computer, PC-9801FA (NEC Co., Japan) to connect AES310 to the Belt Line System. We constructed a 64-point digital I/O board and a four-channel intelligent communication board, and installed them in the computer unit to control the analyzing machines, robot, sensors, and solenoids. In order to organize this complicated control system, we installed OS/2 v. 1.21 as the operating system, and OS/2 Presentation Manager (PM) as the designing user interface. We designed the control program ourselves to attain an interface that is easy to operate.

Testing Procedures.

Preparation by laboratory technicians. Laboratory technicians are responsible for turning the main switch on, supplying five serum trays to the tray supplying machine, and putting control serum into the refrigerator.

Robotic manipulation. After the sample rack is transferred from the Belt Line System, the robot transports the rack to the barcode reader. After the barcode has been scanned, the robot grasps the pipette, inserts a disposable tip, and transfers 50 mL of sample into the grooves of the serum tray. This procedure is repeated for every sample. Control serum is used in grooves 1, 6, and 10. When the serum tray has been filled with 10 samples, the robot inserts the tray into AES310 where samples are blotted on a membrane and the electrophoresis process is completed. After 75 min, test results are printed and reported to the clinicians.

Effectiveness. The robotic system has reduced technician time to less than 10 min per day. The technicians are responsible only for exchanging the electrophoresis buffer, washing the staining tank, and adding the sera.

Accuracy. The accuracy of this system is dependent upon the accuracy of AES310. Using the Sartorius® membrane, the CV is $< 1\%$ for albumin, α_1-, α_2-, β- and γ-globulin tests.

Reproducibility. Reproducibility is also dependent on the accuracy of AES310, and the CV is $< 1\%$.

Processing speed. It takes 4 min for the robot to supply AES310 with a the serum tray containing 10 samples. Processing time for AES310 is seven test tubes per 75 minutes.

Safety. As discussed previously, the risk of disease transmission to technicians has been reduced with the use of the robotic system. The risk of physical injury is very small because of its fully automated construction.

17.7. CONCLUSION

We have described the applications of our robotic system to serum hormone analysis, serological agglutination tests, blood transfusion tests, antibiotic sensitivity tests, and serum electrophoresis. We designed and constructed a computerized system of robotic analyzing machines connected via an automated sample carrying system. Our objective in developing this automated clinical laboratory was to improve the processing speed and accuracy of diagnostic testing while at the same time to reduce the risk of disease transmission and accidental injury to laboratory technicians. We were greatly assisted in this endeavor by the staff at the Kochi Medical School Clinical Laboratory Department; their full cooperation contributed significantly to the success of our accomplishments.

We have not applied to obtain patents for the robotic system in order to allow others the opportunity to benefit from our research and system development. We do request, however, that the designs and innovations described in this chapter not be used for commercial profit.

REFERENCES

1. Sasaki M: Newly built automated laboratory system in Kochi Medical School [abstract]. In Kozakai N, ed: *Proc. 12th World Congress Pathology, Tokyo;* reprinted in *Jpn J Clin Pathol,* 31:518, 1983.

2. Sasaki M: The belt line system—completely automatic clinical laboratory using a sample transportation system. *Jpn J Clin Pathol* 32:119–126, 1984. (In Japanese.)

3. Sasaki M: An innovative conveyor belt system for a clinical laboratory. *Journal of the International Federation of Clinical Chemistry* 3:31–33, 1991.

4. Soini E, Hemmilä I: Fluoroimmunoassay: present status and key problems [review]. *Clin Chem* 25:353–361, 1979.

5. Soini E, Kojola H: Time-resolved fluorometer for lanthanide chelates—a new generation of nonisotopic immunoassay. *Clin Chem* 29:65–68, 1983.

6. Sasaki M, Ogura K: A fully robotic assay for human hormone analysis. *Clin Chem* 36:1567–1571, 1990.

7. Ogura K, Sasaki M, Kataoka H, Nishida M: The innovative robot system for serological examination test and blood transfusion test: Using Seiko RT-3000 robot. *Jpn J Clin Lab Autom* 12:613–618, 1987. (In Japanese.)

8. Sasaki M: How to make and manage clinical laboratory systems using robotic facilities. In Okuda K, ed: *Automation and New Technology in the Clinical Laboratory,* Oxford, UK: Blackwell Scientific Publications, 1990, pp 97–101.

9. Ogura K, Sugihara S, Kataoka H, et al: Development of robotic facility for antibiotic drugs sensitivity tests [abstract]. *Jpn J Clin Lab Autom* 13:519–520, 1988. (In Japanese.)

10. National Committee for Clinical Laboratory Standards: *Methods for Dilution Antimicrobial Susceptibility Tests for Bacteria that Grow Aerobically,* 2nd ed. Villanova, PA: NCCLS, 1990, M7–A2.

11. Ogura K, Sugihara S, Kataoka H, et al: Fully automatic innovation for AES310 type of protein electrophoresis machine [abstract]. *Jpn J Clin Lab Autom* 17:288–289, 1992. (In Japanese.)

12. Markin RS, Sasaki M: A laboratory automation platform: the next robotic step. *MLO: Medical Laboratory Observer* 24: 24–29, 1992.

PART IV

CLINICAL INNOVATION

CHAPTER

18

Strategic Planning for Automation

MARK S. LIFSHITZ AND ROBERT P. DE CRESCE

CONTENTS

Handbook of Clinical Automation, Robotics, and Optimization, Edited by Gerald J. Kost with the collaboration of Judith Welsh.
ISBN 0-471-03179-8 © 1996 John Wiley & Sons, Inc.

18.1. INTRODUCTION

Healthcare has entered into a period of dynamic change at a pace unimaginable even several years ago. The massive and rapid restructuring of this industry, which accounts for about one-seventh of the U.S. economy, has begun to effect every facet of care: direct healthcare providers like hospitals and physicians, secondary vendors such as pharmaceutical companies, and multipurpose hospital suppliers, and finally the end users, consumers. A common goal is to provide more for less, that is, lower costs of care but enhance the quality. Arguably, this rapidly changing environment is best represented by the commercial laboratory industry where lower reimbursement rates (e.g., by Medicare or owing to managed care contracts) have already led to consolidation on a grand scale. Examples include the mergers of megalabs National Health Laboratories (NHL) with Roche Biomedical Laboratories and Corning's MetPath division with Damon Clinical Laboratories to form organizations, each exceeding one billion dollars in annual sales. Hospital laboratories are no less impacted by these same forces, and given their financial resources, may be even more vulnerable than commercial labs. This is because they are part of a larger hospital organization that is being forced to lower its costs but maintain the same level of care. The wave of mergers in the for-profit hospital industry parallels the consolidation that we see in the commercial laboratory sector. For today's laboratory, the message is clear: the environment will continue to rapidly change; to survive and even thrive, a strategic plan is needed to meet these challenges. Once in place, the plan can be used to govern decisions concerning automation (including robotics and instrumentation), facility modernization, and personnel.

18.1.1. The Strategic Planning Process

Strategic planning is a process of (1) deciding on the objectives of the organization and changing or modifying existing objectives; (2) allocating resources used to attain the objectives; and (3) establishing policies that govern the acquisition, use, and disposition of these resources. Decisions affecting services, renovations, equipment purchases, and automation should be done in the context of a total organizational plan; this is particularly important in a hospital where multiple semiautonomous units, such as laboratory, radiology, and nursing, exist.

Strategic planning is best thought of as a four-step process (Fig. 18.1). First, an organization must assess the impact of internal and external environmental factors. This is especially important in an industry like healthcare, which is undergoing a fundamental structural change. In such a rapidly changing environment, proceeding in the wrong direction can be extremely costly. A laboratory's strategic plan is derived largely from that of the parent organization (e.g., hospital), which, in turn, is influenced by the general healthcare environment. For instance, a hospital's decision to become a liver transplant center determines the level of stat service that the lab must provide. Similarly, a hospital's decision to integrate healthcare delivery with other facilities may profoundly effect which

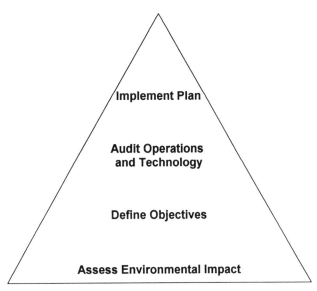

Figure 18.1. The strategic planning process. Note the four steps that begin with assessing environmental impact and end with plan implementation.

tests are performed, when they are done, and how many are ordered. There are also many other external factors such as regulations, reimbursement policies, and staffing. Since the environment affects parts of an organization differently, each area should develop its own strategic plan to cope with its microenvironment.

The second step in strategic planning requires one to define objectives of the organization based on information from the environmental assessment. By analyzing the impact of internal and external environmental forces on each clinical laboratory operation, a blueprint for the future can be developed. For example, if a hospital decides to link services with another facility, the laboratory needs to plan how to consolidate services. Critical to this plan is a list of service standards for both sites. Other objectives, such as cost reductions, must also be considered. Only after this information is defined can the lab review current capabilities and develop a plan for the future.

The third step in planning is to audit laboratory operations and technology. This requires a thorough analysis of the diagnostic testing process, including all preanalytic and postanalytic components. For example, some questions that need to be asked are

When are samples collected?

How are tests ordered?

How are results reported?

Why are tasks done one way instead of another?

In addition, one needs to evaluate current technology (e.g., equipment and methods currently used) and identify future developments that may be applied to the lab. Today's capabilities can then be compared to the objectives developed in the strategic planning process.

The final step is the implementation of a strategic plan, and this requires a close working relationship between the laboratory and other involved parties. Implementation is not simply purchasing equipment or starting a program. It is a detailed plan that identifies resources and uses, develops infrastructure (including software and hardware), initiates processes, and audits and reevaluates the completed plan. For example, a hospital embarking on a point-of-care testing program to complement a patient-focused care model[1] must not only modify facilities and purchase equipment but also establish coordinated laboratory–nursing teams to ensure that the processes is a success.

18.1.2. Strategic Planning and Automation

In the past, most healthcare facilities adopted a short-term approach to total organizational planning. This usually meant planning one year at a time with little or no continuity from one year to the next; so the organization was often pulled in different directions each year. Clinical laboratories, functioning as entities within these organizations, also planned this way. Annual capital equipment requests, the focus of most clinical laboratory planning, were often based on which analyzers needed to be upgraded or replaced and how much funding was anticipated. This approach led to the following: a fragmented method to strategic planning with each department focusing on its own programs; a short-run orientation, typically one year; a focus on annual budgets; small incremental changes from one year to the next; and a reactive approach, responding to short-term problems or opportunities, instead of anticipating them.[2] Personnel decisions were rarely part of the strategic planning process since additional employees could usually be obtained with minimal justification. So, the planning that did take place typically omitted the laboratory's largest expense. In short, this "crisis management" approach encouraged each lab section to develop its own needs without regard for the total laboratory organization. Because cost was rarely an issue, this disjointed approach to planning continued for many years with little if any penalty for failure.

In today's fast-paced healthcare environment, clinical laboratories must adopt a longer-term plan, typically one that spans 3–5 years and one that addresses the needs of the total organization. They need to define their objectives and goals over this period, and not on an annual basis. Needs and opportunities must be anticipated and labs must answer a crucial question: What type of organization do we want to be, what type of services do we want to offer, and how do we want to reach that goal? Of course, the plan must be in keeping with the goals of the total organization. As part of this strategy, laboratories need to consider the role of automation, including instrumentation and robotics, key elements to achieving success in today's extremely cost-conscious environment. In this chapter, the

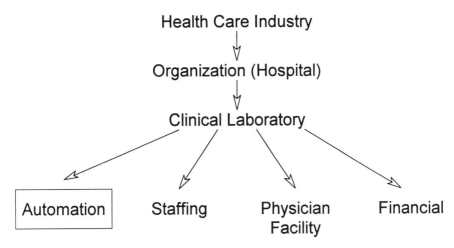

Figure 18.2. The strategic planning tree. Note relationship of automation to internal and external environmental factors.

authors discuss how to approach strategic planning in the clinical laboratory from the perspective of automation. Note that strategic planning for automation is but one component of strategic planning in the laboratory; any plan must consider the complex interrelationships between automation on the one hand and staffing, physical layout, and finance on the other hand. The strategic planning tree (Fig. 18.2) depicts the relationship of automation to the entire strategic planning process.

18.2. ASSESSING THE ENVIRONMENT

Healthcare in the United States is undergoing unprecedented change in several fundamental ways. First, managed care is rapidly transforming the manner in which healthcare is financed through increased competition and global purchasing networks. Medicare and other third-party payers have also initiated cost containment strategies generally manifest as lower reimbursement rates. In addition, every aspect of healthcare delivery is being scrutinized with greater emphasis on medical necessity of care, cost analyses of treatment, and a dominant theme of how to achieve the best outcome at the lowest price. These external environmental factors directly and indirectly influence laboratory automation strategies. The following section explores these influences which are summarized in Table 18.1.

18.2.1. Managed Care

The proportion of insured Americans covered by managed care plans is rapidly growing; by latest estimates it has reached 35.%. Unlike traditional indemnity

TABLE 18.1. Environmental Factors that Impact Planning for Automation

Environmental Factor	Impact
Managed care	More selective use of lab for screening, diagnosis, monitoring, and long-term follow-up when specific indications exist; no more "shotgun" approach to ordering tests
	Growth of outpatient testing at "big three" commercial labs at expense of smaller commercial and hospital labs
Shift to outpatient care	Fewer occupied hospital beds may lead to reduction in lab service needs; growing surplus of beds may also encourage local hospitals to consolidate into one facility
Higher patient acuity	Greater demand on rapid turnaround time and point-of-care testing
Networking	With "hub and spoke" arrangement, networked hospital labs are likely to become "feeder" labs (with less testing done in house) or central facilities (experiencing a growth in testing)
Staffing	Since labor accounts for $\frac{2}{3}$ of a hospital lab budget, it must be considered within an overall cost reduction strategy; more reliance will be placed on automation to achieve labor savings
Reimbursement policy	Fewer outpatient lab tests with emphasis on single tests and small profiles rather than comprehensive panels

insurance plans which provide patients complete freedom to select physicians and hospitals and to receive all care recommended by their physicians, managed care programs contain costs through a primary physician "gatekeeper" who directs care and may restrict access to certain services viewed to be of marginal or no benefit to the patient. Primary-care physicians are typically compensated in a manner that rewards them for keeping down the cost of patient care. Quality is monitored by postservice auditing and evaluation of outcomes versus cost. When the primary physician deems it necessary, patients are sent to preferred specialists who have agreed to provide service as defined by contract with the managed care organization. Noninterventional care is emphasized; procedures are discouraged. Managed care companies reduce costs by centralizing activities in a limited number of facilities; this yields volume discounts and gives them leverage over suppliers. The laboratory, while it represents under 5% of total medical spending, is one area where centralization and volume purchasing have been very popular. This is because the primary provider, specialist, and patient do not perceive significant quality differences among most laboratories. And, laboratory testing can be centralized in an area remote from the patient and still produce timely results in less than 24 h for most tests.

Managed care is focused on total costs, a continuum of care that includes inpatient care, outpatient care, home care, nursing home care, and alternative care. The physician or hospital may be paid one sum to care for all aspects of a patient's condition; laboratory services are usually included in this payment. So the impetus is to eliminate unnecessary tests and delete repetitive tests ordered by different providers caring for the same patient. To accomplish this, laboratories are establishing integrated data networks that provide physicians access to all aspects of their patient's lab work; this, in turn, may be linked to comprehensive patient databases.

Will managed care increase or decrease lab testing? Conventional wisdom suggests that testing will be reduced because there is a financial disincentive to order a test; specifically, it increases costs without increasing revenue. On the other hand, laboratory tests can provide a wealth of information at a relatively low cost, and can often establish a diagnosis without resorting to more expensive procedures. So, cost containment may discourage physicians from bypassing lab tests in the diagnostic workup. Also, managed care emphasizes laboratory tests when valid indications exist for screening, monitoring, and long-term follow-up. For example, cardiac risk assessment and early detection of diabetes mellitus are areas where lab tests are likely to play a major role. On the other hand, random ordering of biochemical profiles or blood counts are unlikely to be supported, even though they are the most frequently ordered tests in today's clinical lab.

18.2.1. Impact of Managed Care on Your Facility

Managed care will likely affect hospital and commercial laboratories differently.[3] The commercial laboratory segment is expected to benefit the most from shifts in testing. Even if the overall volume of testing declines nationally, the commercial sector's percentage will grow. This concentration of business has been an ongoing phenomenon since the early 1970s. Today's megalaboratories are nearly 10 times larger (based on revenue) than similar facilities of 10 years ago. For example, MetPath, a Division of Corning, was an $80 million business in 1985. Today it has sales of over $1 billion. Similarly, Roche Biomedical Labs has grown to over $1 billion in sales from less than $100 million in the same period. Since the average selling price of tests has declined during this time (due to lower reimbursement from Medicare and managed care payers), test volume has increased to an even greater degree than indicated by the revenue figures. As the costs of computer hardware, distribution networks, and other services rise with the demands of managed care, small labs will probably find it difficult to compete and may be acquired by larger competitors or shift focus from routine to specialty testing. More testing and lower reimbursement rates put pressure on labs to reduce costs; automation helps achieve this goal. Large labs can recover the expense of automation more readily since they can amortize fixed costs over a constantly growing test volume.

What will the future hold for hospital laboratories? It is clear that the entire hospital industry and the laboratories that are part of them are in a state of contraction. The easiest way for managed care companies to save money is to reduce hospital utilization, the most expensive part of medical care.

18.2.3. The Shift to Outpatient Care

In the 1970s and 1980s, patients were admitted to the hospital for many conditions now performed on an outpatient basis; a typical hospital stay was 7–10 days. Diagnostic procedures and lab tests were performed without regard to expense since the hospital was reimbursed on a "cost plus" formula. New technologies were immediately implemented since reimbursement was assured. The 1990s have seen a dramatic change in how and where patient care is delivered; this has been fueled by the development of minimally invasive technologies and prospective payment based on diagnosis without regard to cost. The result has been a decline in patient days per thousand population from 400 to under 200 for non-Medicare patients. So, there is a growing surplus of hospital beds that will continue to increase as managed care market penetration grows. Medicare patients have utilization rates of over 1800 patient days per thousand in indemnity settings, while managed care Medicare settings (about 8% of Medicare participants) often approach 1000 patient days per thousand population. What's the impact of this drastic decline in patient days? For one, more testing will be shifted to an outpatient setting where commercial laboratories have traditionally dominated.

18.2.4. Higher Inpatient Acuity

As a result of the shift to outpatient care, hospitals have been left with higher-acuity patients. To meet the demanding and urgent needs of these patients, laboratories will have to move toward providing 24-h full-service operation with greater emphasis on stat and point-of-care (POC) testing. For many tests, turnaround time is likely to be measured in seconds or minutes rather than minutes or hours. Providing "next day" or "several times a week" results may be unacceptable to clinicians. Automation strategies must take into account the volume of testing that will be performed in a POC setting, and the need for rapid testing in the clinical laboratory. It is doubtful that the hospital laboratory will remain a focus of outpatient work as more and more testing is centralized in commercial laboratories. So, the laboratory must carefully analyze the kind of testing it hopes to perform. Tests most likely to remain will be typical rapid turnaround time assays like electrolytes rather than specialized immunoassays (e.g., PTH), which are usually performed on outpatients rather than inpatients.

The focus on rapid turnaround time shapes the need for automation. Many commercial laboratories have embraced automation, but they have the luxury of having 12–18 h to produce results from the time they receive the specimen. So, they can establish the most efficient system to process, transport, and test samples. In a hospital laboratory, the demand for rapid turnaround time, defined as less than one hour for many tests, may preclude a commercial lab approach to automation that emphasizes efficiency rather than turnaround time. A hospital lab will have to use automation and new technology to reduce turnaround time (especially pre- and postanalytic components), in addition to enhancing efficiency.

18.2.5. Reimbursement Policies

In an effort to reduce reimbursement, the Health Care Financing Administration (HCFA) division of the Department of Health and Human Resources (HHS) proposed several initiatives to radically change the way Medicare pays for outpatient automated test profiles. These recommendations may profoundly effect how many and what type of lab tests are ordered in outpatient settings. The first proposal requires that all tests in a profile be medically necessary as a condition for payment; requires labs to document medical necessity when 13 or more tests are ordered in a profile; and establishes a uniform method for incremental payment of tests in excess of a 19-test profile wherein each medically necessary test beyond 19 would be reimbursed at $\frac{1}{19}$th of the profile fee. With an average current allowable charge of $16.03, this would mean each additional test would reimbursed at less than $1, a figure that may be less than cost. If enacted, this proposal would encourage smaller profiles, less testing, and would be a further impetus for labs to lower costs through automation. Another proposal, Ambulatory Patient Groups (APG), would reimburse physicians a lump sum for outpatient visits that would include diagnostic lab tests. Since physicians would have to pay for these services directly, there would be an incentive to lower utilization, namely, reduce lab testing.

18.2.6. Networking

In dense geographic locations it is likely that small ($<$ 100–150-bed) facilities may consolidate or pool resources such as labs. So, a hospital lab's strategic plan needs to identify the very nature of the organization, which can affect the need to automate. Hospital laboratories will be faced with few attractive options and are unlikely to remain independent facilities. Most hospital labs will be part of a network anchored by another hospital or a commercial entity. Will it be a "hub and spoke" arrangement that many institutions are investigating today? If so, will the hospital lab be the "feeder" facility (in which case, testing may diminish) or the "central" receiving facility (in which case, testing may increase)? These decisions dramatically change the amount of space required by the laboratory as well as the type of equipment and level of automation. Hospital labs also need to change their mission to include homecare, POC and alternate-site testing. Technology will also play a role in this transformation. As POC testing becomes more cost effective and grows in popularity, some of the needs for emergency testing in "spoke" facilities will diminish. POC will also lessen the need for rapid-turnaround testing facilities and allow the hospital laboratory to achieve some of the savings realized at commercial labs. With POC testing, hospital labs can better serve home care agencies and nursing homes. This expansion is likely to develop into an extensive electronic network that ties all testing entities together.

18.2.7. Staffing

Staffing and automation are interrelated. Technologist shortages of the 1980s have led to a surplus in the 1990s as the hospital laboratory market contracts. Lower reimbursement has fueled attempts to enhance productivity, often through layoffs, while new technologies have provided the means to achieve this goal. Since labor is by far the largest cost in a hospital ($\sim$ 60%) or a commercial laboratory ($>$ 50% in many cases), reductions in personnel have large paybacks.[4]

Another aspect of staffing is the need to provide a safe workplace for laboratory workers. Procedures that only a few years ago were considered routine, such as open centrifugation, are now considered hazardous. The most labor-intensive portion of laboratory testing, specimen preparation and aliquotting, is a certain candidate for hazard reduction. Thus automation will be driven by both the needs to reduce the labor content of an individual test and the need to reduce the exposure of individuals to potentially hazardous material. The greatest focus in the present and near-term future will be on automating the so-called front end of the laboratory. This is being addressed by vendors at the instrument[5] level and at the laboratorywide level.

18.2.8. Impact on Laboratory Automation

What impact are these environmental changes likely to have on clinical laboratories? This is *the* question that laboratories must ask before they embark on large-scale automation projects. Commercial laboratories are likely to experience continued growth and will need to further lower their direct operating costs to win managed care contracts. As competition increases, these laboratories will be forced to find ways to make themselves more efficient and automation will play an important role.

On the other hand, hospital laboratories may experience growth or reduction in testing needs, depending on their role in the "healthcare network." Either way, hospitals can expect higher-acuity patients with ever-increasing demands on turnaround time. Automation will play an important role in providing faster results in an increasingly decentralized testing environment. Outpatient testing is likely to diminish in hospitals as a result of competitive pressures from managed care.

18.3. DEFINE OBJECTIVES

To make optimal use of automation, one must define objectives. Most projects have uniform goals: reduce costs, improve service, improve quality, and create a safer and more attractive workplace. The benefits of automation vary from one lab to the next. For purposes of this discussion, we have classified labs as either commercial or hospital (Table 18.2). In the latter category, labs may function as a hub in a network (and have many characteristics of a commercial facility) or one of the "spokes" (smaller labs with greater emphasis on rapid turnaround time testing). Instrumentation is considered an integral part of the automation planning for any lab, in fact, in some cases it is desirable to replace existing equipment with new equipment that interfaces with robotic sample-handling systems.

Realistic goals and objectives must be set since automation can require a large capital outlay that takes years to recover through reduced operating expenses. Automation does not have to be "complete" or all-encompassing; it can be implemented selectively or in phases, concentrating on critical segments with the greatest potential payback, specifically, the greatest service benefit for the lowest investment in capital and personnel. We refer to this approach as *focused automation*. Some laboratory tasks can be automated at relatively low cost, yet produce large labor savings. For example, a high-volume facility may benefit from automated aliquotting. A hospital may benefit from a tube transport system that replaces messengers. And, all labs might benefit from consolidating numerous manual and semiautomated procedures onto one fully automated instrument; an approach that has been popular in immunodiagnostics. High-payback projects should be undertaken first. Large projects that entail greater capital costs without proportional savings should be undertaken at a later date, if at all, when the technology is more mature and the risk of failure is lower.

18.3.1. The Commercial Laboratory Model

In the past 10 years the number of commercial laboratories has shrunk from 6500 to 4500. Even more astounding is the consolidation of major labs from eight in 1993 to three in 1995. What happens when a commercial laboratory purchases another laboratory? Typically, the acquirer closes a lab when it identifies a market where two or more of its labs overlap. The remaining facility may

TABLE 18.2. Objectives for Commercial and Hospital Laboratory Models

The commercial laboratory
  Increase utilization of existing capacity
  Decrease sample dwell time in lab
  Improve logistics
  Integrate reference test results with existing databases
The hospital laboratory
  Meet stat testing demand and higher-acuity patient testing needs
  Lower fixed overhead expenses
  Reduce labor component of testing
  Reduce space costs of lab to reflect changed operating environment (maximize space utilization)

double its work overnight, thereby providing an opportunity to automate at a level that may not have been financially feasible beforehand. Full-scale automation is usually considered at a volume of about 10,000 requisitions per day. The commercial laboratory industry has only 25% of its cost in the laboratory. The remaining 75% of costs are in the sales, marketing, logistics, and professional side of the business. Of the 25% lab costs, about 60% (15% of total) is supplies and 40% labor. It is labor costs that automation addresses best.

To justify automation, a commercial laboratory must realize one of three objectives: (1) reduce turnaround time to increase capacity (i.e., process more samples) without incurring additional expense, in contrast to a hospital that is trying to deliver a faster result; (2) reduce cost in the form of lower labor and/or reagent consumption; and (3) increase quality, which prevents reruns and enables a lab to compete more effectively for business. Improved worker safety is also a consideration in front-end automation. Robotics and automation have a bright future in the commercial environment since testing is typically standardized and the high volume justifies large investments in capital equipment.[6] Areas of particular interest are initial specimen handling, aliquotting, and transport of specimens to analyzers. Commercial labs have led the trend to consolidate workstations; by running tests based on technology, not discipline, they have been able to lower operating costs.

18.3.2. The Hospital Laboratory Model

Hospital laboratories are seeking automation strategies for many of the commercial lab reasons. However, commercial lab growth prospects come at the expense of hospital labs. The hospital laboratory must review its test menu. Routine testing may decline as more testing shifts to an outpatient basis where commercial laboratories can compete more effectively. Similarly, esoteric tests will continue to predominate in the outpatient setting, where they often play a role in a diagnostic workup. Investigational assays will remain concentrated at large hospitals and universities but benefit little from automation due to their low volume. The one area that hospitals can anticipate growth is stat testing. Some hospitals will experience growth as mergers and consolidations direct more work to certain facilities. These hospitals will become hybrid facilities with some of the characteristics of a commercial laboratory and the requirements of a hospital-based laboratory. Hospital instrumentation is geared to two functions: rapid turnaround time for critical tests and high-volume production for routine tests. Hospitals have typically used multiple systems dedicated to one or the other purpose. This will undoubtedly change as the nature of hospital labs shifts. Fortunately, instrument vendors have stayed ahead of this trend and have introduced many multimode analyzers.

The growth in stat testing will place a premium on rapid turnaround time. Clearly, one objective of the hospital lab will be to reduce testing time to enable physicians to deal with more acutely ill patients. Reducing turnaround time requires a detailed examination of the entire testing process from sample acqui-

TABLE 18.3. Desirable Features for Automated
Hospital Instruments

Stat interrupt capability
24-h availability
Large on-board menu
Long-term calibration
Random-access processing
Short dwell time
Primary-tube sampling
Bar coding (reagent and sample)
Ease of use
Automatic diagnostics and on-line help
Minimal maintenance, preferably automated

sition to result reporting. Instruments play a pivotal role in this lab service chain. Issues such as sample dwell time, on-board test menu, 24-h availability, and stat interrupt modes are critical factors in instrument selection. Table 18.3 outlines some of the major requirements for hospital lab equipment.

How will hospitals pay for automation? It's doubtful that routine testing revenue will finance automation. However, the cost structure of a hospital laboratory is very different from that of a commercial laboratory. The typical hospital spends about 65% of every dollar on labor and about 35% on supplies. So, proportionately, a hospital has more to save on labor than a commercial lab. Hospital testing is more labor intensive because stats must be run 24 h a day; testing cannot be batched to achieve maximum efficiency. Automation can play a key role in reducing the high cost of stat testing, as can some instruments that combine routine and stat testing capabilities. However, new instrumentation is not the only solution to the very high cost of stat testing. In defining objectives, labs need to also consider the role of POC testing and the long term impact of moving tests from a central location to distributed sites. In the future, laboratory staff will likely spend considerable time servicing and monitoring POC testing.

18.4. AUDIT OPERATIONS AND TECHNOLOGY

An audit of laboratory operations requires a comprehensive analysis of all pre-analytic, analytic, and postanalytic steps (Fig. 18.3) in the context of current and future technology and previously defined objectives. Laboratory instrumentation and its integration within a framework of automation ultimately determines the success of a strategic plan.[7] However, an audit should also evaluate the physical facility and mode of service as it relates to automation. One of the best ways to perform this analysis is to trace the sample flow from test ordering all the way to result reporting and sample storage; this identifies potential bottlenecks and opportunities to improve the process. Without a comprehensive plan to deal

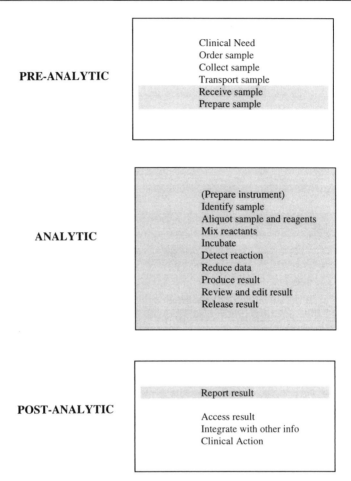

PRE-ANALYTIC

Clinical Need
Order sample
Collect sample
Transport sample
Receive sample
Prepare sample

ANALYTIC

(Prepare instrument)
Identify sample
Aliquot sample and reagents
Mix reactants
Incubate
Detect reaction
Reduce data
Produce result
Review and edit result
Release result

POST-ANALYTIC

Report result

Access result
Integrate with other info
Clinical Action

Figure 18.3. Laboratory testing process: clinical need to clinical action. Shaded areas represent tasks performed by the instrument.

with total sample flow, even labs that automate central operations will not realize all potential savings since in-lab testing is but one component of a larger process. Table 18.4 provides examples of issues that should be considered when auditing operations; these are discussed in greater depth below.

18.4.1. Audit of Preanalytic Operations

18.4.1.1. TEST ORDERING AND COLLECTION. The test order is the first step in any laboratory process; it initiates a chain of events that can be addressed largely through automation. For example, orders generate bar-coded collection labels and analyzers download orders to determine which tests to perform. Automated remote physician ordering (during hospital rounds, or at the office

TABLE 18.4. Some Issues to Consider When Auditing Operations and Technology

Test ordering and collection
   Where are orders placed, in the lab or on the floor?
   Is distributed ordering comtemplated?
   Are samples bar-coded? At the site of collection?
   Does a positive patient ID system exist?
   Who collects samples? When?
Transportation
   How are samples transported? By messenger or automatic system?
   Do all labs participate in the system?
   Are all patient care areas served by the system? Are ICUs served by the system?
   What impact do stat services have on the system?
Identification and centrifugation
   Are samples centrifuged centrally or at site of collection?
   Is there a central processing area?
   Do samples arrive bar-coded?
   How are samples distributed to each lab?
   Does physical layout promote lab efficiency?
Sorting and aliquotting
   Is aliquotting done centrally or in each lab?
   When are samples aliquotted?
   Is a separate sample drawn for each workstation?
   How are samples stored and retrieved?
Reporting
   How are results reported? Through LIS? HIS?
   Are results printed on patient floors? When?
   How are stats reported? How are panic values reported?
   What impact will POC have on reporting?
   Does broadcast paging have a role in reporting?

or home) also ensures that the proper test is selected. In the future, mobile handheld devices might be used to place orders that are then downloaded to the lab's database. Expert systems will also assist physicians with testing algorithms. However, the most automated of systems cannot process tests without an order; this information is required to route and test samples. When tests are performed in a central facility, remote ordering eliminates queuing in the specimen receipt area.

Sample collection can impact total turnaround time to a greater degree than all other components of the testing process. For example, if there is no mechanism for samples to be promptly obtained once orders are written, it is inevitable that long preanalytic delays will occur. Automation cannot solve this problem. Most samples are still collected by venepuncture, although nontraditional sample types (e.g., saliva) and noninvasive monitoring[8] may alter current practices. The sample volume, number, and shape of containers must meet the needs of an automated system. For example: How much sample is needed to centrifuge and aliquot? What container sizes are accommodated in sample processing and analytic equipment? What impact does workstation consolidation have on the number of containers collected per sample? Ideally, bar-coded labels should be produced at bedside (using portable printers storing test orders) or nursing unit. True positive sample identification can be maintained by integrating bar-coded patient identification bracelets into an automatic process that generates labels. This eliminates a source of unexplained laboratory errors that lead to delays.

Commercial laboratories have long understood the benefit of remote ordering and bar-code labeling; it allows a sample to be integrated into a fully automated system as soon as it arrives in the lab. This decreases total processing time, so capacity is increased without additional equipment or space, and economies of scale are realized. An added benefit is improved quality since the paper requisition, a source of error, is eliminated. Remote ordering also allows physicians to create their own practice specific database to which results can be downloaded from the commercial laboratory's host system. The emergence of integrated networks will contribute to remote ordering at the point of care.

18.4.1.2. TRANSPORTATION. How a sample is transported from the collection site to the lab can alter sample integrity and affect turnaround time. Many hospitals use multipurpose, two-way tube transport systems to carry everything from pharmacy supplies to laboratory samples and reports. Transport systems usually have more sending locations (like nursing units) than receiving areas (like lab), so queuing delays may occur at peak periods such as morning phlebotomy. The degree to which this occurs depends on the system's capacity and a variety of other factors: Are all areas served by a tube system? How many samples can each tube hold? Who draws the sample? In a patient-focused care model, several nurses on a unit may be collecting samples instead of a single phlebotomist; so, samples are likely to be sent in separate tubes, thereby increasing "traffic" on the system. Another concern is whether all critical areas are served by the system. Rapid transportation between critical areas and the central lab may eliminate the need for satellite labs; this, in turn, will influence the design of the central lab. Other issues to consider include the frequency with which tubes can be misrouted and the possible implications of transporting potentially biohazardous fluids in the same container as other items such as drugs.

In the future, novel approaches might include a system dedicated to transporting samples from the collection site to the workstation via a carrier, tube, or robot; this would alter the way samples are processed in the lab. Regardless of the approach, tube systems are expensive to install and modify, so they are best designed early in the physical planning process, that is, before a facility is built or renovated. Transportation should be part of an overall strategy to lowering cost and improving turnaround time through automation.

Commercial labs experience even more complex transportation logistics than hospital labs because they are designed around "hub and spoke" branch office networks that typically span a radius of 100 or more miles. To expedite courier dispatch to pick up samples, some labs use the cellular telephone network to track the location of each vehicle. Similarly, by using bar-coded labels affixed at the ordering site, the lab can track the location of each sample in real time.

18.4.1.3. IDENTIFICATION AND CENTRIFUGATION.

When samples arrive in the lab, they must be identified as being "received" and sorted; these tasks can be streamlined by scanning bar-coded tubes automatically or manually. The first significant processing delay usually occurs when serum must be separated for testing. Traditional centrifugation is a multistep batch process, which takes about 10 min. To meet peak demands, most labs require several devices that are staggered in operation. In contrast, continuous centrifugation (e.g., axial centrifugation) holds promise as a more rapid alternative that is easily adapted to a production-line approach since batch processing is eliminated. An alternative to centrifugation is mechanical separation, a batch process that uses filters and/or pumps to yield serum or plasma more rapidly than centrifugation. One drawback to this approach is the cost of disposables.

Centrifugation is a central component to total laboratory automation. However, a focused approach is required since (1) some labs have insufficient volume to justify significant automation, (2) some samples do not require centrifugation, and (3) alternate technologies are emerging that can eliminate the need to separate cells from serum. For example, most POC devices require no sample preparation since they test whole blood.[9] Similar technologies are under development for mainframe systems and may alter the need to centrifuge a large volume of samples. An alternative approach under investigation by a number of vendors is distributed centrifugation wherein the process is integral to the analyzer. One would expect commercial labs to have the greatest need for automated centrifugation. However, this is not the case since most specimens have already been separated by the time they arrive at the commercial lab.

18.4.1.4. ALIQUOTTING AND SORTING.

Most labs still manually aliquot samples in one or more sections. The process consists of uncapping tubes, transferring sample to pouroff tubes, and labeling the tubes. Aliquotting is time-consuming, error-prone, and can create unnecessary exposure to biohazardous material. Early attempts at automating this step were slow and failed to produce bar coded aliquots. These failures occurred because the technology was incapable of fully meeting the real-time needs of the lab. The ideal aliquotting device, of which several are now reaching the market, aspirates sample from a closed container and dispenses it into a bar-code-labeled secondary tube. For this to occur, the primary tube must be bar-coded so the aliquotting device can determine which tests are ordered and what needs to be aliquotted. Aliquot tubes are then sorted by workstation, loaded in rack, and delivered manually or by automated carrier to the appropriate testing area.

Automatic aliquotting is becoming increasingly popular at large commercial facilities since a system in continuous operation can equal the output of up to four workers while also providing greater accuracy and improved safety. However in a hospital lab, the key question to consider is whether automatic aliquoting can save enough labor to justify its acquisition. As workstations are consolidated, there is less need to aliquot; and some facilities find it easier to run a primary tube sequentially on different analyzers than to aliquot sample. On the other hand, aliquotting prolongs sample integrity and storage. It is doubtful that most hospitals will be able to acquire a complete system as they are currently designed. However, they may benefit from integrating specific modules from these systems. Selective automation may be a more economical and practical approach for many hospitals.

18.4.1.5. IN-LAB TRANSPORTATION. After a sample is prepared for testing it must be delivered to the workstation. In hospitals, this task is usually done by lab aides or technologists. However, large commercial labs have developed a variety of automated systems that use special carriers (that course along a track), pneumatic tubes, conveyor belts or shuttles. Some facilities use a robot transport device that is guided down corridors on a scheduled basis. Robotic carts require minimal capital outlay, no alteration to infrastructure (unlike carrier systems) and are easily implemented. However, they are most useful in a commercial setting where there is no immediacy to testing and not in a hospital where stat samples have to be delivered immediately. Regardless of the delivery system, workstation robots can be used to load and unload samples on an instrument. This fully integrated concept is best applicable to large commercial facilities or other high-volume labs. In the future, the need to link transport system and instrument will likely lead vendors to develop standard robotic interfaces instead of today's customized approach.

18.4.2. Audit of Analytic Operations

The central component of any testing process is the analyzer. In many ways, an instrument's design parallels global laboratory operations—it identifies samples, performs tests, and reports results. During the past 10 years, major advances in computers, reagent technology, and robotics[10,11] have led to fewer differentiating features among chemistry analyzers, the largest share of the automated instrument market. To some commercial labs, chemistry systems have approached commodity status with selection criteria based largely on costs. However, differences do exist among analyzers. And while, for the most part, all systems perform as advertised, they may perform differently in various settings. So, from a strategic standpoint the question to ask is not "Does it work?" but "Does it work for me?" For example, a chemistry profiler (e.g., one that runs a specific number of samples per hour) may meet the needs of a high-volume reference lab, but would be inappropriate for a "feeder" hospital running mostly stat tests. Similarly, an instrument with closed-tube chemistry sampling and low throughput may enhance total automation, but it may be the wrong choice for a commercial lab that requires the highest throughput devices.

To select an appropriate analyzer, a laboratory must match strategic objectives with instrument capabilities. Since laboratories have varying needs and analyzers have different strengths and weaknesses, it's helpful to compare attributes among instrument competitors to determine the best "fit(s)." In this section, the authors explore automated instrument characteristics and their relationship to strategic planning.

18.4.2.1. TEST VOLUME. In planning for an instrument, the first issue to consider is test volume. Commercial laboratories typically process large sample batches in a relatively short (8–12-h) period so they need a very-high-throughput analyzer that runs continuously. On the other hand, hospitals have peak periods (usually after the morning collection) followed by low or moderate periods the rest of the day. Hence, appropriate instrumentation differs for these settings.

High-volume systems are usually sample-based, which means that throughput depends on how many samples are processed per unit time regardless of how many tests are run per sample. For example, a 150-sample/h system may produce 3000 results when 20 test profiles are ordered on each sample. However, if two tests are ordered on each sample, throughput plummets to 300 results per hour. Test-based analyzers produce a specific number of results per hour regardless of how many samples are processed. For example, a 600 test/h system can run one test on 600 samples or 20 tests on 30 samples. So, sample density (the number of tests ordered per sample) alters the throughput of sample-based systems but not test-based ones; high density favors sample-based systems and low density favors test-based ones. Commercial labs usually select sample-based systems since most testing is based on profiles; small- to medium-size hospitals usually select test-based systems since emphasis is on single tests and mini- or disease-oriented profiles. Large hospital labs can consider either approach. To evaluate which approach is preferable, the lab should determine sample density and map when samples arrive to ensure that peak demand is also met.

18.4.2.2. TEST MODE. Is most testing stat or routine? Stat testing (found predominantly in hospitals) is very demanding on laboratory operations and instrumentation. Because results are needed immediately, an instrument must be ready to accept a specimen with little delay and minimal queuing. In contrast, routine testing has a much wider window to complete tests, so queuing is less important. While commercial labs usually select a sample-based system to run routine samples, hospitals process tests in stat and routine modes and often consider a test-based system to run both types of tests or a dedicated analyzer for each purpose. Most test-based systems are designed as a compromise; they have adequate throughput for routine testing and a stat interrupt capability; however, frequent stat interrupts may degrade throughput.

18.4.2.3. DWELL TIME. Specimen dwell time (i.e., time from sampling, or sometimes an ID position that precedes sampling, to result availability) is another characteristic related to testing mode and instrument type (sample- or test-based). Dedicated stat systems typically have a dwell time of 1–2 min while test-based systems (for routines and stats) have processing times that range from 2 to 15 min depending on instrument and analyte. Sample-based analyzers have dwell times that range from 12 minutes to 20 minutes depending on sample throughput; faster systems usually have longer dwell times. While dwell time is irrelevant for high-speed analyzers operating in routine mode, it is an important consideration when running stats. In addition to analytic or processing time (i.e., time from sampling to result), the time from bar-code identification to sampling can add to dwell time. On some analyzers, a stat is loaded at the sampling position so it can be processed immediately. On other systems, the stat may have to be placed several positions before the sampling arm so it must wait for preceding samples to be processed; this alters an instrument's ability to meet stat needs regardless of analytic time or throughput. Other instruments can process stats immediately but are unable to read bar codes on these expedited specimens.

18.4.2.4. SAMPLE CONTAINER AND VOLUME. Primary-tube sampling is ideal in hospital and reference labs since it simplifies processing by eliminating aliquoting and sample misidentification that can occur at this step. It's especially useful in chemistry, immunology, and hematology sections where the bulk of automated work occurs. The ability to use a variety of primary-tube types as well as specimen cups is of some importance in hospitals where there is often less control over the collection container than in commercial labs. Sample volume can be an issue in pediatric and oncology settings. Although the analytic sample requirements of most systems is usually in microliters, the "dead" volume of specimen cups can be considerably more. Hematology and blood-gas analyzers also vary in their sample requirements so one must consider how the instrument will be used. Is it for a neonatal intensive care unit (where sample volume is of paramount importance) or adult intensive care units?

18.4.2.5. CLOSED-TUBE SAMPLING. Closed-tube sampling diminishes the effort required to process specimens but more importantly, reduces the risk of blood borne infection for laboratory workers. Hematology analyzers have adopted this feature widely; however, the technology to sample serum/plasma through a closed container has not been as well developed. At this writing, there is only one chemistry system that offers this capability as a fully automated integral part of the sampling unit; however, two other systems offer this feature, one with an off-line preparatory step and another with an on-line step that requires the operator to introduce each tube. Each of these approaches represents a step forward in front-end instrument automation, a process that must integrated with automatic aliquotting and specimen sorting.

18.4.2.6. PROCESSING MODE. Are samples processed in random-access or batch mode? Random-access systems accept samples continuously and process tests in the order that they are requested. Traditional batch systems process many samples for the same test in an effort to produce the most results per unit time; however, new samples cannot be added nor tests initiated once a run begins. Some vendors have designed analyzers with random access and batch features to let the operator run stats in the random access mode and routine samples in the more efficient batch mode. Other systems are "run oriented" in that tests are randomly selected but performed in a batch during which additional tests or samples can't be added. As part of the selection process, a lab should simulate workload on the proposed instrument to determine the impact of processing mode.

18.4.2.7. EASE OF USE. Ease of use is especially important in facilities that operate around the clock. Skills required to run today's systems rely heavily on data management. A uniform vendor interface spanning a family of analyzers can reduce training time for new operators and new systems. Maintenance and complexity also play a role in system usability. Instruments that require long setup times can be suitable for laboratories that process large volumes of tests over a fixed period of time but usually are unacceptable for stat operations that require near-constant instrument availability.

18.4.2.8. REAGENT SYSTEM. Reagents—whether chemistry, immunoassay, hematology, or microbiology—are a major cost component and play a key role in determining overall instrument usability. Reagent systems are "open" or "closed" systems. An open system allows the operator to use reagents that are supplied by both the instrument manufacturer and outside vendors, while a closed system restricts the operator to using an instrument manufacturer's products.

With open systems one can obtain competitive pricing for supplies, which may lead to lower operating costs. And, total costs of operating a system over its lifetime are comprised mainly of reagents, not the instrument capital cost. One problem with using an outside vendor's supplies is that troubleshooting methods may be more complex in that the same vendor is not supporting the instrument and the method. Further, if many outside suppliers are used, the price savings can be negated by the costs associated with ordering and maintaining supplies from different sources and training operators to use different products.

Closed systems, like Ektachem®[12] or Paramax®,[13] use proprietary technology that excludes outside suppliers. In some instances, the reagents are patented; in others, traditional liquid reagents are packaged in a proprietary manner. Closed systems may have higher nominal reagent costs than open systems because of higher production costs and lack of competition. But they usually offer added convenience in the form of minimal reagent preparation and long calibration stability. Some open systems are, in practice, closed because key operating features can be used only with the instrument vendor's reagents. For example, extended calibration, automatic download of reagent parameters, or reagent identification may require the use of the manufacturer's containers or supplies even though the reagents themselves are widely available. This discourages third-party reagents even if it doesn't prevent them.

Most closed systems require no reagent reconstitution since products are packaged in a ready-to-use format. Open systems may require reagent preparation. The key considerations are labor, skill levels, and cost. Keep in mind that reagent preparation may require skilled labor and errors can lead to incorrect results and wasted supplies. Each facility must weigh the convenience of a closed reagent system with the potentially lower nominal costs of an open system. While a large commercial lab may stress lower nominal costs, a hospital lab running 24 h/day may stress convenience.

18.4.3. Audit of Postanalytic Operations

18.4.3.1. SAMPLE STORAGE. After test processing, samples are removed from an analyzer and stored centrally; retrieving a sample can be a monumental task, especially in facilities that process hundreds or thousands of samples each day. Cumbersome manual storage systems are inadequate for large labs; they can benefit from an automated file retrieval system that uses bar codes to track stored samples. In a fully automated approach, samples could be delivered and loaded onto racks identified by x and y coordinates; racks could be loaded into refrigerators and removed when necessary. Sample retrieval is more common in hospitals than commercial labs, in part because physicians are more likely to request that a test be repeated or "added on." So, some degree of retrieval automation could benefit many facilities, even if it only tracked sample storage location.

18.4.3.2. RESULT REPORTING. How results are reported to a physician is an integral part of total laboratory automation; delays in transmitting data can lengthen turnaround time and undermine successful implementation of a strategic plan. For example, a lab that reengineers itself to meet the overwhelming needs of a liver transplant program will meet limited only success if it cannot insure that physicians receive results as quickly as the lab completes them. Laboratories have traditionally relied on hard-copy reports that are either faxed or printed at a remote (e.g., nursing station) or central (e.g., lab) site from which they are distributed. New developments can insure that clinically important results are reported promptly and directly to a clinician; this is an especially important consideration for inpatient testing. One promising approach is to transmit data to personal communicators carried by physicians; data could then be downloaded to a physician's own database for easy recall. Many commercial labs already transmit outpatient data to physician office computers. In another development, information from integrated hospital databases can be displayed at each patient bedside; this promotes patient management at the bedside, including entry of POC test results. When these paperless reporting systems are perfected, there will be little need to transport hard-copy results to a physician, thereby reducing one of the real bottlenecks in the lab process.

18.4.4. Other Considerations

18.4.4.1. PHYSICAL FACILITY. Many labs still have separate sections for chemistry, immunoassay, hematology, microbiology, and blood bank. This can lead to duplication in instrumentation. One should consider whether laboratory disciplines can be consolidated along technological lines. For example, all fully automated analyzers from multiple disciplines (e.g., chemistry, immunoassay, and hematology) may be grouped together. This approach removes artificial barriers that currently exist in many facilities for predominantly historic reasons.

An "open" laboratory—one without physical boundaries—facilitates sample delivery, promotes workstation consolidation and cross-disciplinary testing, and provides the lab with flexibility to adapt its space to ever-changing needs. This design also simplifies the design and implementation of an internal automated sample processing system. In short, "open" labs promote automation; "closed" labs impede it.

18.4.4.2. REMOTE TESTING OPERATIONS. Remote testing operations such as a stat laboratory in the OR or POC testing devices at a nursing station (e.g., glucose meter) or intensive-care unit (e.g., blood gas analyzer) are playing an increasingly important role in most hospitals. The approach to stat labs and remote testing instrumentation must be analyzed in light of recent technological advances since the menu for simple POC testing devices continues to grow.[14,15] For example, a hospital must define current and anticipated remote testing needs: What tests should be done in the intensive care unit or OR? Should blood gases be run in cardiac catheterization or another lab? Should testing be available 24 h? What technology should be used? What is the test volume? What are the costs? All of these issues impact a laboratory's strategic plan for automation. For instance, if all or most chemistry stat testing is moved to remote sites (OR, intensive care unit, etc.), the rapidity with which the central lab's chemistry system performs stats becomes less important; so, a lab may select an analyzer that has a very wide on-board menu despite the long dwell time it may have for stats. Similarly, the decision to run blood gases on traditional equipment versus a handheld device may depend on test volume and who's performing the test.

Robot-controlled stat laboratories[16] allow physicians and nonlaboratory staff to receive immediate results without having to run tests. Sample is placed into a robot, which then introduces the sample to a standard lab analyzer. Robotic laboratories offer the benefit of remote testing and real-time lab monitoring without dedicated on-site staff. In contrast to equipment used in a robotic stat lab, point-of-care testing devices are generally smaller handheld devices that are run by the end user (e.g., physician or nurse). Although this approach eliminates the mechanical complexity of a robot, it offers less real-time lab oversight and relies on the end user to ensure that results are entered in the chart. Planning needs to address how POC testing data can be integrated with other laboratory information.

From a financial perspective, robot-controlled labs are more capital-expensive and require space (albeit minimal); they are best suited to performing repetitive tasks on standard lab equipment and require a moderate volume of testing to justify costs. On the other hand, POC testing, while offering low capital costs, is far more expensive on an operating basis since proprietary (and often unit-dose) reagents are used. However, POC testing is easier for the end user and can be instituted by hospitals with minimal investment of capital and without additional laboratory space.

The integration of point-of-care testing and robotic stat laboratories is key to the long-term automation plan of any laboratory. Laboratories must decide whether it is more efficient to deliver specimens from remote locations to the central lab via a tube transport system or whether it is preferable to establish satellite labs or POC testing to provide rapid turnaround time. These are strategic issues that are not mutually exclusive since automation in the central laboratory combined with point-of-care testing in remote locations can yield an optimal blend: instant results for tests that are required rapidly and longer turnaround time results (usually several hours) for tests run more efficiently and cost-effectively in automated laboratories.

18.5. IMPLEMENTATION

Implementation of your strategic plan is the critical final step in planning for automation in the laboratory. It should also be the simplest if the process has been conducted in a rigorous manner. There are a number of key considerations that can help guarantee success.

The first step is to review all steps in the laboratory associated with a process rather than the particular one that is being considered for automation. This can help eliminate unnecessary steps and prevent rework caused by systematic errors. It is vital that automation change the way the laboratory works rather than merely automate individual steps. Failure to redesign basic processes when a new system is introduced may lead to poor performance. For example, remote ordering should not be limited to entering electronic requisitions; it should be part of a new approach that includes remote bar-code label printers and centrifuges so that samples are completely preprocessed when they arrive in the central laboratory. This redesign must be part of the original project and factored into the anticipated benefits.

The plan should be phased with projects promising the greatest benefit and feasibility started first. A *focused* approach to automation lets a lab automate processes that have a large payback and omit those that are less appropriate because of volume or cost constraints. A good example is specimen transport devices. Few hospitals will ever benefit from a global in-lab automation plan, although almost all can use an automatic tube delivery system. This selective approach also allows the financial benefit to more closely match the laboratory's expenditure. If a modular approach is adopted, additional automation can be considered as instrumentation and/or test volume changes.

Whenever possible, change should be made in a three-step process. Initially all new processes should be conducted in parallel with the existing procedures. Next, a small pilot should be started with the new procedure performed alone. After adequate evaluation and reworking of the new procedure(s), full implementation can begin. Implementation should be phased whenever possible since scaled-up procedures often reveal problems not anticipated or seen in the pilot.

Implementation must be coordinated with departments both inside and outside the laboratory. This is especially important if basic processes are changed. For example, if the laboratory is instituting a POC program, ancillary personnel must be trained to perform the tests, and physicians have to be educated about the new approach. Unless this is properly conducted, the benefits planned from the project will not be obtained. Even when successful, the costs in lost time and credibility can be enormous.

The final implementation step is probably the most important. An audit and reevaluation procedure must be designed before starting the project. Once the new process is under way, it must be periodically reevaluated to ensure that the planned benefits are obtained and, if not, new procedures implemented. A new process cannot be initiated and then ignored for years. For change to be successful, it must be dynamic like strategic planning itself.

REFERENCES

1. Sherer J, Anderson HJ, Lumsdon K: Putting patients first. Hospitals work to define patient-centered care. *Hospitals* 67:14–24, 1993.

2. Holmberg SR: Strategic planning: a management tool for the clinical laboratory. *Clin Lab Management Rev* 2:185–194, 1988.

3. De Cresce RP, Lifshitz MS, Logue LJ: Managed care and the hospital laboratory: survival of the fittest. *Clin Lab Management Rev* 8:472–483, 1994.

4. Benge H, Csako G, Parl FF: A 10-year analysis of "revenue," costs, staffing, and workload in an academic medical center clinical chemistry laboratory. *Clin Chem* 39:1780–1787, 1993.

5. Chow AT, Kegelman JE, Kohli C, et al: Application of existing technology to meet increasing demands for automated sample handling [abstract]. *Clin Chem* 36:1579–1582, 1990.

6. O'Bryan D: Robotics: a way to link the "islands of automation." *Clin Lab Management Rev* 8:446–460, 1994.

7. De Cresce RP, Lifshitz MS: Integrating automation into the clinical laboratory. *Clin Lab Med* 8:759–774, 1988.

8. Ginsberg BH: An overview of minimally invasive technologies. *Clin Chem* 38:1596–1600, 1992.

9. Kost GJ: New whole blood analyzers and their impact on cardiac and critical care. *Crit Rev Clin Lab Sci* 30:153–202, 1993.

10. Lifshitz MS, De Cresce RP: New technologies in chemistry instrumentation: the basis for clinical chemistry automation. *Clin Lab Med* 8:623–632, 1988.

11. Griffiths J: Automation and other recent developments in clinical chemistry. *Am J Clin Pathol* 98(4 Suppl 1):S31–S34, 1992.

12. Shirey TL: Development of a layered-coating technology for clinical chemistry. *Clin Biochem* 16:147–155, 1983.

13. Driscoll RC, Edwards RB, Liston MD, et al: Discrete automated chemistry system with tableted reagents. *Clin Chem* 29:1609–1615, 1983.

14. Lifshitz MS, De Cresce RP: Instrumentation for stat analyses. *Clin Lab Med* 8:689–697, 1988.

15. Jacobs E, Vadasdi E, Sarkozi L, et al: Analytical evaluation of i-stat portable clinical analyzer and use by nonlaboratory health-care professionals. *Clin Chem* 39:1069–1074, 1993.

16. Felder RA, Boyd JC, Savory J, et al: Robots in the clinical laboratory. *Clin Lab Med* 8:699–711, 1988.

19

Workstation Optimization: Need and Steps for Implementation

ROBERT MOORE, KATHLEEN LUCZYK, AND ALAN H. B. WU

CONTENTS

Today, one of the most frequently discussed subjects among laboratorians is the process of workstation consolidation within the clinical laboratory. This topic is of intense interest and represents one of the more difficult problems faced by

Handbook of Clinical Automation, Robotics, and Optimization, Edited by Gerald J. Kost with the collaboration of Judith Welsh.
ISBN 0-471-03179-8 © 1996 John Wiley & Sons, Inc.

laboratory professionals at all levels. The difficulty in resolving this problem is due to at least three factors. First, it requires considerable speculation and subjective assessment of future needs in the clinical laboratory at a time when significant changes are occurring rapidly. Second, the process is being undertaken as a response to events that are beyond the control of the laboratory staff. That is, socioeconomic changes occurring in healthcare are dictating how laboratory medicine is practiced. Third, the laboratory is shifting from a revenue center to a cost center. As such, the laboratory finds itself in the position of having to compete for available business at a time when the demand and reimbursements for laboratory services are decreasing. To be competitive, the laboratory must have tight control over its expenses while at the same time continue to offer a quality product in real time. Although this competition is currently limited to the outpatient market, there are indications that this will be the operating environment of inpatient services where, historically, the clinical laboratory has functioned unchallenged.

In this chapter we will review some of the history that allowed the clinical laboratory to develop its present state and evaluate those factors that are compelling the laboratory to consolidate ("reconfigure" or "reengineer") to meet the challenges of the future. In addition, we will use an example of a large metropolitan laboratory and describe a rational and systematic process that can be implemented in any laboratory to achieve its consolidation goals.

19.1. EARLY GROWTH

Laboratory services began to take a prominent role in patient care several decades ago. Funding of laboratory activities was directly linked to the volume of work. Therefore, money was available to fund technology, research and development, doctoral and postdoctoral training programs, and technical opportunities in the laboratory. The incentive was to do more testing and add esoteric tests to better serve clinical needs.[1,2] This system of increased growth leading to increased revenue made the laboratory a very profitable center in most hospitals. Revenue generated by the laboratory was used to subsidize hospital areas that are clinically necessary but are costly (e.g., dietary, nursing, intensive-care units). The opportunities for profit was also realized by diagnostic companies and instrument manufacturers as equipment was developed to do more testing faster and more conveniently.[1,3]

Automation became very sophisticated. The time required to perform individual tests was reduced to minutes, and it was now realistic to order a chemistry or hematology panel on a patient and have results available in real time for diagnosis and treatment, rather than retrospectively for documenting purposes. Additionally, specimen volume requirements were being reduced, allowing for repetitive testing to actively monitor patient progress. Technology was making faster response times a reasonable expectation, but at an increased cost.

Laboratories were growing in physical size, personnel, and instrumentation at rates faster than other areas in the hospital.[3] This evolution continued with the development of subspecialty laboratories requiring highly trained personnel and sophisticated instrumentation.[4-6] Within the specialty laboratories, a division of labor was created. In the chemistry division of many hospitals, for example, there are separate sections for general chemistry, special chemistry, immunoassays or endocrinology, and toxicology.[7] In hematology, flow cytometric analysis is separate from routine blood counts. This practice has greatly increased the cost of providing laboratory services. The problem now is to reduce these costs while maintaining the high quality of service.

19.2. WORKSTATION OPTIMIZATION PROBLEMS

Table 19.1 lists the various forms of third-party reimbursement. The original fee-for-service system has essentially been discontinued. This was the main source of revenue that allowed laboratory growth as previously described. Today, only a very small percentage of patients receiving laboratory services pay a list fee. This system was replaced by a predetermined fee for service. Under this program a fee would be negotiated in advance and a contractual agreement set up with a responsible party. In this way, laboratory test charges would be known ahead of time, but there were few controls on the number of tests that could be performed. This reduced laboratory revenue some but was still a profitable system.

The government system of diagnosis-related groups (DRGs) was the first serious attempt to contain costs by controlling activity. In this case all similar diagnoses were reimbursed at the same level. This meant that no matter what services were delivered, only a fixed amount would be compensated and if more was spent, the institution suffered the loss, but if you spent less, the institution could keep the total amount of the agreed-on compensation. The incentive was changing from doing more to doing less.[8] Nevertheless, the opportunities for generating revenue still existed because DRGs covered only Medicare patients, which is normally a minority of all patients that a hospital might serve.

The next major attempt to fix the cost of healthcare for third-party payors was the establishment of per diem charges. The rational was to reimburse at a single level for similar procedures on a per day basis and to limit the days of hospital stay. The incentive is to do less and discharge the patient as soon as possible. Under this type of program where the hospital is paid a fixed price for all services rendered, the laboratory becomes a cost center and hence is vulnerable to cost containment programs.

TABLE 19.1. Reimbursement Schedules

Classic fee for service
Predetermined fee for service
DRGs
Per diem
Capitation

Capitation is another of the current approaches to contracted healthcare. An institution must submit a cost "per covered life" without regard to specific services. That is, a dollar amount is paid for the contract period and all healthcare is included in that amount. This places all the risk on the healthcare institution that is awarded the contract.[9] The incentive here is to do the least possible numbers of tests and procedures so as to control expenses more tightly than has ever been required before.

In addition to these basic compensation programs, the awarding of contracts has changed. Contracts are now carrying an exclusivity clause, which stipulates that all the participants (covered lives) in a given insurance program, HMO, PPO, and so on must use specific healthcare providers, including laboratory services for both private outpatients and hospital-based patients. In the past there were significant financial benefits to operating a private for-profit outpatient laboratory while maintaining a separate inpatient laboratory. Under these new compensation and contractual arrangements, institutions can no longer be competitive and maintain this duplication of effort.

As hospitals and outpatient laboratories operate under more stringent reimbursement schedules,[9] survival will require a restructuring of resources. Table 19.2 lists some of the approaches that administrators and external agencies are taking that can have serious implications for the laboratory. All of these efforts are designed to eliminate duplication and costly processes. Smaller and less sophisticated institutions will no longer offer the full array of services as they once did. Networks will be formed to share services. Consequently the more cost-effective operations will increase dramatically in size and scope, while the others will be forced to decrease their operation. For those laboratories whose operations do increase, the challenge will be to assimilate the influx of testing volume at no or very minimal increase in cost. This will put continuous pressure on the workflow patterns that laboratories design and implement.

In addition to sudden changes in volume brought about by administrative arrangements, there will be the issue of flexibility. Any solutions instituted for the current environment must still be flexible enough to adapt to rapid changes that may occur during the next several years. Changes in the physical plant or instrumentation are usually a one-time expenditure but are nevertheless very costly. If flexibility is not part of the plan, then the costs for "reengineering" the laboratory to meet future needs will be prohibitive.[11] This is—and will continue to be—a very dynamic area.

TABLE 19.2. Admionistrative Decisions with Laboratory Service Impact

Corporate acquisitions
Gateway hospitals
National health insurance
Business partnerships
Shared resources

TABLE 19.3. Consolidation Process

1. Evaluate current situation
2. Determine the direction of the laboratory
3. Determine resource availability
4. Evaluate workflow
5. Evaluate physical design
6. Select instrumentation
7. Determine computer capabilities

A simplistic response would be to overbuy or overbuild. The expenses associated with maintenance, consumables, and routine operation as well as other support expenses generally increase as a function of size. It is possible to worsen the laboratory's competitive position with new but oversized additions of space or instrumentation.[12]

Technology continues to evolve, and choices in selecting types of technology can be difficult. There will have to be some risks taken if all the objectives of cost effectiveness, efficiency, low maintenance, and flexibility are to be met. Prudent risks may have a greater return on investments of time and capital than remaining with older technology. Instrumentation has to be evaluated carefully for its future potential as well as its ability to address the immediate challenges.

One approach to laboratory consolidation are the seven steps listed in Table 19.3. Each of these steps has several elements that can be worked on simultaneously. It is important to note that the sequence of events is not critical, and in fact may differ for a given institution. It is also necessary that all the elements are evaluated with objective introspection. The laboratory consolidation process is essentially one of starting with a less efficient, more expensive effort and moving to one of greater efficiency and cost-effectiveness. The route to achieve the final objective is not as important as the achievement of the goal. The overall result of the steps in Table 19.3 is to have at least three definitions. One will define the current laboratory situation exactly. A second will define the position the laboratory wishes to be in after consolidation, and the third will list all changes that are required to achieve that position. Other issues may present themselves as the process continues, but these are the minimum results that should be expected. The last definition may be the most difficult. One change that must be considered will be a reduction in personnel and how to realize that reduction.

19.3. CONSOLIDATION PROCESS

19.3.1. Workflow Analysis and Resources

The objective in workflow analysis is to make the system as tolerant as possible to the requests placed on it. If a principle of "sameness" can be designed into workflow, then there will be a gain in efficiency. Inefficient processes such as STAT analysis, sample splitting, batch testing, specimen transport procedures, and multiple reports violate this sameness principle. Each of these operations creates a special category and handling conditions that will disrupt the normal flow of specimens.

The concept of "STAT" (from Latin *statim,* meaning immediately) tests in a clinical setting is a time-honored tradition. When specimen analysis was slow and tedious, it was logical to give special attention to those specimens that were urgent. Today's technology has made it possible, in many cases, to treat stats as routine specimens, provided the process time is made so short that all results are being returned quickly.

All other sample processing steps should be made as uniform as possible. Anything that requires specimen splitting and relabeling, batch analyzing, or multiple reports should be avoided if at all possible. Figure 19.1 shows how a single hypothetical serum sample requiring general chemistry, hormone, immunoglobulin, and therapeutic drug analysis might be assayed today. Most laboratories would require several workstations to perform the required tests. This is an inefficient process as each workstation requires separate calibrations, controls, maintenance, service, and proficiency testing. The objective of workstation optimization is to consolidate this processing onto a single analyzer if possible, to greatly reduce the effort and costs needed to perform these tests.[12,13]

19.3.2. Instrumentation

Once the number and type of specimens that the laboratory will process have been estimated, instrumentation must be considered. The existing instrumenta-

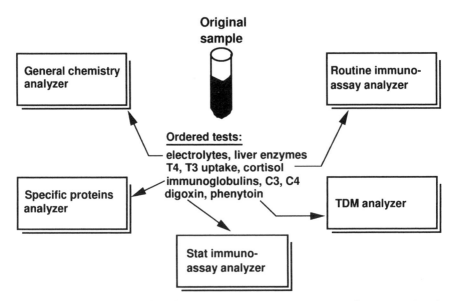

Figure 19.1. Current workflow for a typical sample that has requests for general chemistry, hormones, specific proteins, and therapeutic drugs.

tion must be evaluated in terms of the laboratory's objectives. Features that preclude highly efficient, cost-effective operation must be viewed as serious limitations. If upgrades in hardware and software are not acceptable alternatives, then instrument replacement should be considered.

The reagents used on laboratory instrumentation are an important factor in the laboratory's ability to consolidate workstations. "Closed" systems make use of dry-film reagents or "unitized cartridges" that cannot be modified, altered, or second-sourced. Laboratories are dependent on the priorities of the instrument manufacturer for the introduction of new tests. Most automated immunoassay analyzers are closed systems. Open systems use liquid reagents that can be optimized or replaced by the users. In addition, new assays that may not be important enough for a manufacturer to market can be developed on a "home brew" basis, or adapted through the use of a third-party reagent manufacturer. Competition for reagent contracts between different vendors allow for more aggressive negotiations in the purchase of reagents. In this new environment, a one or two cent reduction in cost per test may be a deciding factor in the laboratory's ability to compete for laboratory services contracts.

19.3.3. Software

Virtually all modern instrumentation has some intrinsic software to handle data and quality-control information. It is a significant advantage if the software can evaluate quality control in real time using some of the generally accepted control rules such as the "Westgard rules."[18] Complete and flexible data reduction algorithms should be available to keep all result calculations as part of the main process. In some instances, off-line calculations are required, but they should be minimized.

Related to the on-board software for data and quality-control evaluation, instruments should have efficient protocols for communicating with other computers. It will be essential to receive demographic and test request information and return results to a host system to keep the flow of specimens and data through the system as uninterrupted as possible.

19.4. THE WORKSTATION OPTIMIZATION MODEL: CASE STUDY

19.4.1. Current Operation and Future Direction

To illustrate the concepts of workstation optimization, we describe efforts currently under way at an 850-bed, private, tertiary-care hospital in the northeastern part of the United States. Table 19.4 lists the features of this facility. All the services listed share the common trait of generating significant numbers of specimens for the pathology laboratory. In evaluating the current situation, and based on 1993 and 1994 occupancy rates, it was apparent that the number of beds would be reduced to 500 or 600. Length of stay (LOS) figures indicated a sharp reduction by 1–2 days, resulting in a LOS from greater than 6 to just over 4

TABLE 19.4. Model Consolidation Laboratory

Private not-for-profit	Pediatric hospital
850 beds	Psychiatic hospital
90 geriatric beds	Corporate hospitals
> 4700 employees	Air ambulance
> 800 physicians	Transplant center
Level 1 trauma center	Dialysis unit
Pediatric trauma center	Oncology center
Outpatient laboratory	20 outpatient clinics
Immediate medical care	

days (a reduction of 17–34%). It is apparent that the use of laboratory services is shifting from primarily inpatient to outpatient locations.

Preadmission lab work and follow-up testing on an outpatient basis is increasing at the institution. Since there is a private, for-profit, outpatient laboratory within the corporate structure, it is logical to combine the laboratories, thereby reducing duplication and achieve maximum cost-effectiveness. Certain components of the outpatient facility such as courier service, specimen processing, and client services would remain intact but the physical testing would be combined with the hospital-based laboratory. This leaves a business structure in place that is capable of marketing all laboratory services responding to client needs and potentially increasing market share without having to increase testing facilities.

Previously the number of employees at both laboratories was at an all-time high and could no longer be supported. One figure that administrators currently use to estimate staffing requirements is four full-time equivalents (FTEs) per bed. This is a total staffing figure, and the laboratory would be allocated on a fraction of this total. Reducing an 850-bed hospital to 600 would mean the elimination of 2300 FTEs from the current staff. There would have to be a significant reduction in FTEs at the outpatient facility, and the remaining personnel would be combined in the single testing laboratory.

There are other hospitals that presently belong to the corporation and negotiations are ongoing for the acquisition of several smaller outlying institutions. These include nursing homes and walkin clinics as well as hospitals. The current approach is to designate these hospitals as "gateway" hospitals. They would treat emergencies and noncomplicated illnesses, but the more seriously ill patients would be transferred to the central institution. Likewise, support services from all institutions, including nonemergency hospital pathology services, would be centralized. Therefore, a significant increase in routine specimens can be anticipated.

Figure 19.2 depicts the changes in patient testing volume with the changes in personnel over a 20-year period for the inpatient laboratory. The fiscal years 1995 and 1996 are projections based on data from those institutions that will be combining services. This reflects only the Division of Chemistry testing, but the trend is similar for other divisions within the Department of Pathology. An

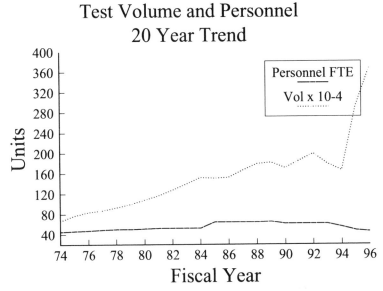

Figure 19.2. Testing volume and personnel beginning in 1974, and projected to 1996 for the hospital used in reorganization model.

anticipated volume of 3 to 4 million chemistry tests per year would exceed the historic high at a time when personnel would be approaching a historic low.

After reviewing the points in Table 19.3, the assessment was as follows:

1. The volume of pathology specimens and testing would continue to grow in a stepwise fashion as centralization of services occurred.
2. Personnel would be reduced by 30–50%.
3. New instrumentation would have to be acquired to meet any of the anticipated demands on pathology services.
4. The laboratory would be expected to support the acquisition of other institutions and the pursuit of healthcare contracts by making cost-effective services available.

19.4.2. Resources and Workflow Analysis

Resources were evaluated in three categories: instrumentation, personnel, and physical plant. Task forces were set up at several administrative levels to determine the current situations required changes if any, and the impact of these changes. The instrumentation that was currently in the laboratory was 10 years old and in need of replacement. The projected increase in volume would have to be considered when selecting replacement equipment. Funds for instrumentation were budgeted before the consolidation study was begun. This is an idiosyncrasy of the capital budgeting process where the budget is submitted 12–18 months before implementation. Minor increases in budgets the first year would be tolerable if the long-term result was a reduction over current spending levels. Overall operating budgets and personnel would be reduced.

The physical workflow of the model workstation consolidation concept is diagrammed in Figure 19.3. Critical to this concept is that specimens move through the system with as little special treatment as possible, irrespective to their labeled status of "ultra-stat," "stat," or simply routine. One way to achieve this is to surround the central receiving and processing station (area 1, Fig. 19.3) of the laboratory with blood-gas analyzers and all routine *high-volume* testing instruments (area 2). The latter category would include analyzers for general chemistry, therapeutic drugs (e.g., theophylline, anticonvulsants, antibiotics), urine screens for drugs of abuse by immunoassay, automated immunoassays (e.g., thyroid function, fertility), routine hematology (blood counts), coagulation (PT, aPTT, fibrinogen, etc.), and urinalysis.

Non-stat, low-volume, or medium-volume tests not available or conveniently assayed on high-volume instruments are placed into area 3 of the design shown in Figure 19.3. Some of the assays and instruments found in that area include serology and autoimmune markers (hepatitis, HIV, TORCH titers, ANA, etc.), specific proteins (prealbumin, IgE, apolipoproteins, etc.), electrophoresis (serum, urine, CSF proteins, hemoglobin, isoenzymes, immunofixation, etc.), low volume therapeutic drugs (cyclosporine, quinidine, methotrexate, ethosuximide, etc.), liquid chromatography (tricyclic antidepressants, urinary porphyrins, urinary catecholamines, etc.), thin-layer chromatography (L/S ratio, drugs-of-abuse testing, amino acids, etc.), and other immunoassays not yet available or unlikely to be available on automated analyzers (tumor markers, parathyroid hormone, insulin, C-peptide, etc.).

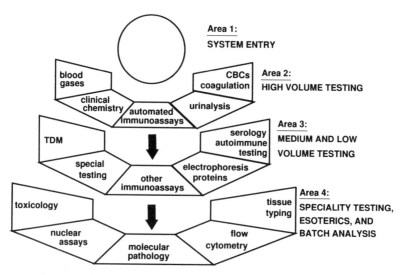

Figure 19.3. Proposed workflow using the optimization model.

Area 4 would be reserved for the esoteric testing, batches, and assays requiring extended processing. These analyses might include forensic toxicology (chain-of-custody documentation, gas chromatography–mass spectrometry, etc.), nuclear assays (estrogen and progesterone receptors, Schilling tests, RBC survival, etc.), molecular pathology (DNA probes, PCR amplification, etc.), flow cytometry for special hematology, special coagulation (factor assays, platelet function tests, etc.), and tissue typing (HLA, paternity, etc.). Few hospitals will be able to offer these highly specialized services in the future environment. For large hospitals and universities, it is quite possible that activities in area 4 could be housed on another floor or another building. Testing that has special considerations such as high security with limited access for chain-of-custody requirements or cleanrooms for DNA procedures may necessarily be isolated. However, unlike areas 2 and 3, where turnaround time is of primary importance, area 4 activities will allow for longer processing times.

The design shown in Figure 19.3 allows a first-in, first-out (FIFO) process to be maintained to utilize a minimum number of processing and laboratory testing personnel. There is an alternative design that may be useful in some special instances. That would be to move specimens vertically rather than horizontally through a system.[14,15] The negative feature of vertical systems is their costs. It usually costs more to move samples to another floor, either mechanically or by people, than it does to move them on the same level. In addition, more technicians and some instrumental duplication will probably be required.

19.4.3. Physical Design

The existing floorplan was not conducive to grouping instrumentation and processes in one general area. The current laboratory has some features—such as a slow tube system for specimen transport from critical-care areas—that are not optimally placed for the new design, but are very expensive to relocate. Consideration was also given to traffic patterns that would develop once couriers with outpatient samples were mixed with delivery procedures for inpatient samples.

A design group was formed that included laboratory directors, administrators, the chief engineer, and an architect from a private consulting group. Several plans were drawn and evaluated as to the objectives and costs.

19.4.4. Instrumentation

The features that were considered a requirement for any selected instrument in the model laboratory are listed in Table 19.5. Although the instruments selected were a chemistry analyzer and an immunoassay analyzer, the requirements are similar for all high-volume automation. For chemistry analyzers it is essential to have a large number of tests on board so that as many routine requests as possible can be completed on a single pass. Combined with reagent systems that have a long on-board shelf life and stable calibration curves, this feature will prove to be very cost-effective. In the example shown in Figure 19.4, new clinical

TABLE 19.5. Instrument Characteristics for Optimum Workstation Consolidation[a]

Random access	Multiple specimen type
High throughput	Multiple container type
Rapid turnaround time	Minimum technologist time
Large on-board inventory of tests	Minimum maintainance
Long stability times for reagents	Low intrinsic cost
Stable calibration curves	Efficient electronic data reduction and QC
Open system	Efficient inter-computer communication protocols

chemistry analyzers now exist that enable all the tests shown to be performed on a single instrument. Homogenous immunoassays such as Enzyme Multiplied Immunoassay Technique (EMIT, Syva Co., Palo Alto, CA),[16] and Cloned Enzyme Donor Immunoassay Technology (CEDIA, Microgenics Corp., Concord, CA)[17] and antibody-based nephelometric assays enable testing for some hormones and proteins, therapeutic drugs, and urine testing for drugs of abuse onto a general chemistry analyzer.

Specific instrument selection was achieved in the model laboratory using the steps listed in Table 19.6. The first step was to evaluate the characteristics of available high-volume instruments and, on the basis of generic information, invite potential vendors to present their product. Flow Diagram 19.1 depicts the

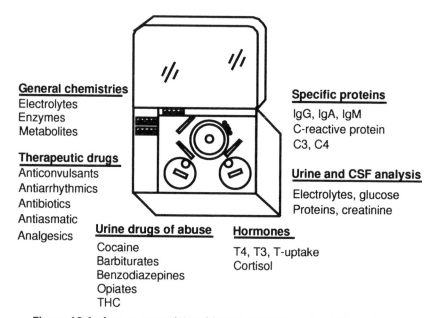

General chemistries
Electrolytes
Enzymes
Metabolites

Therapeutic drugs
Anticonvulsants
Antiarrhythmics
Antibiotics
Antiasmatic
Analgesics

Urine drugs of abuse
Cocaine
Barbiturates
Benzodiazepines
Opiates
THC

Hormones
T4, T3, T-uptake
Cortisol

Specific proteins
IgG, IgA, IgM
C-reactive protein
C3, C4

Urine and CSF analysis
Electrolytes, glucose
Proteins, creatinine

Figure 19.4. Assays compatible with new generation chemistry analyzers.

TABLE 19.6. The Process

Vendor presentations
Initial selection
Site visits
Worksheet and data entry
Detailed analysis
Contract negotiation
Purchase

process of selecting vendors for presentations. The initial phase was to decide whether the instrumentation met some general requirements of the laboratory. That is, would the instrument be compatible with the proposed lab design? Did it meet some preliminary requirements for cost-effectiveness such as competitive pricing on hardware and replacement parts, as well as maintenance agreements? Does the instrument have future potential so obsolescence is not a practical problem?

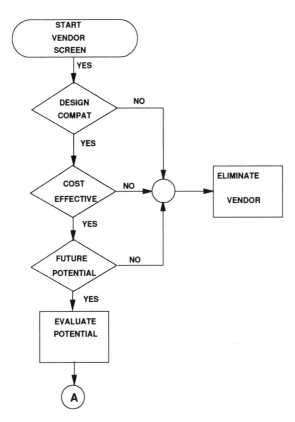

Flow Diagram 19.1.

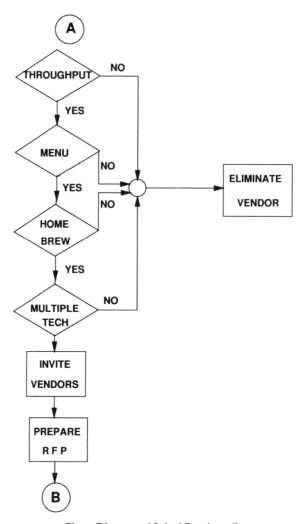

Flow Diagram 19.1. (*Continued*)

Path A defines future potential in terms of throughput capability, menu development, the ability to add our own tests under the "home brew" classification, and whether the instrument is capable of multiple analytic techniques. Can multiple-wavelength spectroscopy be done as well as nephelometry or turbidity? If the answer to any of these questions was "no," then the vendor was eliminated from the screen.

The surviving vendors were invited to give presentations, requests for proposals (RFPs) were prepared, data were collected, and a choice was made as depicted in the last section of Flow Diagram 19.1. If performance were not acceptable, the vendor data would be reevaluated and the second selection made and the process repeated.

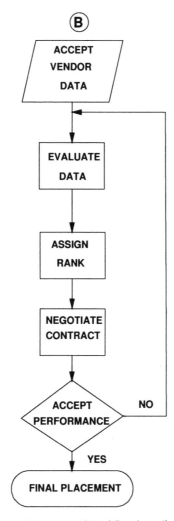

Flow Diagram 19.1. (*Continued*)

There were approximately ten vendors that took part in this initial phase. This presentation lasted about an hour and covered all aspects of the instrument system except cost. Financial data was not a part of the initial presentation since most vendors would not be pursued and the financial workup would take considerable time on the part of all parties.

After the presentations were made, a technical task force reviewed the information and chose the best three candidates. Each of these vendors was contacted, and site visits were arranged at institutions that had volume and test mix conditions similar to those of the selecting institution. It should be pointed out there are at least two caveats with this process. First, the site visit must be to a similar institution. Instruments operating under significantly different condi-

TABLE 19.7. ILAB

Deciding factors
  60 reagent bottles per 900 analyzer
  Open system
  High throughput
  Strong laboratory information system (optional)
  Cost-effective
  Corporate commitment

tions either in terms of volume and mix of samples or in time of operation (e.g., 8 h vs. 24 h) may be misleading in terms of the performance expected at the new site. Second, instruments may be so new that they do not yet have comparable placements in the field. Although this may be a concern and should be evaluated thoroughly, this should not by itself eliminate an analyzer as a potentially valuable instrument. This situation should be evaluated on a case-by-case basis, with consideration given to the resources at the new placement site to support the installation and startup of the instrumentation.

Once the site visits were concluded, all the information for the candidate instruments was compiled in a spreadsheet. The data were entered into a personal computer using a commercial software package. Every aspect of the instruments was listed. Each item was carefully evaluated, and if changes in the laboratory were required to accommodate the instrument, the cost of these changes was estimated by the hospital's engineering group. If any of the candidate instruments was deemed not acceptable, it was eliminated and the remaining vendors were asked to submit precise financial information based on both current and projected volumes of activity.

The task force reviewed this data on a continuing basis and arrived at a decision as to the best fit for the laboratory objectives. Table 19.7 lists the major factors that the ILAB instrument (Instrumentation Laboratory, Lexington, MA 02173) offered the selecting laboratory. It was felt that the significant number of on-board tests represented a major advantage over other instruments. Some of the other points in Table 19.7 are only slightly better than or equal to existing instrumentation. Contract negotiations were conducted to include both on-site and off-site training, biomedical engineer training, costs for an evaluation period, and a "failure to perform" clause. Other issues may be important at other

TABLE 19.8. Projected Impact

Element	Old Lab	New Lab	% Change
FTE	60.8	45	−26.0
Instruments	31	22	−39
Main lab volume	1,286,273	3,668,781	+185.3

TABLE 19.9. Reconfiguration Impact on Testing

System	No. of Tests	% Testing
ILAB	50	80
Immunoassay	25	5

institutions, but it is easier and generally less expensive to determine these issues and have them included in the purchase price or lease/rental agreement.

After the instrumentation was placed and partial implementation of the overall workflow design achieved, the projected savings were reevaluated to determine any significant variance from the original projections. Tables 19.8 and 19.9 list the projected changes. As seen in Table 19.8, the new laboratory configuration should result in a 26% personnel savings coupled with 39% fewer instruments and an increase of 185% in volume of testing. These figures take into account only the high volume testing that would be assigned to area 2 of Figure 19.3. Table 19.9 shows a weighted average for chemistry test orders. When the chemistry analyzer and immunoassay analyzer are combined, a total of 85% of all tests ordered in chemistry can be performed on receipt of the specimen.

Workstation consolidation is a process that all clinical laboratories will be faced with sooner or later.[19] Changes in healthcare delivery, reimbursement, and organizational structures will require the successful laboratory to be work-efficient and cost-effective. Although there are risks with workstation consolidation, the risks associated with doing nothing are considerably worse.

ACKNOWLEDGEMENTS

The authors thank Dr. Pennell Painter, The University of Tennessee Medical Center at Knoxville, for his assistance in providing references.

REFERENCES

1. HEW: *Planning the Laboratory for the General Hospital.* US Dept Health, Education, and Welfare, Public Health Service Publication No. 930-D-10.

2. Melville RS: Automation and its impact on the Clinical laboratory. *RI* (Rhode Island) *Med J* 54:497–520, 1971.

3. Block L: An in-built growth factor is essential in laboratory planning. *Hospitals* 40:103–108, 1966.

4. Owen SE, Finch EP, Byers WH: Good design steps up laboratory production. *Mod Hosp* 91:128–130, 1958.

5. Martina M: Laboratory planning. *Hosp Progress* 41:114, 1961.

6. Armstrong M, Fraser R: Clinical laboratories designed for a teaching hospital. *Can Hosp* 31:41–43, 1954.

7. Wield D: Future planning of pathological facilities. *Br Hosp J Soc Serv Rev* 77:770–772, 1967.

8. American Association for Clinical Chemistry: *The Periodic Report,* Oct 1994.

9. Coile RC: Capitation: the new food chain of HMO-provider payment. *Hosp Strategy Rep* 6:9, July 1994.

10. American Association for Clinical Chemistry: *The Periodic Report,* Sept 1994.

11. Ruys T: Projected need for change. *Lab Management* 8:28–29, 1970.

12. Lifshitz MS, Cresce RP, eds: *Clin Lab Med* 8, 1988; 4:759–774.

13. Castaneda-Mendez K: Re-engineering: is it right for your lab? *Adv Lab* Sept 1994.

14. Clinical Laboratory Automation Solutions by Lab-Interlink, 1011 South Saddle Creek Road, Omaha, NE, 1994.

15. Markin RS: Clinical laboratory automation systems: concepts, designs, and future directions. *Clin Lab Auto* 1–42, July 1, 1994.

16. Rubenstein KE, Schneider RS, Ullman EF: Homogeneous enzyme immunoassay. A new immunological technique. *Biochem Biophys Res Commun* 47:846–852, 1972.

17. Henderson DR, Friedman SB, Harris JD, Manning WB, Zoccoli MA: CEDIA, a new homogenous immunoassay system. *Clin Chem* 32:1637–1641, 1986.

18. Westgard JO, Barry PL, Hant MR, Groth T: A multi-rule shewhart chart for quality control in clinical chemists. *Clin Chem* 27:493–501, 1981.

19. Luczyk K: Preparing the laboratory for the year 2000: workstation consolidation. Paper presented at the Clinical Laboratory Management Association, Orlando, FL, 1994.

CHAPTER

20

Process Control and On-Line Optimization

STEPHEN MIDDLETON AND PAUL MOUNTAIN

CONTENTS

Handbook of Clinical Automation, Robotics, and Optimization, Edited by Gerald J. Kost with the collaboration of Judith Welsh.
ISBN 0-471-03179-8 © 1996 John Wiley & Sons, Inc.

20.1. REDEFINING THE LABORATORY PROCESS

An examination of process control and optimization begins with an understanding of the boundaries of the process. Historically, attempts to improve efficiency and effectiveness have focused on the sequence of events that begins with the arrival of the specimen in the laboratory and concludes once the results are generated by the analytical equipment. When seeking opportunities for optimization, the boundaries must be rethought. In the role of a provider of diagnostic information services, the laboratory's responsibility begins at the time the physician first requests the service and is completed only when the required information is in the hands of the physician. This redefinition of the laboratory is illustrated in Figure 20.1.

Working from the "circle of service" definition illustrated in Figure 20.1, it is evident that an optimized process can be achieved only if all points of interaction and transformation that occur around the circle are examined. The complex and dynamic sequence of events that take place within the walls of the laboratory must be supported by ordering, collection and transportation processes that are optimized to the needs of both the client and the automated laboratory. The real-time monitoring of steps and the production of a specimen suitable for automated handling (i.e., machine-readable label on a standard collection container) should be achieved at the earliest possible point in the cycle. Similarly, the

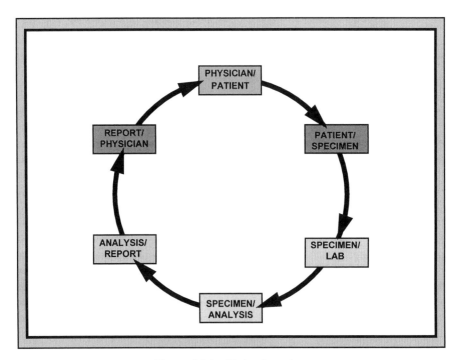

Figure 20.1. Circle of service.

delivery of the information to the physician must include consideration of the total quality of the service. An optimized process will predictably deliver the right information to the right place, at the right time, at the right cost. The "right information" will include the value added through the knowledge embodied in the laboratory worker and designed into the laboratory systems.

An understanding of the scope of our role and the value we expect to add to the diagnostic process should be a living part of the design, implementation, and ongoing operation of the automated laboratory. Working within these terms of reference, we can focus on the complex and challenging task of designing and maintaining an optimal automated laboratory process, without losing sight of the importance of the whole cycle.

At the simplest level, the laboratory can be viewed as a flow of materials, a flow of information, and a series of activities that must be performed to maintain and manage the process. Traditional workflow diagrams combine material, information, and activity to give an overall picture of what happens. For the purposes of automation, although the two are interrelated, the material flow is modeled separately from the information and activity process ("process flow"). A specimen exists in the material flow as an object on which certain actions must be performed (e.g., transport and handling). The same specimen can also be said to exist as a "data store" or repository for information both created and used by the process (e.g., receipt date/time, routing, appearance and volume). Optimal designs for both the material flow and process flow are required. The design must ensure that the right actions are taken at the right time, either automatically or through operator participation or intervention.

20.1.1. Material Flow

The design of an optimal material flow begins with a thorough understanding of the existing flow. This includes creating a map of the current state and identifying the key steps and sequences. The elimination of redundant steps and repetitive loops of activity is an essential procedure when deciding what to automate. The design shown in Figure 20.2 was created by a team of laboratory technologists and technicians (i.e., current state experts), facilitated by experts in systems engineering and process control. The products of material flow design are as varied as the individuals and groups working in the field of laboratory automation. The flow described here is not by any means offered as the one right solution. Rather, it is intended to illustrate the thought process and offer insight into the factors which should be considered when designing a flow that is optimal for your laboratory.

In Figure 20.2, specimens arriving in STS (specimen transport system) boxes have been previously order-entered and bar-code-labeled at the point of collection. At the unpacking station, a decision is made as to the suitability of the specimen (i.e., container type) for automated processing. Specimens classified as "other" typically nonstandard containers, are routed to a manual handling area. All "standard" specimens, as defined by the constraints of the automation, are routed to the automated transport line. In-line quality assurance checks

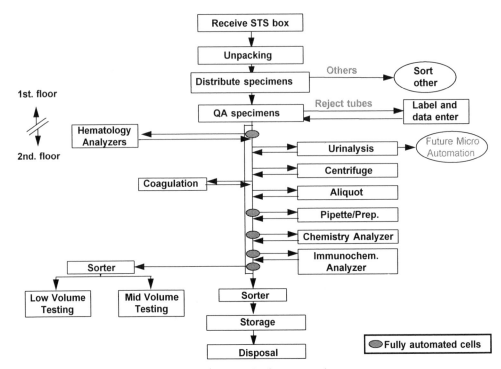

Figure 20.2. Material flow—specimen.

identify problem specimens (e.g., unreadable label) and remove them from the system for operator attention. All specimens allowed to move past this point are suitable for automated handling.

The analytical area of the lab has been designed such that specimens received in a test-ready state (e.g., routine hematology and urinalysis) are diverted off the main transport line at the earliest opportunity. Other automated cells are sequenced in the requisite order: centrifuging must occur prior to the coagulation cell, aliquotting must take place before the specimens can move to the preparation, chemistry, and immunochemistry cells. The pipetting and preparation cell serves two primary functions: the preparation of specimens for HDL cholesterol analysis (the largest volume) and the preparation of any dilutions required for repeat testing. The workcell is positioned to facilitate the largest-volume task. In order to allow specimen movement "back" to previous cells in the line, the transport system is configured as a continuous loop. The loop design also provides flexibility for the addition of future work cells which may not, due to space constraints, be able to be placed in the optimal sequence. Once processing through the automated section is complete, the specimens are routed to one of two sorting stations. Specimens that require testing outside the automated loop are sorted into workstation groups for the low- and mid-volume areas of the lab. Specimens needing no further testing are sorted to storage. In addition to specimens, the flow of reagents, consumables and waste must also be considered. The laboratory model illustrated in Figure 20.2 is complicated by the fact that the operation spans two floors. The problem of completing the materials loop was addressed through the use of a vertical storage carousel system that links the first and second floors. In this way, reagents and consumables can be moved from the loading dock on the first floor directly into the carousel and removed on the second floor as required. Conversely, specimens are placed into storage on the second floor and removed for disposal on the first. The entire system is driven by bar codes and under computer control.

20.1.2. Process Flow

Process flow modeling creates a series of pictures of the various processes through which information is generated and used, and defines the logical relationships between those processes. The models that result are typically much more complex than the material flow models. It is not within the scope of this chapter to provide a detailed description of the modeling process or the use of these tools; for more information, the reader is referred to other sources.[1] Figure 20.3 shows the highest level of process model for our sample automated laboratory. The diagram identifies seven major types of processes or activities

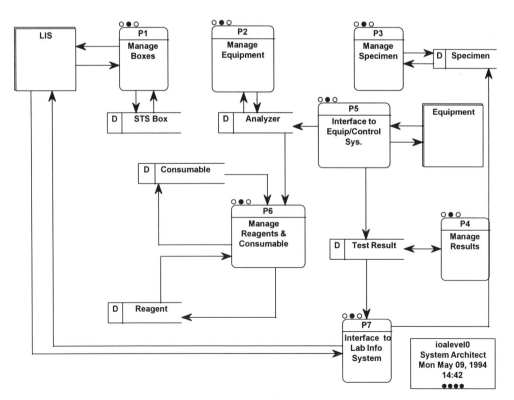

Figure 20.3. Data flow diagram.

(P1–P7) and a variety of data stores (D). The flow of data into or out of a process is indicated by arrows. Moving to an intermediate level of detail (a step called "decomposition"), Figure 20.4 shows the layer behind P3. At this level eight subprocesses (P3.1–3.8) are identified and the associated data flows are labeled. Still more detailed information, called "primitive levels," would be found beneath each intermediate level process.

Ensuring that the process flow is complete and that the logic is intact is both essential to the viability of the final system and at the same time an extremely complex task. The use of a computer-assisted systems engineering (CASE) tool can be invaluable when constructing a complex process model. Such tools help manage and properly identify the multiple levels of the process and check for problems in the logical relationships between the various parts.[2]

20.1.3. Simulations

Computer simulation can provide a sensitive analysis of the proposed automation, allowing the design team to compare performance goals to a prediction of how the system will actually perform once built. There are a number of commer-

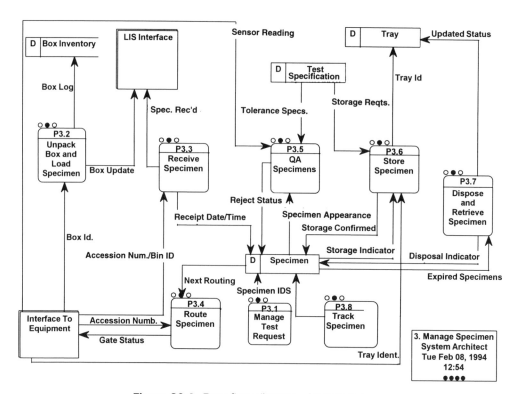

Figure 20.4. Data flow diagram—intermediate.

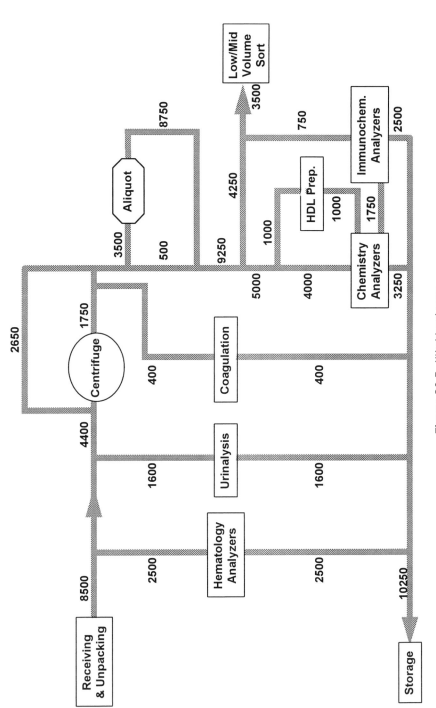

Figure 20.5. Workload map.

cially available simulation packages.[3] Alternatively, the service can be contracted from a consulting group or may be available from the automation vendor. Given the large capital investment required to build an automated system, using simulation to test design assumptions is strongly recommended.

The simulation variables should include, as a minimum, workload distribution (Fig. 20.5), specimen arrival pattern and individual component capacity and availability. The output should include overall specimen dwell time, specific dwell time for various routing patterns and identification of bottle necks. The program should allow various assumptions about future workload increases, changes in arrival patterns, and different component capacities. For a more detailed discussion of simulation modeling, see Chapter 5.

Once an optimally designed process is translated into a real setting and the automated laboratory goes "on line," the operator faces the challenge of maintaining optimal performance. To manage such a complex and dynamic technology based system successfully, an extensive "toolkit" and powerful user interface are required. The process management/control system must enable the operator to manage all components of the automated laboratory effectively. These components can be grouped under three major headings: managing the specimen, managing the equipment and managing the products (includes both quality and results).

20.2. MANAGING THE SPECIMEN

Laboratory information systems typically track patients and tests. However, the specimen is the physical and information entity with which the automated system must deal. Audit trails and tracking mechanisms must uniquely follow and account for each specimen throughout its life cycle. The cycle begins at the time of collection with the assignment of a unique identifier to each specimen container and continues through transport, preparation (during which additional uniquely identified specimens may be created), analysis, archiving and disposal (Fig. 20.6a).

In a traditional laboratory process, the number of available audit points may be as limited as order entry, specimen receipt at the lab, and result release. Only the receipt verification step deals with the actual specimen, while from order entry combined with result release one can conclude that a specimen did in fact exist. In an automated process the goal should be to approach as closely as possible the ideal of continuous tracking. As bar-coded specimens interact with more and more automated modules and thereby generate additional audit points (Fig. 20.6b), we can move closer to this ideal. A process control system, examining this information in real time, can maintain a current-state picture of the status of an individual specimen and provide information about the overall flow. As the theoretical model of what should occur during the specimen cycle is supplemented with actual records of what has occurred, the process control system can extrapolate to provide information about specimen status between

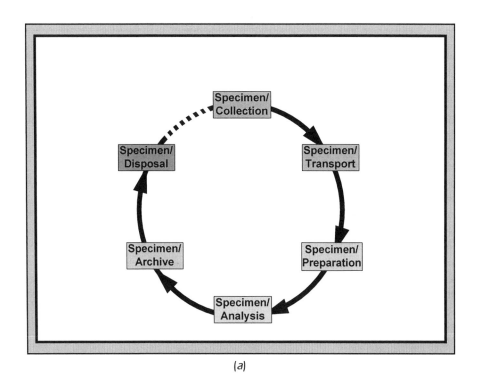

(a)

(b)

Figure 20.6. (a) Specimen life cycle; (b) specimen tracking and audit trail.

audit points. The potential exists to open a virtual window through which the laboratory professional can view the entire process. This capability is a powerful addition to the operator's optimization toolkit.

The specimen tracking and adult trail illustrated in Figure 20.6*b* is broken down as follows (numbers refer to points in Fig. 20.6*b* flow diagram):

1. Request for testing generates bar-code labels in preparation for specimen collection.
2. Labeled primary tubes are ready for transport and/or preanalytical processing.
3. Tubes may be processed on site or transported to another location. Some primary tubes are suitable for direct testing, while others may require centrifugation and separation. The relationship between transport containers, primary tubes, and any newly created secondary tubes is maintained through bar-code labels and tracked by the computer system.
4. Tracking continues through the analytical process by means of bidirectional interfaces.
5. An inventory of stored specimens facilitates recovery for repeat or reflexive testing and the management of specimen disposal.

20.3. MANAGING THE EQUIPMENT

In the past few years the laboratory definition of "automated equipment" has changed. In addition to analytical equipment, we must now include such items as robotics, various transport mechanisms, centrifuges, aliquotters, and pipetting/preparation stations. In current usage, the term "interface" no longer refers only to the transfer of test requests and results between analyzers and the laboratory information system (LIS). All of these automated devices must be able to interact physically with various other components in the system (analyzers with robots, robots with transport mechanisms, etc.), communicate through the process manager with those other components, and receive instructions or commands about interactions.

The operators in automated laboratories will not be able to be continually present at each piece of equipment in order to ensure that all is working as it should. Automated systems must be remotely operable in the sense that any operator must be able to monitor total system status from any process manager terminal—in other words, a true "walkaway" system (Fig. 20.7). Operators will need to know that current instrument status is within specification and be notified immediately of any alarms or alerts that occur. Real time access is required to such information as reagent and waste levels, maintenance status, problem-solving assistance and utilization. Integrating this type of information into process manager displays will allow the operators to be sure that the equipment can handle both the existing and expected workload, that all procedures required to ensure proper function have been carried out, and that events requiring

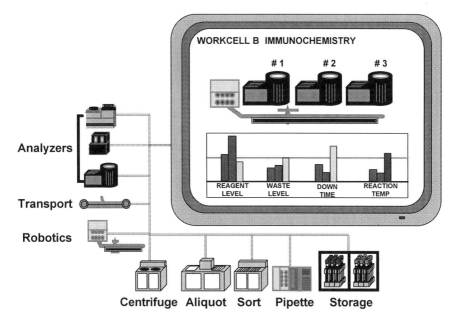

Figure 20.7. Managing the equipment.

intervention (replenish reagent, empty waste, etc.) are identified and acted on before they result in partial or total system shutdown.

20.4. MANAGING THE PRODUCT

20.4.1. Quality

Quality control procedures in a batch environment are typically historical in nature, providing a picture of what has happened over time. From such pictures it is possible to make decisions about the probable reliability and utility of the results produced in a particular time period. With the use of real-time process management technology comes the opportunity to redesign the quality control procedures. The goal now becomes one of supplementing the *what has happened* picture with a continuous view of *what is happening now.* Protocols for automated systems should be flexible (i.e., applicable across a range of methods and disciplines) and provide for real-time analysis so as not to limit the rate of specimen processing.

The automated process utilizes control specimens with known performance characteristics as the first-line validation of instrument performance. The number and frequency of controls is based on the clinical significance of the assay along with the established and observed reliability of the method. Wherever possible, QC specimens should be introduced to the system in bar-coded containers in the same way as patient specimens.

Given that the control sample results are acceptable, ongoing analytical performance can be monitored through the real-time calculation of patient means and the precision of repeated results. If a potential problem is detected, the QC system will alert the operator and call for the introduction of known controls (Fig. 20.8). An optimal combination of controls will be recommended on the basis of the patient result indicators. In order for the mean values of patient results to provide a sensitive indication of system quality, results must be normalized before they are included in the mean calculation. At the time of writing, algorithms are being developed for the selection of "normal" results, the evaluation of population distributions, and the optimized selection of known controls.[4]

Even with automated analysis, known control specimens can only confirm system performance at disparate points in time and provide statistical clues as to the system performance during the time between measurements. The real-time computing power of the process manager provides the opportunity to look in new ways at the quality control information inherent in the most continuous flow of data available—the patient results. Extracting this value in a manual QC process would be simply too costly. The implementation of process management technology provides an opportunity to add quality without adding cost.

20.4.2. Results

Test results are the core of the clinical laboratory's product. Our goal should be to add as much diagnostic value to the results as is reasonably and practically

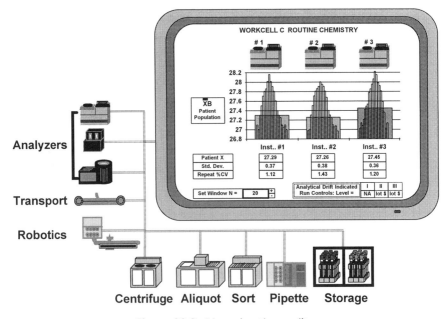

Figure 20.8. Managing the quality.

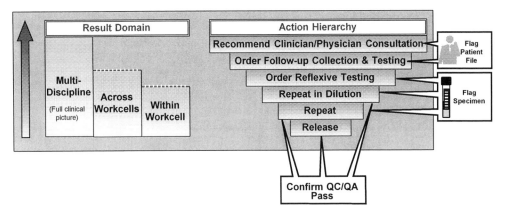

Figure 20.9. Managing the results.

possible before reporting to the physician. The application of expert rules in the process manager will allow a significant expansion of what is considered reasonable, practical and possible. Within its expert knowledge base, the process manager can contain the rules routinely applied (time and workload permitting) by the most expert and experienced of the laboratory's personnel. These rules may cover the relationships expected between results within a particular workcell, results from different workcells connected to the process manager, and results from the patient's previous visits. Before the specimen is released back to the transport system, decisions about reporting, repeating, and repeating in dilution can be made and incorporated into the specimen record and routing instructions. Rules that trigger reflexive testing algorithms, follow-up collection and testing, and physician consultation may also be incorporated (Fig. 20.9).

The power and value of the real-time expert system lies in the rapid and reliable application of rules which cover the routine or predictable decision making required in the laboratory process. The overriding "rule" in all situations is that if the variables observed do not precisely match those designed into the knowledge base, then the process manager alerts the operator and the problem is transferred to the human expert for interpretation. Given this "prime directive", the unmatched speed with which a computer system can appropriately select and apply expert rules offers an exciting, and possibly unparalleled, opportunity to add value to the diagnostic information we provide.

20.5. INTEGRATION AND OPTIMIZATION

All the "techno-tools" and capabilities we have discussed have a single fundamental purpose, which is the provision of high-quality laboratory service at the right cost. The changes resulting from automation are changes of tools and methods, with the major effect being the way in which the human value is added to the service. If there is a single guiding principle, it might be summed up as "people serving people through automation." The value of the technology can be measured in the degree to which it assists people in the application of their knowledge and expertise to the provision of an effective service. The extent to which the automation is successful will be determined largely by the way in which the control and management of the information and materials-handling technologies are integrated in the process manager. Later in this chapter we will discuss the nature of the change experienced by people as the workplace moves from a largely manual to a highly automated environment. It is important to emphasize at this point that while many aspects of the laboratory process become simpler in the automated setting (e.g., the streamlined flow of materials and the elimination of repetitive or redundant steps), the technological environment becomes far more complex. In designing a process manager workstation, which is the operator's window on the technology, the aim must be to render a highly complex system in an intuitive user interface.

Figure 20.10*a* shows the relationship between the pieces of the automated system, the process manager and the laboratory information system. In this design, the process manager is positioned to control all aspects of the automated process. Communication with the LIS consists of receiving orders and sending back reportable results. All analytical, preparation, and handling equipment is interfaced directly to the process manager, replacing the existing bidirectional interfaces between the LIS and analyzers. An architecture could be designed in which the LIS–analyzer interface is maintained for the purpose of transferring orders and results. The positioning of the process manager in the illustrated architecture was driven by the goal of providing the operator with a single integrated tool for the management of specimens, equipment, quality control and results.

Within the automated area, system decisions are made at three levels. At the workcell level, PLCs (programmable logic controllers) or PC controllers make extremely rapid decisions about workcell operation (e.g., the coordination of robot and analyzer movement). In the process controller, decisions may take an order of magnitude longer, perhaps one-tenth of a second (0.1 s). These decisions typically deal with the comparison of monitored variables to acceptable ranges, the detection of unusual events, the triggering of alerts or alarms, and the referral of more complex decisions (e.g., abnormal result analysis) to the expert system. In the expert system layer activity proceeds at a much more leisurely rate and may require 1–5 s for the delivery of a decision. A generic list of functions handled by the process manager is shown in Figure 20.10*b*.

Of particular interest is the availability of real-time expert system products that offer simulation capability and more recently, neural network modules for process control applications. Access to simulation modeling within the process manager represents an optimization tool of great value. It is then possible to ask questions such as "what if next month work load increases 15%" or "what if we install a new analyzer with 20% faster throughput." The application of a neural network, with the ability to identify and learn about relationships between

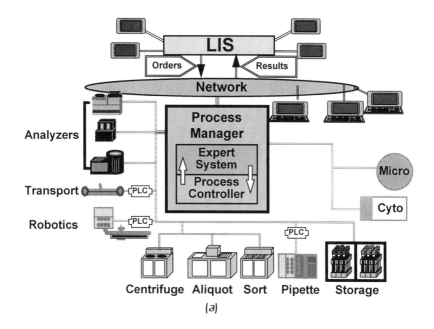

(a)

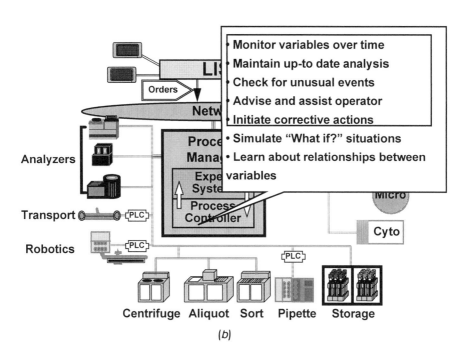

(b)

Figure 20.10. (a) Information control architecture; (b) information control architecture, showing process functions.

highly complex sets of variables, holds such potential as predictive problem identification and targeted preventive action. As the first fully integrated laboratories are commissioned, the investigation and evaluation of these powerful tools promises interesting and exciting possibilities.

The internal structure of the process manager used in the architecture described above is shown in more detail in Figure 20.11. The real-time expert system and process control modules were built using commercially available platforms. Originally, these products were designed for applications such as refinery, high-speed manufacturing and power plant control systems. The interface between the expert system layer and the process controller was available off the shelf, as was the PLC interface required to control the transport and robotic systems. These products also offer interface toolkits which facilitate the development of LIS and analyzer connections. Of special note is the graphical user interface (GUI) toolkit. This feature allows for the rapid development and ongoing live modification and enhancement of user screens. Using this tool, members of the laboratory team operating the automated system will be able to create new displays and continually improve the user interface once the system is in production. This means that as service goals change and/or new key indicators are developed, the operating team can modify the GUI so that it continues to meet their needs.

The integration of specimen, equipment, quality control and result management in the fully operational process manager, is illustrated in Figure 20.12. As illustrated, the process management system is monitoring the status and

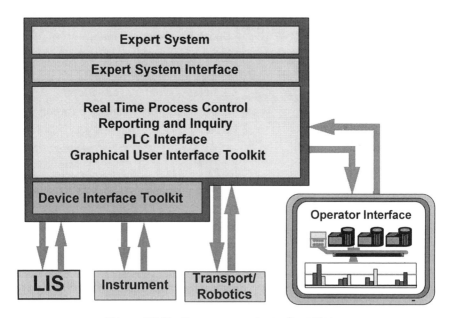

Figure 20.11. Process manager configuration.

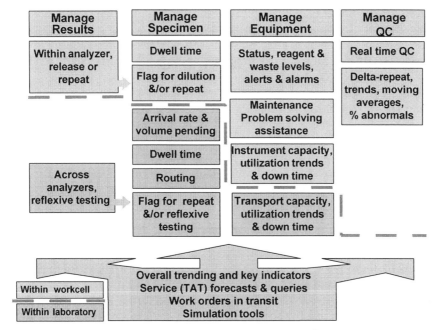

Figure 20.12. Process manager—integrated functions.

controlling the operation of all equipment in the automated line. The operator is kept apprised of the status of key variables and immediately informed if alert or alarm situations occur. The system directs specimen to the appropriate work-cells and instructs analyzers as to the required tests. Decisions about result validity and options to repeat, dilute, or initiate reflexive testing algorithms are made in accordance with the expert system rules. All decisions about continued operation and acceptability of results are made with ongoing reference to the QC parameters. As all the data is consolidated and analyzed, the operator is provided with a real-time picture of the current state of the laboratory operation. Overall trends can be displayed and key indicators calculated on a continuous basis. Forecasting of service level (e.g., average turn-around time) and information about work pending and/or in transit is also available. When the ability to manipulate the current-state information in simulation mode is added, a previously unattainable degree of accuracy in planning for future requirements becomes possible.

20.6. PEOPLE AND TECHNOLOGY—CHANGING THE WAY WE WORK

The way in which people work in the new environment will be a determinant of the extent to which optimization will be achieved. In the past, laboratory workers have been dedicated primarily to the tasks within the analytical workstation to which they were assigned. Functions included the loading and unloading of instruments, the initiation and completion of batches, the transfer of information, and troubleshooting. Only a fraction of available time could be spent in the application of clinical expertise to the interpretation of information, managing the delivery, and improving the quality of laboratory service. In the automated setting, the laboratory worker is no longer dedicated to the manipulation of materials and information within a single workstation. Enabled by the technology, staff can bring their expertise to bear on the full laboratory process. This enlarged scope of activity will necessitate changes in laboratory structure, roles and responsibilities of individuals, and reward and recognition systems. The potential benefits include continuous quality improvement, more effective operations, more challenging jobs, and a higher level of motivation and satisfaction for laboratory professionals.

20.6.1. Focus and Function

Changing the way we work will begin with changes in what we think about in our work. As the tasks that previously occupied the major part of the laboratory worker's time are handled by automation, and the current state is rendered on a second-by-second basis by the process manager, the focus will shift to the importance of trends and patterns of change. With an understanding of how things are changing over time, the operators will be equipped to deal with possible future developments and to participate in planning the changes that will be required to manage those developments (Fig. 20.13). While the changes in the nature of laboratory work promise new and exciting roles in the future, this will not be accomplished without a great deal of stress and dislocation.

Health-care organizations worldwide are experiencing pressure to drive down cost. The indications are quite clear: there will be fewer people working in clinical laboratories in the future. Reduction in cost may be achieved in part through the reduction of service, and where the service is overutilized, this is quite appropriate. However, when the pressure to reduce cost is matched by pressure to improve the quality or accessibility of services, laboratories must look to technology as an enabler.

On the positive side, as traditional laboratory jobs decrease in number, the emerging automation industry is creating new jobs. The design, testing, manufacture, marketing, sales and support of automation technology are all sources of job opportunity. The dislocation arises from the different skills and expertise required to enter these new jobs and the fact that in the near term the rate of job creation will not match the rate of job loss. Over time, new ways of creating value through the application of knowledge will be explored and enabled by technology. The experience gained by laboratory workers who participate in the transformation of the workplace, even as their own roles disappear, will equip them to take advantage of these new opportunities.

Those people who make the transition into new laboratory roles will also experience high levels of stress and a sense of dislocation as the nature of their

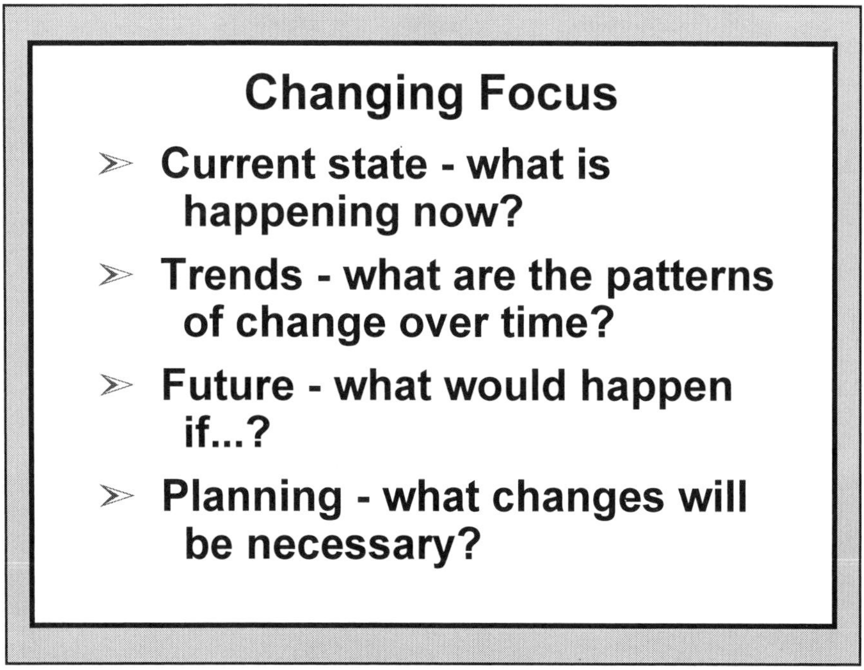

Changing Focus

➢ **Current state - what is happening now?**

➢ **Trends - what are the patterns of change over time?**

➢ **Future - what would happen if...?**

➢ **Planning - what changes will be necessary?**

Figure 20.13. Changing focus.

work changes. Changing from a largely manual to a highly automated environment involves a fundamental change in the nature of work (Figure 20.14). In a manual setting, work is task-based. Experts take action directly on materials and equipment,[5] and the tools or technologies used are typically well understood. When variances occur, the reasons can be determined by reference to the expert's knowledge base[6] (i.e., sum of training and experience). In an automated environment, process expertise is most highly valued. The scope of the technology involved is greater than the knowledge base of any one individual. When variances occur in this setting, they are likely to appear to be random, as they are not clearly a part of a logical cause and effect chain understandable by the operator. In a clinical laboratory, random variances rapidly produce high levels of stress. The role of the expert is to monitor the process and, in response to variance, bring team problem-solving skills to bear. The sum total of the operating team's expertise must be able to identify the source of the variance and initiate corrective action (which may in some instances be a decision to call in outside experts). Given a high degree of reliability in the automated system, these crucial skills must be maintained even though they are used infrequently. The basis for performance measurement will become participation in team problem-solving and decision processes and the interpersonal coordination and communication skills[7] required for effective participation.

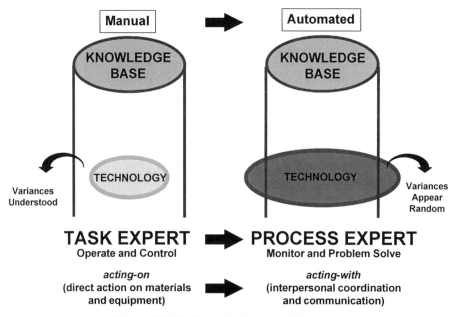

Figure 20.14. Changing focus and function.

20.6.2. Structure

The structure emerging from the examination of the impact of automation on laboratory work is based on teams and functions, as opposed to hierarchy and specialized departments. Multiskilled operating teams, with a high degree of self-direction and a broad range of responsibilities, are essential if the complex technologies and processes of the integrated laboratory are to be managed effectively. A group of laboratory staff involved in designing an automated system produced the original version of Figure 20.15, in an early attempt to communicate some of the magnitude of the coming change. When presenting the drawing to laboratory management and coworkers, they stressed the different nature of the individual responsibilities and organization pictured in the two halves of the diagram. On the left is a traditional laboratory structure and workflow. Specimens are sorted into batches and delivered to various departments. Within departments, there are separate workstations, each with its own staff, equipment and information. Pictured on the right is a laboratory in which specimens are transported discretely in a continuous flow. Instruments that were previously located in separate departments are now integrated into one high-volume production line. There are fewer people, and they are jointly responsible for the operation of a system which crosses several clinical disciplines (i.e., hematology, chemistry, immunochemistry, and specimen receiving and distribution). The implications for the traditional laboratory structure are obvious—this is definitely not only about changes in bench-level jobs! It is worthwhile noting that, in

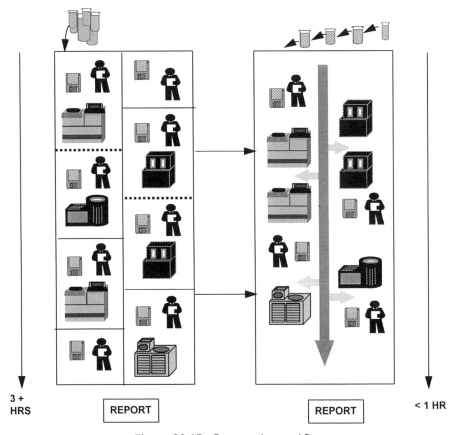

Figure 20.15. Comparative workflow.

addition to the forecast manpower saving, when the continuous-flow model was simulated, specimen dwell time (receipt to result release) in this central reference laboratory, decreased from an average of 3 h to less than 1 h. Also, as a result of the smoothing of workflow through continuous flow, analytical equipment had the capacity to handle double the existing workload.

20.6.3. Roles and Responsibilities

Job and team design must be undertaken in preparation for working in a new structure with new types of responsibilities. The range of skills that will be required by an operating team must be identified and structured into new jobs. The team structure pictured in Figure 20.16 combines core skills with the various types of specialist expertise required to operate an automated laboratory which combines hematology, chemistry and immunochemistry testing. The diagram was created early in the design process for our sample automated facility.

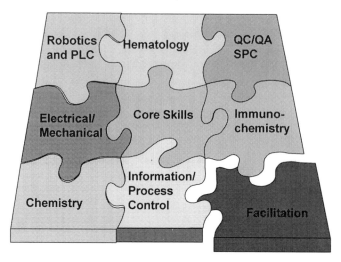

Figure 20.16. The operating team.

Core skills training includes process analysis, teamwork and problem solving, change management and information systems. Ensuring that the team has the specialized clinical skills is a clear requirement. Examination of the team responsibilities identified three additional "specialist" roles. The information and process control specialists are experts in the process management system. They are able to design and develop new user displays and work directly with programmers on more complex system enhancements. This expertise enables the teams to continually improve the tools with which they maintain optimal system performance. The robotics and PLC skills are now included in the Electrical/Mechanical specialists responsibilities. These team members provide the front line service for the materials handling and robotics components of the system. The QC/QA and SPC (statistical process control) skills have been incorporated into the core skills requirements. Facilitation is provided by another specialist position called the "team leader" (a title selected by the staff involved in the design of the teams). The "team leader" position should not be regarded as a reworked senior technologist/technician role, as is illustrated in the following extracts taken from the general overview of team structure and responsibilities, which supplemented the job postings:

- There will be no "rank" on teams.
- Specialists do exactly the same work as anyone else—except that they also lead problem solving in their area of speciality, and sign off as required.
- "Team leaders" are simply "facilitation and communication specialists"— not "the team boss."
- Team members have ongoing and continuous quality improvement projects. There are constant efforts to improve everything.

- The team sets its own priorities. They are guided by a coach, who is responsible for the clear communication of management objectives to the team. However, within those objectives the teams direct themselves.
- No task is too demeaning for any team member. When it is time to dispose of expired specimens, the hematology specialist or team leader is just as likely to be doing the task as anyone else.

20.6.4. Rewards and Recognition

We have seen that automating the laboratory goes far beyond the implementation of transport systems and robots. Roles, responsibilities and expectations change as do the criteria by which we judge an individual's performance and contribution. It follows that the way in which performance and contribution are recognized and rewarded must also change. The difficulty with designing compensation to suit new jobs and new ways of working is the absence of comparators. The first fully integrated automated laboratory systems on line will serve to clarify these issues. We can anticipate that it will take most of the first year of operation to understand the new workplace properly. This time will be used to work through the issues of how to evaluate the performance of individuals and teams, how to value different combinations of skills, and how to relate performance and skill to reward and recognition.

The redesign of reward and recognition systems begins with the hiring process. Understanding the criteria by which people will be judged good candidates for the new jobs is a first major step in understanding what should be valued highly. Also, a significantly different hiring process sends a very clear message that expectations are changing. In the reference laboratory which we are using as an example, all jobs in the automated area were considered to be new positions and were posted as such. All staff were invited to apply. A commitment was made that all positions would be filled by internal applicants and that appropriate training would be provided. This commitment extended to all specialist positions. Figure 20.17 shows the outline of the hiring design created by a project team comprised of staff members and organizational development experts.

The traditional hiring interview focuses primarily on what a candidate says and how it is said. The new process adds direct observation of how a candidate behaves in team problem-solving situations, and how well existing knowledge is applied in new circumstances. As the first teams are hired, the model must deal with the problem of hiring for jobs for which no one has direct previous experience. In these circumstances, the applicants must be judged on their behavior and an assessment of aptitude. The top line of the model describes the three stages of the process leading up to final selection and indicates the two points at which preselection screening of applicants takes place. The boxes below give a general description of the abilities that the section is designed to evaluate. A hiring team typically consists of six to eight people representing the stakeholder groups listed in the model. The same hiring team screens all applicants for a particular position. This model has been successfully used with more

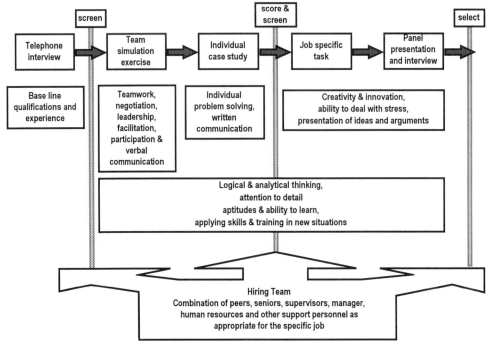

Figure 20.17. The hiring process.

than 120 candidates, most of whom applied for more than one of the available positions.

20.6.5. Motivation and Staff Satisfaction

The years of education and experience, embodied in the skilled laboratory technician or technologist, should not culminate in the manipulation of test tubes or transcription of information. Most of the skilled worker's time is currently spent in what can only be described as "life imitating automation". The value of the human contribution lies in our capacity for critical judgment. Education and experience should find purpose in the application of knowledge to creative decisions and interpretive processes. The implementation of automation technologies has the potential to free workers from the routine and repetitive tasks and provide powerful tools to enhance the application of human knowledge. This result is not, however, a foregone conclusion. Two very different future scenarios have been described. In one possible future, knowledge and control are transferred to the technology "at the expense of human capacity for critical judgment",[8] resulting in loss of meaning and motivation and leading to apathy or adversity. In the alternate vision, "leaders recognize the new forms of skill and knowledge needed to truly exploit the potential of [the new technology]"[9] and the new work provides "unprecedented opportunities for a wide range of employees to add value to products and services".[10]

New technology seems to require a more flexible and self-directed workplace if optimal performance is to be achieved. The technology does not, however, guarantee this result. The outcome is clearly a product of the choices we make when designing and developing the automated workplace. In studying the experiences of workers in a pulp mill during the implementation of computer controlled automation, Zuboff[11] observed significant changes during the time leading up to and following implementation. Beginning in an atmosphere of dread that in the future, the plant would have no roles of value for people, workers developed a sense that the technology was providing access to new types of information and adding a new intellectual dimension to the job. In the authors' experience with a large laboratory automation project staff began with mixed emotions, which included a large proportion of anger and apprehension and some excitement. The anger and apprehension were related to the disruption and uncertainty that the change entailed and the excitement arose from the opportunity to work with the new technology. As the project progressed, a shared sense of pride and accomplishment was described by team members as they began working together, setting and meeting their own goals.

It is possible to create an automated laboratory in which motivated and self-directed teams derive a high level of job satisfaction. To realize this potential, staff motivation and satisfaction must be an integral part of the design. Achieving an optimal laboratory process requires the combination of optimally designed material and data flow systems, with the right roles, responsibilities, and structure. To maintain the process at optimum levels in a dynamic and complex environment, we must add highly motivated staff, with the right combination of skills and abilities, to manage the technology.

REFERENCES AND NOTES

1. Brathwaite KS: *Systems Design in a Database Environment.* New York: Intertext Publications/Multiscience Press, McGraw-Hill, 1989; Kowal JA: *Behaviour Models: Specifying User's Expectations,* Englewood Cliffs, NJ: Prentice-Hall, 1992.
2. Examples of CASE tool software include **System Architect,** Popkin Software and Systems; **IEF,** Texas Instruments; **LBMS,** LBMS Inc.
3. Examples of simulation software include **ProModel,** ProModel Corp, Utah: **Witness,** AT&T ISTEL, UK; **Arena,** Systems Modelling Corp, Philadelphia.
4. MDS Laboratories QC2001 Quality Management Team, with Dr J Westguard. The completed scheme will use an automated version of the Westguard QC Validator product, for control optimization and a real-time statistical process control package, for analysis of patient result data.
5. Zuboff S: *In the Age of the Smart Machine—the Future of Work and Power.* New York: Basic Books, Harper & Collins, 1988.

6. Goodman PS, Sproull LS & Assoc: *Technology and Organizations*. San Francisco: Jossey-Bass Publishers, 1990.

7. Zuboff S: *In the Age of the Smart Machine—the Future of Work and Power*. New York: Basic Books, Harper & Collins, 1988.

8. Ibid.

9. Ibid.

10. Ibid.

11. Ibid.

12. Other technology references: Penzias A: *Ideas and Information—Managing in a High-Tech World*. New York: Norton, 1989; Dreyfus HL, Dreyfus SE: *Mind over Machine—the Power of Human Intuition and Expertise in the Era of the Computer*. New York: The Free Press, Macmillan, Inc., 1986.

CHAPTER

21

Reengineering Clinical Laboratory Processes

RALPH E. FARNSWORTH AND LAWRENCE C. MAGUIRE

CONTENTS

21.1. INTRODUCTION

With the growth of knowledge and technology in medical science there has been a corresponding growth in the number of available options for treating patients. Because this growth has come from a past where we had little knowledge, all improvements were judged to be of value and worthy of use and support. Large sums of money were made available for these improvements. At first, because

Handbook of Clinical Automation, Robotics, and Optimization, Edited by Gerald J. Kost with the collaboration of Judith Welsh.
ISBN 0-471-03179-8 © 1996 John Wiley & Sons, Inc.

there were few new advances, the added costs were small. As knowledge grew and opportunities were seen to make financial gain from new services in healthcare, costs have increased steadily until American society is now unable and/or unwilling to continue to support these escalating costs as they have in the past.

The real question being asked by American society is not whether we should have quality healthcare, but why must it cost so much, and what services and technology offer the best results. These are not easy questions to answer. The people of the United States are now mandating that these issues be addressed. Because they are of such complexity, and there is no one right answer, the government is in conflict as to the right solution. However, major areas of agreement do exist, and healthcare reform will require and include certain features. The new system must (1) be less expensive overall and per unit of service, (2) provide coverage for the entire population, (3) be flexible and fair, and (4) be able to document its value and quality. Our goal is to provide satisfaction for patients, physicians, and third-party payers. Quality, cost and turnaround time are the basis by which the clinical laboratory will be judged.

Laboratories of today cannot expect single instruments or collections of "islands of automation" alone to adequately meet this magnitude of change, but must look to more integrated automated systems that are organized and based on new methods, techniques, and technologies. The principles of total quality management must also be included as intrinsic elements.

Healthcare reform will soon be a reality. If all its elements are not implemented immediately, they will be eventually. Healthcare delivery as we have known it is gone and will never return. Unless we face this reality and work to respond productively, we will be left behind both philosophically and economically. The clinical laboratory can be successful under healthcare reform by using techniques successful in industry, such as "business reengineering."

The clinical laboratory will be challenged with more work at reduced compensation, and as a result, the laboratory must respond with (1) reduced cost per unit test, (2) increased capacity, (3) improved data management, (4) new services, and (5) expanded capabilities.[1,2] Business as usual is doomed. We must reinvent clinical laboratories to compete in the new era of managed care competition and healthcare alliances.

21.2. CLINICAL PROCESS REENGINEERING

These changes are not a reason to be despondent; they are a challenge to those of us in healthcare to preserve from the past what was of most value and use new methods, knowledge, tools, and experience that we as a society have to achieve and exceed the goals the American people have set for us.

As these events are occurring in the healthcare industry, the nation's technology continues to evolve, with particular success in the manufacturing and industrial sectors. The development of industrial technology has been stimulated by foreign competition and the need to provide higher-quality products at a lower cost. The result has been the successful resurgence of those American industries

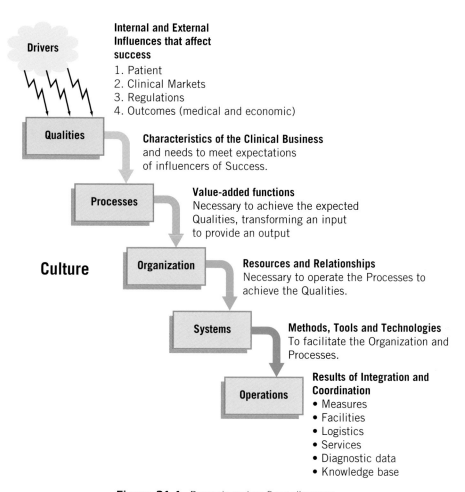

Figure 21.1 Reengineering flow diagram.

that have responded to the challenge by "reengineering" their businesses and processes to optimally take advantage of new technologies and techniques (see Fig. 21.1, color plate).

Advances made in industry can and should be applied to develop and deliver a more cost-effective healthcare system.

21.2.1. Reengineering Defined

Business reengineering is the fundamental rethinking and radical redesigning of business processes to achieve dramatic improvements in critical contemporary measures of performance, such as cost, quality, service, and speed.[3] To provide true success in the automation of the clinical laboratory it is necessary to approach the problem through *total quality reengineering*. This process initiates a critical look at the real needs and goals of the laboratory, based on (1) business drivers, (2) strategic objectives, and (3) goals for ongoing improvement.

21.2.2. The Clinical Laboratory Business

In the healthcare industry, clinical laboratories are the most similar in their structure, functions, inputs, and outputs to existing industrial enterprises. An input (specimen) is collected, processed (material handling), work (analysis) is performed on it, and a finished product (reliable data) is distributed to the customer. A good portion of the work performed in the laboratory is labor-intensive materials handling, sample separation, redistribution, analysis, quality control, waste management, and the acceptance and distribution of data.

Strategic business reengineering must be driven by laboratory personnel, but with the total support of top management, by demonstrating the vision and leadership necessary to accomplish organizational effectiveness and attain substantial advantage. The clinical laboratory is an area with great potential for dramatic improvement in costs, quality, efficiency, and capacity while reducing the exposure of hazardous clinical specimens to healthcare workers. Ideally, a unified system of specimen handling integrated with analysis and the laboratory information system is needed to provide specimen transportation, tracking, manipulation, analysis, and reporting. All this can be accomplished without human intervention or exposure (see Fig. 21.2).

21.2.3. Clinical Process Reengineering

A major lesson learned from industry is that *a successful business is constantly challenged to overcome the habits that have lead to success in the past.* Future success is assured by using a process that structures goals and plans to objectively discover fresh ideas, processes, and methods.

Achieving competitive success will depend on transforming the laboratory's core processes into strategic capabilities that consistently provide *superior value to the customer.* This requires identifying "customers" (Fig. 21.3), and develop-

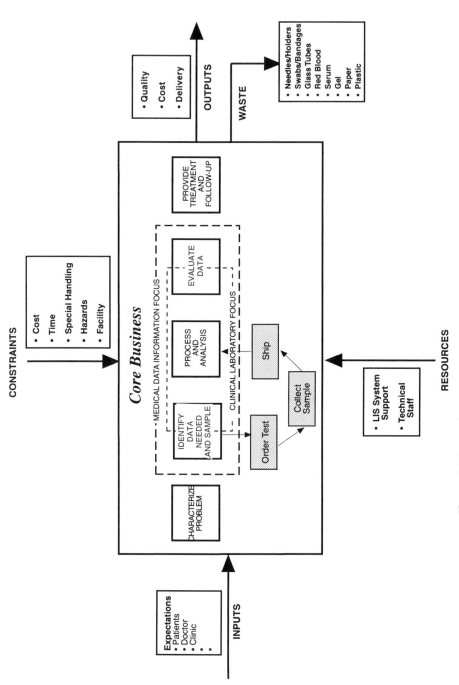

Figure 21.2. Medical specimen processing system life cycle.

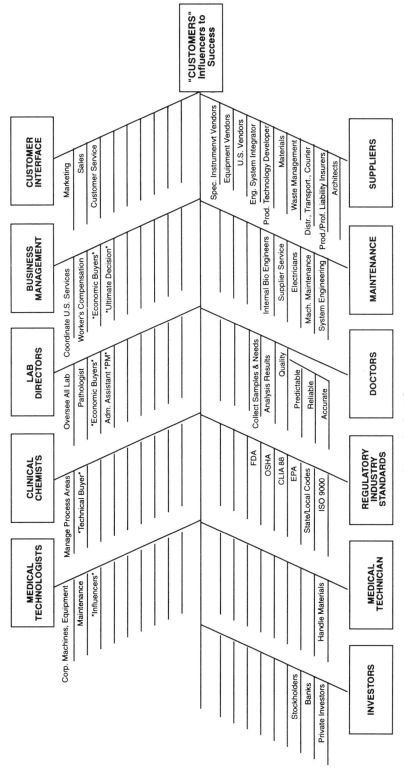

Figure 21.3. Influencers to success.

545

ing and analyzing the core process beginning with customer expectations and ending with customer satisfaction (Fig. 21.4). Clinical process reengineering looks at the business core process, and develops ways to offer innovative services that achieve physician and patient satisfaction, and at the same time provide dramatic improvements in the laboratory. Possibilities include:

1. Information systems that provide total customer service needs, including sample tracking, customer requirements, and billing.
2. Artificial intelligence (AI) software to determine required tests, specimen draw requirements, and other decision-making operations.
3. Automated transport modes within the facility, and AI packages to select best transportation methods for commercial laboratories.
4. Automated central processing and analysis.
5. Instrument interface, including automatic protocol and data reduction.
6. Specimen tracking and status availability.
7. Automated distribution of results, and suggested options.
8. Automated storage and retrieval systems.
9. Waste management systems.

Each of these possibilities already exists and is being used daily in the manufacturing and industrial sector. All that remains is to integrate these advances into the clinical laboratory. Start by thinking in terms of fresh ideas, processes, and methods. Industry has learned that what you do first is important, but what you don't do becomes critical.

Although much has been written in the last 2 years on reengineering as a concept and a desirable goal, little has been written about a methodology or means for accomplishing the conceptual goals. Most has been written about the successes of businesses that have *focused change on the processes* of their business and brought new technology to improve them.[4] Little has been written specifically about how success is achieved and failure avoided. As a result, there is appearing in literature reports "failures" of "reengineering" projects. Many of these failures are due to projects that do not meet the definition of reengineering, or to a lack of practical implementation. Some failures are due to a correct beginning made with the help of consultants, but cannot be completed because of the inadequacies of consultants to provide design, build, and implementation. Success requires not only the correct conceptual approach, but also the ability *to bring the improvements in processes and culture to reality.*

21.2.4. Reengineering Methodology

The remainder of this chapter focuses on a methodology that has been developed for implementing reengineering, and the current concepts of quality as an intrinsic element and its emphasis on application for the clinical laboratory. Reengineering efforts require certain prerequisites. A successful effort *must be*

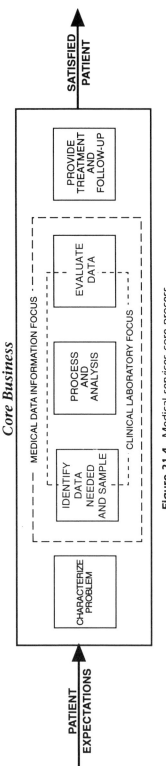

Figure 21.4. Medical services core process.

driven and supported by top management. Anything less will fail and is best not undertaken. It requires thinking "outside the box" and a willingness to look at a business from the ground up, and the intimate and dedicated involvement of the "best and brightest" in a business, those with experience and credibility in the business. The primary requirement is a "reengineering team" made up of top management, process owners, and facilitators dedicated to lead the effort through to implementation (see Fig. 21.5).

The *total quality business process reengineering* approach is structured through the following steps derived from "business drivers." Reengineering is a logical framework for change focused on implementation. It involves six basic elements, each related in a logical and hierarchical manner:

1. *Drivers.* The internal and external influences that effect the success of the business. Drivers are the forces that characterize the world in which the business exists and must function. Most fall into one of seven categories: (1) culture, (2) demographics, (3) business environment, (4) new markets, (5) competitive advantage, (6) technology, and (7) government (see Fig. 21.6).

2. *Qualities.* Clarify the intent of the business. Qualities are expected by all customers in the life cycle of the business. There are five key qualities needed for a business: (1) *vision*—a statement that gives guidance in building a culture, the most desirable future state, a long-term focus that is not judged for possibility; (2) *mission*—the core purpose or reason for existence today; (3) *fundamental objectives*—strategic "how-to"s that help achieve the vision; (4) *business values*—beliefs that drive behavior (degree of excellence, relative worth, utility or importance of activities, and efforts); (5) *leadership style*—the style manage-

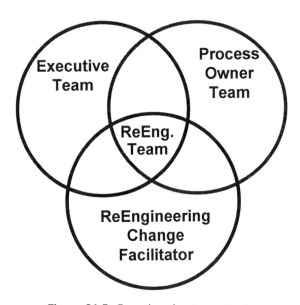

Figure 21.5. Reengineering team structure.

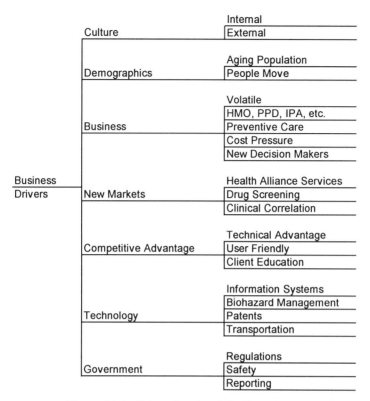

Figure 21.6. Drivers for the clinical laboratory.

ment uses to run the business (this may be dictatorial, autocratic, participative, etc.). Together, these qualities determine the direction of the business in the long and near term as well as the approach that will be taken to achieve the goals.

3. *Processes*. To improve, it is necessary to understand the current process. Mapping the present process is done by recording the step-by-step activities involved in a clinical laboratory from order origination to reporting the result. This should include all elements of material handling, analysis, information management, and specimen storage or disposal, and should be done at a level that captures major steps and activities but does not get bogged down in unnecessary detail. The qualities defined at a conceptual level describe the *ideal future state* and provide the basis for mapping the future process plan. With these two processes defined, and by identifying the *gaps* that exist between the present and the future state, process changes needed to meet the goals of the business are identified. It is *implementing* these changes that results in the benefit of reengineering.

4. *Organization*. Resources and relationships are necessary to operate the future process to achieve the qualities. The structure of the business and its people required to meet the needs of the process.

5. *Systems.* Methods, technology, and tools to facilitate the organization and processes. Includes not only computer systems, but all systems and tools involved in the processes (supply systems, analysis equipment and techniques, storage systems, etc.).

6. *Operations.* Integration and logistics of the business elements. After all the preceding elements and definitions have been realized or implemented, the *operations* (the final element) are determined to deliver the results of the process. Operations are the result of integration and logistics of the business elements, including measures, products, services, and facilities. Most businesses focus on operational issues without consideration for their relationship to other elements or the process of their business. As a result, buildings, equipment, support services, training, sales, and other activities lack integration or coordination within the business or with their customers and products. This fragmentation and lack of coordination were survivable in the past but are lethal in this new world of healthcare reform.

7. *Culture.* All of these elements occur in the overall context of the culture and people of a business. Reengineering requires as much effort and focus on planned beneficial *cultural* change as on change of business's structural elements and equipment changes. Lack of attention to the culture of the business may result in rejection of the improved process by employees and the failure of the project. Cultural reengineering is done by direct involvement at all levels in the organization throughout the reengineering effort. This allows critical input and alignment.

21.2.5. Three-Phase Approach to Systems Integration

Providing a fully integrated laboratory with operations, systems, and organizations developed to meet defined processes derived from fundamental objectives and goals is achievable with today's technology. A three-phased approach is recommended.

21.2.5.1. PHASE I: CONCEPTUAL DESIGN. This design utilizes process reengineering methods, tools, and techniques to translate the guiding principles of these elements into needed changes at the conceptual level. Start by identifying customers (influencers of success) and their needs and the goals to be put in place to achieve them. Phase I would typically involve a workshop with the reengineering team and others (including top management) from the laboratory, and professional facilitators skilled in strategic business process reengineering methods. The workshop objectives include team alignment and clarification of scope, opportunities, and issues. Over the next few weeks, ongoing interaction will develop the following deliverables:

1. Organized and distilled workshop data
2. Background data summary

3. Detailed customer definition.
   a. Intent of business
      i. Business drivers, trends, opportunities, and goals
      ii. Vision, mission, and fundamental objectives
      iii. Technology needed in terms of products, services, or performance
      iv. Leadership needed to champion and reinforce goals
   b. Processes
      i. Process goals
      ii. Core process
      iii. Support processes
   c. Organization
      i. Organization goals
      ii. Functions and capabilities needed
   d. Systems and integration architecture to streamline the organizational effort
   e. Operations needed
   f. Simulation to validate performance and optimize processes
4. Total cost and benefits analysis, including an options assessment ladder

21.2.5.2. PHASE II: SCHEMATIC DESIGN. This design converts the conceptual requirements into detailed engineering specifications, and develops a commitment plan to meet or exceed goals and expectations. Emphasis is placed on project success factors, specifications, project schedule, milestones, and benefits and/or savings, and cost estimates will be refined.

Phase II might take several months depending on the complexity of the project. Supplementary engineering personnel will be required to provide detail to areas involving technical expertise. Deliverables include

1. Functional diagrams
   a. Component positions
   b. Resource profile
   c. Risk summary
   d. Constraints
   e. Input/output requirements
   f. Waste factors
2. System design package
3. System block diagram (capacity and timing)
4. Equipment list
5. Block layout and space requirements
6. Data management requirements
7. Phase III implementation proposal
8. Cost/benefit estimates

21.2.5.3. PHASE III: DETAILED DESIGN AND IMPLEMENTATION. This phase includes the detailed design, fabrication, installation, validation, and startup of the automated laboratory, and monitoring the execution to ensure that goals and expectations are met. All available commercial products appropriate to the project goals would be purchased and installed. Some refinement or customization of existing equipment and laboratory systems may be required. Phase III deliverables include the following:

1. Creation and startup of a fully integrated clinical laboratory
    a. Technical requirements
    b. Engineering design
    c. Drawings and documents
    d. Complete specifications
    e. Equipment fabrication and assembly
    f. Project control and management
2. Facility and systems construction
3. Equipment installation
4. System verification
5. Subsystem test and verification
6. Business operations
    a. Operator and maintenance training
    b. Function output and performance evaluation
    c. Design and technical manuals
    d. Audit checklists
    e. Archiving of all project documentation
7. Final acceptance and production startup

21.2.6. Benefits

The total quality approach to clinical process reengineering provides in-depth assessment of progress and establishes a baseline from which to measure processes over time. Most importantly, it identifies an organization's strongest areas and areas with greatest need for improvement. It will improve customer satisfaction and key business performance by aligning technology to the performance gaps in critical areas.

Clinical laboratories must look beyond the elimination of FTEs as the only benefit of integrated automation. Clinical process reengineering will provide the means to identify and quantify all costs and savings in the laboratory. The integrated laboratory automation benefits checklist (see Fig. 21.7) is an example of the identifiable benefits and savings that can be achieved.

Success in achieving and sustaining total quality performance can be measured by three essential criteria:

1. *Value : Price Ratio.* Defined by the customer, in terms of their perception, this ratio is a measure of customer satisfaction.
2. *Value : Cost Ratio.* The basic element of financial success, and with value-based pricing, this ratio is a cornerstone of world class performance.

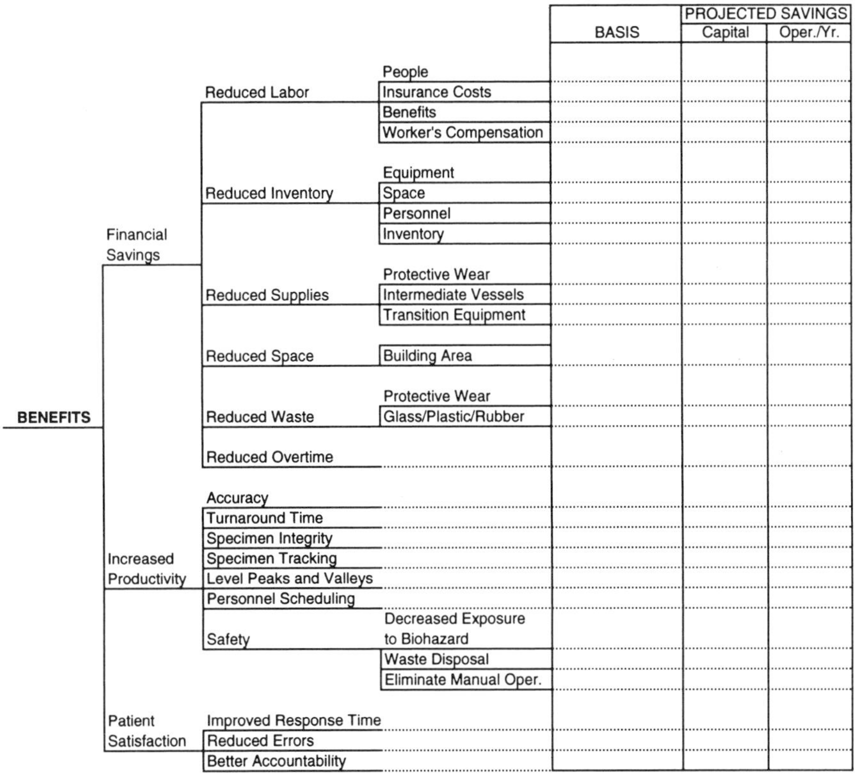

BENEFITS			BASIS	PROJECTED SAVINGS Capital	Oper./Yr.
Financial Savings	Reduced Labor	People			
		Insurance Costs			
		Benefits			
		Worker's Compensation			
	Reduced Inventory	Equipment			
		Space			
		Personnel			
		Inventory			
	Reduced Supplies	Protective Wear			
		Intermediate Vessels			
		Transition Equipment			
	Reduced Space	Building Area			
	Reduced Waste	Protective Wear			
		Glass/Plastic/Rubber			
	Reduced Overtime				
Increased Productivity	Accuracy				
	Turnaround Time				
	Specimen Integrity				
	Specimen Tracking				
	Level Peaks and Valleys				
	Personnel Scheduling				
	Safety	Decreased Exposure to Biohazard			
		Waste Disposal			
		Eliminate Manual Oper.			
Patient Satisfaction	Improved Response Time				
	Reduced Errors				
	Better Accountability				

Figure 21.7. Integrated laboratory automation—benefits checklist.

3. *Error-Free Performance.* This basic element of quality as traditionally defined measures the cost of nonconformance.

21.3. SUMMARY

The provision of universal healthcare at a time the nation is constrained by the economy has put extreme pressure on the healthcare industry to provide higher-quality, lower-cost services. These are the same challenges that our manufacturing industries have met and responded to by *reengineering* their businesses through strategic planning based on customer needs, and by taking advantage of new techniques and technology. The healthcare industry has the opportunity to utilize industry's "lessons learned" and provide value beyond present-day expectations.

Our industrial and manufacturing industries have suffered a long and painful learning curve. Implementing change has become the primary skill for survival and gain in competitive advantage. Advances made in industry can and must be applied to the healthcare services industry to develop and improve a more cost-effective healthcare system. The clinical laboratory seems to be an ideal place to start.

The successful laboratories of tomorrow will not be satisfied with single instruments that improve part of their current processes, but rather, fully integrated automatic systems focused on new methods and processes. We must team together to critically explore laboratory strategies and business goals to identify core processes and *identify core processes* in order to design and build an integrated system based on *strategic business goals* and *fundamental objectives*.

Clinical process reengineering has begun in several laboratories: large reference laboratories, university medical center labs, and pharmaceutical research laboratories. Total quality reengineering is a logical, orderly approach for change in a business or laboratory. It is a powerful tool for orderly, rational, beneficial, and dramatic improvement. It requires a new, novel, and logical way to see ourselves and our activities. This approach to change has features similar to scientific methodology, but it is applied to the laboratory in a business sense.

The three-phase approach provides the logical steps to implementation, but we must keep in mind that this is not the end of the reengineering effort. Just as in other quality programs, there is a continued need for improvement. Business drivers, qualities, processes, organization, systems, and operations must be reexamined regularly for changes that occur in healthcare. This will provide a means for rapid reaction to changes, and the ability to stay ahead of the competition.

Reengineering offers a logical, dramatic, and effective method for change. Successful reengineering projects must focus and combine equally on changes in culture and people as well as hardware and software in order to be successful. Clinical process reengineering offers an ideal means to respond to the current and future changes in healthcare.

In this era of healthcare reform, we are forced to look beyond the present and the past if we are to be successful.

> One of the greatest risk we have is from the *successes* of the past: they can blind us from recognizing *possibilities* for the future.

REFERENCES

1. Buchner WF, Brown JW: The impact of health care reform on the clinical laboratory. *MLO* 26:30–35, 1994.

2. Bissell MG: Health care reform and the clinical laboratory. *MIO* 25:24–29, 1993.

3. Hammer M, Champy J: *Reengineering the Corporation*. New York: Harper Business, 1993.

4. Morris D, Brandon J: *Reengineering your Business*. New York: McGraw-Hill, 1993.

22

Cost-Effectiveness and Benefits of Automation and Robotics

GEOFFREY F. AUCHINLECK, ROGER B. LINES, AND
WILLIAM J. GODOLPHIN

CONTENTS

Handbook of Clinical Automation, Robotics, and Optimization, Edited by Gerald J. Kost with the
collaboration of Judith Welsh.
ISBN 0-471-03179-8 © 1996 John Wiley & Sons, Inc.

22.1. INDUSTRIAL AUTOMATION FOR COST REDUCTION FOLLOWS A FAMILIAR PATTERN

Since the turn of the century, many industries have applied automation and mechanization, but it was not until after World War II with the growth of mass production, the implementation of assembly lines and the invention of the micro chip, that industry implemented the modern definition of automation. Starting in the 1950s, a well-defined pattern has emerged for cost justification of industrial automation.

When first introduced, industrial automation technology was very costly. For example, in 1959 the Sperry Rand Corporation acquired a new computer prompting the report: "Although it will cost over six million dollars (or rent for more than \$135,000 per month) the company claims it is the fastest and most advanced machine of its kind in the world."[1] The computer could calculate a company payroll in 15 h. Large institutions could afford the capital outlay, but the high cost severely handicapped wide spread introduction of the technology.

As costs fell, industries undergoing growth were able to implement automation. Automation allowed businesses such as telephone and oil companies to expand rapidly, increasing revenue and employment to meet accelerating demands for their services:

> The productivity increases resulting from automation are astounding. It used to take the Ford Motor Company twenty-four hours to produce an engine block from a rough casting. With automation, it takes 14.6 minutes.[1]

Increased manufacturing capacity justified automation implemented during this period.

By the 1970s, both office and manufacturing automation had strong footholds in many of the top U.S. industrial companies, but was still found mostly in the domain of high-volume production. Competing to reduce product pricing and struggling for market share, industry justified automation by reducing the direct and indirect labor costs associated with their products. The labor component of manufacturing costs dropped dramatically. This was confirmed in a recent study of leading industrial companies that have a substantial level of automation. This study found that "the average product cost percentages of about 54 percent for direct materials, 13 percent for direct labor, and 33 percent for manufacturing overhead do represent a substantial shift of production costs from direct labor to fixed overhead costs."[2]

In the last decade, smaller businesses have been able to automate using new technology and flexibly designed equipment. Justification of the capital cost of automation through labor savings alone is difficult for small companies. Consequently automation purchases are now being justified by accounting for not only labor costs, but also lower scrap and material costs, lower inventories, reduced manufacturing cycle time, and improved quality and competitive position.

Although the technology and processes of the clinical laboratory are unique, automation of laboratories is following a pattern parallel to industrial automation. Figure 22.1 illustrates the effect of automation on staffing, and shows how this pattern might apply to clinical laboratories. Automated analysis was initially

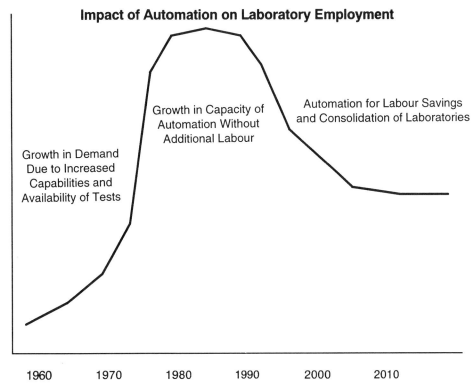

Figure 22.1. Typical employment trends in industries undergoing automation, as applied to the clinical laboratory. Employment grew rapidly in the 1960s and 1970s as automated analysis created an increased demand for tests. Employment is now declining as automation replaces laboratory staff and laboratories consolidate to reduce costs.

beyond the reach of most laboratories. As costs fell, clinical laboratories grew rapidly in size and capacity. Over a period of approximately 30 years, staffing levels burgeoned and turnaround times plummeted as demand for more and better tests rose as fast as automation and new technology made them available.[3,4]

Economic, political, and regulatory pressures are now driving clinical labs to be more efficient and cost-effective. Increased competition and limited budgets are forcing labs to find ways to reduce their costs. As in other industries, laboratories are now looking to automation to address their needs. Cost justification for new automation will quickly focus on direct and measurable cost savings, usually through the labor savings.[5] This trend is so widespread that it will substantially change many aspects of laboratory operations. An immediate result is the consolidation of laboratories into regional centers that can effectively make use of automation technologies and other economies of scale.[3]

Smaller labs and those that have already introduced islands of automation[6] will ultimately need to use more subjective cost justifications for automation. These justifications will likely include the following:[7]

1. Increased safety for laboratory staff through reduced contact with specimens, resulting in lower costs for sick time and disability
2. Fewer transcription and sample mis-placement errors, resulting in direct savings to the laboratory
3. Better turnaround times, permitting more flexible staff allocation and possibly a competitive advantage.

22.2. AUTOMATION CAN BE APPLIED THROUGHOUT THE CLINICAL LABORATORY

Although the general pattern of cost justifications for automation in the clinical laboratory is familiar, the automation technology, its application, and the benefits to be realized are unique. To properly evaluate the cost effectiveness and other benefits of automation in the clinical laboratory, the process between collection of a sample and delivery of results to the physician must be examined in detail. This will highlight the areas of opportunity for automation in the laboratory.

22.2.1. Sample Collection

Sample collection includes all the activities that must be performed to cause a specimen to arrive in the laboratory. This includes the capture of the test request information from the physician, collection of the specimen, labeling of the collection tube, collection of patient information and transport of the specimen, test request information, and patient information to the laboratory in a suitable form.

Sample collection may seem to be unsuited to automation, yet it does provide some interesting opportunities. For example, although there is nothing immediately available to automate the actual drawing of a blood sample, the steps of preparing and labeling the collection tube, entering the test request information and patient demographics, and transport of the sample to the laboratory can be automated with currently available technology.

Commercial products to address some of these automation opportunities are well developed and available. Several manufacturers offer transportation systems for delivering samples to laboratories, ranging from tried and true pneumatic tube systems (Metsec Industries, Pevco Systems International) to electric transport systems and state of the art autonomous guided vehicles (Translogic, TELE-engineering, AutoTech). Advanced data management systems (described below) can be used to collect test and patient information on the ward or at the collection site to minimize transcription of data.

Some newer ideas for increasing the level of automation of the sample collection step are not yet commercially available, but have been successfully demonstrated. Dr. Kenneth Whisler of St. Luke's Presbyterian Hospital in Chicago has developed a system in which a portable device is used to read a barcode on the patient's wristband and directly link the demographic information to the bar code label on the blood collection tube.[8] This eliminates a data entry step and has the added benefit of eliminating transcription errors. Dr. Whisler says "Our approach was to try to create a seamless communications pathway that quickly transfers information from its collection point to its ultimate destination in the computer system."

22.2.2. Data Entry and Management

Data entry and management include all those activities required to collect, analyze, organize, and present information associated with and derived from a specimen. No automation effort can succeed without recognizing that data management is at least half of what a laboratory does. Without accurate and efficient handling of information about the specimen, patient, and test results, no amount of sample handling produces anything of value.

The use of computers to automate the management of data in the laboratory is well established. Many companies offer commercial software packages to the laboratory (Antrim, Baxter Healthcare, Citation Computer Systems, Compulab Healthcare Systems, Creative Computer Applications, Diamond Computing, HBO & Company, Health Science Systems, IDX Systems, Meditech, NLFC, Terrano, and many others). Many of these systems offer integration with bar code printers and readers to simplify the identification of samples. A full implementation of such a laboratory information system can also include collection of patient information and test requests at or near the patient, use of a bar-code label on the specimen tube linked to data in the computer to eliminate the need for handling paper, and automatic reporting of results to the physician through fax or terminal connections.

Automation technologies that are just beginning to enter the clinical laboratory environment include document scanners and voice-recognition systems. (Diamond Computing Company, MedPlus Inc.). Even in labs that use very advanced laboratory information systems, a significant amount of labor is dedicated to data entry. Simplifying and speeding up this step, or eliminating it wherever possible would have some benefit.

22.2.3. Specimen Preparation

Specimen preparation includes all those activities that are required to get a sample into a condition suitable for analysis. This includes centrifuging, aliquotting, pipetting, dilution, and sorting of the specimens into batches for introduction to automated analyzers.

The specimen preparation step has attracted considerable academic and commercial attention in recent years.[5,7,9,10] Several companies are now offering automation systems and components to automate all or part of these processes. Automated pipetting machines are the best developed of these components, but automated centrifuges, aliquotters, and sorting machines are now entering the market from a number of suppliers (AutoMed, Coulter, Olympus).

Some of the commercially available specimen preparation systems offer standalone devices that perform a certain function, operating much like a conventional automated analyzer in that specimens must be manually loaded into the machine and manually unloaded once processing is complete. Most manufacturers are moving away from this concept to offer machines that can be linked together as a system providing automatic processing and transport of samples through all the specimen preparation steps.[11] This distinction is important, as it has considerable impact on the way a laboratory introduces and grows its automation system.

Although there is still considerable academic and precommercial work being done on specimen preparation automation, all the specimen preparation functions can already be achieved with commercially available automation.

22.2.4. Interface to Automated Analyzers

Interfacing to analyzers includes the activities of preparing worklists for the analyzer, transporting the sample to and from the instrument and the actual loading and unloading of the sample. These activities are recognized as being separate from specimen preparation as they are usually dependent on the requirements of the individual analyzer and are more closely associated with the analysis step than the preparation step.

Commercial products to automate these functions are just beginning to enter the market (AutoLab, Coulter, Lab Interlink, Labotix). Most of these products are centered around conveying systems of various types, which automate the transport of samples to and from the analyzers. Conveying technology is well established in other industries and should easily adapt to the clinical lab setting.

Some commercial systems are beginning to directly address the loading and unloading of analyzers and automatic worklist generation (Coulter, Sysmex). Incompatibility among sample carriers for various analyzers has made this a particularly difficult task, and as a result, there is no single system currently available that will automatically load and unload all types of analyzers.

A number of automation systems at the precommercial stage will address the analyzer loading and unloading problem. These systems, usually based on a commercial robot arm (e.g., the Hewlett-Packard ORCA™ system), will likely be the solution of choice for the interim period until standard sample carriers are adopted by instrument manufacturers.

22.2.5. Analysis

Analysis of the sample, or determination of a specimen's physical and chemical characteristics, is the functional focus of the clinical laboratory and as a result has traditionally been the focus of automation in the laboratory. Automated analyzers are commonly available for all except the most esoteric tests and have deeply penetrated the clinical laboratory environment. These machines continue to evolve to reduce operating costs, offer more test options and provide more efficient ways to deliver test result data. They are available from a large number of commercial suppliers. This form of automation is extremely mature and well developed.

In situations where an automated analyzer is not available due to the esoteric nature of the test, automation systems are also commercially available. These systems provide simple functional building blocks that can be assembled together to perform a huge variety of tests (Zymark, Hewlett-Packard). The systems are usually based on a robotic arm that moves a specimen from one functional block to the next. Using this approach, highly unusual and specialized tests have been successfully automated.

22.2.6. Postanalysis

Postanalytic functions include storage and retrieval of samples after analysis and disposal of wastes. Often, these "tail end" activities are overlooked in considering automation, although they can contribute significant costs to the operation of a laboratory.

Very few automation products are commercially available for these functions. Some basic functional blocks, such as refrigeration systems that include inventory tracking and locating functions to the level of individual shelves have been constructed. These include storage systems that can be linked directly to a conveying system or robotic loading device, so that individual samples can be directly and automatically retrieved from storage.[3]

One example is an automated sample tracking system in use at Rush-Presbyterian-St. Luke's Medical Center in Chicago.[8] This system records the location of up to 7000 samples in a computer so that the refrigerator, shelf, rack and storage slot for a particular sample can be retrieved.

22.3. THE BENEFITS OF AUTOMATION ARE GREATER IN SOME AREAS THAN OTHERS

We have seen that each of the processing steps identified can be automated to a greater or lesser extent. The benefits of automation will similarly vary with each step of the process. To evaluate these benefits, the impact of automating each step must be estimated. Cost savings is usually the focus of such estimations. Ideally, the operating costs of laboratories that have already introduced automation should be used to develop these estimates, but this is practical in only one step of the process.

The analysis of specimens has traditionally been recognized as the most labor-intensive and expensive part of the clinical laboratory's operation. This is probably why most efforts at introducing automation have addressed analysis. This focus has resulted in a vast number of automated analyzers, which have improved in efficiency over the years. Continued competition by instrument manufacturers will no doubt result in incremental improvements in analyzers, but are unlikely to provide dramatic cost reductions. It would appear that the point of diminishing returns has been reached for automation in this area.

With the exception of computerized data management, very little experience has yet been gained in automating the remaining processing steps. Although many new technologies are beginning to enter the market, there is little data available to measure the impact of these technologies in North American laboratories. The most advanced laboratories in terms of automation, operating in Japan, were built with considerable government support, making it very difficult to evaluate the economic impact of automation of the individual process steps.[9] Therefore, evaluation of the cost benefits of these new automation technologies is necessarily speculative.

Without relevant experience to use as a model, another way to evaluate the cost benefits of automation is required. Miles Diagnostics has presented an approach based on the relative cost of each process step.[12] Their analysis is based on breaking down the cost of analyzing a single specimen (Fig. 22.2). Their results show that specimen collection, including blood drawing, transport to the laboratory and data entry contributes 9% of the cost. Specimen preparation, including centrifuging, aliquotting, sorting, and consumable costs contributes 19%. Interface with the instrument, including worklist generation, data entry into the instrument, transport of sample to and from the instrument, and operation of the instrument contributes 28%. The instrument processing step, including capital cost, reagent cost, controls and repeats, contributes 35%. Finally, disposal and results reporting, including archiving and transport of finished samples, contribute the remaining 9%. By this analysis, the logical places to look for maximum cost benefit are in the sample preparation and instrument interface steps.

The large cost component associated with sample preparation has attracted a high level of attention from equipment suppliers and laboratories. Most current automation developments are focused on this area, including the steps of cen-

Contributions to Cost of Testing

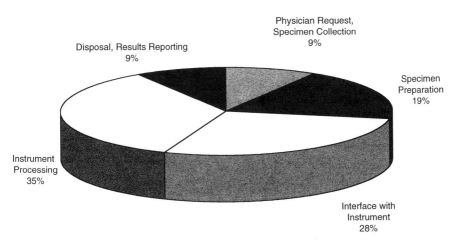

Figure 22.2. Contributions of various processing steps to the total cost of analyzing a specimen. "Physician request and specimen collection" includes venipuncture, data collection, and transport of the specimen to the laboratory. "Specimen preparation" includes data entry, aliquotting, sorting, and centrifuging and consumables cost. "Interface with instrument" includes worklist generation, and transport to and from the instrument. "Instrument processing" includes capital equipment cost, reagents, controls, and repeats. "Disposal and results reporting" includes archiving, transport, disposal, and distribution of results. [Data courtesy of Miles Diagnostics (Canada).]

trifuging, aliquotting, worklist automation, conveying and automated loading and unloading of instruments. It seems clear that equipment suppliers believe that cost benefit analysis will drive the marketplace to adopt automation in these areas.

22.4. THE BENEFITS OF AUTOMATION CAN BE MEASURED IN TERMS OTHER THAN COST SAVINGS

Cost benefits are not the only considerations in automation of the clinical lab. Although more subjective in value, analysis of other benefits is also important and may be particularly important in justifying automation in smaller laboratories. One way of evaluating these benefits is to identify the potential advantages of automation and then see what steps in the process can make best use of these advantages. In some cases, it is possible to define a measurable parameter related to the desired benefit and evaluate the impact of automation on this parameter. This approach helps remove some of the subjectivity in the analysis and provides a means for validating the impact of automation when it is in use.

22.4.1. Safety of Laboratory Personnel

The most obvious hazard to laboratory staff is the manual handling of samples that may be infectious. The most direct way to reduce this hazard is to eliminate, wherever possible, direct contact with the samples. Unfortunately, this is close to impossible at the collection step (unless patients can be taught to draw their own blood), but throughout the rest of the process steps can be taken to minimize exposure.

Certain process steps are recognized as particularly risky in terms of exposure. These include aliquotting and pipetting, and may include centrifuge unloading in the event that a tube has broken in the centrifuge, a not uncommon occurrence. Certainly the requirement to remove the cap of a specimen tube to pour off or pipette liquid is a particularly unacceptable hazard. For these reasons, automation of the sample preparation steps would seem to have the greatest safety benefits.

22.4.2. Improved Turnaround Time

Improved turnaround time is an example of a benefit that can be related to measurable parameters. To evaluate the possible impact of automation on turnaround time in the lab, the amount of time currently spent on different parts of the analysis process in the lab can be analyzed. A study done by Godolphin et al.[13] shows that the largest component of the turnaround time (37%) for a typical sample is the accessioning process, which includes sample log-in, centrifugation, and aliquotting (Fig. 22.3). The next largest components are run time (or sample analysis) at 25% and receive (time between venipuncture until the sample is received in the lab) at 20%. From this analysis, it is clear that the greatest reduction in turnaround time can be achieved in the accessioning step.

22.4.3. Reduced and Simplified Repeated Tests

Another benefit of automation may be the reduction of repeat tests. The best opportunity for achieving such reduction is through eliminating as much variability in sample preparation as possible. With time, consistent preparation should result in a better understanding of the variables in the test process and reduce the requirement for repeats.

A more direct benefit can be realized through reducing the amount of time spent locating and retrieving additional sample material to repeat a test. Automated sample preparation will reduce the amount of specimen prepared for each test by using only the exact amount required. The remaining specimen can be placed in storage for any additional tests. If the amount of specimen available is measured prior to storage, searches for samples which are not available will be eliminated.

Searching for additional sample material can be greatly simplified through automating storage of specimens. A system that permits direct location of sam-

Distribution of Times for Testing

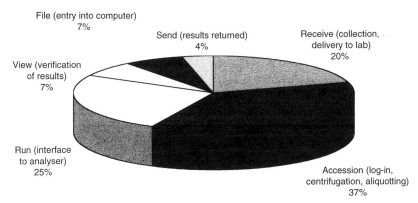

Figure 22.3. Distribution of time required for each major step in the procurement, processing, analysis, and reporting of a test result in a clinical chemistry laboratory. "Receive" is the elapsed time form venipuncture until the specimen is received in the laboratory; "accession" is the time required for preanalytical processing such as log-in, centrifugation, and aliquotting; "run" is the time from the completion of aliquotting until the analytical result has been produced; "view" is the time required for verification of the result (including checking the quality control results); "file" is the time until the verified result has been entered into the laboratory computer system; and "send" is the time to inform the ward, nurse, or physician of the result by either telephone or computer terminal, or the time until the result would be available to them by these means. (Data drawn from Ref. 13.)

ples wherever they are stored would eliminate a considerable amount of searching.

22.4.4. Other Benefits

For each process step in the clinical laboratory, a number of other benefits might be realized through automation. These benefits are difficult to quantify in a meaningful way, as they relate more often to a "gut feeling" that there "should be a better way." In a very interesting survey performed by Boehringer Mannheim, an attempt was made to quantify this "gut feeling" by asking 245 clinicians from throughout Europe and North America to evaluate sample handling steps on a scale ranging from 0 (no difficulty) to 2 (difficult). The results of this unpublished study are shown in Figure 22.4.[14] Although the results of this study are less clearly defined than cost and turnaround time analysis, the perception that sample transport and preparation are particularly troublesome is supported.

Perceived Difficulty of Process Steps

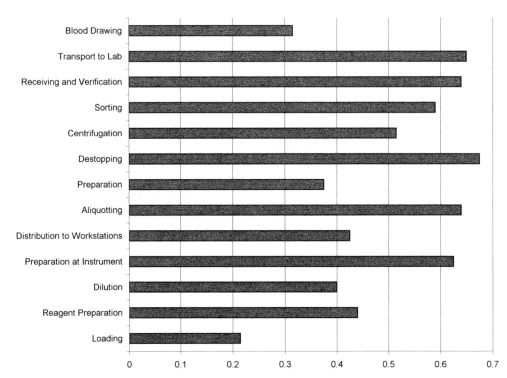

Figure 22.4. Results of a survey of 245 clinicians who were asked to rate each of the sample handling steps shown in terms of "difficulty of step—(bottleneck/labor intensive)." The rating scale was either 0 (no difficulty) 1, or 2 (most difficulty). Respondents were drawn from Germany, France, Spain, Italy, USA, and Canada. (Data courtesy of Boeringer Mannheim.)

22.5. APPROACHES TO AUTOMATION

We have seen that automation can be applied to virtually every part of the clinical laboratory and that various approaches can be used to evaluate the benefit of such automation. Another consideration in such a project is the scope of automation that should be attempted. For very large laboratories, automation of process steps for which cost reductions are small may still make sense because of the high volume of processing done by the laboratory. In smaller labs, only those areas in which substantial cost savings can be realized will provide a reasonable return on the capital investment.

Some laboratories, notably in Japan, have had success in attempting to totally automate the laboratory and "do it all at once." In these laboratories, everything that can conceivably be automated has been automated and the implementation was simultaneous and sweeping. These labs represent extreme examples of automation approaches and are as close to the ultimate "lab in a box" as can be achieved with modern technology.

Some large North American labs are also attempting broad automation approaches in which large parts of the laboratory are automated simultaneously. These efforts are not as extensive as the Japanese examples, as the attention is focused only on the very high-volume areas of the lab, but within these areas the automation is as intensive as possible.

These broad ranging automation projects are intended to automate as much as possible all at once, in order to obtain the maximum benefit available in the areas automated. This approach is predicated on the assumption that cost reduction and other benefits are captured in certain lab areas and that these areas are best treated as monolithic entities that are wholly replaced by automated systems. This approach naturally leads to a focus on automation of high-volume areas of the lab first, as these areas can more easily justify the large capital investment required for automation. This appropriately recognizes that the cost benefit of automation varies widely for different parts of the lab.

The alternative approach to automation is the piecemeal "do a bit at a time" concept. Rather than looking at various areas of the lab as monolithic blocks, certain functions are selected for automation based on their perceived benefits. This approach requires more modular automation devices to be used, so that the cost benefits of each automation module can be maximized. Although this approach has the advantage of minimizing initial capital outlay and permitting the choice of automation devices that will most easily be cost justified, it can result in a disconnected and incoherent automation system composed of mutually incompatible components that will frustrate future efforts to automate intervening processes. This risk aside, modular automation of selected laboratory functions is probably the most beneficial approach for all but the largest laboratories.

If a stepwise approach to automation is selected, the choice of which steps to automate and the order in which to automate them can be based directly on perceived cost benefit at each stage. From the analysis of the availability and benefit of automating each stage in the process presented above, a reasonable approach to automation is to start with automated specimen preparation, followed by automated analyzer loading and unloading. Finally, transport systems for moving samples around the laboratory would round out the automation of the main functions of the lab. Automation of other functions would be taken on only if and when the cost benefit was justified.

22.6. OTHER IMPLICATIONS OF AUTOMATION IN THE CLINICAL LABORATORY

Although we have concentrated on analyzing the impact of automation on the operations of laboratories as they are currently run, it is important to recognize that automation will fundamentally change the way laboratories operate. To make best use of the capital investment required to install automation, there will be a tendency to maximize the use of the equipment through consolidation of laboratory functions. This will eliminate the unnecessary duplication of automation systems in the lab, and will break down the divisions between lab departments. The end result will be a move toward an open lab layout in which lab staff handle a much wider variety of samples and tests than is currently the norm.

22.7. SOME EXAMPLES OF LABORATORY AUTOMATION PROJECTS

Very few North American laboratories have implemented automation outside the analysis step; hence each example given below is, at least in part, speculative. The very nature of the rapid changes being experienced by laboratories makes it very difficult to analyze the real impact of such systems.

22.7.1. A Theoretical Example Utilizing Modular Automation

Miles Diagnostics has published an automation example based on actual information from a major North American hospital laboratory serving a hospital of 850 beds.[12] In this example, 1200 specimens per day are collected, with three or four tubes of blood being collected per specimen. On average eight tests are performed on each patient, which requires 50% of the specimens to be aliquotted into three aliquots. In this example, the laboratory employs 80 FTEs, 30 of whom are in specimen processing.

The model laboratory was analyzed before and after the introduction of automation for centrifuging, aliquotting, and sorting. No specific automation equipment was specified in this example, although a modular, incremental approach is described. Based on this approach to automation, a direct reduction of 10 FTEs in specimen processing was deemed to be possible. Additional benefits that might be possible with automation included a reduction in the average number of primary tubes required due to more accurate aliquotting, a reduction in the number of repeats and errors, and even a reduction in length of hospital stay due to improved turnaround time of test results.

This analysis gave a theoretical realizable cost savings of $216,160 per year, which includes a reduction of 10 FTEs, a slight reduction in the cost of consumables and repeat tests, and increased capital and maintenance costs of $217,000 per year.

22.7.2. Another Theoretical Example Using Broader Applications of Automation

The Coulter Corporation has published a workflow case study for another hospital laboratory very similar to the one in the Miles study.[15] Once again, the data for the workflow study is drawn from an actual hospital laboratory in North America.

In this example, the lab collects 800 chemistry and 400 hematology samples per day. Prior to automation, the laboratory employs 27 FTEs in specimen processing, chemistry, and hematology.

The Coulter analysis presumes full automation of the sample preparation, hematology, and chemistry areas of the lab, including automated transfer to and from the analyzers, automated aliquotting and centrifuging, automated slide making and staining, and even an automated refrigerated storage locker for automatic storage and retrieval of chemistry samples. The Coulter laboratory automation system implementation which is the basis of the analysis is shown in Figure 22.5.

By analyzing the workflow after automation, Coulter is able to demonstrate a reduction of 12.5 FTEs, for a direct cost savings through labor reduction alone of $317,393 per year. This is similar to results obtained in Japanese laboratories utilizing similar technology, which have reported "labor cost savings of 30% to 50% and/or workload increases of up to 200% without additional staffing.[16] Coulter's analysis also notes that "in addition to the financial benefits of automation, there is also a reduction in exposure of personnel to potentially biohazardous specimens, an improvement in quality control, and more time to devote to abnormal results."[15]

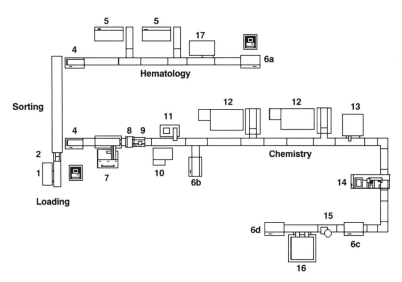

Figure 22.5. An example of a Coulter laboratory automation system implementation. Components are (1) inlet unit, (2) bar-code verification/H-lane, (3) sorting station, (4) sample transfer robot, (5) STKS connection, (6) outlet unit, (7) centrifuge, (8) serum level detector, (9) cap removal unit, (10) secondary-tube labeler, (11) aliquotting unit, (12) instrument connection, (13) stockyard, (14) pipetting station, (15) cap replacement unit, (16) storage locker, and (17) slide maker/stainer. (Drawing courtesy of Coulter Corp.)

22.7.3. A System under Development: MDS Laboratories (Toronto, Ontario, Canada)

The principal MDS laboratory in Toronto is a very large commercial laboratory performing about 12 million tests per year and serving about 10,000 physicians.[17] This laboratory draws samples from a huge area; some samples travel as much as 1000 miles to reach the laboratory. On a daily basis, the laboratory processes more than 12,000 specimens with an average turnaround time of about 3 h. Samples are drawn at a large number of collection points where they are centrifuged and labeled. Test request data is entered into a central computer system at the time of the draw.

Planning for automation of this laboratory began in 1988. The current automation program will see full automation of all the high-volume areas of the lab, beginning with high-volume chemistry in 1994. Within the high-volume area, virtually all processing is automated, including the control of the process itself through the use of an expert system. The layout of the laboratory floor of the MDS automated laboratory is shown in Figure 22.6.

HIGH VOLUME PRODUCTION LOOP
MDS Toronto

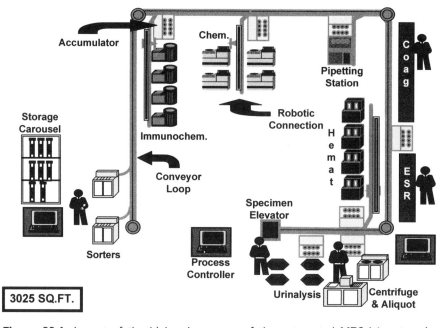

Figure 22.6. Layout of the high-volume area of the automated MDS laboratory in Toronto. Specimens are received one floor below the laboratory and are introduced onto the conveyor belt. An elevator mechanism lifts the samples up to the laboratory floor. (Drawing courtesy of AutoLab systems.)

The automated laboratory includes an extensive conveying system that is loaded with samples in a receiving area of the laboratory building. The conveying system delivers samples to a number of automated workcells that deliver samples to and from a variety of analyzers, automated aliquotters, and pipetting stations. After passing through the high-volume process area, samples are sorted automatically to low- or midvolume testing areas in which manual processes are still used. When all tests are completed, the original sample is sorted for storage in a computerized refrigeration system that permits automatic relocation of any sample for retrieval.

The MDS laboratory automation project is a good example of the approach of choosing a high-volume area of the laboratory and attempting to automate that part of the lab entirely. For a laboratory comparable in size to MDS, this approach seems to have considerable merit and value. This approach to automation was developed by MDS through their AutoLab Systems division, which integrated sample handling equipment manufactured by AutoMed Corporation, conveying systems developed by Labotix Automation Inc. and software developed by AutoLab.

Although implementation of this automation system is not yet complete, MDS estimates that the full automation system will significantly reduce their direct test costs. In addition, detailed simulation of the operation of the automated lab has demonstrated that turnaround time for test results should drop to one hour, with stats completed in about 20 min.

22.7.4. Mayo Clinic (Rochester, Minnesota)

The Mayo Clinic laboratory in Rochester serves the 1950 beds of the two major Mayo Clinic hospitals as well as a large outpatient client base. The Mayo Clinic laboratory tests more than 1.2 million blood specimens per year. The lab employs 191 phlebotomists and offers more than 900 different tests. All blood samples are prepared for analysis in a central processing area that employs 21 people. The peak arrival rate of samples is 1400 per hour, with about 3500 samples processed per day.[5,18]

Mayo's approach to automation is much more conservative than that taken by MDS, in that only one carefully chosen area of the lab has been targeted for automation. Mayo's approach is to automate only the central processing area of the lab, and within the central processing, only the preparation of samples for routine testing. Their strategy involves automation of single functions in the laboratory, consistent with a long-term strategy of extensive automation across the entire laboratory.

In the current stage of automation, Mayo has chosen to automate the centrifuging, aliquotting, and sorting of routine samples using two AutoMed Sample Handling Systems (shown in Fig. 22.7). This limited approach still has considerable benefit for the laboratory, with a direct savings of 70% of the manual labor or about 9 FTEs expected when the automation system is fully operating.[10]

Additional benefits which the Mayo Clinic anticipates include reduced tran-

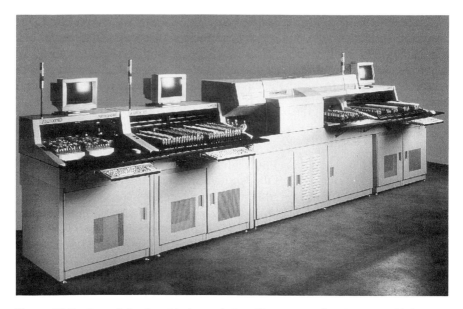

Figure 22.7. One of the AutoMed sample-handling systems for the Mayo Clinic. Each system includes a loader module, a presort module, an automated centrifuge (not shown), an aliquotter, and a final sort module. Samples are manually unloaded from the sort modules and carried to the next processing step. (Photograph courtesy of AutoMed Corp.)

scription and transposition errors, reduced batching of samples and increased ability to handle a varying number of samples with the same staffing level. Mayo also feels that automated aliquotting will permit the drawing of a minimum amount of blood, which is particularly important for extremely ill patients. Reduced exposure to biohazards is also perceived to be a great benefit.[10]

22.8. SUMMARY: METHODOLOGY FOR EVALUATING LABORATORY AUTOMATION BENEFITS

Although cost–benefit analysis is at present the most common tool for evaluating the benefits of applying automation to various parts of the clinical laboratory, it provides an incomplete representation of the range of benefits that may be realized. As laboratory automation develops, we can expect that laboratories, like other industries before them, will need to evaluate benefits other than direct cost savings to justify investment in automation.

To evaluate potential benefits other than cost savings through labor reduction, and to isolate those areas in which automation can have the greatest impact, another approach to analysis is required. One such approach is to identify a possible benefit to the operation of the laboratory, establish a metric relevant to

TABLE 22.1. Approaches to Evaluating Laboratory Automation

Method	Advantages	Disadvantages
Direct cost analysis based on FTE count before and after automation	Provides direct cost arguments for capital investment decisions	A cost argument alone may not fully justify automation and many possible benefits are missed by a cost analysis alone
Identification of desirable benefit and development of a representative metric	Focuses on specific desired results	Does not provide capital investment justification based on realizable cost savings
Qualitative analysis of problem areas in the laboratory operation	Captures problem areas and potential benefits not recognized by other methods	Provides no real quantitative analysis; a very subjective measure

that benefit and review the operation of the laboratory prior to automation to see where gains can best be realized. We have seen how this approach is used with respect to turnaround time.

Another evaluation approach is to quantify the relative difficulty of each process step in the laboratory based on the "gut feeling" of those working in the laboratory setting. Although much less definitive than the cost or specific metric approach, this purely qualitative approach offers some insights into the benefits of automation.

Each of the three evaluation approaches shown in Table 22.1 will provide different insights to the benefits of automation of the clinical laboratory. A complete benefits analysis should include some aspects of all three methods so that a deeper understanding of the impact of automation can be realized prior to implementation.

REFERENCES

1. Buckingham W: *Automation, Its Impact on Business and People.* New York: Harper & Row, 1961.
2. Riley FJ: *Assembly Automation: A Management Handbook.* New York: Industrial Press, 1983.
3. O'Bryan D: Robotics: A way to link the "islands of automation." *Clin Lab Management Rev* 5:446–460, 1994.
4. Godolphin W, Lines RB, Bodtker K: Automated sample handling in the clinical laboratory. *Abstracts, 3rd Internatl Conf Symposium Automation, Robotics and Artificial Intelligence Applied to Analytical Chemistry and Laboratory Medicine, Jan 25–28, 1994.* Elsevier, San Diego, 1994.

5. Bennet KE, Scheetz KJ, O'Sullivan MB, Moyer TP: Automation strategies of the Mayo Clinic. *In* Eggert AA, Ross PJ, Sobocinski PZ, Tomar RH, Westgard JO, eds: *Proc Clinical Laboratory Automation Workshop, June 6–8, 1993.* Madison: University of Wisconsin, 1993, pp. 59–66.

6. Middleton S, Mountain P, Kemp A: Laboratory automation: a model. *Leadership: Can Hosp Assoc* 2:20–24, 1993.

7. Maclin E: Riding the next wave of laboratory automation. *Clin Chem News* 2:11, Dec 1993.

8. Whisler KE: Major steps in automation of the specimen handling process. *In* Eggert AA, Ross PJ, Sobocinski PZ, Tomar RH, Westgard JO, eds: *Proc Clinical Laboratory Automation Workshop, June 6–8, 1993.* Madison: University of Wisconsin, 1993, pp. 105–111.

9. Skjei E: Front-end automation: the last hurdle. *CAP* (College of American Pathologists) *Today* 8:1,12,14,16–17, 1994.

10. Bennet KE, Dale JC, Moyer TP: Analysis of automation for pre-analytical medical laboratory specimen preparation. *Abstracts, 3rd Internatl Conf Automation, Robotics and Artificial Intelligence Applied to Analytical Chemistry and Laboratory Medicine, Jan 25–28 1994.* Elsevier, San Diego, 1994.

11. Skjei E: Re-Engineering the lab. *CAP Today* 8:1, 1994.

12. Nicolin M: Workflow and productivity. Etobicoke, Ontario: Miles Diagnostics (Canada) Inc., 1994. (Personal communication.)

13. Godolphin W, Bodtker K, Uyeno D, Goh LO: Automated blood-sample handling in the clinical laboratory. *Clin Chem* 36:1551–1555, 1990.

14. Hoffmann G, Holtkotte H, Retterath M: Laboratory integration study. Mannheim, Tutzing, Germany: Boeringer GmbH, Dec 1992. (Personal communication.)

15. Wills SD: Workflow case study. Miami: Coulter Corp, 1994. (Personal communication.)

16. Wills SD: An integrated system for automation of the clinical laboratory. *Abstracts, 3rd Internatl Conf Automation, Robotics and Artificial Intelligence Applied to Analytical Chemistry and Laboratory Medicine, Jan 25–28, 1994.* Elsevier, San Diego, 1994.

17. Mountain PJ, Middleton SR: People, information, & automation—a fully integrated approach. *In* Eggert AA, Ross PJ, Sobocinski PZ, Tomar RH, Westgard JO, eds: *Proc of the Clinical Laboratory Automation Workshop, June 6–8, 1993.* Madison: University of Wisconsin, 1993, pp. 121–125.

18. Dankbar GC, Shellum JL, Bennet KE: The use of simulation to evaluate automated equipment for a clinical processing laboratory. *Proc 1992 Winter Simulation Conference,* Arlington, Virginia, 1992.

POINT-OF-CARE TESTING

CHAPTER

23

The Economic Aspects of New Delivery Options for Diagnostic Testing

JOSEPH H. KEFFER

CONTENTS

23.1. INTRODUCTION

Clinical laboratory testing is being driven by reform of the healthcare delivery system, changes in the science of medicine, and advances in testing technology. Describing the need for management response to accelerated change, Tom

Handbook of Clinical Automation, Robotics, and Optimization, Edited by Gerald J. Kost with the collaboration of Judith Welsh.
ISBN 0-471-03179-8 © 1996 John Wiley & Sons, Inc.

Peters recommends the following: "Ready?—Fire!—Aim!"[1] This advice may or may not be appropriate for healthcare institutions. On one hand, providers of clinical laboratory services might appropriately heed this advice as they respond to requests for point-of-care testing (POCT). ON the other hand, fearing the potential increased costs of rampant decentralized testing, we are cautioned by more traditional advice: "No margin—no mission." It is intuitively apparent that the cost per result for POCT will generally be higher than batch testing on highly automated instruments that capture economy of scale efficiencies. This chapter addresses relevant issues with emphasis on the economic aspects of POCT advocating a "total economics" perspective. I advocate incorporation of comprehensive assessment of costs in context, rather than a limited focus on cost per test result and report the limitations of existing cost-effectiveness studies.

Assessment of the advantage of POCT should involve evaluation of efficacy, medical need, and responsibility for implementation. One should also incorporate some form of cost appraisal. Implicit in this and all such analyses is the need to compare and contrast the advantages of several options, each of which acknowledges limited resources.

23.2. EFFICACY OF TESTING

Although efficacy is not the principal focus of this review, an illustration of what is meant by efficacy seems appropriate. The first question should be whether a proposed intervention will achieve the goal intended. In a recent study of a proposal to install a stat laboratory in an emergency room (ER) of a large public hospital, it was determined that of the three phases of testing, preanalytical, analytical, and postanalytical, factors associated with the preanalytical and postanalytical phases contributed the most to increased turnaround time (TAT) of patient's laboratory results and were responsible for the majority of delay.[2] Creation of a satellite laboratory to alter the "dwell time" for the analytic phase of testing would not significantly improve the outcome—that is, the turnaround time—and thus, did not meet the standard required for efficacy.

The efficacy associated with placing limited function laboratories in surgical suites has been described by Kost.[3] A comparable contribution has been reported by Despotis[4] with regard to reduction of transfusion requirements as a consequence of providing on-site coagulation testing for cardiovascular surgery. Regardless of the reader's judgment on the degree of persuasion contributed by these analyses, they represent the type of evaluation appropriate for documentation of efficacy.

23.3. IMPLEMENTATION OF POINT-OF-CARE TESTING (POCT)

Faced with the challenge of expanding POCT, reviews have generally identified the conflicts. Cost and medical justification remain concerns and hard data is lacking with regard to "cost-effectiveness." Stimulated by the Clinical Laboratory

Improvement Act of 1988 (CLIA '88),[5] our laboratory has established a range of POCT at a variety of sites using a wide array of personnel (Table 23.1). Each application reflects review and appraisal of the appropriateness of the testing chosen to be performed at each location. In no case did we perform a complete and formal cost-effectiveness/cost-benefit analysis. The guidelines we used to guide our decision making are listed in Table 23.2.

These guidelines have functioned effectively and are self-explanatory. Clinical staff and allied health personnel have responded to them and are supportive of their implementation. They acknowledge them as a requirement for both the medical and scientific validity of POCT as well as compliance with accreditation and regulatory requirements. It is clear that the decision to introduce testing must be based on a combination of medical and management judgment in lieu of available formal cost-effectiveness analysis. A "total economics" perspective is essential.

TABLE 23.1. Point-of-Care Testing at Parkland Memorial Hospital

Location	Test(s)
Arthritis clinic	Joint fluid exam[a,b]
Dermatology clinic	Tzanck prep, Koh prep[a,b]
Urology clinic	Urine dipstick and sediment exam[a,b]
OB/ER	Dark-field exams[a]
Diabetic unit	Glucose quantitative serum[a–c]
Special-care nursery	Blood gases[g]
Neurology–stroke clinic	Whole-blood Prothrombin time[c]
Acute dialysis	Activated clotting time (ACT)[c]
Chronic dialysis	Activated clotting time[c]
Operating room	ACT,[b] "physiologic profile-9"—for blood gases, HCT, lactate and ionized calcium, electrolytes[e]
Cardiac catheterization lab	Oxygen saturation,[c] activated clotting time[c]
GI LAB	Helicobacter biopsy test[a,b]
OB/ER	Urinalysis, glucose, HCT, HGB, pregnancy test, (HGC) specific gravity[c,f]
Ambulatory-care clinic	Urinalysis, glucose, HCT, HGB, pregnancy test, (HGC) specific gravity[c,f]
OB screening	Urine dipstick, pregnancy test[c,f]
Employee physician office	Urine dipstick, glucose, HGB, pregnancy test, specific gravity, strep screen, occult blood, KOH prep[a,c]
Medicine clinic; diabetes clinic	Whole-blood HCT, NA, K, Cl, BUN, glucose[d,f]

[a]Staff physician.
[b]Resident physician.
[c]Registered nurse.
[d]Medical technologist (B.S.) or Technician (MT, MLT).
[e]Licensed vocational nurse.
[f]Medical laboratory assistant (physician office assistant).
[g]Respiratory therapist.
[h]Perfusionist.

TABLE 23.2. Guidelines for Initiating POCT

Laboratory testing performed outside the central lab that falls into the CLIA '88 moderate or high complexity category must meet the following guidelines. Under these conditions, the laboratory will cooperate with and assist clinical services in initiation and operation of POCT. The Department of Pathology accepts responsibility for and remains accountable for the quality of tests selected for POCT.

1. There should be a medical justification based on the need for the information in a timeframe appropriate to influencing significant patient care decisions.
2. The quality of the laboratory information must support quality medical care. Inaccurate and unreliable laboratory data are worse than no data.
3. The method must be such that nonlaboratory personnel can consistently perform the test, even if infrequently given the opportunity to do so.
4. The laboratory method and instrumentation should be selected by or approved by the laboratory expert appropriate to that field. The laboratory should provide and update standard operating procedures for the POCT site as well as for the laboratory. The laboratory should develop the documentation procedure for capturing patient results and oversee the process of transmitting the results to the laboratory information system for patient chart entry and billing purposes.
5. Laboratory personnel should provide training and certify personnel selected to perform laboratory testing.
6. To be certified, personnel performing POCT should be well trained, and demonstrate the ability to reproduce appropriate test results.
7. Only personnel who have been identified, trained, and certified by the laboratory are authorized to perform such testing procedures.
8. Basic routine maintenance should be the responsibility of testing personnel. Troubleshooting, and any maintenance considered complex, should be the responsibility of central laboratory personnel.
9. Quality control (QC) data should be collected in the routine course of performance of laboratory testing *by those personnel normally producing the results in the patient-care setting.*
10. The central laboratory should periodically monitor the proficiency of those performing testing using unknown samples that simulate true patient sample data.
11. The central laboratory personnel should provide continuing critical review of QC and proficiency testing data with feedback to the appropriate responsible authority on the ward.
12. Flagrant disregard or disinterest in these standards should be recognized as contrary to the best interest of patient care. Under these circumstances, POCT should be halted.

23.4. RATIONALE FOR POCT

Providing laboratory services associated with POCT is driven fundamentally by the perceived or real requirements for improved turnaround time (TAT) of patient test results. In a recent survey,[6] 91% of the respondents established the preeminence of turnaround time. Patient satisfaction followed at 34%. Jahn described a "disappointment index"[7] that noted the disparity between the shorter TAT expectations of physicians and nurses as contrasted with laboratorians' longer projections regarding acceptable turnaround time; thus, there is a guaranteed "disappointment" among the individuals served by the clinical laboratory. This may be explained further by data generated by Pellar and co-workers[8] describing TAT performance in terms of percentiles. There is a tendency among the laboratory staff to focus on their average performance or best performance rather than the poorest percentile, and more narrowly on the specimen dwell time within the laboratory. The clinician judges laboratory performance on the basis of "vein to brain" turnaround time. Reality reminds us that we are judged by our worst performance percentile rather than by our optimal performance. The i-STAT®, a portable chemistry analyzer, clinically and commercially available and approved by the U.S. Food and Drug Administration (FDA) illustrates the type of technology permitting POCT to reduce TAT to the ultimate irreducible minimum, testing at the source of the question: the patient. Carried to the next level, continuous intravascular biosensor monitoring is a developing technology driven by the perceived need for constant monitoring of vital functions.[9] It is the biochemical analogy to continuous monitoring of electrocardiographic events.

23.5. ECONOMIC PRINCIPLES RELATED TO POCT AND COST-EFFECTIVENESS ANALYSIS

Economics is defined here as the attempt to bring scientific method to bear on an appropriate investment of resources in order to gain benefits. This has been phrased well by Weinstein and Stason:[10] "for any given level of resources available, society (or the decision making jurisdiction involved) wishes to maximize the total aggregate health benefits conferred." In other words, the thrust of economic assessment is to prudently invest limited resources for maximum benefit. Weinstein states further: "the available database on the effectiveness of most clinical procedures is distressingly limited. Nevertheless, the tendency among health professionals to demand objective, scientifically valid proof, though laudable, begs the necessity to use the best available evidence no matter how uncertain, to make today's resource allocation decisions."[10] His words remain correct today.

It is essential to understand the use of the terms cost-effectiveness (CEA) and cost benefit analysis (CBA). They are fundamentally about comparisons. There is always, at least, a comparison between the status quo and the proposed intervention. As noted by Naylor et al.,[11] such analysis warrants caution: "we urge physicians and policy makers to regard economic evaluation as a technology—promising, clearly helpful, still in need of refinement and open like any new technology, to both wise use and well-intentioned abuse." Let us take a closer look in order to apply economics intelligently.

In an excellent review of CEA and CBA, Udvarhelyi et al.[12] defined CEA as a tool which "compares the net monetary costs of a health care intervention with some measure of clinical outcome or effectiveness such as mortality rates or life years saved." The authors proceed to contrast this with CBA, which they describe as "the costs of a health care intervention . . . assessed the same way as in cost effectiveness analysis but (in which) measures of clinical outcomes or effectiveness are typically converted into monetary units as well." These are the fundamental similarities and differences. Both must capture all costs. Appropriate values must be assigned for the range of benefits measured as the result of the investment. The difference is the assignment of some form of dollar value to the outcome, typically converting the number of years of life extension into a formula that includes quality of life and assigns a value to each quality-adjusted life year (QALY). Udvarhelyi reviewed published articles in the medical literature purporting to address these subjects and evaluated them against widely accepted criteria considered essential for CEA and CBA. Six principles, derived from Weinstein,[10] which are the hallmarks of CEA were applied:

Principle 1. "an explicit statement of a perspective for the analysis should be provided."[12] For example, the analysis defines cost and benefits based on who pays the bill. This might be the individual, physician, the hospital, or society. Clearly, the analysis will differ depending on the perspective of each. A decision to resuscitate a low-birth-weight infant has a short-term impact on the attending physician and the hospital. It has a potentially long-term impact on society resulting from long term morbidity.

Principle 2. "An explicit description of the benefits of the program or technology being studied should be provided."[12] The benefits are often assumed. To provide clarity, and to achieve common understanding for those reviewing the cost analysis, the benefits should be made explicit. This includes evidence for the efficacy of the proposed technology.

Principle 3. "Investigators should specify what types of costs were used or considered in their analysis."[12] Costs are invariably diverse having variable magnitude depending on the site and institution and depending on the perspective alluded to above. Costs of side effects should be included as well as costs averted.

Principle 4. "If costs and benefits accrue during different periods, discounting should be used to adjust for the differential timing."[12] Discounting has two aspects, one is the inflationary impact. If one invests current dollars and the benefit derived is in the distant future, then the costs are greater in terms of current dollars because of the inflationary erosion associated with the later dollars gained. Examples of this are the costs of immunization programs which avoid future costs of disease. A second and important aspect of discounting, often overlooked, is consideration of alternative options such as the "opportunity costs" of investing comparable dollars in a different resource. One might consider the alternative of investing in a satellite laboratory with the associated capital investment required, or alternatively an investment in ultrasound equipment for an obstetrical unit that might create a different revenue stream.

Principle 5. "Sensitivity analyses should be done to test important assumptions"[12] This term refers to the inherent uncertainties associated with valuation of both the costs and the benefits. If projections rather than actual measurements are used to predict and approximate the unit costs of testing or the value of the benefit projected, then it is appropriate to make a series of formulations based on different assumptions (e.g., higher or lower costs) that are explicit rather than implicit. This approach provides some measure of validity to the summary assessment of the analysis. In other words "sensitivity analysis can be used to demonstrate whether a conclusion is robust over a range of plausible assumptions or whether it hinges on the accuracy of a particular assumption."[12]

Principle 6. "A summary measurement of efficiency such as a cost benefit or cost effectiveness ratio should be calculated and preferably expressed in marginal or incremental terms unless one alternative or strategy is dominant."[12] In other words, one concludes the study by placing the costs in the numerator and the benefit in the denominator. This provides a comparison ratio for options that have been entertained and may include the existing status quo and alternative proposed interventions. Consider the option of serving the ER or intensive care unit by creation of a satellite laboratory with all of the overhead of capital equipment and staffing, contrasted with introduction of a pneumatic-tube system or handheld testing devices used by nursing staff. These are suitably predisposed to review by creation of an appropriate ratio of the costs to the benefits and comparison of the options.

23.6. LIMITATIONS OF ECONOMIC STUDIES OF POCT

Udvarhelyi and associates[12] used a computer program that identified journal articles in the Medline database pertaining to cost-effectiveness in the general medical literature during several selected time periods. They identified 304 such articles and eliminated all except those which were truly focused on cost-effectiveness. This process then led to 77 articles that were reviewed with the ultimate conclusion that only three met all six of the criteria listed above. They concluded that numerous reports alleging cost-effectiveness analysis are incomplete and inadequate. Similar findings are reported by Lee and Sanchez.[13]

The limitations of CEA have received considerable attention recently. This has been made more urgent by the growing tendency of government payers to apply

CEA to policy making as described by Laupacis et al.[14] In response, Gafni[15] describes the variables and limitations associated with CEA emphasizing the limitations of the use of QALYs. In particular, they emphasize the uniqueness of the assignment of values both for cost and benefit relating to the "very special circumstances" that they assert do not usually apply in practice. We are reminded of Weinstein's excellent description of QALYs.[10] In converting an extension of life into a dollar value, it is necessary to develop a product $[Y \times \gamma]$ where Y represents the years gained and γ represents a corresponding weight assigned by the analyst or reviewer: "each definable health status, ranging from death to coma to varying degrees of disability and discomfort to full health, and accounting for age differences, is assigned a weight from zero to one and the number of years spent at a given status, Y_s, is multiplied by the corresponding weight, γ_s, to yield a number, $Y_s\gamma_s$, that might be thought of as an equivalent number of years with full health—a number of quality adjusted life years (QALYs). The source of these weights is ultimately subjective."[10] While such analysis is distant from a decision whether to provide POCT in a proposed model, one can readily see that true and thorough CEA may not be appropriate for many decisions. Inherent in CEA is the assumption that one knows the outcome impact in terms of the change in survival years. Rarely are long-term survival gains in person-years known and short-term effects are often projected into life years.[11] Finally, subjectivity impacts the values assigned related to both the ethical and economic perspective of the source. As a consequence, the cost effectiveness ratio may vary dramatically as assigned by different individuals and is highly variable and subjective rather than mathematically robust hard data.

As we consider CEA of POCT, we should explicitly identify costs and benefits associated with intervention options. In my quest for guidelines and previous experience, my search of the Medline database between 1976 and July 1994 revealed 8788 articles alleging to address CBA and 3075 articles that were separately listed under the category "diagnosis, laboratory." Combining the two categories revealed only 69 articles that characterized CBA relating to diagnostic laboratory testing. Many of these were excluded as nonrelevant to the clinical laboratory. None of the articles approached the fulfillment of the six principles described by Weinstein[10] and more explicitly by Udvarhelyi.[12] Nevertheless, I have assembled a list of cost categories (Table 23.3) and benefits (Table 23.4) derived from our experience and a wide array of literature sources that are appropriate for economic assessment of POCT.

Some of the listings in Tables 23.3 and 23.4 may be irrelevant or redundant for one application or another. They will vary from case to case and are offered to stimulate consideration. Conventional, all-inclusive categories such as preanalytical, analytical, and postanalytical costs serve a purpose and are valid. However, they do not facilitate preconsideration and capture of all the costs and associated benefits. The lists are offered to be more comprehensive and explicit in order to focus on decision making with regard to POCT. In short, it may be a useful checklist.

TABLE 23.3. Positive and Negative Costs Associated with POCT

1. Cost of CEA/CBA study including design, implementation, data capture and analysis.
2. Cost of the intervention or technology proposed (with emphasis directed toward comparisons for POCT):
   A. Preanalytic costs: specimen acquisition including order entry, phlebotomy/fingerstick, transportation, centrifugation, breakage in centrifuge, pouring off, and distribution.
   B. Analytic costs: production costs including capital equipment (purchase or lease), space, disposables, reagents, operator time, training time, supervision time, troubleshooting, and professional review.
   C. Quality component or prevention costs: including training and retraining, continuing education, quality control, quality assurance, proficiency testing, preventive maintenance, service contracts, costs of repeat testing, dilution of high values, and associated costs.
   D. Postanalytic costs: the costs of data capture and data transmission to the recipient including documentation in the medical record and long-term storage of laboratory reports according to regulatory requirements.
   E. Miscellaneous costs:
      1. Variable costs associated with unique institution/site/proposed intervention.
         a. Indirect cost for overhead including heat, electricity, institutional support.
         b. Institutional debt impact (significantly different for investment costs in an institution that is debt-free vs. debt-laden).
         c. Alternatives for resource investment, for example, to include the revenue stream which could be generated by an alternative investment of dollar resources.
         d. Variable associated costs depending on who performs the test, for example, physicians, physician assistants, nurses, clerks, or medical technologists. Costs associated with "base staffing" of the laboratory, including coverage for vacations, illness, and holidays, as well as reagent costs, and the impact of test volume.
      2. Cost of the side effects or morbidity of option A versus intervention B.
      3. Induced cost associated with additional healthcare or support for individuals who benefit from the technology, including for purposes of illustration, prolongation of life by successful treatment of a fatal disease resulting in future hospitalization rather than death, a perspective variable with the analyst.
      4. Negative cost consisting of costs that are averted, for example, cost of illness avoided by successful immunization and prevention (actually a benefit).
      5. Cost of discounting for current dollars versus inflationary dollars in the cost/benefit mismatch of time and cost of lost opportunity for alternative investment.
      6. Impact of economy of scale resulting in marginal test cost changes, for example, by decentralizing blood glucose testing, the unit cost per test in the main laboratory is increased.

TABLE 23.4. POCT Benefits for the CEA Equation

1. Improved turnaround time.
2. Improved patient management—improved patient satisfaction, for example avoidance of 5:00 a.m. early wakeup for blood glucose in diabetics and substitution of 7:00 a.m. bedside glucose.[19]
3. Resultant improved productivity, for example, increased throughput in the clinic or emergency facility with constant staffing.
4. Physician/nurse job satisfaction enhancement through "empowerment" with resultant decrease in employee "burnout" and turnover.
5. Improved relations between the laboratory and the clinical personnel with reversal of the "disappointment index."
6. Increased efficiency in patient throughput resulting from shorter waiting time in the ER improved "word of mouth" reputation and increased patient flow.
7. Decreased errors:
   a. Transcription of orders
   b. Clerical transfer
   c. Transportation
   d. Breaking (centrifuge or dropping)
   e. Sample repeats and dilutions
8. Improved communications:
   a. Immediate test reporting
   b. Direct specimen handling and barcoding on site with fewer intervening links (time cost of personnel)
   c. Decreased errors and resultant cost of correction
   d. Decreased phone time: waiting and being "handed off" to second and third parties in either the laboratory or ward while reporting results
9. Decreased physician "mental switching" with immediate disposition of an assessment of a patient problem by continuous focus of the mental stream stimulated from history and physical exam. Immediate provision of a potassium value with disposition of the diuretic treated patient. Contrast this with the usual scenario of the physician "switching off" to attend another patient while awaiting a 90-min potassium turnaround time, then refocusing on the former patient's problem.[16]
10. Decreased transfusion in cardiovascular surgery resulting from decreased platelets, component therapy, blood loss, and reoperation with risk of infection from reexploration.[4]
11. Decreased operating room (OR) time and staff overtime awaiting stat laboratory testing during surgery.[16]
12. Decreased dietetic services for customized service and decreased floor nurse time associated with special meals awaiting blood glucose testing results in the morning.[17]
13. Improved outcomes:
    a. Morbidity and mortality QALYs $(Y_s \times \gamma_s)$[10]
    b. Overcome short supply of medical technologists
    c. Benefit of alternate investment opportunities
14. Decreased testing cost opportunities using only needed tests (e.g., hematocrit, and potassium/BUN) in place of complete blood count and multitest biochemical profile.

23.7. LITERATURE REVIEW OF THE ECONOMIC ASSESSMENT OF POCT

Search of the laboratory medicine literature on POCT reveals preoccupation with the economics of bedside glucose testing in monitoring diabetics. POCT should be divided into bedside glucose and "all others" from consideration of the sheer magnitude of the former and heterogeneity of the latter. An excellent study documents continued improvement in analytical tools for POCT of glucose and substantial caution and guidance with regard to minimizing improper performance.[17] Regardless of whether one considers the Diabetes Control and Complications Trial (DCCT) to be definitive from the standpoint of cost justification,[18] fingerstick glucose testing has become the standard of care. In spite of the limitations with regard to precision measurements of glucose, Watts[19] has appropriately quoted Voltaire, "the best is the enemy of the good." POCT decisions should be based on a total economics assessment and CBA, regardless of compromised assay precision, and in spite of the higher cost per test result that is not only intuitive, but also generally provable.[20] Nosanchuk presents excellent observations with regard to alternative test costs for POCT and central laboratory glucose testing.[21] He assigns data for an optimized air-tube transfer strategy and central laboratory testing and contrasts this with POCT. No data is presented on the costs associated with delays in testing, the actual percentile performance of central laboratory testing on a 24-h basis, or costs and benefits achievable by decreasing central laboratory testing such as reduction in staffing, or diminished contention among specimens competing for the same analytical time.[21] Bedside glucose testing represents the standard of care for diabetics as recommended by the American Diabetes Association.[22] Yet, "we do not yet know whether bedside testing in the hospital, when compared to centralized testing with rapid turnaround, results in more rapid stabilization of glucose concentration, fewer complications, or reduced hospital stay."[23,24] Nor are such studies likely to be forthcoming. Since POCT glucose testing is already the standard, our option is to continue to optimize it. This will require innovation with a variety of solutions in various environs.

Reviewing the cost of POCT in a large hospital, Handorf[25] reported hypothetical costs associated with the alternatives of central laboratory testing for glucose versus bedside testing. It is notable that the cost of decentralized testing in this calculation was made apparently justifiable on the basis of assignment of "external failure costs" that represented wasted, inappropriate, or duplicative pharmacy and dietary services due to slow turnaround of glucose levels on diabetic patients. The reader might conclude that this is a subjective, site-specific judgment, which would appear to justify the apparent precise cost effectiveness. While this is so for that postulated example, it may not be the case in another institution.

In another example, Statland and Brzys[26] describe a mathematical model, "calculating amortized laboratory costs" (CALC), for comparing bedside testing and creation of a new stat lab for provision of blood gases and related testing in an intensive-care unit. In describing the satellite lab option, Statland and Brzys assign the costs of amortization for a totally new laboratory fully loaded with capital equipment and 24-h staffing. This results in total costs of $202,800 versus bedside testing of $7703. There is an alleged difference in labor cost of $150,000, which they used to effectively, "validate" the assessment. In reality, this analysis suffers from two of the common shortcomings of these studies: comparing only two options when there may well be a third (such as the installation of a pneumatic tube or limited shift staffing) and undervaluing the labor cost of nurse performed testing. Again, the point is clear that one would expect an analysis to be highly variable depending on the site and location and unique aspects associated with each institution. Consequently, one should recognize that a technology, although proven by others to be "cost-effective," may not be cost-effective for you.

By contrast, Jacobs[27] reported consolidation of stat laboratories appropriately contrasting a series of options for costing. Typically, the range of alternatives are not explicitly considered in most studies, and hypothetical, unsupported labor costs are usually questionable.

A current influence on decentralized testing that can be described as a "movement" is the model identified as the "patient-focused hospital" patient-care concept.[28] The essential elements of this model include cross-training of nursing personnel with a multidisciplinary competence resulting in decentralization of ancillary services to the floors and integration of a computerized medical record. The implications for the central laboratory are a fairly radical reallocation of laboratory resources to the wards. In describing this model, Kost and Lathrop[28] provide very little financial information, but they report that "studies of hospitals that have restructured show that personnel related costs can be reduced 20% to 30% hospital-wide, and that overall operating costs are reduced 10% with a return within 2 to 3 years." This is an impressive statement, although hard data do not yet exist to support this assertion. The authors' model has great intuitive benefit; however, it is important to recognize that hard data in the field of economic assessment of POCT is substantially limited. Our own experience is informative.

Recently, we attempted a prospective, randomized, case-controlled study to validate the contribution of POCT in a trauma intensive-care unit (ICU). We sought to test the hypothesis that the availability of acute physiologic monitoring using the Nova® Stat Profile-9 providing capability for blood gases, electrolytes, hematocrit, lactate, glucose, and ionized calcium, would affect the morbidity and mortality of these patients by providing immediate test results in contrast with the existing support from the central laboratory. The study design included assignment of alternate patients admitted to the ICU to either the existing standard of care using the central laboratory or the augmented service. Nurses on the unit were intensively trained over a period of months to ensure that all personnel were competent to perform the necessary steps and to have confidence that the system was operating effectively. A formal protocol was approved by the Institutional Review Board, and the following outcomes were to be recorded: mortality, time to intubation, time to extubation, total time on ventilation, C-pap trials, and hyperventilation therapy for increased CNS pressure (elapsed time to stabilization). Difficulties encountered in the study included nurse turnover requiring retraining, data capture requiring interface of the instrument to the laboratory computer, cumbersome nurse–computer interaction, and the maintenance of appropriate records. All of these obstacles were overcome. However, in the ongoing study, it became apparent that the patients to be compared, and alternately assigned to the study group or the control group, included numerous variables that would impact the outcomes studied. Consider comparing patients with femoral fractures and crushed-chest injuries to those with head injury, either alone or in combination with pelvic fractures. We became persuaded that the range of morbidity was so varied that conclusions with regard to the contribution of the intervention strategy would be unconvincing. Anecdotal support for POCT was quite clear with regard to individual needs and interventions, although strict scientific conclusions were not warranted on the basis of assignment via a single variable. Nevertheless, we believe that this intervention made sense in this acute-care environment in spite of the lack of hard data. We continue to hold this position.

The lessons we have learned indicate that in order to have a scientifically valid study for proving cost-effectiveness based on improved morbidity or mortality, it is probably essential to have a homogeneous patient population such as might be encountered in renal dialysis or in coronary artery bypass graft surgery wherein age and prior clinical status can be standardized better than in our heterogeneous trauma study group. In many medical cases, we conclude that truly controlled studies of the contribution of decentralized testing are not readily feasible in view of the complexities of the models studied. But this is not unique to POCT. Consider the enormous costs associated with treatment of myocardial infarction. There are considerable variations in the intensity of treatment and the degrees of resource commitment including the use of invasive procedures associated with various practice patterns.[29] In responding to commentary regarding the limitations of this study and others, Mark and coworkers observed, "We believe that in the absence of data from such a randomized trial, our observational comparisons generate useful questions about the effectiveness and efficiency of care after myocardial infarction."[30] Alternative strategies must be adopted employing judgment in order to guide decisions with regard to initiation of decentralized testing in the absence of hard data.

23.8. COST-EFFECTIVENESS JUDGMENTS

We recently decided to consider introduction of POCT into two settings. By contrast with the foregoing case, these may be of use in illustrating alternative courses of decision making in the absence of detailed CEA and complete cost studies. The first example represents replacement of an outmoded, poorly performing blood gas instrument from a "research laboratory" in the major operating suite of Parkland Hospital. It became apparent that this was an inadequate and poorly maintained source of testing in a busy operating room requiring extensive blood gas support and related testing for acute trauma cases, cardiovascular and thoracic surgery. Support from the central lab averaged 30 minutes with a poor performance for the worst percentiles in contrast with another hospital's reported 5–6 min.[31] In collaboration with our anesthesiology colleagues, we chose to place a Stat Profile-9® (Nova Biomedical) in the operating room, using laboratory support and training for this mission. Anesthesia staff, in the form of licensed vocational nurses, were provided, and after a period of intensive training culminating in certification, the system was placed in service. The laboratory personnel continue to play a support role for troubleshooting and ongoing training, and to provide direction for quality control performed by nursing personnel (as described in Table 23.2). Rational judgment was substituted for hard data to drive this implementation. Assessment of its efficacy and cost-effectiveness, albeit subjective, is unquestioned.

A second example relates to the outpatient arena. Our medical clinics are severely congested and patients are typically scheduled to arrive at either 7:30 a.m. or 1:00 p.m. as a group. Formerly, each would have a CBC and chemistry profile performed. They waited in a queue for phlebotomy, followed by further waiting in the clinic to be seen after test results are reported. We introduced the use of the i-STAT® instrument[32] in several of these heavily populated clinics. We had previously decentralized phlebotomy to the clinic area. We then implemented on-site limited testing using the i-STAT® [i.e., hematocrit, substituted for a CBC, and in place of the 18-test chemistry profile, we performed a BUN (blood urea nitrogen), glucose, and electrolyte testing]. As a result, patients can be seen promptly with far less waiting. This further decongests the phlebotomy waiting area near the central laboratory permitting other clinic patients to have more prompt service. Additional benefits appear to be the future opportunity to reschedule patients at more appropriate intervals, thus improving patient satisfaction as well as physician care. Physicians have indicated that they had previously ordered the more extensive complete blood count and comprehensive chemistry profile "since the blood was going to the lab, anyway." We therefore entertained the possibility that costs of testing per "laboratory encounter" will measurably diminish, not increase. We have not waited for a full cost analysis in view of the immediate gains and in spite of the apparent increase in the cost per test result of this testing modality. The overall benefits are compelling. Again, rational judgment was substituted for the missing hard data. Eventually, if urgent clinic needs are satisfied by POCT, we may close the dedicated clinic laboratory, which duplicates much of the central laboratory at high aggregate cost.

Recently, as reported earlier, Saxena and Wong described a detailed analysis of the turnaround time problems in an emergency room.[2] We experienced similar problems and agree that their resolution requires analysis and separation of the variables associated with preanalytical, analytical, and postanalytical testing. As in their report of a comparable hospital, we found the preanalytical and postanalytical times to be the major variables rather than the dwell time in the laboratory for analytical testing. In addition, we learned that the preanalytical time was particularly prolonged as a result of clinical errors originating in the emergency room, inappropriate test code ordering by computer, lack of bar coding, mismatch of tube placement in "baggies" with a different patient's requisition slip, and the like. There were demands for development of a laboratory in the emergency room. We addressed this by placing our laboratory clerk in the emergency room to immediately facilitate the process from the moment the blood is drawn through computer entry of the orders into the lab system, printing of a bar-code label, proper troubleshooting and avoidance of error at the "front end," transshipment to the lab, and finally delivery of the electronically printed result to the physicians and nurses for whom they are intended. The "perceptions" of the nurse and physician staff in the emergency room are that the central laboratory has been totally renovated and they assume acquisition of new laboratory instrumentation. In fact, the perceived turnaround time has dropped from 90 min to 20 min, while the actual performance of testing in the main laboratory remains unchanged. The entire improved outcome resulted from a "front to back end" "reengineering" of the process.

Overall, we have concluded that examples of formal CEA applied to POCT do not exist in the literature sufficient to significantly influence our decision making. Moreover, they are unlikely to appear in the near future for all of the reasons previously discussed. We have adopted a policy of making a "cost effectiveness judgment" that is based on the best available evidence and the appropriate proportion of resources required to achieve the intended goal. It is not a question of doing CEA or not; rather, it is a question of assessing the extent to which it should be done. One should not be immobilized by waiting for exhaustive data. Consider the cost of performing an exhaustive CEA and then contrast this with determining the proportionate benefit likely to be derived prior to proceeding. We adapted a graphic illustration of this from Laupacis (Fig. 23.1).[14] It can be seen that if a proposed intervention is obviously less costly and yet more

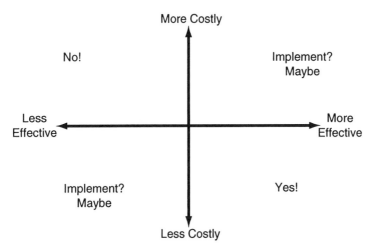

Figure 23.1. Economics of point-of-care testing. [Reprinted from *Laupacis*[14] by permission of the publisher, *Can Med Assoc J* 1992; 146(4):473–481.]

effective, then it should be adopted as common sense would dictate. Conversely, if something is obviously more costly and less effective, one would clearly not elect to introduce this. The difficulties are in the areas where testing may be variably more costly and the benefits vary in effectiveness. In short, there will necessarily be a requirement for continuing to apply rational judgment.

As we move forward into this rapidly changing era, decision making with regard to change will be urgent and compelling. We must change rapidly, basing this on making rational judgments rather than conducting time-consuming and exhaustive formal CEA/CBA studies in an effort to provide hard data.

23.9. POCT AND THE NEW TAT-DRIVEN CATEGORIES OF LABORATORY TESTING

Laboratory testing has been conveniently categorized in the past as "in-patient, out-patient, or reference laboratory testing." We propose that testing be classified as "immediate, urgent, discretionary, or esoteric." Immediate need would require POCT in either the inpatient or outpatient arena for a variety of reasons defining that need. They exist and will become more compelling. In the outpatient arena, we recognize increasingly that in the managed care paradigm, if a physician can make disposition of the patient's problem with one visit, this is to be desired over a return visit principally required to review results from laboratory testing prior to making final disposition. We illustrate this using an urgent care setting. In the future, TAT-driven categories will include "urgent" testing (i.e., TAT of test results 4–8 h) such as may be performed in a central hospital laboratory, "discretionary" testing (24–72-h TAT), and finally, esoteric testing involving extremely challenging testing or testing for extremely rare analytes that would be optimally performed in a true esoteric reference laboratory. We believe that this will result in a more limited menu of laboratory tests performed in the acute-care setting. Options will exist to perform the 8-h and discretionary tests stimulating an efficient regional network of laboratories. Such a model exists and is being facilitated in our setting by the electronic infrastructure provided by the esoteric reference laboratory partner, The Mayo Reference Laboratory. In our university, we are linking our six affiliated hospital laboratories and specialized esoteric pathology laboratories through the computer linkage facilitated by this system. This system provides the necessary infrastructure and encourages division of labor and sharing of expertise while simultaneously reducing costs for each member laboratory and creating a unified array of laboratory services. It efficiently and economically minimizes redundancy extending from the bedside and intensive care to electron microscopy. The relevance for this discussion is that it will free existing resources to enhance decentralized testing contributions in an economically relevant context. In turn, as POCT becomes technologically more advanced, the network interplay will more extensively contribute.

23.10. CONCLUSIONS

What lessons have we learned regarding CEA? We conclude that there will be a continuing need for both medical and management judgment. It is appropriate to integrate proportionate cost detail to the extent required for the rational judgment. Evidence for decision making should be in the context of total benefits; therefore, total economic considerations. The first question is whether CEA should be a routine part of POCT assessment. The answer is invariably "yes." The second question is to what extent. Tom Peters admonition "Ready?—Fire!—Aim!" can be balanced now by the appropriate context. It is not only appropriate, but may be essential for survival. But, CEA demands that the management team have appropriate expertise, prior experience, motivation driven by quality of care, and exercise true collaboration for the process engaged. Tom Peters has quoted Henry Mintzberg[33] as saying, "while hard data may inform the intellect, it is largely soft data that generates wisdom." We agree with this and recognize that while data is king, the absence of data is not justification to avoid change. Recall Naylor's caution:[11] "we urge physicians and policy makers to regard economic evaluation as a technology—promising, clearly helpful, still in need of refinement and open like any new technology to both wise use and well intentioned abuse." Finally, we return to Weinstein's conclusions in his superb primer regarding CEA for health and medical practices.[10] He discusses the reality that such analyses are frequently uncertain and founded on questionable data resulting in cautions for individuals that prompt reluctance to act. He counsels: "nevertheless, resource allocation decisions do have to be made and the choice is often between relying upon a responsible analysis with all its imperfections and no analysis at all."[10] This is the reality that we must ultimately confront. CEA/CBA studies described in the existing medical literature do not provide sufficient accuracy or detail to guide others. More importantly, the perspective of the individual laboratory and institution varies considerably as well as the actual costs experienced and the value of the benefits derived. Nevertheless . . . act we must!

REFERENCES

1. Peters T: Embracing chaos, audiotape series. Niles, IL: Nightingale-Conant, 1992.

2. Saxena S, Wong ET: Does the emergency department need a dedicated stat laboratory? *Am J Clin Pathol* 100:606–610, 1993.

3. Kost GJ: New whole blood analyzers and their impact on cardiac and critical care. *Crit Rev Clin Lab Sci* 30:153–202, 1993.

4. Despotis GJ, Santoro SA, Spitznagel E, Kater KM, Cox JL, Barnes P, et al: Prospective evaluation and clinical utility of on-site monitoring of coagulation in patients undergoing cardiac operation. *J Thorac Cardiovasc Surg* 107:271–279, 1994.

5. Clinical Laboratory Improvement Amendments of 1988. 42 USC 201, Public Law 100-578, Oct 31, 1988.

6. Bickford GR: Decentralized testing in the nineties: a survey of U.S. hospitals. *Clin Lab Management Rev* 8:327–338, 1994.

7. Jahn M: Turnaround time down sharply, yet clients want results faster. *MLO* 25(9):24–30, Sept 1993.

8. Pellar TG, Ward PJ, Tuckerman JF, Henderson AR: The freckle plot (daily turnaround time chart): a technique for timely and effective quality improvement of test turnaround time. *Clin Chem* 39:1054–1059, 1993.

9. Venkatesh B, Brock TH, Hendry SP: A multiparameter sensor for continuous intraarterial blood gas monitoring: a prospective evaluation. *Crit Care Med* 22:588–594, 1994.

10. Weinstein MC, Stason WB: Foundations of cost-effectiveness analysis for health and medical practices. *N Engl J Med* 296:716–721, 1977.

11. Naylor CD, Williams JI, Basinski A, Goel V: Technology assessment and cost-effectiveness analysis: misguided guidelines? *Can Med Assoc J* 148:921–924, 1993.

12. Udvarhelyi IS, Colditz GA, Epstein AM: Cost-effectiveness and cost-benefit analyses in the medical literature. *Ann Intern Med* 116:238–244, 1992.

13. Lee JT, Sanchez LA: Letter to the editor. *Ann Intern Med* 117:172, 1992.

14. Laupacis A, Feeny D, Detshy AS, Tugwell PX: How attractive does a new technology have to be to warrant adoption and utilization? Tentative guidelines for using clinical and economic evaluation. *Can Med Assoc J* 146:473–481, 1992.

15. Gafni A, Birch S: Guidelines for the adoption of new technologies: a prescription for uncontrolled growth in expenditures and how to avoid the problem. *Can Med Assoc J* 148:913–917, 1993.

16. Popper C: Using cost-effectiveness analysis to weigh testing decisions. *MLO* 24(Suppl): 29–35, Sept 1992.

17. Nichols JH, Howard C, Loman K, Miller C, Nyberg D, Chan DW: Laboratory and beside evaluation of portable glucose meters. *Am J Clin Pathol* 103:244–251, 1995.

18. Diabetes Control and Complications Trial Research Group: The effect of intensive treatment of diabetes on the development and progression of long-term complications in insulin-dependent diabetes mellitus. *N Engl J Med* 329:977–986, 1993.

19. Watts NB: Bedside monitoring of blood glucose in hospitals: speed vs. precision and accuracy. *Arch Pathol Lab Med* 117:1078–1079, 1993.

20. Jones BA, Bachner P, Howanitz PJ: Bedside glucose monitoring: a College of American Pathologists Q-probes study of the program characteristics and performance in 605 institutions. *Arch Pathol Lab Med* 117:1080–1087, 1993.

21. Nosanchuk JS: Keefner R: Cost analysis of point-of-care laboratory testing in a community hospital. *Am J Clin Pathol* 103:240–243, 1995.

22. American Diabetes Association: Bedside blood glucose monitoring in hospitals. *Diabetes Care* 9:89, 1986.

23. Rainey PM, Jatlow P: Monitoring blood glucose meters. *Am J Clin Pathol* 103:125–126, 1995.

24. Jatlow P: Point of care testing in the emergency department. *Am J Clin Pathol* 100:591, 1993.

25. Handorf CR: POC testing: Must quality cost more? *MLO* 25(Suppl):28–33, Sept 1993.

26. Statland BE, Brzys K: Evaluating stat testing alternatives by calculating annual laboratory costs. *Chest* 97(Suppl): 198S–203S, 1990.

27. Jacobs E: What is the correct means of cost accounting patient focused testing? Philadelphia: National Academy of Clinical Biochemistry, May 1994.

28. Kost GJ, Lathrop JP: Designing diagnostic testing for patient-focused care. *MLO* 25(Suppl):16–26, Sept 1993.

29. Mark DB, Naylor CD, Hlatky MA, et al: Use of medical resources and quality of life after myocardial infarction in Canada and the United States. *N Engl J Med* 331:1130–1135, 1994.

30. Mark DB, Naylor CD, Armstrong PW: [Letter]. *N Engl J Med* 332:471–472, 1994.

31. Winkelman JW, Wybenga DR: Quantification of medical and operational factors determining central versus satellite laboratory testing of blood gases. *Am J Clin Pathol* 102:7–10, 1994.

32. Woo J, McCabe JB, Chauncey D, Schug T, Haney JB: The evaluation of a portable clinical analyzer in the emergency department. *Am J Clin Pathol* 100:599–605, 1993.

33. Peters T: Death to strategic plans. *CAP Today* 62, May 1994.

24

Robotic Automation of Near-Patient Testing

ROBIN A. FELDER

CONTENTS

Handbook of Clinical Automation, Robotics, and Optimization, Edited by Gerald J. Kost with the collaboration of Judith Welsh.
ISBN 0-471-03179-8 © 1996 John Wiley & Sons, Inc.

24.1. INTRODUCTION

Near-patient testing is necessary to provide analytical results to critically ill patients in timely fashion. Near-patient testing can be provided in a variety of ways, including rapid specimen transportation, placing analytical instruments in the hands of physicians, or handheld analytical devices. Each of these methods can be used effectively to provide the necessary medical information; however, each comes with a price in either turnaround time, quality of service, or cost. Ideally, what is needed is a system that combines the best features of all these methods. This chapter will review some currently available technology for point-of-care testing and compare and contrast their relative effectiveness. The need for near-patient testing is still under debate. Several recent conferences have focused on the medical relevance of rapid analytical testing. However, there is no clear consensus on situations where near-patient testing is needed because definitive outcome studies have not been conducted. Studies currently under way will define the benefits of testing performed for physician convenience versus testing necessary to improve patient outcome. In order to provide the best quality laboratory services at the lowest cost, we created a remotely controlled clinical laboratory that provides whole-blood analysis of blood gases (p_{CO_2}, p_{O_2}), pH, electrolytes (Na, K, Cl), glucose, and hemoglobin near the patient bedside yet maintains the distinct advantage of central laboratory control. The automated remote laboratory provides extremely rapid turnaround, eliminates the cost of labor for specimen processing, reduces the risk from contaminated specimens, reduces staff training, and results in improved patient care.

24.1.1. Incentives for Cost Containment

The advent of managed care and possibly a nationalized healthcare plan has caused healthcare providers to focus on controlling costs. The laboratory is a favorite target for the hospital administrator's budget axe because it is viewed as a cost center, not a revenue generator. Since reimbursements by insurance companies is based primarily on diagnosis related groups (a hospital is given a fixed reimbursement to treat a specific disease, not on the actual costs accrued per patient), there is a disincentive to increase the numbers of laboratory tests. Many laboratories are in the process of centralizing services and consolidating facilities to survive the anticipated reduction in reimbursements to laboratories. These events are likely to have a major impact on laboratories by eliminating those that do not remain cost-competitive. Yet, it is interesting that at a time when laboratories are consolidating and downsizing there are projections that the diagnostics industry will grow to $38 billion dollars by 1996.

Various methods are being used to control costs, such as eliminating redundancy in instrumentation, increasing the productivity of existing staff, reducing administrative costs, and reducing the duplication and unnecessary tests ordered from the laboratory. However, these formulas can be best applied to large-volume laboratories that perform routing testing. Assessing the economics of point-of-care testing requires the use of different cost-accounting formulas.

At a time when laboratories are consolidating their services, surveys have indicated that near-patient testing is on the increase.[1] This increase in costly testing results from the need for rapid turnaround, which is essential to proper patient management.[6] Blood gas, electrolyte, and glucose analyses are used in critically ill patients with respiratory and circulatory collapse. Disorders requiring blood gas and electrolyte analyses are usually life-threatening; therefore rapid results are necessary to assess their respiratory and electrolyte status, guide in the prescription of medications, and aid in the administration of therapy. Critical care tests are perceived as important for patient management; in fact, these tests account for 58% of the tests performed in a typical neonatal intensive care unit over a one-year period.[6] A recent survey of physicians at The University of Virginia revealed the turnaround time expected by physicians for certain stat and routine tests (Table 24.1). Point of care testing primarily arises from the need to deliver arterial blood gases in less than 15 min. However, at the University of Virginia, most physicians would prefer to have a wider menu of analytical tests available at the point of care and in less than 15 min.

Ideal laboratory turn around times were also the subject of a recent report from the College of American Pathologists (CAP) Q-probes program (Q-probes 93-04, prepared by S. Steindel and P. Howanitz). The CAP recommendation was 90% of orders returned within 45 min, while emergency-room physicians actu-

TABLE 24.1. Perceived Minimal Turnaround Times for Selected Analytes

Test	TAT
Stat	
Arterial blood gas	0–15 min
Stat complete blood count (CBC)	0–30 min
Stat chem 7	0–45 min
Stat toxicology	0–45 min
Qualitative hCG	0–45 min
Routine	
CBC	2 h
CBC with differential	2 h
EKG (ECG)	2 h
Chemistry (general)	2 h
Metabolic profile	2 h

ally prefer 100% in less than 30 min. Surgeons, on the other hand, had set turnaround goals that were unrealistic.

While it is generally agreed that rapid results improve patient health, there is little data to support this notion. The literature is full of anecdotal evidence.[8] For example, the length of stay for patients in the critical care unit usually decreases in concert with the decrease in turnaround time for analytical tests. There is a need for additional carefully planned studies to quantitate the benefits of point-of-care testing.

24.1.2. Lowering Costs in Critical Care

Intensive-care units are notoriously expensive, accounting for over 50% of the costs of a hospital stay for a critically ill patient. Of these costs, laboratory services are the most expensive.[7] Therefore, hospitals are most profitable when patients are sent home as soon as possible. Laboratory tests that provide more rapid diagnosis for the patient usually result in improved patient outcome[10,21] and quicker discharge. However, providing the critical care ward with rapid analytical results is also costly. A balance must be met between providing convenient service to the critically ill patient and physician and controlling laboratory costs. However, critical care laboratory services do not easily lend themselves to the cost to conservation. The need to provide rapid (<5 min) and inexpensive laboratory testing to critically ill patients has prompted the development of a number of novel technologies.

Two options for providing critical care analytical testing include centralizing laboratory services or decentralizing laboratories to provide service near the patient's bedside. Centralization of laboratories has the advantage of reducing staff needs as well as the number of analyzers required to provide the service. However, delays often occur in most transportation systems that are required to move the specimen to the laboratory. These delays can frequently lead to increased pre-analytical error.[20] Delays are not always due to the transportation method alone. There are many steps required in the preparation of a specimen for transportation, for example, calling the messenger, putting ice in a bag, labeling, and waiting for the transportation messenger. On the other hand, the decentralized laboratory option includes the use of a satellite laboratory or the newer handheld analytical instruments.

24.1.3. Specimen Transportation Options for Rapid Turnaround Time

Numerous methods are currently available to provide rapid transportation of critical specimens to the central laboratory, which is often located several hundred yards away from the patient. In most institutions several of the options listed in Table 24.2 are installed and working in concert. Providing a means to move the specimen from the patient to the laboratory requires an ongoing expense. For example, at the University of Virginia we spend in excess of one

TABLE 24.2. Specimen Transportation Options

Human messengers
Installed conveyance—pneumatic tube, electric cart
Mobile robotics

million dollars a year moving medical specimens around the hospital using human messengers.

Human messengers, while often quite reliable, have some drawbacks. Human delivery is inherently a batch process. Roving messengers will service a critical care unit only at discrete times. Furthermore, the time required to call a stat messenger adds costs to the analytical process and further delays the reporting of results. Even with careful handling of specimens we have experienced tube breakage or misplacement several times each year in the medical center. The average cost of human messengers on the East Coast of the United States is approximately $16,000 per year.

Other transportation options include installed conveyance devices. For example, pneumatic tubes or electric carts that travel through the walls. Pneumatic tubes have the advantage that transportation is rapid. For point-to-point pneumatic-tube systems there are few reports of systems failures. User satisfaction is generally lower when switching mechanisms are installed that are capable of sending the carrier to various locations. Some hospitals rely on pneumatic tubes for long-distance transportation; for example, the Mayo Clinic in Rochester, Minnesota has several systems that transport specimens over long distances (greater than a mile). Pneumatic tube systems have limited carrying capacity, therefore, only a few specimens may be sent at one time. For critical care specimens the limited cylinder capacity is sufficient. However, when both a tube system and a messenger system have to be operated coincidentally in order to have a method to transport larger specimens (e.g., 24-h urines), then the redundant systems become less cost-effective. Another drawback of pneumatic tubes are reports of the accelerations encountered in tube systems causing changes in some serum analytes. For example, Ellis Jacobs from Mt. Sinai Medical Center (New York, NY) described a study where 30% of neonatal heparinized specimens were clotted as a result of pneumatic tube transportation.[9]

Electric carts were developed in response to the limited transportation capacity of pneumatic-tube systems. Not only do they have increased capacity, but some will also maintain the cargo compartment in an upright position through the use of a gimbling mechanism. The cart systems come at a higher cost and also require a larger station where they can be loaded and unloaded. In fact, it is the necessity for additional staff to unload these carts and then transport the contents to their final destination that has obviated their use in many institutions. The ideal transportation system will pick up the material to be transported and then drop it off at its final destination. Mobile robots have been developed in response to this need for unattended pickup and delivery.

Mobile robots have been reviewed in Chapter 12. However, it must be mentioned in relation to this chapter that there are no successful examples of the use of mobile robotics to transport specimens for critically ill patients. Mobile robotics have yet to reach the degree of sophistication and speed necessary for reliable stat delivery.

It is the inability of transportation systems to adequately provide consistently fast delivery that has prevented the commercial laboratories from penetrating the critical care market. Hospitals and clinics must provide their own laboratory services if they desire rapid turnaround.

24.2. OPTIONS FOR POINT-OF-CARE LABORATORIES

The need for rapid analytical results for the management of critically ill patients is well documented,[2,15,24] yet many institutions which perform critical analytical tests in their central laboratory have turnaround times that exceed 20 min. As a solution, many medical institutions use staffed point-of-care laboratories to improve analytical turnaround times. For example, in 19 states, over 85% of 33 surveyed hospitals having more than 450 beds have fully staffed point-of-care testing laboratories.[19] However, point-of-care laboratories require at least one full-time technologist at all times. Five technologists are required to staff a point-of-care laboratory in order to maintain 24-h service. Therefore, various alternative approaches to providing point-of-care laboratories are being considered (Table 24.3).

24.2.1. Physician- and Nurse-Operated Laboratories

One alternative to a costly fully staffed laboratory is to place an analytical instrument in critical care areas to be operated by the medical staff. This approach has not completely eliminated the need for additional medical technologists. Additional laboratory staff are needed to regularly run quality control checks, maintain the instrumentation, and perform the training of nurses and physicians. Instrument malfunctions and errors are not always monitored by the nontechnically oriented users. Regularly scheduled maintenance and training is a daily exercise to assure proper instrument use. Furthermore, the Clinical Laboratory Improvement Act of 1988 (CLIA '88) may preclude the operation of analytical instruments by nontechnologist operators. Blood gas analysis is considered

TABLE 24.3. Point-of-Care Laboratory Options

Staffed laboratory
Instrument operated by physician or nurse
Mobile laboratory
Handheld analyzer
Biosensors
Remote automated laboratory system

a moderately complex test that will require the operator to be a certified medical technologist or trained physician.

Newer, easy-to-use instruments will facilitate this approach to point-of-care laboratories. For example, th Mallinkrodt Gem Systems blood gas analyzers have been engineered for simplicity, accuracy, and robustness in the hands of non-laboratory personnel. On-board quality control and totally replaceable fluid and electrode packs virtually eliminate maintenance problems. Similar simple-to-operate instruments are being offered by Diametrics (St. Paul, MN). The IRMA (Immediate Response Mobile Analyzer) is a portable instrument capable of measuring pH, p_{CO_2}, and p_{O_2}. A quality-assurance (QA) menu is built into the software to meet quality-control (QC) regulations. The 5-lb instrument can be transported to a patient's bedside where it operates from self-contained batteries.

More sophisticated analytical instruments are available that can reliably measure a wide variety of analytes, for example, the Ciba Corning 800 series instruments. This system redefines the versatility and automation of whole-blood analysis. Its modular design allows the addition of bar-code scanning, additional analytes, or software upgrades at any time. The manufacture (Ciba Corning Diagnostics Corporation, East Walpole, MA) has provided RS-232 ports as well as a network port on the back of the instrument to allow data transmission to the LIS. It automatically determines the type of specimen that has been placed in the sample port and draws only the amount of blood required. This type of next-generation instrument will improve the reliability of nurse or physician-operated instrumentation. However, more confidence can be gained by coupling this analyzer to a RALS or robotic RALS described below.

Blood gas analyzers that are operated by the medical staff spend most of their time beyond the control of the medical laboratory. Even instruments that provide a method to record quality control provide only a retrospective record of instrument performance. Furthermore, staff members who are uncertain about the instrument operation have no immediate access to knowledgeable technologists. Therefore, this approach to near-patient testing may result in more errors than systems in which the entire analytical procedure is supervised by trained medical technologists.

24.2.2. Mobile Laboratories

Moving the specimen to the laboratory results in delay of critical tests in some instances; thus some groups have suggested moving the laboratory closer to the patient. For example, Luckey et al. at the Baptist Memorial Hospital used a cart to hold an activated clotting-time analyzer so that it can be moved around the operating suite as needed.[11] Another scheme, Mobile Lab, was developed by Travers and others at the Veterans Administration.[23] Blood gas, coagulation, and complete blood count instrumentation are placed on a rolling table. A computer is used to gather all the instrument data and provide the modem link with which to transmit data to the central laboratory. When laboratory services are needed in outpatient clinics, critical care units, or emergency room, the Mobile Lab™ can be dispatched to the site. Mobile Lab takes approximately one hour to set up in order to be ready to provide analytical results. Mobile Lab could be used in a clinic in the morning and then moved to a new location in the afternoon. Duplication of instrumentation is therefore unnecessary. With a simple telephone hookup, Mobile Lab can send analytical results or QC data to the central laboratory where the results can be entered into the LIS for billing and monitoring of quality control.

Data presented by Travers et al. demonstrate a reduction in turnaround time, duplicate test ordering, and non-revenue-generating tasks with the use of Mobile Lab.[23] The overall FTE savings were 0.22 per 966 tests or 9 h per week (20% of an FTE). Further benefits were quoted as providing less "switching time." Switching time is the time required for physicians to reconcentrate on a patient once they have moved to the next patient. Rapid turnaround will help ensure that all the test results are available at the time the physician is performing a physical exam and formulating a diagnosis.

One of the first examples of placing an analytical instrument on a cart was provided by Nova Biomedical. The Stat Profile series of instruments can be mounted on a rolling cart equipped with a battery and an uninterrupted power supply (UPS). This configuration of laboratory has the advantage over the Mobile Lab concept of providing continuous uptime so that the cart may be quickly taken to a site where emergency laboratory medicine may be needed.

24.2.3. Bedside Handheld Instruments

Bedside testing using handheld analytical instruments[5] has had limited success because of issues related to accuracy, precision, and the high cost of analytical reagents. High costs associated with stocking portable analyzers, reagents, and the training necessary to assure proper utilization have also been a deterrent to their use. CLIA '88 regulations may also have a negative impact on the successful introduction of handheld bedside analyzers into the medical environment. The problems associated with bedside glucose testing will only be compounded by analyzers offering a wider menu of analytes.

Recently, technological improvements have provided more reliable handheld analytical devices. The i-STAT System (i-STAT Corp., Princeton, NJ) has created a handheld device that performs blood gases, electrolytes (Na^+, K^+, Cl^-, Ca^{2+}), hematocrit (conductometrically), pH, p_{CO_2}, p_{O_2}, BUN, and glucose[18] (see Chapter 27). A variety of calculated parameters based on the measured analytes are also provided. The i-STAT handheld unit contains the electronics, while disposable cartridges contain the microfabricated thin-film electrodes and immobilized enzymes. The user chooses a cartridge, places several drops of whole blood on the cartridge receiving area, and places the cartridge into the handheld unit. Calibration fluid is automatically flooded over the electrodes, followed by the whole blood. After the analysis is complete, the data is displayed on a LCD (liquid-crystal-display) screen and stored in the unit for transfer to the LIS via infrared or wire connections. Quality control is performed on several cartridges in each box; otherwise no other QC is performed on the units since they have built-in self-diagnosis.

24.2.4. Remote Automated Laboratory System

In order to address the need for rapid turnaround at reduced cost while maintaining high quality, we have invented a novel method of providing near-patient laboratory services.[13] Remote control of laboratory instruments has allowed us to keep our medical technologists in the central laboratory while they operate clinical analyzers that remain near the patient's bedside. Two versions of remotely controlled laboratories have been developed. The manually operated version allows nurses to present the specimen to the sample port of the instrument. The use of laboratory robots has also been developed as an alternative to human-operated sampling. The use of remote control to perform critical care testing is attractive because it reduces the major cost of operating satellite laboratories, provides the rapid turnaround necessary for critical specimens, and maintains laboratory quality in the hands of the trained professionals. Therefore, the goal of our clinical laboratory robotics research project has been to provide the medical staff with blood gas and electrolyte analyses in an unmanned robotically operated satellite laboratory.

Our first challenge was to establish reliable computer control of a commercial blood gas analyzer (Nova Stat Profile 5, Nova Biomedical, Boston, MA). We designed an instrument interface that allowed bi-directional communication between instrument and host computer.[12] Furthermore, the interface did not alter instrument function and required attachment only to the output port. Analytical instrument control signals vary from instrument to instrument and from vendor to vendor. In order to maintain compatibility of any instrument with our remote control system, all signals were translated on an erasable/programmable read-only memory (EPROM) chip contained on an interface card. The signals were then available in a standardized format that was compatible with signals used in the remote laboratory system. This translation allowed rapid interfacing of a variety of analytical instruments incorporated into the robotics laboratory, but also allowed us the capability to change to a different brand of analytical instrument with minimal changes to the robotic lab hardware. The remote control interface allowed us access to monitor all calibration cycles, chamber evacuations, washes and sampling mode, retrieval of patient and calibration results, initiation of instrument settings for the patient's temperature and hemoglobin concentration, and barometric pressure, as well as time and date.

RALS communicated through a network server attached to a central monitoring station (satellite central) equipped with an IBM/PS2 50 personal computer, and a remote computer that communicated directly with the analytical instrument. Communication with the central laboratory was established through a conventional Novell™ local-area network (LAN). Satellite central was equipped with a touch-screen monitor that allowed selection of operating parameters without the need for a keyboard.[14] Color cues were used extensively to convey information. Arterial specimens were displayed in red numbers and venous specimens in blue numbers. Flashing numbers indicated that the results were out of the reference range. The last 10 analyses obtained on the patient could be displayed in tabular form to facilitate interpretation of out of range results or establish trends. If a pending result was not verified within 10 s, the satellite central computer sounded a loud alarm that required touch-screen interaction to eliminate.

The remote laboratory was also operated through a touch-screen interface similar to that of satellite central. Through the touch screen, the operator had access to patient demographics, a menu of analytical tests available at that location, indications of instrument malfunctions, and a countdown timer to indicate time to completion of the analysis. The analysis of whole-blood electrolytes (sodium, potassium, chloride, ionized calcium), oxygen, carbon dioxide, pH, glucose, and hemoglobin can be performed in our RALS laboratories. The following is a stepwise description of the analytical sequence:

1. The nurse, physician, or medical student draws a sample of arterial or venous blood and places a cap on the syringe. The specimen is then transported immediately to the RALS system (Fig. 24.1).

2. A member of the clinical staff approaches the "user interaction station" (UIS) to request a laboratory analysis. The UIS was designed as a touch-

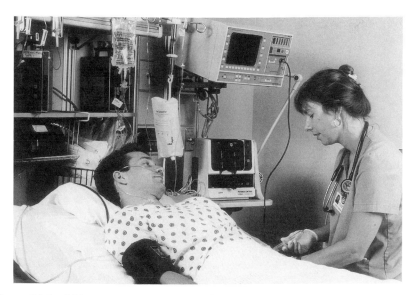

Figure 24.1. Critical care laboratory analysis begins with the drawing of blood from a patient in the critical care unit.

screen interface allowing users to interact with the system without removing their gloves. Initially, the screen allows the user to indicate the patient's location (Fig. 24.2). All the patients in the hospital are available in the RALS system. After identification of the patient's location, a list is generated on the touch screen, from which the patient may be selected (Fig. 24.3). The patient list is continuously updated from the hospital information system (HIS). Alternatively, patient demographics can be entered directly from the touch screen. The next step involves indicating patient information such as temperature and Fi_{O_2} (since these parameters affect the calculated blood gas results) (Fig. 24.4).

3. After patient demographics are entered and the analytes requested are chosen (Fig. 24.5) and verified by the requesting staff member, the UIS computer instructs the staff member to uncap the syringe and place the open end into a receptacle on the instrument (Fig. 24.6). After the instrument aspirates the required whole blood for analysis, the user is instructed to remove and discard the specimen.

4. A countdown timer is displayed on the touch screen indicating the time necessary until the analysis is complete.

5. After the analyzer has completed its analysis, the results are transmitted to the main laboratory over a LAN. A technologist is alerted to the arrival of patient analytical data by an alarm sounding from a touch screen posi-

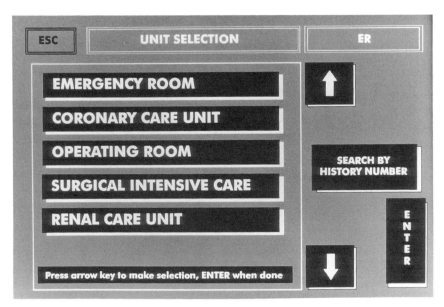

Figure 24.2. Using a special computer monitor, the patient location is selected by touching the area on the screen indicating the unit where the patient is being treated. Alternatively, patients may be located by entering the history number.

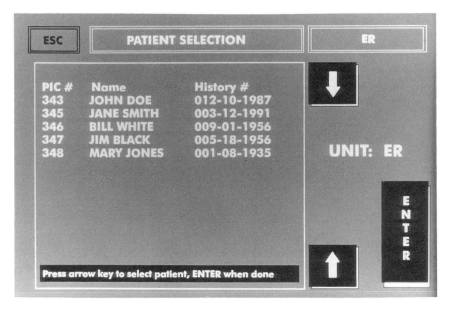

Figure 24.3. Patients are selected from a list presented to the user by the computer using the touch-screen interface. Even gloved fingers can be used on the touch screen.

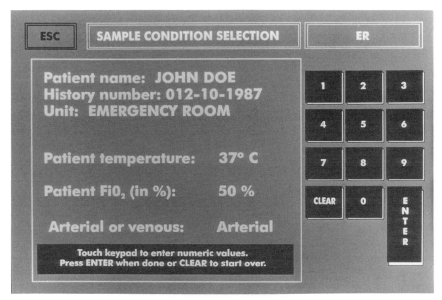

Figure 24.4. Patient temperature, Fi_{O_2}, and the source of the specimen (arterial or venous blood) are then selected from the next touch screen. The screens are automatically presented to the user in a logical sequential fashion.

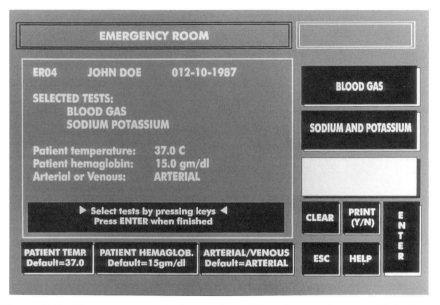

Figure 24.5. The analyses required are selected from the touch screen. Only those analytes selected are sent to the LIS for billing.

tioned over the laboratory bench. The technologist can then review the results and review previous results from the same patient by addressing a database (Fig. 24.7). Color cues are used to facilitate a quick review of the analytical results. The technologist has the choice of requesting a reanalysis of the specimen, in which case the entire analytical sequence is repeated. Alternately, the laboratory can be shut down electronically and a repair technologist dispatched to the laboratory. Usually, the results are acceptable and "accept" is pressed on the screen, following which the results are immediately available on the UIS in the critical care unit (Fig. 24.8).

24.2.5. Robot-Operated Analytical Sequence

An alternate configuration of automated laboratory has been configured that uses a commercially available robot arm to do many of the functions normally performed by the staff member (Fig. 24.9). The use of the robot arm allows rapid entry of multiple specimens as well as totally unattended operation.

The robot used was a CRS (CRS Plus, Toronto, Canada). Additional components of the robot included the robot controller and host microcomputer. In addition the robot came equipped with gripper sensors that gave feedback indication of the forces applied by the robot fingers. Gripper sensors provide simple touch sensing that can detect the presence or absence of an object in the robot end effectors.

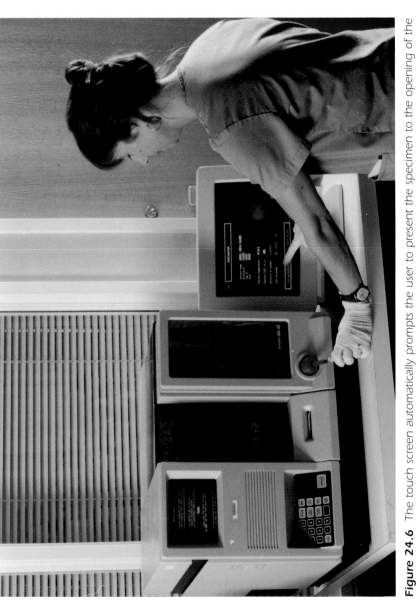

Figure 24.6 The touch screen automatically prompts the user to present the specimen to the opening of the red sampling port on the NOVA Biomedical Stat Profile instrument. The correct placement of the specimen as well as sampling are automatically initiated by the RALS system.

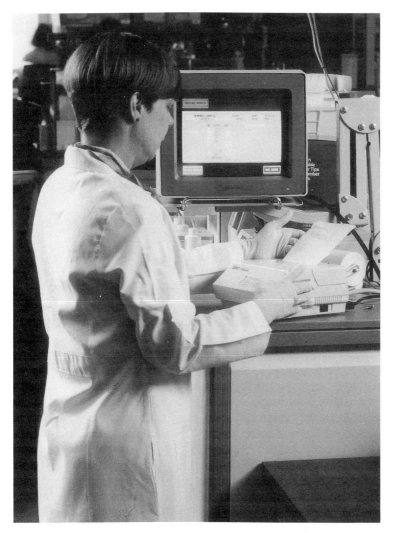

Figure 24.7. Once the analysis is complete, the results are automatically transmitted to the central laboratory, where a medical technologist reviews the analysis, instrument functions, and any errors that might have occurred.

The robot was programmed to perform simple, "pick–place" operations on 3-mL plastic syringes containing whole blood. The robot was trained to use several peripheral tools designed to assist the robot in complex procedures such as cap removal and replacement, specimen mixing, and air-bubble removal ("burper"). The CRS arm is capable of a high degree of repetitive movement precision (repeatability of 0.05 mm); however, an orientation device was incorporated into the design of the robot environment to allow the robot to recalibrate its location should it become disoriented.

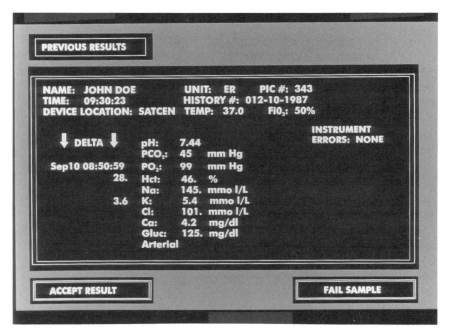

Figure 24.8. In <15 s the technologist reviews the results, appends an electronic signature, and transmits the data back to the critical care unit UIS, where the results are available for review. Simultaneously, the results are also sent to the LIS for archiving and billing.

The use of the robot results in an alternate analytical sequence:

1. The use of the UIS is identical in the robotic laboratory as compared to the nonrobotic laboratory.

2. After identifying the patient and selecting the analytical profile, the requesting staff member selects, "accept" from the touch screen. The UIS then initiates a request to the robot computer to open a door driven by a pneumatic cylinder. The user is presented with a single-sample receptacle in which the syringe is placed and then the user removes his/her hand from the door, followed by verification of the request on the UIS. The UIS communicates the verified request to the robot computer, closes the door, and instructs the robot to begin working.

3. The robot lowers its actuators (fingers), grasps the syringe, and moves it to a mixing chilling chamber. Following a 30-s mixing–chilling cycle, the syringe is removed from the mixer by the robot, which then places it in a pneumatically driven uncapping device. The host computer determines whether there is sufficient sample volume for an accurate blood gas analysis. If all system checks are acceptable, the robot closes its end effectors to grasp the syringe at the proper location for accurate insertion into the

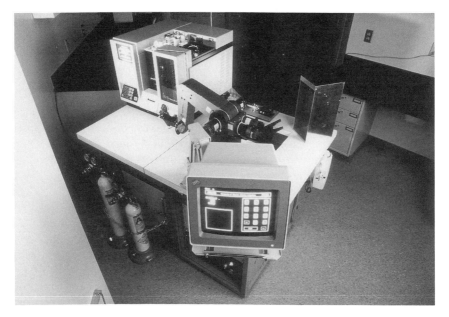

Figure 24.9. A second version of RALS has been in clinical service for several years. A robot arm performs many of the functions of the user in the critical care unit such as cap removal, sampling, air-bubble removal, recapping, and storage for potential reanalysis.

instrument. The entry port of the instrument was modified to facilitate specimen placement, and to reduce the risk to the user.[4]

4. The robot controller then checks electronically whether the blood gas analyzer is ready to accept a specimen. If the instrument is calibrated and in the ready mode, the robot places the syringe into the sample port of the instrument. A conical syringe luer tip guide was engineered to facilitate the robot in hitting its target.

5. The instrument aspirates the required whole blood for analysis and initiates analysis. After the analysis is complete, the robot removes the specimen, now containing a small air bubble where the whole blood was removed. The robot then positions the syringe in a "burper" that ejects the air bubble by advancing the syringe plunger and simultaneously washes the tip.

6. Subsequently, the robot recaps the syringe at the decapping station and then returns the syringe to the mixer–chiller to maintain specimen integrity.

7. The robot removes the syringe from storage and drops it into a contaminated waste receptacle.

Analytical results obtained by robots were compared to those obtained via manual introduction of specimens. The use of the robot was not predicted to interfere with the analytical results. Deming regression of data obtained manually and by robot yielded similar results.

24.2.6. Speed and Utilization

The use of the remote-controlled clinical laboratory has reduced the average turnaround time for analyses from 20 min ± 10 (n = 200) to 4.2 min ± 0.3 (n = 200). Readily available blood gas analysis through the use of near-patient laboratories is thought to increase utilization, which quickly increases costs. Other studies have demonstrated that removing impediments to obtaining blood gas results usually results in test overutilization. The presence of an arterial line in critically ill patients was demonstrated to increase the frequency of blood gas determinations.[17] Therefore, the effect of easy obtainable on-site blood gas determinations on utilization was measured. However, we found that RALS did not result in an increase in blood gas utilization. In our own TCV unit, over a 6-month period prior to the installation of the automated laboratory (Jan.–March 1991) we performed 1417 blood gas analyses per month. During a 6-month period after the initiation of operation of the automated laboratory (Jan.–March 1992) there was no increase in blood gas utilization: 1777 blood gas analyses per month. The apparent increase was due to an increased patient census of 275 versus 333 during that same period. Furthermore, we had more critically ill patients on the unit during the second data gathering period when the remote-controlled laboratory was installed (25 critically ill vs. 5 for the previous year). Therefore, there was no increase in blood gas utilization after the installation of the remote-control system. One explanation for this phenomenon is the use of blood gas utilization guidelines within our institution.[3]

24.2.7. Cost Savings

The utilization of the remote-control laboratory concept has resulted in the following cost savings: messenger time $19,500, nursing time $22,750, supplies $3,900, and less maintenance—$7500, resulting in a total savings of $38,650 in the first year. This savings did not take into account the savings that would result if a RALS laboratory replaced a fully staffed satellite laboratory. In this case a conservative estimate of the annual savings would be $219,000. Cost savings are realized by the elimination of the messenger, and savings on nursing time used to order, prepare, and give the specimen to the stat messenger, as well as supplies associated with bagging the specimen for transportation. The number of steps involved with human-assisted transportation versus RALS is considerably smaller (Fig. 24.10).

24.2.8. Advantages

The major advantage of remotely controlled laboratories is that the technologist in the central laboratory remains responsible for verification of the final result as well as operation of the analytical instrument. The healthcare personnel who

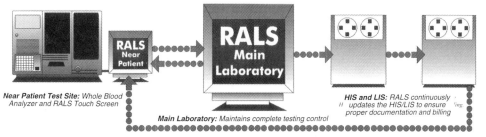

Figure 24.10. The flow of data begins with obtaining patient demographics from the HIS. These data are stored in the RALS system. Patient results are shared between the near-patient test site and the central laboratory. Completed results are then made available to the LIS and the HIS if necessary. Within seconds, all data storage systems are kept up to date.

introduce the specimen into the remote-control laboratory are delivering the specimen to the analytical instrument, and are not responsible for successful completion of the analytical procedure. CLIA-certified technologists remain in control of the operation and maintenance of the analyzer and reporting of results through a dynamic interface.

24.2.9. Clinical Justification

Rapid blood gas determinations reduce the average stay of patients in the critical care ward. In the thoracic and cardiovascular postoperative unit (TCV), weaning of patients from the ventilator requires frequent blood gases.[22] Ventilator settings cannot be adjusted until ABG results are obtained from the laboratory. More rapid turnaround of analytical blood gas resulted in reduced average weaning time and hence reduced cost of critical care services.

24.2.10. Interfacing to the HIS

Laboratories have improved efficiency of data management through the use of dynamic interfaces between LISs and each clinical analyzer. Bidirectional interfaces have typically allowed the exchange of patient identification, date and time of test, and final results. However, detailed information about instrument function and the ability to remotely control an analytical instrument is seldom included in instrument output. The unique feature of the remote-control laboratory is the full bidirectional interface allowing total access to patient demographics, analytical results, as well as all instrument functions. Furthermore, by gaining access to the instrument data bus, we can also read instrument error codes generated during component malfunction as well as monitor informative parameters such as electrode drift. Detailed analysis of instrument function allows a proactive approach to instrument maintenance that would predict component failure, enabling replacement before failure.

A dynamic link must be established between the LIS, HIS, near-patient UIS,

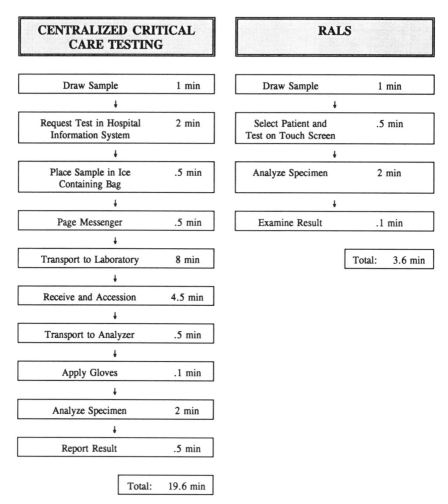

Figure 24.11. Timing studies demonstrate the many steps required to perform messenger-assisted blood gas analysis. The RALS system, on the other hand, requires many fewer steps and shorter turnaround time.

and the central laboratory (Fig. 24.11). Only downloading is necessary from the central laboratory to the LIS and then to the HIS in turn. Full bidirectional communication is necessary between the near-patient RALS installation and the central laboratory. Interfaces between the hospital information system (HIS) and LIS facilitate demographic downloading and request uploading. All registered patients are listed in the touch-screen database at all times. Therefore, we have eliminated the need to use a keyboard for patient demographic entry since each patient can be identified by a touch to the computer screen. During an emergency, valuable time can be lost requesting a blood gas analysis in the HIS. We have eliminated this step by designing an interface that allows the specimen to be requested in the HIS postanalysis by computer. Interface design is a major time-saving component in laboratory analysis. The laboratory alone generates approximately 50% of the data transactions in a hospital.[16] Therefore, the use of local task-specific databases and the use of touch-screen technology has reduced the clerical tasks associated with satellite testing.

24.2.11. Reliability

The RALS system, after the initial years when it was under development, has become quite reliable. Estimated breakdowns per 1000 tests on parts of the system other than the instrument average less than 0.01%. The instrument accounts for the highest percentage of breakdowns, due to its complexity and the complexity of the sample matrix (whole blood) that is being aspirated by the instrument. Some of the instrument malfunctions are reduced by requiring standardized heparinized tubes in the critical care network that are compatible with the RALS system. The second source of malfunctions is the network connection. Critical care networks are still not viewed by hospital administrations as essential expenses. However, when you consider that a student browsing the Internet is on the same network as a patient on a respirator, the need for a separate and secure critical care network becomes readily apparent. The third source of malfunctions is severe power fluctuations that are a product of the local power vendor in Virginia. Uninterruptable power supplies have obviated these problems.

24.2.12. Training

The remote-control laboratories were designed to work effectively in a decentralized location by healthcare personnel who did not receive formal laboratory training. The UIS was designed as a user-friendly touch-screen device with similar features as an automated bank teller. We thought that much of the hesitation to interact with a computer could be overcome by using technology already familiar to many people. Interaction through the UIS was designed by technologists; therefore it is direct and intuitive. The first screen simply asks for the identification number of the person requesting access to the system. The second screen requests the patient demographics to be entered. This screen is followed by a menu choice of the tests offered in the robotic laboratory. Alterations to the default values for patient temperature and hemoglobin concentration follow the test selection. Finally, the user input is summarized for verification and then the user is prompted to place the sample into the robot lab.

Following a brief training session, each user is required to sign a checklist indicating they have learned or understood six items:

1. The user should be able to select a patient from a list.
2. The user should be able to modify patient temperature and Fi_{O_2}.

3. The user should be able to mix and hold a specimen in the sampling port.

4. The user should be able to retrieve the finished results from the touch screen.

5. The user must be aware that the instrument does not check for hemolysis, which can raise plasma potassium.

6. The user must be aware that all air must be absent from the specimen for an accurate blood gas result.

24.2.13. Fault-Tolerant Design

Analytical equipment that performs critical care services must be designed to minimize failure and loss of patient results. We have incorporated fault-tolerant design into our robotic system. Communication between the UIS, the host robot computer, satellite central (computer which is monitored by the technologist), and the network sever computer is through a LAN (3Comm, New York, NY). All patient information is stored immediately after entry in files that are maintained in the host computer and network server. Should a power failure interrupt operation of the robot laboratory, the information on each specimen such as storage rack position, demographic information, and analytical results can be retrieved.

24.2.14. Maintenance

The presence of a remote laboratory in a critical care unit quickly becomes essential to patient care. However, all instruments either malfunction and must be shut down for repair. In addition, preventative maintenance is performed daily and a more extensive maintenance is performed weekly. Proper scheduling of preventative maintenance can obviate problems with availability of analytical results when critically ill patients are on the ward. The software in the RALS system can quickly determine patient census on the ward and indicate to the medical technologist the appropriate time to come to the unit for service. The computer can also predict and inform the technologist at satellite central of upcoming low demand hours. Unfortunately, malfunctions cannot be scheduled. Through the touch screen, RALS can direct users to other RALS systems that are functional. Also, depending on the malfunction, the RALS computer will be able to estimate, based on past experience, the number of minutes required to repair the instrument.

24.2.15. Safety

Specimens containing biohazardous substances have always been a danger in medical laboratories. Hepatitis virus types A, B, and C have been known for many years, yet only recently have laboratory procedures been under more stringent scrutiny from regulatory agencies (Public Law 100-578, 100th Congress, Clinical

Laboratory Improvement Amendments of 1988; Oct. 31, 1988). The increased emphasis on laboratory safety has been brought about, in part, by the recent appearance of HIV. Current clinical whole-blood analyzers of either the direct injection type (e.g., Corning 288) or the specimen aspiration type (e.g., Nova Biomedical Stat Profiles) present a significant hazard to the operator.[4] Injection of specimens into a clotted analyzer has the potential hazard of specimen splash-back onto the operator, while the aspiration type presents a probe during aspiration that could potentially puncture an operator's skin. We have modified the entry port of our aspiration type analyzer with a special sensor containing a conical port to eliminate the potential for puncture wounds. Furthermore, using the robot has obviated the possibility of puncture wounds.

24.2.16. Government Regulations

Point-of-care laboratory work must be done under a Clinical Laboratory Improvement Act (CLIA) certificate and accredited by a regulatory agency such as the College of American Pathologists (CAP) and Joint Commission for Accreditation of Health Care Organizations (JCAHO). These agencies dictate requirements concerning quality control, personnel qualifications, documentation, and training. Point-of-care testing must be done under a state license as well. The testing must be under the supervision of a technical director, who must be a trained Ph.D. or physician. Technologists performing most point-of-care testing must have a high-school diploma and 2 years of appropriate experience as a medical technologist. Technologists must demonstrate documented proficiency in each moderately complex test they perform. Written directions must be followed, including quality control. Remedial action must be documented for all aberrant tests. The need for the laboratory to supervise the adherence to correct procedures while satisfying government regulations has necessitated the development of the RALS system. In particular, there is a need to follow a proficiency testing protocol that establishes policies for acceptable and unacceptable specimens and how to deal with them.

24.3. SUMMARY

The value of point-of-care testing in the total quality management of medical treatment is just beginning to be measured and understood. Rapid turnaround provides a higher-quality specimen and therefore could reduce laboratory errors and repeats. Fewer repeats could also reduce iatrogenic blood loss. Studies are also under way to determine the efficacy of delivery options. Furthermore, determining the best menu of analytical tests to be included in a rapid turnaround panel and for what medical conditions are beginning to be defined. Assessing the impact of point-of-care testing for physician convenience is also an important area of study. Does providing services for physician convenience result in improved patient outcome and reduced costs? Will rapid turnaround lower costs by obviating the need for patients to be recalled when laboratory results are ready after an office visit?

Methods or providing point-of-care testing are varied, but most emphasize the need for reducing specimen transportation and increasing the test menu available on analytical instruments near the patient. The best methods for point-of-care testing are those that allow the physician and laboratory to cooperate in the diagnostic process. The RALS system provides the analytical tests at the earliest possible time point, but only after the laboratory has provided the necessary profession expertise.

REFERENCES

1. Barman MR: Alternative-site testing: mixed feelings about the inevitable. MLO: *Med Lab Observ* 22(12):22–29, Dec 1990.

2. Belsey R, Baer D, Sewell D: Laboratory test analysis near the patient. *JAMA* 255:775–786, 1986.

3. Browning JA, Kaiser DL, Durbin CG: The effect of guidelines on the appropriate use of arterial blood gas analysis in the intensive care unit. *Resp Care* 34:269–276, 1989.

4. ECR1: Evaluation: blood gas analyzers. *Health Devices,* 18:245, 1989 (Plymouth Meeting, PA). Emergency Care Research Institute.

5. Erickson KA, Wilding P: Evaluation of a novel point-of-care system, the i-STAT portable clinical analyzer. *Clin Chem* 39(2):283–287, 1993.

6. Fletcher AB: The essential role of the laboratory in the optimal care of the sick neonate. *J Internatl Fed Clin Chem* 2:166–172, 1990.

7. Girotti MJ, Brown SJL: Reducing the cost of an ICU admission in Canada without diagnosis-related or case-mix groupings. *Can Anaesth Soc J* 33:765–762, 1986.

8. Graham JE: The challenge of labs without walls. *MLO* 26(Suppl)(9S):10–14, 1994.

9. Jacobs E: Economics of delivery options. Paper presented at conference entitled Medical Economic, and Regulatory Issues Affecting Point-of-Care Testing. Philadelphia, May 6–7, 1994, The National Academy of Clinical Biochemistry.

10. Knaus WA, Draper EA, Wagner DP, et al: An evaluation of outcome from intensive care in major medical centers. *Ann Intern Med* 104:410–418, 1986.

11. Luckey L, Carey S, Hathorn G: POCT for coronary bypass patients: fast results without bypassing quality. *MLO* 26(Suppl)(9S):31–35, 1994.

12. Margrey KS, Martinez A, Vaughn DP, Felder RA: Standardizing robotic laboratory instrument interface techniques through microcomputer applications. *In* Strimaitis JR, Hawk GL, eds: Zymark Corp., Hopkinton, Mass. *Advances in Laboratory Automation, Robotics,* Vol. 5, 1988.

13. Margrey K, Martinez A, Roberts J, Holman W, Felder RA, Boyd JC, Savory J: US Patent 5,366,896, Robotically Operated Laboratory System, Nov 22, 1994.

14. Martinez A, Vaughn DP, Margrey KS, Felder RA: Touch screen/graphics interface technology for a remotely monitored, robotic clinical laboratory. *In* Strimaitis JR, Hawk GL, eds: Zymark Corp., Hopkinton, Mass. *Advances in Laboratory Automation, Robotics,* Vol. 5, 1988.

15. Mikkelsen DJ, James KR, Dohrman DH: Experience with laboratory instrumentation placed in critical care situations over a seven year period. *NZ Med J* 100(835): 686–688, 1987.

16. Mishelevich DJ, Teufel BG: Capacity planning guide for mainframes running the IBM patient care system (PCS). *Comput Hosp* 19–25, Sept/Oct 1981.

17. Muakkassa FF, Rutledge R, Fakhry SM, Meyer AA, Sheldon GF: ABGs and arterial lines: the relationship to unnecessarily drawn arterial blood gas samples. *J Trauma* 30:1087–1095, 1990.

18. Perkins S, Shields J, Broer H, Jaciow D: Implementing cross-department use of a point-of-care system. *Am Clin Lab* 9–11, Nov 1993.

19. Riley JB, Burgess BM, Smith CA, Crowley JC, Soronen SW: In vitro measurement of the accuracy of a new patient side blood gas pH, hematocrit and electrolyte monitor. *J Extra Corporeal Technol* 19:322–329, 1987.

20. Salem M, Chernow B, Burke R, Stacey J, Stogoff M, Sood S: Beside diagnostic blood testing, it accuracy, rapidity, and utility in blood conservation. *JAMA* 266:382–389, 1991.

21. Schroeder SA, Showstack JA, Schwartz J: Survival of adult high-cost patients. *JAMA* 245:1449–1449, 1981.

22. Tong DA: Weaning patients from mechanical ventilation. A knowledge-based system approach. *Comput Meth Programs Biomed* 35:267–278, 1991.

23. Travers EM, Wolke JC, Johnson R, Brown L, Lijewski R, Pinkos A, Trost A: Changing the way lab medicine is practiced at the point of care. *MLO* 26:33–40, 1994.

24. Zaloga GP, Hill TR, Strickland RA, et al: Bedside blood gas and electrolyte monitoring in critically ill patients. *Crit Care Med* 17:920–925, 1989.

25

Information Integration for Point-of-Care and Satellite Testing

ELLIS JACOBS

CONTENTS

25.1. Introduction
25.2. Mechanisms for Providing Critical Care Services
25.3. Point-of-Care Testing Systems
25.4. Integrating Data into the Medical Record
25.5. The Future
References

25.1. INTRODUCTION

Advances in science and technology are enabling the decentralization and distribution of clinical diagnostic procedures with the ability to produce results with equivalent validity as central laboratory procedures. Decentralized testing sites include satellite laboratories as well as bedside or point-of-care (POC) testing. Point-of-care testing provides distinct advantages over central laboratory and satellite lab services for both the patient and ordering physician. However, if data

Handbook of Clinical Automation, Robotics, and Optimization, Edited by Gerald J. Kost with the collaboration of Judith Welsh.
ISBN 0-471-03179-8 © 1996 John Wiley & Sons, Inc.

generated in these various decentralized testing sites are not integrated into the medical information system, whether a hospital information system (HIS) or an integrated healthcare information system as described by Korpman,[1] then various problems with the utilization of this data are created.[2] Despite extraordinary advances in diagnostic and therapeutic modalities, because of the lack of information integration, improvements in the optimal use of medical information have lagged significantly.

The general flow of the creation of laboratory knowledge (i.e., data) from time of perceived need to when the healthcare provider has it to act on [e.g., total or therapeutic turnaround time (TTAT)] is depicted in Figure 25.1. However, with POC and satellite lab testing, this flow is altered (Fig. 25.2). This is due to the critical nature of such testing and the need for rapid TTAT. Specimen transit and result reporting times are minimized because of the proximity of the testing site to patient-care activities. In this arena a major concern is not with how fast the healthcare provider obtains the results, but rather whether the data is getting into the medical record to be officially recorded and for others to have access to. In fact, the rapid availability of results creates a quality-assurance dilemma. It is possible for data to be seen and acted on before any quality-control checks or other external mechanisms of assuring test result reliability can be applied to the analytical systems. Therefore, it is critical that these POC testing devices have built-in quality control/quality assurance (QC/AQ) systems (Table 25.1). These automatic functions prevent erroneous data from being seen by the healthcare provider.

The driving forces behind distributed or POC testing have been previously

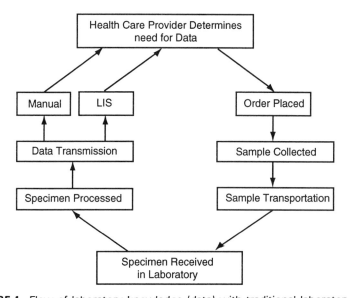

Figure 25.1. Flow of laboratory knowledge (data) with traditional laboratory testing.

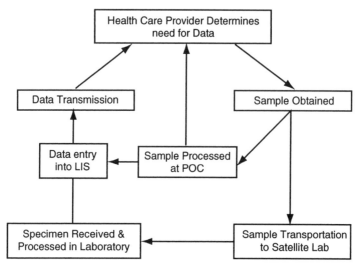

Figure 25.2. Flow of laboratory knowledge (data) with POC and satellite laboratory testing.

well documented[3,4] and include benefits for all involved: patient, physician, laboratory, and administrator. In general, faster TTAT of critical lab results is better for the immediate medical management of critically ill patients. However, it is still necessary to get this data into the information systems for overall coordination of medical care and follow through. Information saturation and the inability to use the information available, because of both lack of organization and sheer data volume, is beginning to haunt every aspect of modern life.[5] Medicine is no exception to this trend of information overload and is, in fact, significantly affected by it.

With the development of distributed testing systems, there has been a development of isolated packets of clinical information scattered throughout the

---

TABLE 25.1. POC Analyzer Automatic QC/QA Functions

Automatic calibration
System lockouts and/or suppression if
    QC not performed within specified time interval
    QC results out of acceptable range
    Patient identification not entered
    Valid operator identification not entered
Data management function
    Patient result logs
    QC/QA logs
    Maintenance logs

medical landscape, including laboratory information system (LIS) records, private clinic records, and physician progress notes. It is important for all this information to be linked together; otherwise it does not serve all who may need access to it for various reasons. Clinical workstations, such as bedside terminals, are the ultimate mechanism of data integration.[6] These devices allow not only for the two-way flow of clinical data between the healthcare professional and the electronic medical record but also for the integration and presentation of medical knowledge. Bedside access to information systems allows for both accurate recording of clinical data and the more efficient use of the healthcare providers' time on clinical care rather than clerical duties.[7]

25.2. MECHANISM FOR PROVIDING CRITICAL CARE SERVICE

There are various means by which critical care laboratory services can be provided; the most common is the processing of stat specimens within the main laboratories.[8,9] In some settings satellite laboratories and/or the use of POC testing devices have been implemented to meet specific rapid TTAT needs for diagnostic information. It must be remembered that the primary purpose of any of these systems is the delivery of data, not specimen transport or the physical performance of the analytical procedure. How this data delivery function is met varies, and the characteristics of each one represents a unique challenge to data integration.

There are two basic types of satellite laboratories: those staffed with laboratory personnel and those that use automation. The remote automation laboratory is discussed in Chapter 12. Samples are analyzed at remote locations through the use of robotics, and the data is automatically transmitted to the central laboratory for review by a medical technologist via the Remote Automated Laboratory System (RALS™) (Medical Automation Systems, Inc., Charlottesville, VA) (Fig. 25.3). The system, through a touch-screen user interface, monitors all analyzer functions, outputs actual as well as calculated values, and provides real-time reporting of results. All results are compared to critical value ranges and, if they exceed these limits, are displayed as blinking values. Delta checks are performed by comparing the current values to the most recent test results. Previous patient results can be immediately recalled by touching the appropriate button.

On review and verification by the medical technologist in the central laboratory, the results are sent back to the patient site where they can be viewed and printed by the requesting physician and/or other healthcare professionals. Simultaneously, the results are uploaded to the LIS, which ensures proper tracking of patient data and patient billing. The downloading function of the system allows patient demographics to be transferred to RALS™ in order to "tag" a patient. In this setting there is not a problem with data integration since the RALS™ system interfaces with both the LIS and hospital information system (HIS) and thereby ensures complete capture of data as well as physical control of the test process by the central laboratory.

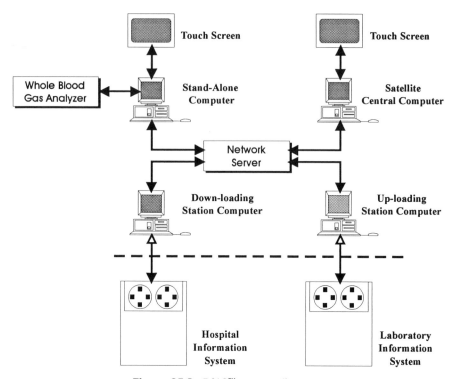

Figure 25.3. RALS™ system diagram.

Satellite laboratories are smaller versions of main labs and as such have equipment that may or may not be interfaceable with the LIS. With utilization of a stat broadcast function in the LIS, data can be rapidly transmitted to the ordering physician. The data flow in the Stat Laboratory at The Mount Sinai Medical Center is depicted in Figure 25.4.[9] All the major equipment in the laboratory is directly interfaced with the LIS. When testing is completed, identification and result data are automatically transmitted to the LIS via the interfaces or manually entered, where they are held for verification. Some of the instrument interfaces are personnel computer (PC)-based. This allows for data buffering and, when necessary, retransmission of results. Within 1–2 min of verification in the LIS, Stat laboratory results are sent to the ordering units.

Depending on the ordering location, the stat lab results will appear on either physiological monitors at the anesthesiologist's workstation in the OR, bedside stat printers in the cardiothoracic intensive care units (ICUs), or unit stat printers in the other ICUs. Through a LIS linkage with the computer controlling the anesthesiology mass spectrometer systems, test results appear in a window that opens on the anesthesiology physiological monitors and is automatically entered in the anesthesiology OR case records. Therefore, through this linkage of a basic stat broadcast function of the LIS and a data input function of the anesthesiology mass spectrometer, not only was total turnaround time reduced by rapidly closing the loop associated with result reporting, but another function of the OR record keeping system was automated.

In point-of-care testing, instruments are either brought to or kept at the patient's locations. Often the systems are operated by non–traditionally laboratory-trained individuals. From the laboratorian's perspective, there is a loss of control of data in the point-of-care setting versus central and satellite labs. In the latter, data is not seen by the healthcare provider without specific quality control and quality assurance requirements being met. However, with bedside systems the data is immediately available to anyone walking by. Another problem is that due to the sense of "immediacy of results"; once the individual has the data, there is little regard for getting it into the data management system. Hence, the best POC testing systems are those that automate these functions.

Quality-assurance software is available in some POC instrumentation, which allows for the automatic record keeping of QC results, patient samples, maintenance, calibrations, and so on. Ideally these systems could automatically transmit these logs to a central location, such as a PC, where the information can be collated and the results forwarded on to the LIS for integration with other laboratory results and proper recording in the medical record. In this manner, the problem of individuals forgetting to properly record the data, with the excuse that they are too busy with patient care or any other reason, is eliminated. Additionally, if set up correctly, once built-in QC/QA requirements have been met, the data could flow unattended on a continuous basis. This would allow access to the data, throughout the LIS/HIS system, on almost the same timeframe as that of the caregiver who is performing the procedure.

An alternative solution to this problem of lack of control and inconsistent entry of POC testing data into the medical record is similar to the RALS™ system. The Remote Lab Supervision (RLS™) (Nova Biomedical, Waltham, MA) software allows the central laboratory to manage and control POC testing. When an analysis is initiated, the operator ID and test results are transmitted to the central laboratory for review, verification, and acceptance or rejection. Abnormal and

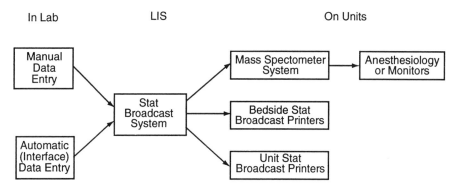

Figure 25.4. Data transmission in Stat Laboratory at The Mount Sinai Medical Center.

alert values are flagged for the laboratory reviewer and the instrument operator. The results can be stored on disc or transmitted to the LIS for entry into the patient record and billing system.

25.3. POINT-OF-CARE TESTING SYSTEMS

There are different types of analytical systems utilized at the point of care. Most of them are noninstrument, qualitative assays that utilize either competitive or noncompetitive immunoassays with a visually read positive/negative answer. The only way information from these various noninstrumental based devices can be input into the medical record is manually.

One way to classify the various instrument-based POC systems is according to degree of portability (Table 25.2). The handheld and small, battery-powered portable systems are, because of their flexibility of use, very dependent on manual operations to get the data into the LIS. This is in contrast to the analytical systems in main and satellite laboratories that are hard-wired into the LIS. Transportables typically are compact whole-blood analyzers that are transported to the point of need. An example would be a blood gas, electrolyte, or glucose analyzer placed on a cart with a battery backup power supply to keep the system energized during transport. *Ex vivo* and *in vivo* systems are physically attached to the patient. Most *ex vivo* blood gas and electrolyte systems withdraw specimen for analysis and then return it to the patient. *In-vivo,* catheter-based systems analyze on both "point in time" and continuous bases, whereas the *ex vivo* systems generally perform assays only at specific time points.

TABLE 25.2. Classification of POC Instrumentation by Portability

Type	Example
Transportables	Stat Profile 5[a]
Portables	Gem Premier[b], Piccolo[c]
Handheld	PCA[d], IRMA[e]
Ex vivo	Gem Stat with extracorporeal circuit[b]
In vivo	Paratrend 7[f]
Noninvasive	Pulse oximeters

[a]NOVA Biomedical (Waltham, MA).
[b]Mallinckrodt Sensor Systems, Inc. (Ann Arbor, MI).
[c]Abaxis, Ind. (Sunnyvale, CA).
[d]i-Stat Corp. (Princeton, NJ).
[e]Diametric Medical, Inc. (St. Paul, MN).
[f]Pfizer Biomedical Sensors (Malvern, PA).
See Chapter 27 for additional details regarding biosensor systems.

25.4. INTEGRATING DATA INTO THE MEDICAL RECORD

Various forms of data output (Table 25.3) are associated with POC testing systems. This allows for a variety of means by which data gets into the system. They range from manual entry of qualitative results from visually read devices to wireless automatic transmission and autoverification of quantitative results from a bedside analyzer. Infrared wireless communication has limited applications; it is effective only for short distances. However, the frequency of radio signal transmissions can be adjusted to maximize penetration of the environment. Figure 25.5 illustrates a wireless pen-based portable computer that uses spread spectrum radio transmission.

Hand entry into the medical chart is the only viable mechanisms for non-instrument-based systems. However, if an institution has implemented ward ordering of test requests, these results can be entered into the LIS from the floor. If the tests are made as "answer on ordering" type, then, when the healthcare professional places a test order in the system, there is an immediate request for the result to be entered.

For some of the various analytical POC testing systems the best interface would be a direct linkage into the LIS, whereas others require an intermittent linkage, due to needs for mobility. Similar to main laboratory equipment, POC testing systems can be hard-wired into the communication network. However, this requires that they be relatively stationary. Each instrument could be directly linked into the LIS, or multiple units could be linked to a central (network) computer, which, in turn, is connected to the LIS. In the latter, the network PC could, via an autoscripting program, log onto the LIS and order, transmit, and verify test results. A variant on the latter would be the use of radio signals to transmit the results to a central receiving station, which is then subsequently linked to the LIS.

Transportable Units. An example is the Stat Profile 5. There are several ways these analyzers can be integrated into the medical information network. Many LIS interfaces use a PC to capture, buffer, and reformat the instrument data stream for transmission to LIS. Data is stored on the hard drive and can be

TABLE 25.3. Types of Data Output Devices Utilized in POC Testing Systems

Visual readings
Display screens
Printers
RS-232 ports
Infrared beams
Radio signals
Modems

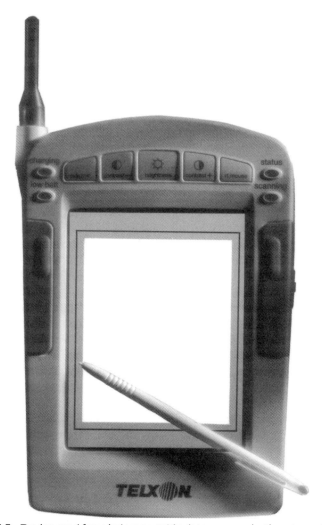

Figure 25.5. Device used for wireless portable data communications to and from the LIS (PTC-1134, TELXON, Akron, OH: Virtual Lab,™ Cerner Corporation, Kansas City, MO).

retransmitted at a later time if the LIS connection was down when the data was originally generated. Therefore, this type of PC based system could be used for the transportables. Data is captured on the hard drive as if the system were interfaced but had a communication line failure. At a LIS terminal, the tests can be requested on a patient to obtain an accession number. This number can then be entered into the analyzer, or PC, to be attached to the results when they are transmitted to the LIS. The PC is connected to a LIS port, and the stored results are then transmitted for entry into the patient record and billing system. Alternatively, if the system is stationary, it could use either the RALS™ or RLS™ systems previously described.

Portable Units. Examples are Gem Premier and Picollo; both these systems have formatted data output to RS-232 data ports. However, the Picollo system has been demonstrated with radio transmission. We are developing a program that will allow multiple Premier units to be linked to central PC. This central computer will gather patient data and analyze QC data. If all QC rules are passed, in a real-time mode, the PC will log onto the LIS and, through an autoscripting program, order, transmit, and verify test data into the laboratory information system. This is similar in concept to the automatic remote lab functions of the RALS™ or RLS™ systems.

Handheld Units. An example is the portable clinical analyzer (PCA) which stores patient data and identity within itself. At a docking station, through an IR linkage, the data can be printed or transmitted into a notebook PC. Several units can be networked to the same PC. In turn, this PC can store the data for later transmission to the LIS or, if permanently connected to the LIS, send data on a real-time basis.

Ex Vivo, In Vivo, and Noninvasive Systems. Data integration for *ex vivo, in vivo,* and noninvasive systems is, in concept, no different than for any other instrument based POC analytical system. *In vivo* and noninvasive systems have the ability to produce continuous data output, as well as specific point-in-time determinations. Specific point determination can easily be entered into the LIS through any of the mechanisms previously described (hand entry, direct or indirect LIS linkage through RS-232 ports, etc.). Because of their continuous data output, *in vivo* and noninvasive systems are often utilized as trend monitors. Currently there is increasing need to get these trend graphs into the electronic medical record, since they should be accessible for the immediate medical management of the critically ill patient.

25.5. THE FUTURE

As point-of-care and satellite testing becomes more of a standard in the general practice of medicine, elimination of the scattered caches of data and integration into a laboratory database increases in importance. Patient-centered integration is the key to a successful healthcare information system.[10] Information systems must be integrated around information units, not geopolitical units. Since hospitals are oriented around patient care, their information systems should be similarly focused.

Clinical workstations are more than data recording and display devices; they include a variety of applications for processing that data to assist patient care.

Clinical workstations offer multiple views of patient data and medical knowledge for multiple users.[11] They will function as an interface between the user and the patient data as well as interfacing pertinent medical knowledge. A system has been developed that receives stat results from the LIS, prints a report in the ICU, and captures that data for review in a custom spreadsheet format at color terminals in the ICUs.[12] Available services include a reference nomogram plot of arterial blood gas data, automated access to the clinical information system, and a Medline database.

As the production of information becomes more diffuse (distributed), the ability to integrate it becomes more difficult. A key to the future success of any POC/satellite testing system will be how easily it can be integrated into the medical information network.

REFERENCES

1. Korpman RA: Health care information systems: patient-centered integration is the key. *Clin Lab Med* 11:203–220, 1991.
2. Friedman BA, Mitchell W: Integrating information from decentralized laboratory testing sites. *Am J Clin Pathol* 99:637–642, 1993.
3. Rock RC: Why testing is being moved to the site of patient care. *MLO* 23(9S):2–5, 1991.
4. Jacobs E: TQM and POC testing. *MLO* 25(9S):2–6, 1993.
5. Naisbett J: *Megatrends.* New York: Warren Books, 1982.
6. Cimino JJ: Data storage and knowledge representation for clinical workstations. *Internatl J Bio-Med Comput* 34:185–194, 1994.
7. Korpman RA: Bedside terminals can improve nursing efficiency. *Healthcare Finance Management* 4:48–59, 1991.
8. Fleisher M, Schwartz MK: Strategies of organization and service for the critical care laboratory. *Clin Chem* 36:1557B–1561B, 1990.
9. Jacobs E, Sarkozi L, Coleman N: A centralized critical care (stat) laboratory: The Mount Sinai experience. *Crit Care Rep* 2:397–405, 1991.
10. Korpman RA: Health care information systems—patient centered integration is the key. *Clin Lab Med* 11:203–220, 1991.
11. Chute CG, Cesnik B, van Bemmel JH: Medical data and knowledge management by integrated medical workstations: summary and recommendations. *Internatl J Bio-Med Comput* 34:175–183, 1994.
12. Barrows RC, Allen B, Fink DJ: An X window system for stat lab result reporting. *Proc Annu Symp Comp Appl Med Care,* Institute of Electrical and Electronics Engineers, 1993, pp. 331–335.

CHAPTER

26

New Developments and Clinical Impact of Noninvasive Monitoring

MARK A. ARNOLD

CONTENTS

26.1. INTRODUCTION

The concept of noninvasive clinical measurements is straightforward. First, a selected beam of electromagnetic radiation is transmitted through a vascular region of the body, and then the resulting spectral information is used to compute the concentration of a desired chemical constituent. Such a measurement is termed "noninvasive" because there is no need to invade the body to collect a sample of fluid or tissue for the analysis. Of course, the electromagnetic radia-

Handbook of Clinical Automation, Robotics, and Optimization, Edited by Gerald J. Kost with the collaboration of Judith Welsh.
ISBN 0-471-03179-8 © 1996 John Wiley & Sons, Inc.

tion invades the body, but this invasion is both painless and harmless to the patient.

Interest in noninvasive clinical monitoring has been fueled by the success of pulse oximetry in monitoring oxygen saturation levels.[1] In pulse oximetry, two specific wavelengths of near-infrared radiation are sequentially, and repeatedly, transmitted into the body by a small pair of light-emitting diodes (LEDs). A fraction of these incident beams are backreflected and detected by a silicon diode detector. One of these wavelengths corresponds to light absorbed by the deoxygenated form of hemoglobin. The other wavelength is equally sensitive to all forms of hemoglobin and, thereby, provides a reference signal against which the deoxyhemoglobin-based light intensity can be judged. The final result is a small, lightweight device that can be easily strapped onto the fingertip of an adult or child, or the heel of an infant and the healthcare personnel receives a continuous readout of oxygen saturation. The continuous nature of this device permits monitoring the progress of a patient without the unpleasantness and expense of drawing and analyzing multiple blood samples. The hope is to expand this measurement concept and to provide continuous analytical information for a variety of clinically relevant blood constituents.

Several unique approaches have been proposed and are being pursued to achieve noninvasive measurements of clinically relevant compounds in the human body. The most studied approach, and that presently receiving the greatest attention, is based on near-infrared (NIR) absorption spectroscopy. Although this chapter focuses on the basic features of NIR spectroscopy for noninvasive sensing, approaches based on nuclear magnetic resonance[2,3] spectroscopy are also being evaluated.

Monitors for the noninvasive measurement of blood glucose have received considerable research attention in recent years because of the clinical needs for reliable home blood glucose monitor technology. Results of the recently concluded DCCT study[4] clearly demonstrate the clinical benefits of maintaining tight control of blood glucose levels. Ideally, diabetic patients measure their blood glucose levels multiple times each day and, in response, inject the required amount of insulin needed to maintain the glucose concentration within a relatively tight tolerance range. A major limitation of this treatment plan is the unwillingness of many diabetic patients to prick their fingers multiple times a day in order to collect the blood samples needed for measurement. A noninvasive blood glucose monitor would effectively eliminate the pain barrier responsible for the reluctance to make multiple daily measurements. The large numbers of type I diabetics, who would directly benefit from a noninvasive blood glucose measurement technology, stimulate research activity in this area.

Regardless of the analyte of interest, glucose, cholesterol, or oxygen saturation, the analyte must selectively interact with the incident radiation. In fact, the underlying premise of noninvasive monitoring is predicated on the hypothesis that each chemical constituent of interest will absorb unique portions of the transmitted radiation and that the magnitude of light absorption is related to concentration. The key is to select a wavelength region within the NIR spectrum where the chemical constituents of interest absorb.

26.2. THE NIR SPECTRUM

The NIR region of the electromagnetic spectrum extends from the red side of the visible spectrum (700 nm) to the beginning of the midinfrared region of the spectrum (2500 nm). This spectral range can also be described in wavenumbers, where wavenumber is the reciprocal of wavelength converted to units of reciprocal centimeters (cm^{-1}). Both wavelength and wavenumber are used in the literature, which can be confusing. Nevertheless, the NIR spectrum extends from 14,286 to 4000 cm^{-1} or from 0.7 to 2.5 μm.

Molecular transitions that occur within the NIR spectrum are associated primarily with overtones and combinations of fundamental CH, NH, and OH vibrational transitions. The fundamental transitions are much stronger and appear in the midinfrared spectrum. Unfortunately, water strongly absorbs midinfrared radiation, which limits the depth of penetration into the human body to only a few hundred micrometers, which is not compatible with noninvasive monitoring. The fact that CH, NH, and OH stretches can be observed in the NIR spectrum is good because essentially every clinically relevant compound possesses these functional groups. Thus, NIR spectroscopy, and noninvasive monitoring, has the potential to be general in nature and applicable to a wide variety of analytes.

In practice, th NIR spectrum is limited to a few regions where water does not absorb. The NIR spectrum of water is well characterized with two large water-absorption features centered at 5200 and 7600 cm^{-1}. In addition, there is a third strong water absorbance band that is centered in the midinfrared region at 3800 cm^{-1}. These water-absorption features define three spectral windows that are available for noninvasive spectroscopy. These ranges are 4000–5000 cm^{-1}, 5500–6500 cm^{-1}, and 8500–14,000 cm^{-1}. This first region, termed the *combination region,* corresponds to the combination of fundamental stretching and bending vibrational transitions that occur nominally at 1500 and 3000 cm^{-1}, respectively. The second region corresponds to the overtone region for the fundamental bending vibrational transitions. The last region contains molecular information corresponding to higher orders of these combination and overtone transitions.

The spectrum shown in Figure 26.1 is an example of a NIR spectrum of an aqueous solution. This particular spectrum is for a 0.5 M glucose solution prepared in a 0.1 M phosphate buffer adjusted to pH 7.0. The three open spectral windows mentioned above are evident in this spectrum. In addition, three unique types of spectral features can be identified. First, the noisy regions correspond to strong water absorption. So much of the light is absorbed by the water, essentially no photons are transmitted through the sample and detector noise is observed. The second type of spectral feature is the negative deviations from the baseline. These negative deviations also indicate regions where water absorbs, but the absorption is weaker compared to the noisy regions. Positive deviations correspond to glucose absorbance features.

The spectrum in Figure 26.1 clearly illustrates that no glucose absorbance features are present at wavenumbers larger than 6500 cm^{-1}, but there are several weak water-absorbance features evident in this long-wavenumber (short-

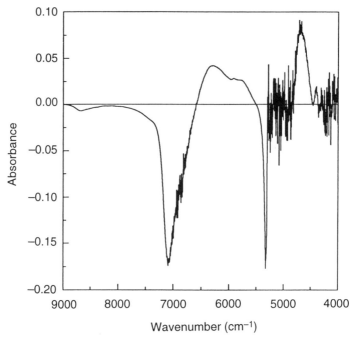

Figure 26.1. Near-infrared absorbance spectrum for 0.5 M glucose in a 0.1 M, pH 7.0 phosphate buffer.

wavelength) region. Several preliminary accounts[5,6] claim success in extracting glucose information from this short-wavelength NIR region. Unfortunately, these claims are essentially unsubstantiated with sound scientific documentation, which makes it impossible to understand the origin of the glucose-dependent information. One possibility can be obtained by looking at the detailed work by Brown and coworkers.[7-9] This group has documented that multivariate calibration methods can be used in combination with short-wavelength NIR spectroscopy to measure numerous chemical and physical properties of aqueous solutions. In the Brown work, both the chemical and physical information is presumably obtained from alterations in the position and shape of the water-absorbance bands located in this region of the spectrum. This analysis opens the speculation that glucose can be quantified in aqueous media based on the interactions between glucose and water and the corresponding alterations of the water absorbance bands. To date, no detailed reports have been published that prove the existence of reliable glucose information in the short-wavelength region of the NIR spectrum.

In contrast, absorbance features directly associated with the glucose molecule are clearly evident in the long-wavelength portion of the NIR spectrum (see Fig. 26.1). These features represent overtone and combination bands associated with CH vibrations within the glucose molecule. Relative to the overtone region, the spectral information in the combination region is characterized by higher absorptivities and sharper and better-defined absorbance bands. These features make the combination region preferred in terms of potential measurement sensitivity and selectivity. The remainder of this chapter will focus on the measurement of clinically relevant compounds based on absorbance spectroscopy over the combination region ($5000-4000$ cm^{-1}).

26.3. MULTIVARIATE CALIBRATION METHODS

From an analytical standpoint, the success of noninvasive clinical monitoring is limited by the ability to extract the analyte concentration information from the spectral information in a selective and reliable manner. A noninvasive monitoring scheme demands that the measurement be made in the absence of any chemical reagents or physical separations to enhance the selectivity and accuracy of the measurement. All the analytical information must be obtained from the spectral information. The principal challenge is to develop spectral processing algorithms that are capable of selectively extracting the analyte information in the presence of many other spectral features that include noise, baseline variations, and absorbance features associated with other molecular components in the sample matrix. A critical aspect of this challenge is to develop spectroscopic instrumentation capable of providing high-quality NIR spectra that contain spectroscopic information affiliated with the analyte molecule and that minimizes noise and baseline variations. No spectral processing algorithm can extract analytical information that is not present in the spectra or that is severely overshadowed by noise.

Relatively simple univariate calibration methods can be used to relate a single, specific spectral feature to the analyte concentration when a simple matrix is involved. The measurement of glucose in a simple phosphate-buffered aqueous solution is an example of a successful univariate calibration scheme.[10] For the most part, however, matrix complexity demands the use of multivariate calibration procedures where information associated with multiple analyte-dependent features within the spectrum is used to develop the working relationship between the spectral information and analyte concentration. For example, the addition of protein to a phosphate-buffered aqueous matrix requires multivariate calibration methods to successfully quantify glucose at clinically relevant concentrations.[11]

Partial least-squares (PLS) regression generally outperforms other multivariate methods such as multilinear regression and principal-components regression (PCR). The basic features of PLS are presented elsewhere.[12] The power of PLS is based on its ability to correlate minute spectral variations to analyte concentration variations. The procedure of developing a PLS calibration model requires a set of training spectra that encodes spectral and analyte concentration information into the algorithm. The major weakness of the PLS algorithm is the tendency to overmodel the data by incorporating noise within the training set in to the calibration model. Overmodeling can be difficult to detect and generally requires the use of a second independent data set that is used for prediction. All PLS calibration models must be tested by predicting the analyte concentration from a series of independent spectra. Often times a training set can lead to an apparently valid calibration model only to find that this model cannot predict from independent spectra. The key experimental parameters for the PLS algorithm are the spectral range and the number of PLS factors.[10-12]

Multivariate calibration models are needed to account for the high degree of overlap between spectral features for each molecule in the matrix. An example is the measurement of glucose in the presence of glutamine.[13] These two organic compounds represent the combination of a carbohydrate and an amino acid, which differ considerably in terms of their chemical properties, but which are similar from a NIR spectroscopic standpoint. The spectra presented in Figure 26.2 shows the NIR spectral features for aqueous solutions of glucose and glutamine, individually. Each spectrum is characterized by unique positions and widths of the absorbance bands. These differences in the spectral bands provide the information needed to selectively measure glucose in the presence of glutamine, as well as the selective measure of glutamine in the presence of glucose. The overlap in these spectral features, however, demands the incorporation of multiple spectral features into the calibration in order to provide selectivity for

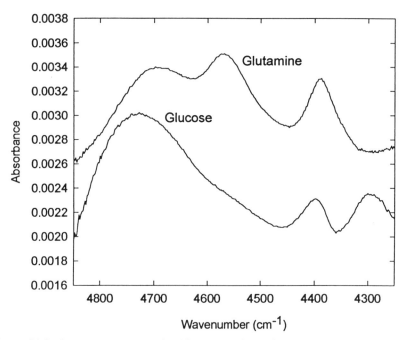

Figure 26.2. Absorbance spectra for 10 mM solutions of glucose and glutamine.

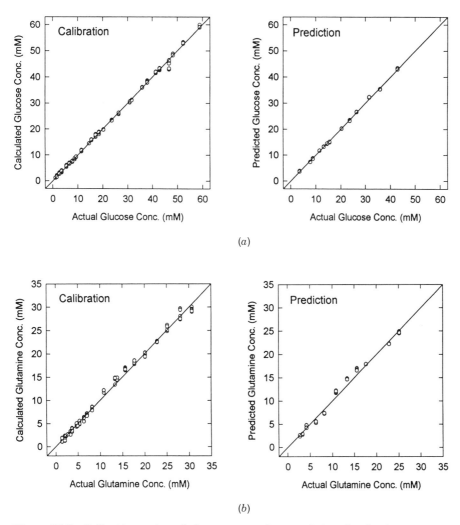

Figure 26.3. Calibration and prediction concentration correlation plots for the measurement of glucose (a) and glutamine (b).

these measurements. In effect, the absorbance at a single wavenumber is not adequate to selectively measure one species over the other.

A PLS calibration model for glucose can be constructed by analyzing a training set of spectra that incorporates NIR spectra measured from unique mixtures of glucose and glutamine. Results of such a model are presented as two concentration correlation plots presented in Figure 26.3. The first plot shows the calibration data where the glucose value computed from the calibration model is plotted relative to the known glucose concentration in the standard solution. The second plot shows the predicted glucose concentrations relative to known values in the prediction data set. The unity line, which is also shown, represents the ideal response. For both calibration and prediction values, the data points fall along the unity line. Compliance of the prediction data set is especially noteworthy, because this type of response demonstrates the ability of the model to predict, thus validating the utility of the entire calibration and measurement procedure. The mean percent error of prediction (MPEP), standard error of prediction (SEP), and standard error of calibration (SEC) parameters are 2.21%, 0.41 mM, and 0.64 mM, respectively.

Figure 26.3 also shows the corresponding calibration and prediction plots for the measurement of glutamine. Again, both calibration and prediction points fall on the unity line. The computed MPEP, SEP, and SEC are 8.17%, 0.80 mM, and 0.67 mM, respectively, for glutamine. These data indicate that the ability to measure glutamine is not as good as for glucose. The key thing to note, however, is that multiple analytes can be determined from a single NIR spectrum which expands the analytical utility of the method.

26.4. SPECTRAL QUALITY

It is important to realize that the analytical information is obtained from an absorbance measurement that relies on differentiating small differences between the incident and transmitted intensities. The noise of the spectrum must be sufficiently low that this difference is actually quantifiable. The requirement for low noise is particularly critical at low concentrations of a weak NIR-absorbing molecule, such as glucose, because the amount of light absorbed is small and the difference in intensity can be easily lost in the noise.

An excellent example of how an enhancement in spectrometer quality can dramatically improve analytical performance involves the measurement of glucose in a whole, undiluted blood matrix.[14] In this experiment, a large volume of whole blood was obtained from a single cow during slaughter, with EDTA added to prevent coagulation. Different glucose levels were obtained by adding solid glucose to aliquots of the blood. The actual glucose level was measured at the time the NIR spectrum was collected by analyzing a small volume of the sample with a Yellowsprings Instruments Model 2300 blood glucose analyzer.[15] Two independent data sets were collected. NIR spectra and the corresponding glucose concentrations were measured for 65 individual samples in data set 1 and 79 samples in data set 2. In both cases, training and prediction data subsets were established with all spectra associated with a given sample being placed in one subset or the other.

The concentration correlation plot for the best calibration model for data set 1 is shown in Figure 26.4. Both the calibration and prediction data points are plotted. Both types of data follow the unity line and the prediction data fall within the scatter of the calibration data. The scatter of the data is quite large, however, and the limit of detection for glucose is well above the normal range.

The spectrometer was modified between the collection of data sets 1 and 2. A Nicolet 740 Fourier transform spectrometer was used for both experiments. For

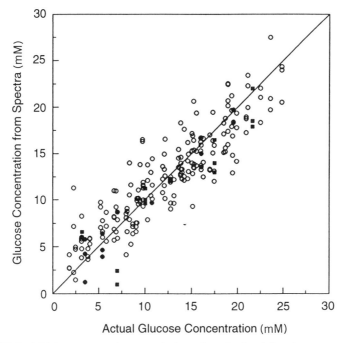

Figure 26.4. Initial concentration correlation plot obtained for the measurement of glucose in undiluted whole blood with limited signal-to-noise ratio.

data set 1, however, the spectrometer was equipped with a 150-W tungsten—halogen light source, calcium fluoride beamsplitter, and liquid nitrogen–cooled InSb detector. For data set 2, the source power was increased and a backreflecting mirror was added to the source housing in order to present a double image of the source filament through the spectrometer. The result is more light reaching the detector, which enhances the signal-to-noise ratio (SNR) of the spectra.

Figure 26.5 shows the concentration correlation plot for the second whole-blood matrix experiment where the spectra were collected with the upgraded spectrometer. The improvement in analytical performance is striking. By getting more light to the detector, the SNR of the measurement is enhanced by a factor of 3.4, which clearly has a major impact on the quality of the calibration model. All points, calibration and prediction, fall tightly around the ideal unity line. The SEP decreases from 2.3 to 0.4 mM.

Besides noise, variations in the baseline of a spectrum degrades spectral quality and can significantly reduce analytical performance. Baseline variations are generally caused by changes in the experimental parameters between collection of the reference and sample spectra. Slight alterations in spectrometer alignment can be a source of baseline movement. In addition, changes in temperature represent a major source of baseline variation. The effect of temperature is especially significant with water-based samples because of shifts in the

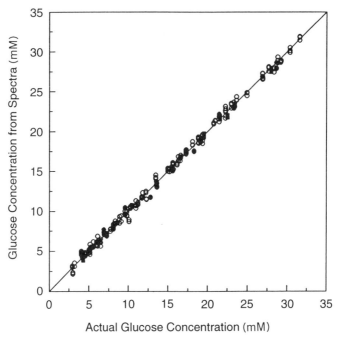

Figure 26.5. *Improved calibration model for measuring glucose in undiluted whole blood resulting from enhanced signal-to-noise ratio.*

water absorption bands as a function of temperature. Several raw absorbance spectra for a sample of 9.2 mM glucose are presented in Figure 26.6. These spectra were collected at the indicated temperatures, while the reference spectrum was collected at 37°C. The spectral features represent baseline variations caused by slight changes in the position and shape of the water-absorbance bands, nominally centered at 3800 and 5200 cm⁻¹.[10] Although these changes are small relative to the overall magnitude of the water absorbance, they are larger than the entire glucose absorbance features used for the analysis.

The effects of baseline variation can be reduced by treating the spectrum with a digital Fourier filtering step. The procedures for implementing this software process are detailed elsewhere.[12] Briefly, a Fourier transformation is computed for the raw absorbance spectrum. The Fourier transform algorithm treats the spectrum as a superposition of sinewaves. These various sinewaves are separated by their frequencies (termed digital frequency, f) by the Fourier transformation. The digital frequencies associated with the analyte bands can be selectively extracted by multiplying the Fourier transformed spectrum by a Gaussian-shape function. This multiplication step effectively weights the digital frequencies under the Gaussian curve while eliminating all other digital frequencies. After this multiplication step, the spectrum is returned to the original data domain by performing an inverse Fourier transform. The result is a dramatic decrease in the high-frequency, choppy noise and a reduction in baseline variation. In this

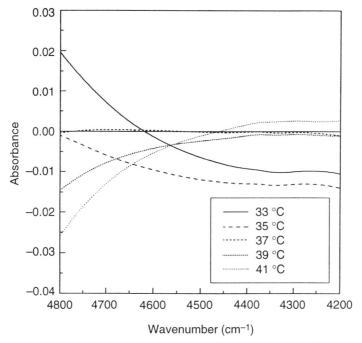

Figure 26.6. Near-infrared spectra collected for 9.2 mM glucose at different temperatures.

scheme, the choppy noise corresponds to high digital frequencies, and baseline variations are low digital frequencies.

The key to a successful digital filtering step is the proper assignment of the Gaussian filter response function. The Gaussian curve is defined by the position along the digital frequency axis and the width of the curve. The mean and standard deviation establish the position and width of the Gaussian curve, respectively. If the curve is placed in the wrong position along the digital frequency axis, the sinewaves that define the shape of the analyte absorbance band will not be weighted heavily and will be eliminated. If the Gaussian curve is too wide, undesirable noise will pass through the filter, and, if the curve is too narrow, useful analytical information will be lost. Strategies to identify the ideal mean and standard deviation for the Gaussian response function have been detailed in a recent report.[10,12] Basically, all combinations of mean and standard deviation are used to filter spectra in the training data set and in a monitoring data set. PLS calibration models are prepared after implementing each filter. Spectra in the monitoring data set are used to test the prediction ability of each calibration model. A surface is then constructed by plotting a response function defined as the reciprocal of the sum of the mean square error of calibration and the mean square error of prediction [1/(MSEC + MSEP)] as functions of the mean and standard deviation values. The ideal mean and standard deviation can be identified as the combination of values that gives the highest value for this response function.

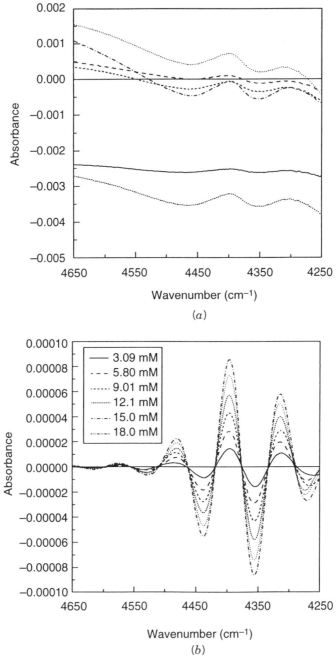

Figure 26.7. Raw (*a*) and Fourier filtered (*b*) spectra for glucose solutions at different temperatures.

The effectiveness of the Fourier digital filtering is demonstrated in Figure 26.7, where a series of raw and filtered absorbance spectra are presented. These spectra correspond to aqueous solutions with different glucose concentrations. In addition, the temperature for the sample and reference spectra were 41 and 37°C, respectively. Baseline variations represent the predominant features in these spectra, not glucose concentration variations. The lower set of spectra are obtained after filtering the raw spectra with a digital Fourier filter. After filtering, the resulting spectral features are centered around the 4400-cm^{-1} glucose absorption band and the magnitude of this feature correlates with glucose concentration. Clearly, the adverse effects of baseline variation have been effectively eliminated by the filtering step.

The practical benefit of using Fourier filtering to eliminate baseline variation is illustrated in the ability to predict accurately from spectra collected at temperatures not represented in the calibration model. This ability has been evaluated[16] by building a calibration model with training and monitoring data sets that consisted of spectra collected only at 37°C and then testing the ability of this model to predict from spectra collected at temperatures ranging from 33 to 41°C. The resulting concentration correlation plot is presented in Figure 26.8.

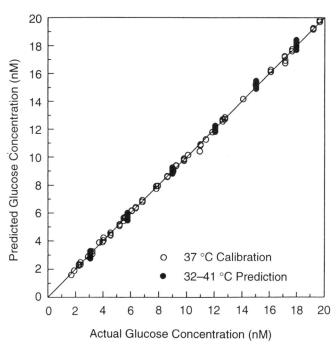

Figure 26.8. Concentration correlation plot showing both calibration (open circles) and prediction (closed circles) results where the calibration model is computed with spectra collected at 37°C and the prediction data set contains spectra collected at different temperatures ranging from 32 to 41°C.

There is essentially no temperature-dependent difference in the prediction ability of this model. The overall SEP is 0.14 mM across all temperatures compared to a SEC of 0.11 mM for only 37°C.

26.5. MULTIPLE ANALYTES

A powerful potential feature of NIR spectroscopy is the ability to measure the concentration of numerous analytes in a sample based on the analysis of a single spectrum. This concept was presented above for the simultaneous determination of glucose and glutamine with PLS regression analysis of NIR spectra. This idea can be extended further. In fact, recent results indicate the possibility of measuring glucose, glutamine, lactate, glutamate, and ammonia simultaneously from a single NIR spectrum.[17] Five individual calibration models are constructed and then used to provide the analytical information.

From a clinical standpoint, the concept of determining multiple analytes from a single serum, plasma, or whole-blood sample is attractive. Indeed, the feasibility of such measurements has been demonstrated by successfully measuring

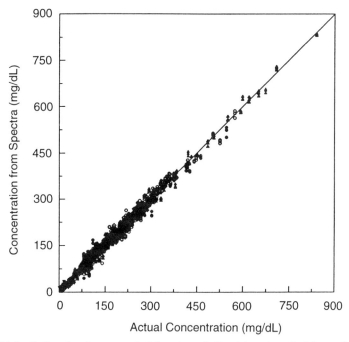

Figure 26.9. Calibration (open symbols) and prediction (closed symbols) correlation plot for multicomponent analysis of undiluted human serum samples for triglycerides (up-triangles), cholesterol (diamonds), urea (squares), glucose (circle) and lactate (down-triangles).

albumin, globulin, total protein, cholesterol, triglycerides, urea, and glucose from a single NIR spectrum as analyzed by individual calibration models.[18–20] Figure 26.9 provides an example of the measurement of triglycerides, cholesterol, urea, glucose and lactate in undiluted human serum samples.[20] Both predicted and actual concentrations are plotted for each analyte. The correlation between prediction and actual concentrations is excellent for all of these analytes, except for lactate. Closer inspection of the lactate response reveals that the calibration model is incapable of providing sufficient accuracy for clinical chemistry measurements. In general, the ability to measure any analyte diminishes considerably as the analyte concentration approaches millimolar concentration levels.

26.6. FUTURE PROSPECTS

As work toward noninvasive clinical measurements progresses, the analytical utility of NIR spectroscopy for clinical and biomedical applications is being established. The concept of a reagentless clinical chemistry analyzer is an excellent example of how NIR spectroscopy may develop and advance technology in the clinical chemistry laboratory. Current progress indicates that NIR spectroscopy can be used to measure multiple analytes in clinical samples without destroying or altering the sample and without the need for expensive reagents. Alternatively, NIR spectroscopy might be used to continuously monitor soluble chemical species in bioreactors or cell cultures. Whatever the application, the principal limitation of current NIR measurements in aqueous solutions is a millimolar limit of detection.

It must be stressed that, despite numerous claims in the mass media, no one has ever successfully demonstrated an ability to measure *in vivo* glucose levels in a noninvasive manner. A preliminary report by Haaland and coworkers[21] suggests that glucose information is present in NIR spectra collected across human fingertips. Nevertheless, all results to date indicate that the major obstacles to success are related to the quality of spectra that can be obtained with present optical components. The weak absorptivities of the glucose molecule make accurate absorbance measurements extremely difficult. Essentially, the problem is to measure small differences in light intensity caused by a weak absorber located in a highly scattering matrix. A novel approach, coined Kromoscopic analysis, has been offered[22] to measure such small light intensity differences by analyzing signals obtained from a series of detectors with unique spectral response curves. This format offers the feature of using each detector under high-SNR conditions, which should enhance the analytical performance of the measurement. Unfortunately, the ability to measure clinically relevant levels of glucose in a plain aqueous medium could not be demonstrated in preliminary investigations.[22] Nevertheless, the Kromoscopy approach stressed the need to acquire high-quality spectra that actually contain the chemical information needed for the analysis. Issues of absorptivity, signal, and noise must be considered. Although noninvasive measurements of clinically and biomedically important substances are not yet possible, the tremendous potential of this approach will continue to drive advancements in both spectroscopic and computer-based data analysis technologies.

In the near future, the impact of noninvasive biosensing technology will be particularly significant in the general area of biomedical research. The availability of an analytical device capable of providing selective concentration information in a continuous manner will permit detailed investigations that are simply not possible with current state-of-the-art technology. For example, researchers are interested in monitoring *in situ* blood glucose levels during periods of sleep. Nocturnal hypoglycemia is a problem that cannot be examined in an efficient manner given the present limitations pertaining to sample collection requirements. Furthermore, noninvasive biosensing technology will revolutionize drug delivery and drug transport studies by providing a means to spatially resolve the drug molecules within a test system and then to follow directly the transport of this species within the human body as a function of time.

The clinical impact of noninvasive biosensing technology will be equally significant based on the potential to perform *in situ,* reagentless, and continuous clinical measurements. Sample-free, clinical measurements can be envisioned in numerous healthcare settings. Indeed, noninvasive biosensing is ideally suited for near-patient testing in operating rooms, emergency rooms, intensive care units, neonatal clinics, and even in physician offices. Furthermore, scaled-down devices could be useful in ambulatory settings and for patient home testing situations. The reagentless feature of this technology makes it ideally suited for monitoring chemical substances during numerous medical procedures. The principal utility of this technology will be the ability to monitor the *in vivo* chemistry of a patient in a point-of-care fashion. Such a capability has the potential to impact essentially all areas of medical science and all clinical specialties.

REFERENCES

1. Wraith A: A review of pulse oximetry. *SAAD Digest* 10:22–29, 1993.

2. Beckmann N, Fried R, Turkalj I, Seelig J, Keller U, Stalder G: Noninvasive observation of hepatic glycogen formation in man by 13C MRS after oral and intravenous glucose administration. *Mag Res Med* 29:583–590, 1993.

3. Nakada T, Kwee IL: Noninvasive analysis of aldose reductase activities in rat testis: 3-FDG NMR spectroscopy and imaging. *Mag Res Med* 29:543–545, 1993.

4. Diabetes Control and Complications Trail Research Group: The effect of intensive treatment of diabetes on the development and progression of long-term complications in insulin-dependent diabetes mellitus. *N Engl J Med* 329:977–986, 1993.

5. Rosenthal RD, Paynte LN, Mackie LH: Noninvasive measurement of blood glucose. US Patent 5,086,229, Feb 4, 1992.

6. Barnes RH, Brasch JW: Noninvasive determination of glucose concentration in body of patients. US Patent 5,070,874, Dec 10, 1991.

7. Lin J, Brown CW: Near-IR fiber optic probe for electrolytes in aqueous solutions. *Anal Chem* 65:287–292, 1993.

8. Lin J, Brown CW: Near-IR fiber optic temperature sensor. *Applied Spectroscopy* 47:62–68, 1993.

9. Lin J, Brown CW: Universal approach for determination of physical and chemical properties of water by near-IR spectroscopy. *Applied Spectroscopy* 47:1720–1727, 1993.

10. Arnold MA, Small GW: Determination of physiological levels of glucose in an aqueous matrix with digitally filtered Fourier transform near-infrared spectra. *Anal Chem* 62:1457–1464, 1990.

11. Marquardt LA, Arnold MA, Small GW: Near infrared spectroscopic measurement of glucose in a protein matrix. *Anal Chem* 65:3271–3278, 1993.

12. Small GW, Marquardt LA, Arnold MA: Strategies for coupling Fourier filtering and partial least-squares regression: Application to the determination of glucose in plasma by Fourier transform near-infrared spectroscopy. *Anal Chem* 65:3279–3289, 1993.

13. Chung H, Arnold MA, Rhiel M, Murhammer DW: Simultaneous measurement of glucose and glutamine in aqueous solutions by near infrared spectroscopy. *Appl Biochem Biotech,* 50:109–125, 1995.

14. Hazen KK, Arnold MA, Small GW: Near-Infrared Spectroscopic Measurement of Glucose in Multiple Matrices of Whole Blood. submitted for publication.

15. Burmeister JJ, Arnold MA: Accuracy of the YSI Stat Plus analyzer for glucose and lactate. *Anal Lett,* 28:581–592, 1995.

16. Hazen KK, Arnold MA, Small GW: Temperature insensitive near infrared measurements of glucose in aqueous matrices. *Applied Spectroscopy* 48:477–483, 1994.

17. Chung H, Arnold MA, Rhiel M, Murhammer DW: Simultaneous measurement of glucose, glutamine, glutamate, lactate and ammonia in aqueous samples by near infrared spectroscopy. submitted for publication.

18. Hall JW, Pollard A: Near-infrared spectrophotometry: a new dimension in clinical chemistry. *Clin Chem* 38:1623–1631, 1992.

19. Hall JW, Pollard A: Near-infrared spectroscopic determination of serum total protein, albumin, globulins, and urea. *Clin Biochem* 26:483–490, 1993.

20. Hazen KK, Arnold MA, Small GW: Near infrared spectroscopic measurement of multiple components in undiluted human serum samples. (Unpublished results.)

21. Robinson MR, Eaton RP, Haaland DM, et al: Noninvasive glucose monitoring in diabetic patients: a preliminary evaluation. *Clin Chem* 38:1616–1622, 1992.

22. Sodickson LA, Block MJ: Kromoscopic analysis: a possible alternative to spectroscopic analysis for noninvasive measurements of analytes in vivo. *Clin Chem* 40:1838–1844, 1994.

CHAPTER

27

In Vitro, Ex Vivo, and In Vivo Biosensor Systems

GERALD J. KOST AND CLIFFORD HAGUE

CONTENTS

Handbook of Clinical Automation, Robotics, and Optimization, Edited by Gerald J. Kost with the collaboration of Judith Welsh.
ISBN 0-471-03179-8 © 1996 John Wiley & Sons, Inc.

27.1. FOCUS

In the past decade, point-of-care testing emerged to improve patient outcomes in the operating room, emergency department, and intensive care unit.[90–96,454] Biosensor-based whole blood analyzers enabled this paradigm shift in diagnostic testing to occur.[97,98] In critical care settings, the medical efficacy of point-of-care testing is well established.[97] Eventually, most rapid response testing will be performed at the point of care. *Ex vivo* and *in vivo* biosensor systems will accelerate this trend. An exciting future is ahead—one where these monitoring systems will augment, complement, and replace *in vitro* testing during at least the initial stages of critical illness. After briefly introducing the principles of whole-blood biosensors and *in vitro* systems, we assess *ex vivo* and *in vivo* biosensor systems from a clinical perspective. Schematics and photographs of actual systems give the reader an opportunity to study the progress of patient monitoring systems. Many references are cited in the text. A topical bibliography concentrating on the past 5 years provides additional resources. Ultimately, *ex vivo* and *in vivo* monitoring will have a profound impact on critical care and will substantially improve patient outcomes.

27.2. PRINCIPLES OF WHOLE-BLOOD BIOSENSORS

27.2.1. Background

Figure 27.1 outlines common measurements and principles currently used *in vitro* for whole-blood analysis. Biosensors found in whole-blood analyzers include the ion-selective electrode (ISE), substrate-specific electrode (SSE), analyte-specific optical sensor (ASOS), and electrical conductance sensor (ECS). Ionized calcium (Ca^{2+}) and ionized magnesium (Mg^{2+}) are important and rela-

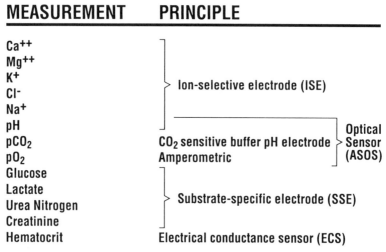

Figure 27.1. Whole-blood measurements and biosensor principles.[98]

tively new clinical measurements (please see recent reviews[454,537]). Figure 27.2*a* is a schematic of a Mg^{2+} ISE. The acronym ISE refers to measurement of cations (e.g., K^+) as well as anions (e.g., Cl^-). Figure 27.2*b* is a drawing of a glucose SSE. Figure 27.2*c* shows a lactate SSE. The acronym SSE was introduced in 1991[283] and refers to the measurement of glucose, lactate, urea nitrogen, creatinine, and other metabolites. The acronym ASOS was introduced recently[391] to describe clinical optical sensors. Most point-of-care testing instruments also include hematocrit measurement performed with an electrical conductance sensor (ECS). *In vitro* instruments use these biosensors to measure several analytes simultaneously and quickly. Speed and efficiency are major advantages in critical care settings.

Ex vivo and *in vivo* blood chemistry monitoring systems generally are limited to relatively few analytes, primarily those that vary rapidly and require fast response or frequent measurements. These analytes include glucose, blood gases (p_{O_2}, p_{CO_2}), pH, potassium, sodium, ionized calcium, hematocrit, oxygen saturation, and to a lesser extent urea, creatinine, and lactate.[173,397,483] Temperature must either be measured or controlled. Most effort has been devoted to the development of *ex vivo* and *in vivo* systems that monitor these analytes in the hospital environment, particularly the operating room and intensive care unit. Glucose is also the focus of ongoing attempts to develop a wearable or implantable monitoring system for outpatient use by diabetics.[50,65,234,282,313] We will briefly discuss the measurement principles of electrochemical, fiber optic, and relatively new fiber optic chemical sensors. Miniaturized electrochemical and fiber optic sensors are used in several of the intermittent and continuous monitoring systems presented below.

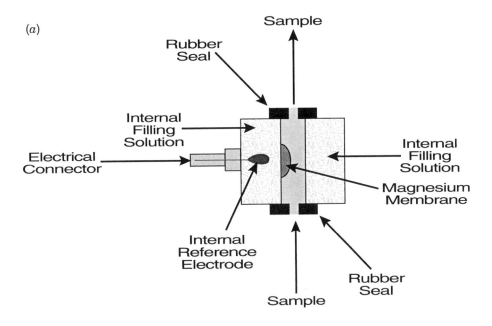

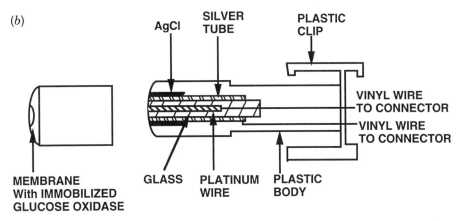

Figure 27.2. Biosensors for whole-blood measurement. (*a*) An ion-selective electrode (ISE) for the measurement of ionized magnesium. The external reference electrode (not shown) is located in the sample flow path (see Fig. 27.3). (*b*) A substrate-specific electrode (SSE) for the measurement of glucose. The anode and cathode are at the tip under the membrane within this enzyme-based amperometric sensor. (*c*) An SSE for lactate. (Courtesy of NOVA Biomedical.)

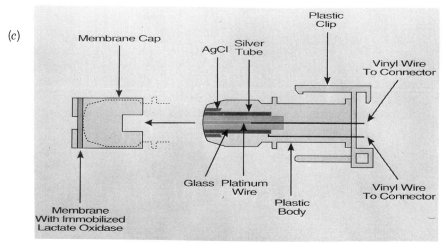

Figure 27.2. (*Continued*)

27.2.2. Electrochemical Sensors (ISE and SSE)

Electrochemical sensors fall into two categories: (1) potentiometric and (2) amperometric. Most potentiometric sensors use an ion-selective membrane that incorporates a specific ionophore into the membrane matrix. The membrane functions as the biodetector of the electrode. When in contact with blood or other body fluid, the ionophore selectively interacts with a target ion species and creates an electrical potential across the membrane (see Fig. 27.2*a*). This potential is measured between the internal and the external reference electrodes. The potential is logarithmically proportional to the activity of the ion that is being measured in the sample. In some systems, measurements must be corrected for interference (e.g., correction of Mg^{2+} for Na^+, Ca^{2+}, and pH in the sample). Whole-blood analyzers commonly use ion-selective electrodes (ISEs) for the measurement of electrolytes and pH *in vitro*.[187,454] Figure 27.3 illustrates the placement of electrodes in a sample flowpath and the position of the external reference electrode. A modification of the basic potentiometric sensor, the Stowe–Severinghaus electrode, is used to measure p_{CO_2}.[488] In this electrode,

---

Figure 27.3. Modular biosensors for Stat Profile series whole-blood analyzers. (NOVA Biomedical.) (*a*) The Plus 9. The sample first flows through the preheater. Then, it flows through the plastic block in the "zig-zag" capillary, where it contacts the sensors. The reflection on the left shows the location of the sensor tips where the electrodes (on the right) fit into the cylindrical receptacles. Electrochemical measurements include (top to bottom) Cl^-, Na^+, Ca^{2+}, K^+, glucose, lactate, pH, p_{CO_2}, and p_{O_2}. Hematocrit is measured by conductance (ECS) and is Na^+-corrected. The reference electrode ("R") also is in the flow path. After analysis the sample flows into a biohazard container via the waste ("W") channel. (*b*) The Ultra. Electrode block and O_2 saturation sensor. (See Table 27.3 for measurement ranges.) (Courtesy of NOVA Biomedical.)

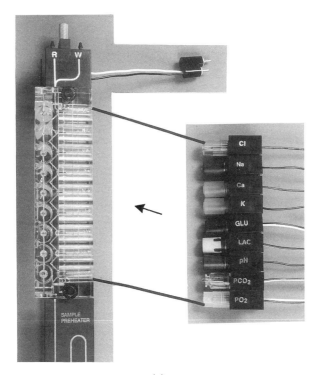

(a)

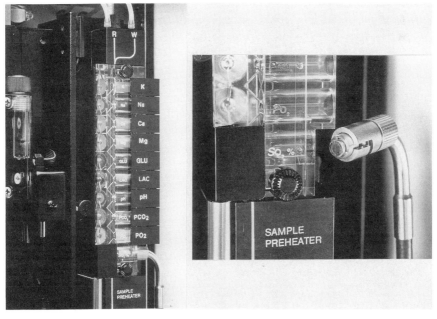

(b)

CO_2 from the sample being measured diffuses across a CO_2-permeable membrane into a bicarbonate buffer that is in contact with a pH sensor. When the CO_2 reaches equilibrium in the bicarbonate buffer, the p_{CO_2} of the sample can be calculated based on the pH measured in the buffer.

The response of potentiometric sensors is logarithmic. Therefore, small errors in the measured potential produce large errors in the results. These errors will affect both accuracy and precision. If there is a change in activity from a_1 to a_2, there will be a corresponding change in the sensor potential. If $\Delta E = E_2 - E_1$, it follows from the Nernst equation that $\Delta E = [(RT \ln 10)/(ZF)]\log[\text{ratio of the activities}]$. When ΔE is 1 mV, T is 310.15 K (37°C), and Z is 1, the ratio of the activities will be equal to $\log^{-1}[(\Delta E)/((RT \ln 10)/(ZF))] \approx \log^{-1}[1 \text{ mV}/61.54 \text{ mV}] = 1.038$. Hence, a ± 1-mV change in the measured potential is equivalent to approximately a $\pm 4\%$ change in the reported value. The reference electrode alone can introduce uncertainty of up to ± 0.5 mV from junction potential, sample matrix, and boundary-layer phenomena where the electrolyte enters the sample flowpath. This is equivalent to a change in accuracy of approximately $\pm 2\%$ for monovalent ions [i.e., $Z = 1$ and $\log^{-1}(0.5 \text{ mV}/61.54 \text{ mV}) \approx 1.019$] or approximately $\pm 4\%$ for divalent ions (i.e., $Z = 2$ and $\log^{-1}[0.5 \text{ mV}/30.77 \text{ mV}] \approx 1.038$). Instabilities during the electronic measurement of the potential of the sensor electrochemical cell (ISE::reference electrode) and electrical noise coming from sensor modules or *in vivo* probes detract from the precision of the analyte readings. Inaccuracy and imprecision combine to produce time-variant changes in calibration. As a consequence, *ex vivo* and *in vivo* monitors must either be designed for very high stability or else incorporate periodic recalibrations to correct for this drift.

Amperometric sensors used in monitoring systems generally are based on the Clark-type oxygen electrode.[423] A barrier membrane placed over the sensing electrode allows oxygen from the sample to diffuse to the electrode, but excludes chemical species that potentially could interfere with electrode function. A voltage applied across the sensing and reference electrodes reduces oxygen and at steady state, generates an electrical current that is linearly proportional to the p_{O_2} in the sample. A common enzyme-based amperometric sensor is the glucose SSE (see Fig. 27.2*b*). Immobilized glucose oxidase oxidizes the glucose substrate. Several different approaches have been used to quantitate this oxidation reaction and to determine substrate concentration. These include oxygen consumption, which requires an additional reference oxygen sensor, and hydrogen peroxide generation, which does not.[321] Measurement of the latter is more practical, in view of sensor space constraints. There are many different glucose SSE designs. Some use other electron acceptors to reduce dependence on O_2. Barrier membranes of various configurations are used to exclude interfering species, select for the target substrate, and control the rate of diffusion of the substrate into the sensor. For amperometric sensors in general, slight changes in membrane permeability or in the electrodes over time can cause drift in the output current. Therefore, for monitoring applications, SSEs also must be designed for high stability or be recalibrated periodically.

27.2.3 Electrical Conductance Sensor (ECS)

Electrical conductance sensors involve applying an alternating voltage across two or more electrodes in contact with the fluid sample and measuring impedance (conductance) to the resulting current flow. This method is used to determine the hematocrit in whole blood. The conductivity is dependent on the volume of relatively nonconductive blood cells between the electrodes and on the electrolyte concentration in the blood. A correction for the electrolyte concentration can be approximated by the simultaneous measurement of the whole-blood sodium level to produce a more accurate estimate of hematocrit.[173] Measurement of hematocrit by conductivity has been reported to produce falsely low values under conditions where plasma has been replaced with crystalloid, such as in patients receiving large transfusions of processed autologous blood.[540]

27.2.4. Fiber Optic Sensors

Fiber optic sensors have been used to differentiate oxygenated blood from deoxygenated blood by spectrophotometry.[430] A narrow-waveband light source generates light that is transmitted down one or more optic fibers to the tip of a catheter. Light reflects from the blood back through one or more optic fibers to a photodetector. Several wavelengths are chosen such that the differential absorption characteristics of oxyhemoglobin and hemoglobin allow determination of the ratio between the two.

27.2.5. Fiber Optic Chemical Sensors

Fiber optic chemical sensors, also referred to as *optodes,*[461] have received considerable attention as a technology that has potential advantages over more conventional electrochemical sensors for automated monitoring. Optodes can be made very small, require no direct electrical connection to the patient, are free from electromagnetic interference, and can incorporate internal referencing to reduce or eliminate drift.[190,514] On the other hand, commercial experience to date has shown that they can be difficult and costly to manufacture and have low production yields.[76] Four basic approaches to fiber optic chemical sensors have been described, including absorption, fluorescence intensity, fluorescence lifetime, and surface enhanced Raman spectroscopy (SERS).[514] Commercial systems are based primarily on either absorption or fluorescence intensity. With both approaches, light is passed through an optic fiber in the catheter to the sensor that contains an indicator. In absorption sensors, the target analyte is measured by the intensity of the color of the indicator, which changes in proportion to the analyte concentration. In fluorescence intensity sensors, it is the intensity of a lower wavelength light reemitted by an indicator that changes in proportion to the analyte concentration. Most developmental work with optodes has focused on p_{O_2}, p_{CO_2}, and pH, although fiber optic chemical sensors for electrolytes and glucose also have been described.[331,419]

27.3. TRANSPORTABLE, PORTABLE, AND HANDHELD *IN VITRO* WHOLE-BLOOD ANALYZERS

27.3.1. Clinical Rationale and Significance of Point-of-Care Testing— Synopsis

Whole-blood analyzers, critical medical indications, and rising expectations of patients and physicians have shifted laboratory diagnostics to the point of care (see detailed discussion[97]). Expanding transplantation and intensive care are increasing the need for rapid test results and immediate medical decisions. Whole-blood analysis improves accuracy, eliminates centrifugation, reduces response time, and conserves blood volume. Whole-blood analyzers simultaneously measure several vital function indicators (e.g., Ca^{2+}, Mg^{2+}, K^+, Cl^-, Na^+, pH, p_{CO_2}, p_{CO_2}, glucose, lactate, urea nitrogen, creatinine, O_2 saturation or hematocrit) in <2 min with one 200 μL (or less) whole-blood sample. Several handheld, portable, and transportable point-of-care instruments are available. Table 27.1 summarizes biosensor-based tests available on instruments from different manufacturers. Urea nitrogen, lactate, ionized magnesium, creatinine, and total CO_2 are some of the most recent additions to whole-blood test menus. Other whole-blood *in vitro* tests are available (β-hydroxybutyrate, hemoglobin, thrombosis, and hemostasis indices) or under development (HCO_3^-, phosphorus). The clinical impact of point-of-care testing is demonstrated by ionized calcium, now established in importance for cardiac and neurologic problems, by lactate and ionized magnesium, promising new point-of-care measurements, and by other analytes needed in critical-care settings.[454] The hybrid laboratory[92–94] and knowledge optimization[97] facilitate the optimal support of cardiac and critical care for improved patient outcomes.

27.3.2. Selection and Performance Evaluation of Whole-Blood Analyzers

Excellent on-site performance is essential if whole-blood analyzers are to be clinically effective. Table 27.2 outlines criteria for the selection and performance evaluation of *in vitro* whole-blood biosensor systems. Important criteria for instrument evaluation include test cluster, point-of-care, and patient-focusing features. Security, ease of operation, and speed in the intended clinical setting are essential. The design of a point-of-care instrument should be ergonomic. Operation should be straightforward. For example, in an emergency the operator should be able to interrupt an automatic two-point calibration to save time. The one-point calibration cycle should be short. Calibration drift should be minimal. The biosensors should not be sensitive to operator technique or to the type of clinical application (e.g., resuscitation, point-of-care, or satellite laboratory). Throughput must match clinical input, especially during emergencies. Handheld and portable instruments should be efficient, reliable, durable, com-

TABLE 27.1. Representative *In Vitro* Biosensor Systems—Whole-Blood Tests

Whole-Blood Instrument(s); Manufacturer, Location	Biosensor-Based Tests[a] [Other Tests]
988, 995, and COMPACT Series;	Ca^{2+}, K^+, Na^+, Mg^{2+}, p_{O_2}, p_{CO_2}, pH
OMNI Series;	Ca^{2+}, K^+, Na^+, Cl^-, p_{O_2}, p_{CO_2}, pH, glucose, lactate, urea nitrogen, [hematocrit, hemoglobin], [CO-oximetry]
OPTI 1;[b] AVL, Roswell, GA	p_{O_2}, p_{CO_2}, pH
800 Series; Ciba-Corning, Norwood, MA	Ca^{2+}, K^+, Na^+, Cl^-, p_{O_2}, p_{CO_2}, pH, glucose, lactate [CO-oximetry]
IRMA; Diametrics, St. Paul, MN	Ca^{2+}, K^+, Na^+, p_{O_2}, p_{CO_2}, pH, [hematocrit]
1600 Series (1630/40, 1650); Instrumentation Laboratory, Lexington, MA	Ca^{2+}, K^+, Na^+, Cl^-, p_{O_2}, p_{CO_2}, pH, [hematocrit]
i-STAT Series; i-STAT, Princeton, NJ	Ca^{2+}, K^+, Na^+, Cl^-, p_{O_2}, p_{CO_2}, pH, glucose, urea nitrogen, [hematocrit]
GEM Premier, Stat, and 6 Plus; Mallinckrodt Sensor Systems, Ann Arbor, MI	Ca^{2+}, K^+, Na^+, p_{O_2}, p_{CO_2}, pH, [hematocrit]
Stat Profile and NOVA Series; NOVA Biomedical, Waltham, MA	Ca^{2+}, K^+, Na^+, Cl^-, Mg^{2+}, p_{O_2}, p_{CO_2}, pH, glucose, lactate, urea nitrogen, creatinine, total CO_2, [O_2 saturation, hematocrit]
StatPal II, III; UniFET, La Jolla, CA	Ca^{2+}, K^+, Na^+, p_{O_2}, p_{CO_2}, pH, [hematocrit]
ABL 620; Radiometer America, Cleveland, OH	Ca^{2+}, K^+, Na^+, Cl^-, p_{O_2}, p_{CO_2}, pH, [CO-oximetry]
2300 STAT Plus; YSI, Yellow Springs, OH	Glucose, lactate

[a]*Notes:*

1. Some tests may be under development; others are added as test menus expand.
2. Some manufacturers offer a free-standing, attachable, or built-in CO-oximeter; new technologies (e.g., AVL PolyOx multiwavelength CCD video) may be used; and other tests may be added in addition to hemoglobin parameters.
3. Glucose meters were omitted from the table; for details of instruments and performance, please see the references under the topic heading "Glucose" (Refs. 205–371). For information on the Abaxis whole-blood analyzer, please see Reference 485a.

[b]Optical fluorescence technology—ASOSs are used to measure p_{O_2}, p_{CO_2}, and pH.

TABLE 27.2. Criteria for the Selection and Performance Evaluation of *In Vitro* Whole-Blood Biosensor Systems

Test cluster, point-of-care, and patient-focusing features
  Appropriate and complete test clusters
    Critical-care profile—number and selection of tests
    Test clusters that match clinical objectives
    Modularity of biosensors and adaptability of test menus
    New biosensors, exchangeability, and upgrade capacity
  Specimen volume, type, and matrices accepted
  Ergonomics and simplicity
    Compactness, weight, power efficiency, and battery option
    Speed, ease, and security of operation
    Operator identification, validation, and notification system
    Automated calibration cycle, duration, number of points, and user
      modifications; microprocessor control of detection system
    Analysis cycle, emergency interrupt, throughput, and data archiving
    Biohazard control and containment
  Reliability, durability, and validation for the intended level and modality of clinical application
    Point-of-care, satellite, or remote review sites with network interfacing
    Transportable (mobile cart), portable, or hand-held
    Critical care, hospital, clinic, ambulance, aircraft, helicopter, site of rescue, or home
System performance (technical and clinical)
  Results consistent and compatible with other *in vitro, ex vivo,* and *in vivo* whole-blood systems
  Accuracy, precision, bias, resolution, and response time
  Performance in the high and low extremes of measurements
  Linear over the clinical range, the span from low to high critical limits, and anticipated levels for quality control and proficiency testing
  Biosensor reproducibility for exact measurements (vs. trend monitoring)
  Stability (drift) of biosensors at the site of use, idle, or in storage
Performance maps, quality paths, and outcome indicators
  Cost-effectiveness, number and efficiency of process steps, medically useful half-life of test results, number of instrument errors, and impact on length of critical care or hospitalization
  Prefessional productivity and satisfaction of physicians, care teams, and patients
  Quality path performance optimization
  Patient outcomes (prospects)
Manufacturer, government, and accreditation agency factors
  Training software programs and educational materials (e.g., videos)
  Resources for point-of-care operator credentials
  Costs of instruments, consumables, and maintenance
  Quality control, quality assurance, proficiency testing, and continuous quality improvement

(continued)

TABLE 27.2. (*continued*)

Compliance with state and federal regulations
Acceptability for accreditation agencies (e.g., CAP and JCAHO)
Knowledge optimization[97]
  Outcomes optimizer functions (physicial capture)
  Temporal optimization
  Diagnostic–therapeutic process optimization
Integration
  Robotics and remote review capabilities
  FAST QC, quality pattern recognition, and patient diagnostic patterns
  Alarms, critical limits storage, and critical results notification
  Information integration
    Storage and archiving capacities
    Computerized information systems (LIS and HIS)
    Workstation integration with other critical-care areas (LAN or WAN)
    Personal data communications (e.g., wireless)

pact, and lightweight, with streamlined requirements for reagents, maintenance, biohazard disposal, and quality control. Programmability, self-diagnostics, data management, and simplicity are important, since operators with different levels of experience perform measurements. Operation of transportable instruments from a main laboratory with fast specimen transport and results reporting, a carefully placed satellite laboratory, a bedside workstation, or a mobile cart generally is clinically effective. One must cautiously balance the quality of measurements, size format of the instrument, and operating expenses.

The accuracy, precision, and linearity of whole-blood analyzers must be (1) excellent in the near-normal ranges, (2) acceptable in the high and low extremes, and (3) comparable for the same analytes measured on different instruments. Several investigators and professional organizations are working toward consistency and standardization of whole-blood methods and of biosensor measurements (see "Guidelines" section[372–404] in the bibliography). If feasible, use of the identical biosensor technology in several clinical sites facilitates consistency. System performance depends on biosensor stability and reproducibility. Trend monitoring may be adequate in certain clinical settings, while others require exact measurements. A designated reference instrument (e.g., on a mobile cart) can be moved on site for side-by-side anaerobic split-sample comparisons. Transporting and then analyzing whole-blood samples for comparison studies performed at distant sites may introduce preanalytical errors and is inadvisable. Individual instrument histories, tracking records, and comprehensive quality assurance are essential. The relative performance of operators and instruments can be assessed with pattern recognition techniques[390] using control materials, blind samples, and whole-blood clinical specimens. Other new approaches to quality control and quality assurance are needed for single-use biosensor cartridges and *ex vivo* and *in vivo* systems.

Inconsistent results due to instrument-specific normal reference intervals or measurement inaccuracies become apparent as unexpected shifts that confound accurate and swift diagnosis as, for example, the patient is transferred from the emergency department to the operating room and subsequently, to the intensive care unit or patient-focused care center. Seamless information processing and pattern recognition techniques can help eliminate inconsistencies. Significant progress has been made with bar coding, reagent efficiency, and menu-driven touch screens, while the integration of information and interlinking of satellite sites are not yet developed adequately. Small bench instruments are used frequently in satellite laboratories in operating rooms, emergency departments, and intensive care units. These instruments allow flexible selection of test menus and usually can be interfaced with computerized laboratory information systems through RS-232 ports. A smart printer, magnetic storage, and interfacing capability are important. Instrument interfacing should be designed for rapid information exchange with the laboratory information system (LIS) and the hospital information system (HIS). The consolidation of cabling from several bedside instruments and critical care monitors remains a problem. Remote review systems[78] are invaluable and should be anticipated at the time of instrument selection. Fiber optic networks, electronic mail, facsimile (FAX) machines, beepers (pagers), two-way radios, and cellular phones can help facilitate communications. In the future, patient results should be communicated to a base station by telemetry and wireless communication systems.

The effective communication of patient results is essential. For example, the risk of miscommunication of actionable results during a fast-paced patient resuscitation is great. The datastream of results flows so quickly that assimilation into the patient record, a legal necessity, often lags behind real-time care and can impair the clinical impact of whole blood tests. This situation calls for the increasing use of robotics, remote review, artificial intelligence, and intelligent decision systems.[454] Manufacturers and vendors should work to reduce the direct costs of equipment, consumables, and maintenance and should support on-site training programs for point-of-care operators. Some vendors and hospitals have developed videos to educate operators with different clinical expertise and to explain documentation requirements for quality assurance. Besides the ability to quickly and reliably communicate patient results and quality records, one of the criteria for the purchase of a point-of-care instrument should be the provision of instruction programs and plans for operator training that satisfy federal, state, and professional accreditation requirements.

27.3.3. Relevance of Critical Limits to the Measurement Ranges of Biosensors

Critical limits define the boundaries of the low and high life-threatening values of diagnostic test results.[532–537] Critical limit frequencies suggest test priorities

TABLE 27.3. Comparison of Measurement Ranges of Whole-Blood Analyzers with Critical Limits[98]

Measurements	Transportable			Portable	Handheld	Critical Limits[a] (mean low, mean high)	
	Stat Profile Ultra	Stat Profile 9	Stat Profile 10	GEM Premier	i-STAT	Adult	Pediatric
Test Selection	Customized	One menu	One menu	Cartridge-based groups	Cartridge-based groups		
Max. Tests[b]	11	10	10	7	8		
pH	6.50–8.00	6.50–8.00	6.50–8.00	6.80–7.80	6.80–8.00	7.21, 7.59	7.21, 7.59
P_{CO_2}[c] (mm Hg)	3.0–200	3.0–200	3.0–200	5–99	10–100	19, 67	21, 66
P_{O_2} (mm Hg)	0–800	0–800	0–800	0–760	0–800	43, NA	45, 124
Ca^{2+} (mmol/L)	0.1–4.9	0.1–4.9		0.1–5.0	0.25–2.50	0.82, 1.55	0.85, 1.53
K^+ (mmol/L)	1.0–20.0	1.0–20.0	1.0–20.0	0.1–9.9	2–9	2.8, 6.2	2.8, 6.4
Na^+ (mmol/L)	80–200	80–200	80–200	100–200	100–180	120, 158	121, 156
Cl^- (mmol/L)	50–200	50–200	50–200		65–140	75, 126	77, 121
Glucose (mg/dL)	15–500	15–500	15–500		20–450	46, 484	46, 445
Urea Nitrogen[c] (mmol/L)	3.0–100		3.0–100		3–140	NA, 104	NA, 55
Lactate (mmol/L)	0.3–20.0	0.3–20.0	0.3–20.0	15–52		NA, 30.6	NA, 36.9
Hematocrit (%)	12–70	12–70	12–70		10–75	18, 61	20, 62
Mg^{2+} (mmol/L)	0.1–3.0						
O_2 Saturation (%)	30–100						

Notes

[a] Critical limits [532–537] are from national surveys of U.S. medical centers [533] and children's hospitals [534] and for ionized calcium, from a special national survey of both types of hospitals.[537]

[b] Maximum number of simultaneous measurements on one whole-blood sample.

[c] Total CO_2 and creatinine measurements in whole blood are available on the NOVA-16 along with Na^+, K^+, Cl^-, glucose, urea nitrogen, and hematocrit, a total of eight tests. The Stat Profile Ultra has the most extensive menu of up to 11 measurements in test clusters selected by the user; a CO-oximeter can be used with it.

and can assist in the selection of biosensor systems and test clusters for effectiveness in different critical-care settings. Table 27.3 compares the biosensor measurement ranges of three instruments of different formats (transportable, portable, and handheld) to the mean low and mean high critical limits at United States medical centers and children's hospitals.[533,534,537] Critical results that arise during medical emergencies in the operating room, intensive care unit, or emergency room, may fall outside the high and low critical limits. Critical results also will occur during emergency resuscitation, transport, and field rescue. Therefore, it is important that the measurement ranges of biosensors in *in vitro* systems span the range of critical limits and critical results that one expects to encounter clinically. The measurement ranges also should cover analyte levels anticipated in the course of quality-control evaluations and proficiency testing. These principles also apply to *ex vivo* and *in vivo* monitoring systems, although even wider measurement ranges may be required for some diagnostic problems or special treatment protocols.

27.3.4. Survey of *In Vitro* Biosensor Systems

Instrument formats include[454] (1) compact models (e.g., Stat Profile Plus and Ultra series, NOVA series; NOVA Biomedical, Waltham, MA) that are transportable for use at the bedside, in the operating room, or during emergencies; (2) portable models (e.g., GEM Premier; Mallinckrodt Sensor Systems, Ann Arbor, MI) that have self-contained cartridges for measurement of electrolytes and blood gases; and (3) handheld models (e.g., i-STAT series; i-STAT, Princeton, NJ) that can be used in flight and field rescues.[84] We illustrate each of these three formats, starting first with a compact whole-blood analyzer (Fig. 27.4). This format can be transported on a cart for mobile operation (Fig. 27.5). Figure 27.6 illustrates a portable whole-blood analyzer. This instrument uses the multiple sample self-contained cartridge in Figure 27.7. Figure 27.8 is a schematic illustrating the arrangement of electrochemical sensors, pumping mechanism, and prepackaged calibration solutions in the cartridge. Figure 27.9 shows a handheld instrument with a cartridge ready for insertion. Figure 27.10 illustrates the method of filling the cartridge with a whole-blood sample. The cartridge components are assembled as shown in Figure 27.11a. Figure 27.11b is a diagram of one of the biosensor chips in the disposable cartridge. These three instruments perform the measurements listed in Table 27.3, which also gives the measurement ranges of the biosensors. Generally, manufacturers continuously strive to expand test menus and to extend linear ranges of the biosensors to better cover clinically critical events. For example, United States medical centers and children's hospitals require emergency physician notification of glucose levels exceeding 450–500 mg/dL.[532–537] If a glucose biosensor is inaccurate, imprecise, or nonlinear in that range, both medical and legal problems may arise, especially in patients unaware of de novo onset diabetic ketoacidosis.

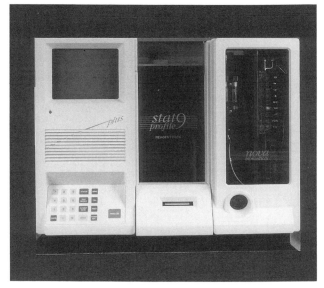

(a)

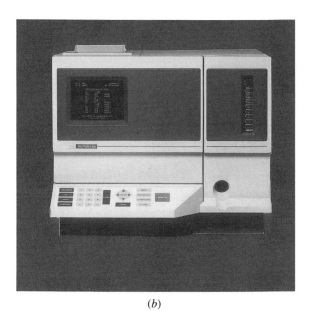

(b)

Figure 27.4. Stat Profile series whole-blood analyzers. (a) The "Plus 9" biosensor block (shown in Fig. 27.3) is in the cabinet to the right. (b) The "Ultra" also measures Mg^{2+} and O_2 saturation. (Courtesy of NOVA Biomedical.)

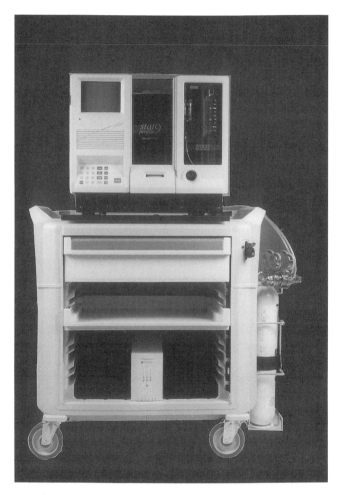

Figure 27.5. Illustration of a *transportable* format. First introduced in 1989, this type of cart has gas supplies and a 30-min power supply for transportable operation of the Stat Profile and NOVA series whole-blood analyzers. Mobile formats were introduced over 15 years ago. For example, carts were used to transport instruments and microcomputer workstations to the patient's bedside for monitoring.[556,562,564,565] Transportable analyzers also have been used in several medical centers to assist surgical procedures, transplants, and resuscitations. Recently, carts have been developed for the transport of roving laboratories.[506] (Courtesy of NOVA Biomedical.)

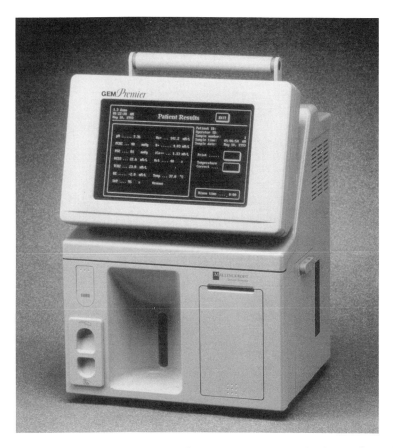

Figure 27.6. Illustration of a *portable* format. The GEM Premier is a self-contained whole-blood analyzer that performs Ca^{2+}, K^+, Na^+, p_{O_2}, p_{CO_2}, pH and hematocrit testing. (Courtesy of Mallinckrodt Sensor Systems.)

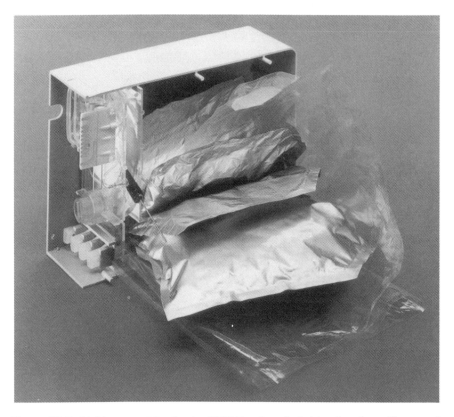

Figure 27.7. Multiuse cartridge for the GEM Premier whole-blood analyzer. The capacity is either 150 or 300 sets of measurements. The cartridge is disposable and houses the biosensors (top), calibrants, sealed waste container, and other components identified in Figure 27.8. (Courtesy of Mallinckrodt Sensor Systems.)

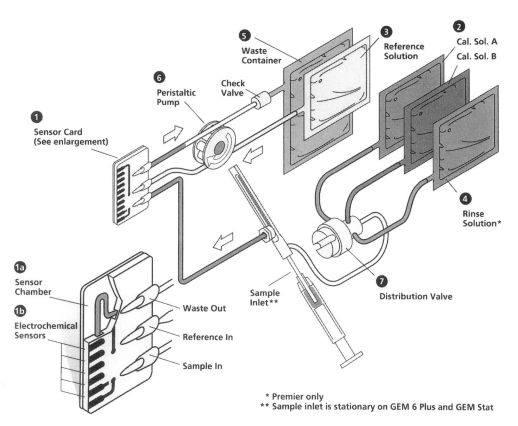

Figure 27.8. Schematic of the biosensor card and fluidics system for the GEM Premier disposable cartridge. Components are as follows: (1) Biosensor card. A 0.1-mL gastight chamber, 1*a*, houses the array of electrochemical sensors, 1*b*, that generate results in 92 s. (2) Calibration solutions. Flexible gas-impermeable bags with no dead space allow calibration, including p_{O_2} and p_{CO_2}, in different ambient conditions. (3) Reference solution. (4) Rinse solution. (5) Waste container. A one-way check valve between the pump and the waste container traps biohazards in the waste container. (6) Peristaltic pump. Blood samples are pumped to the biosensor card for analysis and then to the waste container. (7) Distribution valve. The valve selects calibrant, sample, or rinse solution for pumping through the biosensor card. (Courtesy of Mallinckrodt Sensor Systems.)

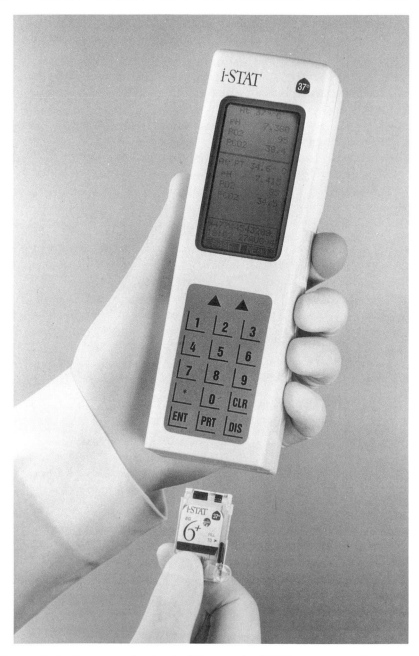

Figure 27.9. Illustration of a *handheld* format. The i-STAT system uses disposable cartridges. This single-use cartridge ($^{EG}6^+$) requires temperature regulation (37°C) for measurements of p_{O_2}, p_{CO_2}, and pH. It also includes measurements of electrolytes (Na$^+$, K$^+$) and hematocrit (Courtesy of i-STAT.)

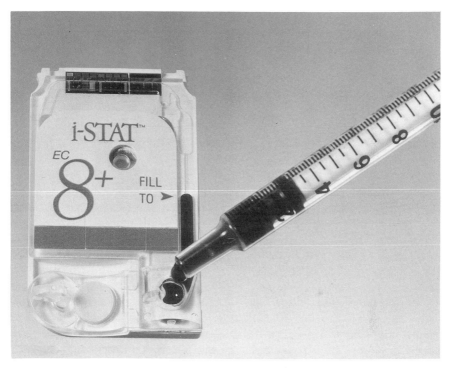

Figure 27.10. i-STAT sample application. Blood is applied to the sample well, enters the fluid channel, and then comes in contact with the biosensor chips (see Fig. 27.11). This cartridge ($^{EC}8+$) provides measurements of Na^+, K^+, Cl^-, pH, p_{CO_2}, urea nitrogen, glucose, and hematocrit. (Courtesy of i-STAT.)

(*a*)

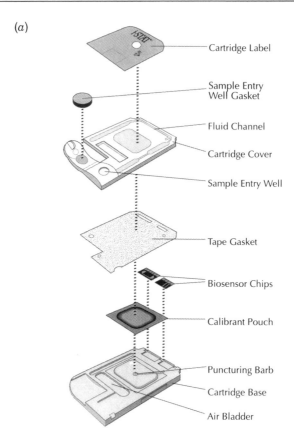

Cartridge Label

Sample Entry
Well Gasket

Fluid Channel

Cartridge Cover

Sample Entry Well

Tape Gasket

Biosensor Chips

Calibrant Pouch

Puncturing Barb

Cartridge Base

Air Bladder

Figure 27.11. i-STAT cartridge. (*a*) The schematic of the cartridge components and assembly. (*b*) A biosensor chip with a detailed enlargement of the microfabrication of the
urea sensor. (Courtesy of i-STAT.)

Figures 27.12–27.14 compare two different designs for portable instruments.
Both of these began commercially as portable blood gas instruments for use in
critical care settings. One is based on a single-use cartridge with self-contained
calibrants (Fig. 27.13). The other (Fig. 27.14) uses a disposable multisample
module and requires external calibration by the operator. These manufacturers
are adding electrolytes and metabolites to the test menus and therefore, improving versatility. Multisample instruments can use traditional quality control protocols. However, single–use cartridges and cassettes call for non–traditional quality control. Figure 27.15 is a photograph of a portable instrument that uses fiber
optics and the cassette shown in Figure 27.16. The trend toward miniaturization
is increasing the availability of these smaller modular instruments with inter-

(b)

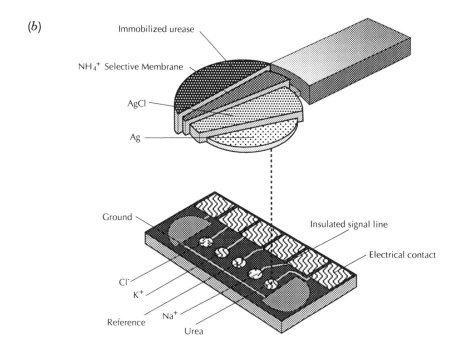

Figure 27.11. (*Continued*)

changeable cartridges. The nanofabrication of biosensors will enable the selection of multiple test menus and eventually, up to 30 or 40 tests on one instrument platform. Currently, the most common hand-held instrument is the glucose meter (Fig. 27.17), which is used by diabetics for self-monitoring of capillary blood glucose levels to help guide insulin therapy. This glucose meter uses an electrochemical biosensor strip (Fig. 27.18). The manufacturer currently is developing a glucose dehydrogenase method for glucose measurement that is not sensitive to oxygen tension and therefore can be used with other types of blood samples. As microfabrication hurdles are overcome and manufacturing costs decrease, more disposable sensors will appear for tiny digital instruments like this glucose meter.

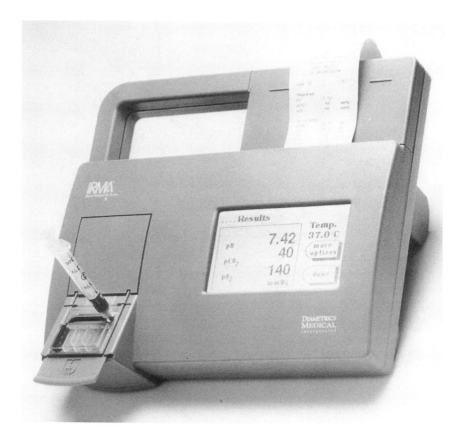

Figure 27.12. IRMA (Immediate Response Mobile Analysis) instrument. This portable whole-blood analyzer measures blood gases, pH, and other analytes. Features include an interactive touch-screen display, automatic measurement of barometric pressure, quality-assurance menu, data management, CLIA compatibility (moderate complexity), battery power (≤3 h), 37°C operation, and self-calibrating disposable cartridge (see Fig. 27.13). (Courtesy of Diametrics Medical.)

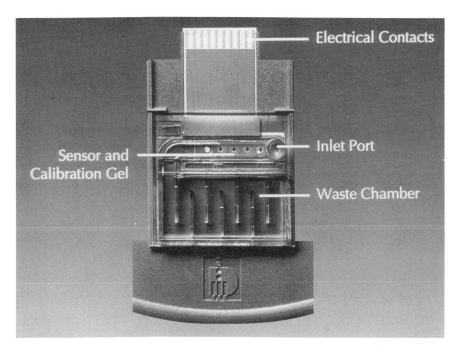

Figure 27.13. IRMA disposable single-use cartridge. The sensors, located to the left of the inlet port, include, from left to right, the reference electrode, pH, p_{CO_2}, K^+ (planned), and p_{O_2}. The blood sample (200 μL) displaces the calibration gel, flows over the sensors, and then is trapped in the waste chamber. Measurement ranges are as follows: pH, 6.80–7.80; p_{CO_2}, 4–200 mm Hg; and p_{O_2}, 20–700 mm Hg. Analytes planned for other cartridge configurations and their ranges are Ca^{2+}, 0.2–5.0 mmol/L; K^+, 1.0–20.0 mmol/L; Na^+, 80–200 mmol/L; and hematocrit, 10–80%. (Courtesy of Diametrics Medical.)

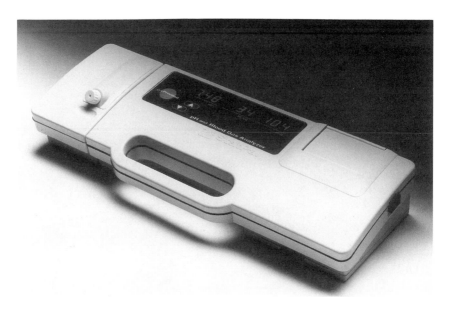

Figure 27.14. StatPal II blood gas analysis system. This portable instrument uses a disposable multi-use module (on the left) for 8, 15, or 30 samples and provides measurements of pH, p_{CO_2}, and p_{O_2}. User calibration is performed prior to each set of analyses. Measurement ranges are pH, 6.80–7.80; p_{CO_2}, 1–99 mm Hg; and p_{O_2}, 0–600 mm Hg. A novel portable model that includes electrolyte and hematocrit measurements with facsimile/modem and radiofrequency telecommunications will be introduced. (Courtesy of PPG Medical Sensors–UniFET/CIRRUS MEDICAL.)

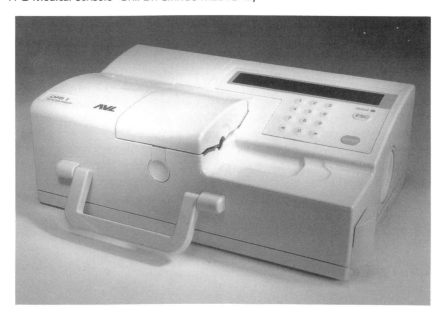

Figure 27.15. OPTI 1 blood gas analyzer. Features include optical fluorescence sensor technology, multilingual software, and a self-calibrating, self-contained cassette (illustrated in Fig. 27.16). The rechargeable battery pack lasts 6–8 h. The CLIA complexity level is moderate. (Courtesy of AVL Scientific.)

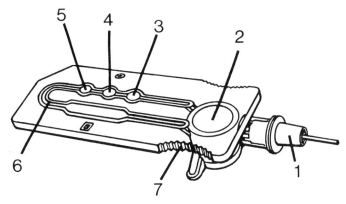

Figure 27.16. Drawing of the disposable cassette for the OPTI 1. The schematic shows the following: A syringe adapter (1). When removed, a capillary sample can be inserted into this port. Buffer storage (2). Optodes for p_{O_2} (3), p_{CO_2} (4), and pH (5). The sample flow path (6) and chamber. Grips (7) for insertion of the cassette into the OPTI 1 cradle that has light path couplings for the optical measurements. Sample volume is 80 μL. Analysis requires less than 2 min. Measurement ranges are p_{O_2}, 20–500 mm Hg; p_{CO_2}, 10–100 mm Hg; and pH, 6.90–7.70. (Courtesy of AVL Scientific.)

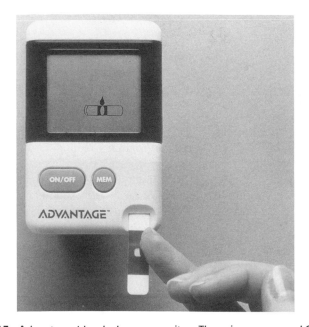

Figure 27.17. Advantage blood glucose monitor. The microprocessor LCD cues user steps. Here, it calls for a blood sample (13–50 μL), which is being applied to the electro-chemical sensor strip (see Fig. 27.18). The memory capacity is 100 glucose results with time and date of each. The monitor uses a plug-in code key for calibration information on sensor strips. Two-level quality control checks are provided. The power supply is two 3-V lithium coin cell batteries. (Courtesy of Boehringer Mannheim.)

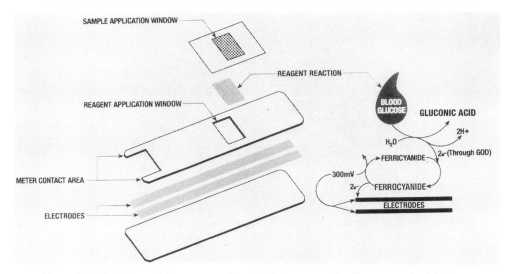

Figure 27.18. Glucose biosensor used on the Advantage. The diagram on the left shows the strip construction. The diagram on the right shows the reaction sequence and electrochemical principle. Glucose is measured electronically in whole blood by determining the current (e⁻) shuttled by ferrocyanide/ferricyanide when coupled with glucose oxidase-catalyzed oxidation of glucose to gluconic acid. The glucose measurement range is 20–600 mg/dL. (Courtesy of Boehringer Mannheim.)

27.4. *EX VIVO* AND *IN VIVO* MONITORING

27.4.1. Introduction and Definitions

It was not many years ago that blood pressure measurements and electrocardiograms were conducted on an intermittent basis. A nurse with a blood pressure cuff or a technician with an electrocardiogram machine would come to the patient's bedside at periodic intervals or on stat orders. Today, the majority of critical care patients are monitored continuously for these physiological observations for at least a portion of their hospital stay. The continuity of the measurements is considered medically indispensable. Blood chemistries, on the other hand, are virtually all still measured on an intermittent basis. Although point-of-care testing is a rapidly growing trend, most blood chemistry measurements are also still made at a location remote from the patient. Over the past 20 years there have been many efforts to develop monitoring systems to automate the measurement of various blood chemistry parameters, with relatively few commercial successes. We discuss next the reasons behind the effort to develop blood chemistry monitoring technology, the requirements for successful monitoring systems, current monitoring methods, and potential future directions.

Before proceeding, however, several definitions are necessary. Various terminology is used to describe invasive blood chemistry monitoring systems, including extracorporeal, paracorporeal, extravascular, extraarterial, intraarterial, subcutaneous, on-line, in-line, indwelling, *ex vivo,* and *in vivo.*[60,173,397,493,500,509] Indeed, even the term "monitor" has been used in varying ways and according to at least one author, excludes any device which permanently removes blood from the patient.[493] For the purposes of the following discussion, however, a monitor is defined as a system that is attached in some way to a patient and that provides information to the clinician regarding one or more analytes either continuously, intermittently, or on demand. The two major categories of invasive blood chemistry monitoring systems are (1) *ex vivo*—any automated or semiautomated monitor that involves invasive physical communication with the patient in some way and for which the sensors are located external to the body and (2) *in vivo*— any automated monitor for which the sensors themselves are physically located within the body. We will discuss noninvasive transcutaneous monitoring briefly here. Noninvasive monitoring is discussed in greater detail elsewhere (see Arnold[132]).

27.4.2. Potential Benefits of Monitoring

Blood chemistry monitoring offers a number of potential benefits over *in vitro* testing. Table 27.4 lists these benefits, several of which we discuss below.

27.4.2.1. IMMEDIATE INFORMATION ON PATIENT STATUS. Perhaps the greatest driving force for monitoring is the compelling need to provide immediate information on patient status. Major process steps in diagnostic testing include (1) test is ordered, (2) blood sample is drawn and labeled, (3) packaged sample is transported to the laboratory, (4) analyses are performed, (5) test results are communicated to the patient site, and (6) therapeutic decisions are

TABLE 27.4. Benefits of *Ex Vivo* and *In Vivo* Monitoring

Immediate, continuous, serial, or as-needed data instead of historical information
Detection of unexpected or rapid changes missed between *in vitro* measurements
Interrelationships of biochemical and physiological variables and phenomena
Data for closed-loop physiological control systems (e.g., oxygenation–ventilation[408])
Expanded clinical knowledge base and basic understanding of pathophysiology
Blood conservation, reduced iatrogenic transfusions, and decreased transfusion
    complications
Trend monitoring to anticipate change rather than react to out-of-control conditions
Elimination of *in vitro* sampling, preanalytical, and postanalytical errors
Decreased risk of transmission of bloodborne diseases to care team or other patients
Reduction in nosocomial infections due to contaminated sampling lines or
    venipuncture devices
Elimination of costs for additional *in vitro* measurements over the time period of
    monitoring
Cost reduction (direct, annual) through improved outcomes compared with current
    practice
Timely therapeutic intervention leading to improved clinical outcomes

made. With *in vitro* testing, the clinician receives historical information on the patient's condition when the information is minutes or even hours old. For example, Zaloga et al.[129] reported that the processing time for stat electrolytes in an intensive care unit at a teaching hospital was an average of 7 min for laboratory time (laboratory receipt to results generation), 90 min for testing time (test ordering to results receipt at the patient site), and 150 min for therapeutic time (test ordering to therapeutic decision). A 1992 national survey of 24 hospitals[100] revealed that the average time between sampling and receipt of results for stat blood gases was approximately 20 min, with a typical range of 5–60 minutes. In another recent study comparing turnaround time between a central laboratory and a point-of-care analyzer,[428] the turnaround time for the central laboratory averaged 30 min (range 10–123), while the turnaround time for the point-of-care analyzer averaged 18 min (range 8–89). The turnaround time for the point-of-care analyzer was longer than expected based on the instrument analysis time of approximately 1–2 min[421] and potential response time of only 5 min for whole-blood analyzers. Queuing and interruptions in a critical care unit may explain the delays. *Therapeutic turnaround time* (the time from test ordering to treatment[90–98,391,454]) frequently is prolonged because physicians leave the patient area before test results are received, become busy with other patients, or repeat tests because the delay in finding and reviewing results casts doubt on whether they still reflect current patient condition.[129,130] The therapeutic turnaround time clearly is an important performance indicator for the assessment or comparison of *in vitro, ex vivo,* and *in vivo* biosensor systems used to support critical care.

Monitoring compresses turnaround time into instrument analysis time, which generally does not exceed more than 1 or 2 min, and provides much more frequent information on blood chemistry status than is possible with conventional manual measurements. This immediate and frequent information is important in the detection of unexpected or rapid changes in biochemical variables when these changes occur during intervals between intermittent *in vitro* measurements. Immediate feedback from monitors also can lead to the rapid detection of problems with life-sustaining equipment, such as malfunctioning oxygenators, gas valves, or gas filters that otherwise might lead to compromised patient care. It has been proposed that this capability alone may lead to the adoption of monitoring as a standard of care with certain high-risk procedures such as cardiopulmonary bypass, spurred on by the likelihood of high-profile medical malpractice judgments in cases where monitoring might have prevented either complications or death.[484] Finally, because monitoring is generally automated, the availability of patient blood chemistry data is not dependent on a clinician's judgment as to when measurements are necessary. The data are immediately visible to the critical care nurse, who can initiate corrective measures. This paradigm fits the modern view of critical care as a collaborative process overseen by a performance team that continuously improves the quality of patient care and patient outcomes.[97]

27.4.2.2. DETECTION OF TRENDS. Monitoring provides a better basis for detecting trends and modifying therapy to maintain control, rather than correcting changes after patient variables have exceeded clinical targets. Trend monitoring can be accomplished with *in vitro* measurements, but practical limitations on the frequency of measurements can lead to misinterpretation of actual trends. For example, Figure 27.19 shows a 72-h glucose profile based on output from a monitor taking automatic measurements every 30 min.[251] Superimposed on this profile is a second profile based on a typical *in vitro* measurement frequency of four glucose tests per day. As can be seen from the two profiles, significantly different conclusions could be made regarding the percent of time the patient's blood glucose levels were within target control limits.

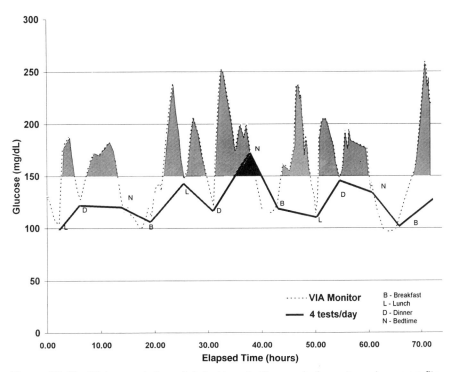

Figure 27.19. Misinterpretation of clinical trends. The graph shows two glucose profiles acquired during the same time period from a diabetic patient. The dashed line shows results generated every 30 min by the VIA *ex vivo* blood chemistry monitor. The solid line shows results from a typical *in vitro* testing protocol with one measurement before each meal and one at bedtime. Periods when the glucose results exceeded the patient's upper target control limit, 150 mg/dL, are shaded. Significantly different clinical conclusions could be drawn regarding both the time above the target control limit and the direction of change at the time of *in vitro* testing (Adapted from Ref. 251.)

27.4.2.3. MORE TIMELY THERAPEUTIC INTERVENTION.   Short response time, high frequency of information, and the ability to identify trends through automated monitoring may lead to more timely therapeutic intervention, with better clinical outcomes as a result. Although this assumption remains to be demonstrated with blood chemistry monitors due to their recent availability, clinical experiences with noninvasive *in vivo* transcutaneous monitoring[555–559,562,564,565,568–570] (Fig. 27.20) and pulse oximetry have provided some documentation in this area.

27.4.2.4. REDUCTION IN TESTING ERRORS.   Since monitoring is generally technique- and operator-independent, sample errors common to *in vitro* measurement are avoided. These include preanalytic errors such as sample contamination with ambient O_2 and CO_2, anticoagulants, or flush solutions, and sample degradation due to sample aging, storage conditions, mixups, and loss.[374,382]

27.4.2.5. DECREASED BLOOD HANDLING.   Blood handling, from drawing the sample at the patient bedside to placing it into the analyzer, is reduced or eliminated by monitoring. This issue has become increasingly important to hospitals in recent years because of the growing risks of human immunodeficiency virus, hepatitis, and other bloodborne diseases. Millions of dollars are being spent converting equipment and clinical practice to reduce these risks. The potential exposure to contaminated blood by needle sticks or various blood handling tasks is perhaps greatest for the clinician, but patients also can be at risk. In one study, 26 adult patients contracted acute hepatitis B infections via percutaneous transmission from a spring-loaded lancet device that was used to obtain fingerstick blood samples for the measurement of blood glucose.[545] The transmission of the virus was not due to reuse of lancet blades, but apparently caused by residual blood on the platform of the device following use on a patient who was a carrier of hepatitis B virus.

27.4.2.6. REDUCED BLOOD LOSS.   Many monitoring approaches eliminate the blood loss associated with blood chemistry measurements. One of the major causes of blood loss in hospitalized patients is sampling for laboratory testing,[525,526,530,551] which has been shown to be a significant and independent predictor of the decline in patient hemoglobin levels.[544] Critical care patients, who can least afford it, have larger volumes of blood drawn than patients who are stable,[546] a situation particularly true and disadvantageous for small or vulnerable patients. Blood loss due to laboratory tests is a well-documented cause of anemia in neonatal patients[524,531,542] and has been reported to be the single largest factor leading to anemia in premature infants.[524] Because the neonate's blood volume is so low, typically 80–110 mL/kg,[528] even small losses necessitate blood replacement. Typically, guidelines will trigger transfusions if the neonate's hematocrit drops below 35%, if accumulated blood loss equals 10 mL, or if 5–10% of the total blood volume is removed.[523,529,541] Since blood gas measurements are sometimes required as frequently as every 30 min,[554] and most blood gas analyzers require a minimum of 0.1–0.25 mL or more per sample,[421] these recommendations could result in frequent—even as often as daily—transfusions in some critically ill neonates. Blood loss from sampling for laboratory tests also can lead to increased transfusion requirements in adults. In one study, patients in the intensive care unit who had arterial lines had an average of 944 mL of blood withdrawn for laboratory tests.[551] The authors concluded that of 36 patients who received transfusions, the blood loss secondary to laboratory testing contributed to the need for transfusions in seventeen (46%).[551] Clearly, a blood chemistry monitor that could eliminate or reduce blood sampling for *in vitro* laboratory testing would be of profound benefit to certain groups of critically ill patients, independently of any additional value related to faster and more frequent results.

27.4.2.7. REDUCED LINE CONTAMINATION.   Another potential benefit from automated monitoring is a reduction in line contamination. Each time blood is drawn from an existing vascular access line for an *in vitro* sample, the integrity of that line is broken and there is a finite risk of infection. Several studies have reported significant levels of bacterial contamination of lines and sampling ports used for drawing blood samples.[522,527,548] Because monitoring reduces the need to draw blood samples, there may be a concomitant reduction in the risk of related nosocomial infections, including more virulent hospital-acquired organisms. Of course, the ideal way to manage this risk would be by performing noninvasive monitoring (see Arnold[132]).

27.4.2.8. COST-EFFECTIVENESS.   Cost-effectiveness is an issue of increasing importance when considering any new technology.[69–130] With published prices of single-patient use blood gas sensors in the range of $150–$300 each,[72] the costs of monitoring versus *in vitro* testing can raise significant questions. In some cases, monitoring may provide unambiguous cost savings over current practices. For certain diagnosis-related groups (DRGs) (e.g., liver transplant, neonatal respiratory distress syndrome, and tracheostomy), the average number of arterial blood gas tests can range from 30 to as high as 50 per stay.[86] With the reported direct costs for *in vitro* blood gas studies ranging $9–$19 per test,[100,115,120] monitoring clearly provides an economical alternative. Another example is the reduction in the need for transfusions that monitoring can provide, particularly in the case of neonates. A recent European study estimated that the true cost per transfusion in low-birth-weight infants, including average treatment cost for the complications due to transfusions, was $1203 (U.S. dollars).[538] Although the authors noted that materials costs and complication rates of transfusions can vary from center to center and from country to country, the costs of transfusions are so high that a monitoring system that reduces transfusion requirements in neonatal patients can be readily shown to be cost-effective.

For cases that are less clear, one can perform direct-cost analysis that compares current *in vitro* methods with monitoring and include items that contribute to the variable cost for each *in vitro* test, such as gloves, syringes, specimen

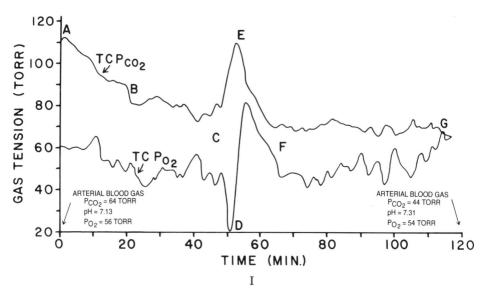

Figure 27.20. (*I*) The significance of *in vivo* monitoring. Continuous monitoring reveals clinically significant fluctuations that may be missed by *in vitro* testing. Transcutaneous (TC) p_{CO_2} monitoring assisted the management of respiratory acidosis (*A*) in a premature infant with respiratory distress syndrome.[564] The ventilator rate was adjusted to decrease TC p_{CO_2} (*B*). Then, it appeared safe to suction the patient (*C*). Suctioning resulted in a pronounced drop in TC p_{O_2} (*D*) and a rise in TC p_{CO_2} (*E*). Suctioning was discontinued (*F*), and the ventilator was adjusted to decrease p_{CO_2} and increase p_{O_2} (*F*). There was progressive reduction in TC p_{CO_2} with relief of the respiratory acidosis over the 2-h monitoring period. This case illustrates how *in vivo* monitoring facilitated temporal optimization.[97] At the end of the session (*G*), *in vitro* testing showed that arterial p_{CO_2} dropped to 44 mm Hg with a pH of 7.31, compared with values of 64 mm Hg and 7.13, respectively, at the start of monitoring. (Reproduced with permission of the *American Journal of Clinical Pathology,* Volume 80, page 835, 1983.) (*II–IV*) Discrimination interval analysis of noninvasive *in vivo* monitoring. (*II*) The discrimination band quantifies the reliability of inverse estimates of the independent variable obtained from values of the dependent variable and the calibration (regression) line relating the two. (*III*) For transcutaneous p_{CO_2} (dependent variable) and arterial p_{CO_2} (independent variable), the width of the discrimination interval (solid black lines) ranges from 10 to 50 torr (mm Hg), depending on the values of the statistical parameters, P and α. The dotted line gives the width of a single inverse estimate for $P = 0.95$. (*IV*) This is the least-squares calibration line for TC p_{CO_2} data from 70 neonatal intensive care unit infants with average gestational age of 30 (SD 3) weeks and average birth weight of 1383 (SD 609) g.[565] Inverse estimates are more reliable near the means (the "V"s) of the pairs of observations. The statistical bands are *A,* Working–Hotelling; *B,* standard error of estimate; *C,* single inverse estimate; and *D,* unlimited simultaneous discrimination, for $P = 0.95$ and $\alpha = 0.05$. For additional details, see Reference 389a. (Reproduced with permission from GJ Kost: Discrimination and other statistical intervals for the interpretation of *in vivo* patient monitoring data. *Statistics in Medicine* 5:347–354, 1986.)

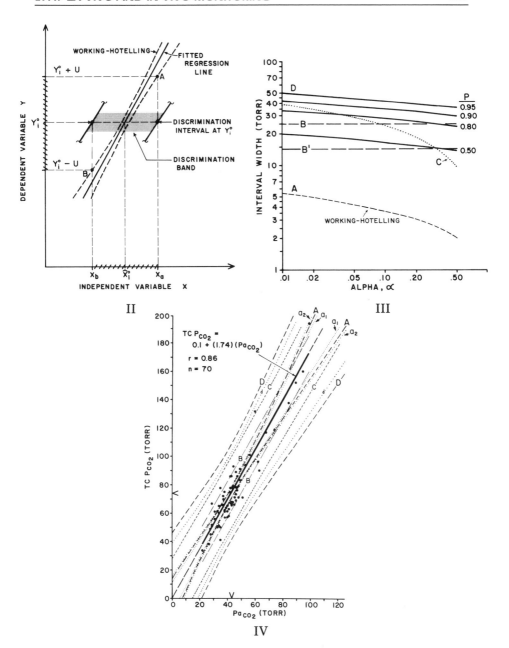

Figure 27.20. (*Continued*)

tubes, labels, *in vitro* sensors, and labor, to arrive at a direct cost per test. This then can be compared with the costs of monitoring per patient, all of which can be considered variable, since each monitor is dedicated to a single patient when in use, to arrive at a break-even point in numbers of tests. For clinical applications that involve more *in vitro* tests per stay than the break-even point, monitoring is clearly cost-effective and should be considered on the basis of cost alone. Because blood chemistry monitoring systems are a relatively new technology, this break-even point is likely to decrease over time as economies of scale reduce the cost of manufacturing sensors. Another factor that affects direct-cost analysis is the number of analytes measured by the monitor. If the monitor measures only p_{O_2}, for example, it may provide no direct-cost savings at all if *in vitro* p_{CO_2} and pH measurements are still obtained at the same frequency as before, since blood gas analyzers provide p_{O_2} as well as p_{CO_2} and pH. In general, the more analytes the monitor measures, the more *in vitro* tests it will displace, and the lower the break-even point is likely to be.

Direct-cost comparison, however, leaves out consideration of other potential cost savings that may occur by incorporating monitoring into the total (hybrid) laboratory program.[92–96] These include potential staff reductions, elimination of night shifts, reduction in maintenance and total capital costs, and transfer of costs between departments. These factors can be better accounted for in the assessment of annual costs[114,120] and the use of cost accounting methodologies for the assessment of true costs per test, such as those recommended by the National Committee for Clinical Laboratory Standards (NCCLS).[106] In addition, a recent study by the Canadian government separated all laboratory tests into two groups, one with tests that could affect immediate clinical decisions and one with tests that would not. One conclusion of the study was that the optimal cost strategy is to eliminate hospital-dedicated central laboratories, conduct all immediate tests at or near the point-of-care, and send all other diagnostic tests to regional laboratories.[99,112,124] Under such a scenario, the incorporation of monitoring into the point-of-care testing program conceivably could play a significant role in the overall laboratory cost reduction and the integrated economic success of the managed healthcare system.

27.4.2.9. CLINICAL OUTCOMES. The greatest potential cost savings from monitoring, however, does not come from direct comparison with *in vitro* testing, but rather from the possibility of improving clinical outcomes (Table 27.5). Since monitoring technologies are relatively new, most research studies to date have focused on comparing system performance to laboratory analyzers rather than on measuring clinical outcomes. Outcome studies, however, will be conducted much more frequently in the future as the incentives associated with healthcare reform stimulate the evaluation and reevaluation of all types of diagnostic procedures. Outcome parameters that may be positively impacted by monitoring include objective measurements such as hours spent on ventilation, hours in the intensive care unit, length of hospital stay, mortality rate, readmission rate, number of transfusions required, and the frequency and severity of

TABLE 27.5. Outcome Parameters Potentially Affected by Monitoring

Volume of tests performed in the conventional laboratory
Number and type of transfusions required
Titration of ventilator care and cardiopulmonary therapies
Time on ventilation or other life-support devices
Hours or days in the operating room or recovery unit
Length and costs of critical care or hospital stay
Frequency and severity of complications
Morbidity and mortality rates
Readmission and relapse rates
Subjective outcomes (QALY saved, HYE—see text)
Patient care quality indicators (e.g., frequency of surgical procedures and inpatient
   utilization)
Comparative data ("report cards") and competitive success in managed care

complications. In addition, the consideration of subjective outcomes in evaluating diagnostic technology, such as quality adjusted life years (QALYs) saved and healthy-year equivalents (HYE), has also been stressed.[127] A formal approach to outcomes optimization is described elsewhere.[97]

27.4.3. When Not to Monitor

There are also reasons why monitoring may not be the technology of choice (Table 27.6). If monitoring places the patient at higher risk for complications than *in vitro* testing, it will probably not make sense to monitor except under special circumstances. For example, a sensor system that requires an extracorporeal blood loop with the consequent need for systemic heparinization is unlikely to be used due to the associated risks except where such loops are implemented for other reasons, such as during cardiopulmonary bypass.[173] A patient undergoing bypass surgery where frequent blood gas measurements are necessary may justify use of a blood gas monitor, whereas a routine abdominal surgery case where a single blood gas measurement is considered adequate

TABLE 27.6. Reasons for Not Monitoring

Space constraints at the patient's bedside or elsewhere (e.g., emergency transport)
Problems with initiation (e.g., vascular access) or removal of vascular lines
Target analyte is stable and likely to remain so, or is not available with current
   biosensors
Excessive time lag in the sensor measurement cycle reduces clinical effectiveness
Possibility of data overload or of overtreatment
Higher risk for the patient with monitoring than with *in vitro* testing
Higher true cost than *in vitro* testing
No significant difference in outcomes between monitoring and *in vitro* testing

would not. Monitoring also is not necessary when the target analytes are stable and likely to remain so, or when infrequent testing is adequate.

Cases where monitoring is clearly more costly than *in vitro* testing also will impact the decision to use a monitor. As discussed earlier, this is complicated by determination of true costs and may be profoundly affected by differences in clinical outcomes. Continuous monitoring in some cases may also cause "data overload"[494] and reveal underlying variability in analyte levels that does not ultimately affect clinical outcomes, but may result in treatment modifications or additional procedures and their associated costs. In these cases, intermittent monitoring or *in vitro* testing may be the preferred approach. Finally, monitoring means another piece of equipment attached to the patient. In some cases space constraints may play a role in the decision regarding whether or not to monitor. Some blood gas monitors, for example, weigh close to 100 lb and would not be feasible to use in emergency transport vehicles or even some crowded operating rooms and intensive care units. Second- and third-generation monitoring systems that are smaller or integrated with other bedside systems are likely to render this consideration less important.

Blood chemistry monitoring is still in its infancy, and few systems are in clinical use. The potential benefits of monitoring are many, but its ultimate adoption as a standard tool in the arsenal of diagnostic medicine will depend on a number of factors. These are discussed in the next section.

27.4.4. Clinical Requirements for Monitoring Systems

Investigators have defined a number of requirements for blood chemistry monitoring systems.[397,471,493,500] Table 27.7 provides a summary of issues that should be considered in the development or evaluation of automated monitors for general clinical use.

27.4.4.1. REQUIREMENTS RELATED TO THE POTENTIAL BENEFITS OF MONITORING.
The most important requirements are those that relate to the potential benefits monitoring provides. For immediate information, rapid biosensor response time is essential. For example, some early blood gas sensors required many minutes to reach equilibrium with arterial blood, thereby compromising their potential utility. In general, the objective for monitor response time should be similar to the analysis time for *in vitro* analyzers, typically 1 or 2 min. To detect rapid or unexpected changes, generate meaningful trend information, and enable more timely therapeutic intervention, monitors should provide for frequent measurements. How frequent depends on the particular analytes being monitored and the specific clinical application. Perhaps ideally this should be continuous, but even systems that conduct only hourly automatic measurements could potentially provide clinicians with far more cost-effective and outcome-oriented data than is generally available from a main laboratory. The question to ask is not what is the ideal measurement frequency, but instead what measurement frequency is adequate to provide a cost-effective level of

TABLE 27.7. Clinical Requirements for an Automated Monitoring System

Requirements related to the potential benefits of monitoring
  Rapid response time—preferably within 1 or 2 min
  Capable of frequent serial or continuous measurements
  Little or no blood handling by the care team
  Little or no patient blood loss
  Closed system with no waste or removal of waste in an enclosed container
  Cost-effective, with greater benefits than risks to patient
Basic operating requirements
  Simple setup, operation, maintenance, and if needed, electronic calibration
  Small enough to transport easily and fit next to the patient's bed
  Battery power and memory backup, with a "low battery" alarm
  Fault detection and reporting capabilities
  Preferably automatic—no operator action required to generate measurements
  Clamps to an intravenous infusion pole or integrates with other bedside
    equipment
  Withstands the rigors of hospital use, including fluids, electrostatic discharge,
    electromagnetic interference, mechanical shock, and vibration
  Operated by respiratory technician, nurse, anesthesiologist, physician, or other
    professional
Information handling
  Visual display, ideally both numerical and graphical
  Ability to generate printed results report
  Alarms, alerts, advisories, algorithmic analyses, and programmability
  Ability to connect to patient data management systems or other external equipment
    via an RS-232 port
Quality of measurements
  Satisfactory accuracy, bias, and precision compared with laboratory analyzers
  Stability over desired period of use or else correctable through automatic
    calibration
  High specificity, not affected by potential interfering agents
  Nonthrombogenic and not affected by ambient conditions
  Operation and results unaffected by patient changes (blood flow, temperature, and
    hemodynamic fluctuations)
  Within the "limits of agreement" (Bland and Altman[375]) or reserved for trending
    only [329a]
  Performance consistent with peers or minimum standards established by
    multicenter studies

improvement in patient care. Recently, it has been suggested that even with blood gas monitors, the assumption that intermittent monitoring is less desirable than continuous monitoring may be incorrect, if the intermittent monitor is associated with lower costs and higher reliability.[494]

To reduce transmission of bloodborne diseases, monitors should involve no blood handling by the clinician, or at the very least, measurably less than with _in vitro_ sampling. To reduce the need for transfusions, little or no blood should be consumed in the measurement process. To meet these demands and to reduce the risks of nosocomial infections associated with sampling lines, monitors should be "closed" systems and either generate no waste or dispose of all biohazard waste in an enclosed container. Historically, the direction of many monitor development projects was set by asking clinicians what they would ideally want in a monitor, rather than what the minimum requirements might be. As a consequence, most commercial efforts have been directed at continuous *in vivo* monitoring, which has proven to be a difficult technical challenge (see 27.4.5., "Technical Challenges of Monitoring"). Finally, as discussed earlier, documentation of cost-effectiveness is required, and the benefits of monitoring clearly must outweigh the risks to the patient.

27.4.4.2. BASIC OPERATING REQUIREMENTS FOR MONITORS.

Monitoring systems also must meet basic operating requirements for bedside instrumentation (see Table 27.2 regarding *in vitro* devices). *Ex vivo* and *in vivo* systems must be simple to set up, operate, and maintain. If they cannot be quickly mastered by nurses, respiratory care practitioners, anesthesiologists, or other clinicians who will use them on a routine basis, they will not be implemented successfully. Although it is advisable that clinical laboratory personnel participate in the evaluation and management of patient-attached blood chemistry monitors, it is unlikely that laboratory technologists will play any greater role in the actual daily use of these systems than they do with pulse oximeters or bedside glucose meters. However, participation of clinical laboratory staff in quality assurance and proficiency testing would help ensure that monitoring systems produce diagnostic results that are consistent with *in vitro* test results obtained at the point of care or in the main laboratory.

Monitors should provide for automatic operation that preferably does not require operator action to generate measurements. For intermittent monitoring systems, the ability to acquire an on-demand measurement also is necessary. Systems should be small enough for easy transport and should fit easily at the patient bedside. This can be accomplished with a dedicated stand, a means of clamping to an existing intravenous infusion pole or to a cart, or through integration with other equipment like bedside cardiac monitors. Battery power with memory backup, and the ability to withstand the rigors of hospital use, including fluid spills, electrostatic discharge (ESD), electromagnetic interference (EMI), and the shock and vibration encountered by rolling across rough surfaces and bumping into walls, are also important requirements. Finally, fault detection and reporting capabilities must be an integral part of the system design, both to prevent the generation of erroneous measurements and to assist in troubleshooting and maintenance.

27.4.4.3. INFORMATION HANDLING.

Monitoring provides several opportunities to optimize knowledge of patient status. Blood chemistry observations are available faster and more frequently. With the abundant data generated by monitors, conventional charting no longer provides optimal methods for presenting or reviewing the information. In addition to numerical output, the real-time graphical display of biochemical variables provides significant information that is useful in assessing trends. Another opportunity to optimize knowledge of patient condition is automatic exception reporting. Range checks and other analyses can be conducted on data as acquired. Automatic alerts can be generated when clinical intervention is needed. Advisories can warn the care team not only when variables rise above or fall below a target range but also by means of more sophisticated algorithms, when the rate of change, duration of change, or a combination of changes signal certain physiological events. Finally, automated monitoring provides a means for integration of blood chemistry results with other patient-care databases. This could include local direct connection to bedside cardiac monitors or more general integration with institutionwide systems for patient outcomes management.[97] Real-time data in graphical format then would be available to physicians at system terminals throughout the hospital. All these features facilitate the temporal optimization of critical care.[97]

27.4.4.4. QUALITY OF MEASUREMENTS.   Monitoring presents challenges to the traditional methods employed with laboratory analyzers in both the assessment of accuracy and precision of measurements, as well as ongoing quality control and proficiency testing. This has been recognized implicitly by the specific exclusion of blood chemistry monitors from regulation by the Clinical Laboratory Improvement Admendments (CLIA) of 1988: "Until definitional and technical issues have been resolved, *in vivo* and externally attached patient dedicated monitoring is not subject to CLIA. Should it be determined at a later date that it is subject to CLIA, proper notice and opportunity for public comment will be provided."[379] Although this exclusion potentially simplifies some issues in the adoption and management of monitoring systems within a hospital, the tasks of assessing performance, providing continuous quality improvement, and reconciling some types of monitoring data with physiological variables remain.

The first step in assessing performance is the determination of how well results obtained with the monitoring system agree with those obtained with conventional technology, preferably a gold standard if available. This comparison is necessary to demonstrate that the monitor provides output adequate enough in quality and consistency to replace *in vitro* testing. In principle, this is accomplished by determining the accuracy and precision of the monitor's measurements against known standards and comparing the performance with conventional laboratory analyzers. Bias represents the average difference between the values measured by the monitor and the "true" values. In terms of the same paired difference data, precision is the standard deviation of the differences. Precision reflects the consistency or reproducibility of the measurements. Correlation coefficients and regression analysis also are used to compare two methods of clinical measurement, but relying solely on these measures may be misleading or even inappropriate,[375,392] depending on the application and type of regression analysis (e.g., linear least-squares regression versus Deming regression[390a]).

Assessing performance in the clinical setting often is complicated by a lack of knowledge of the "true" value of the analyte being measured. With *in vitro* blood gases and pH, for example, the clinical accuracy and reproducibility of laboratory analyzers cannot be quantified precisely.[115] Differences in performance between different commercial analyzers, preanalytic errors with *in vitro* measurements, variability of blood gas values over short periods of time in stable patients,[399,401] and problems associated with the precise timing of comparison samples all add to the difficulty of assessing agreement. Noninvasive monitoring introduces even greater uncertainty. For example, heating, skin thickness, vascularity, and other factors fundamentally affect the values generated by noninvasive transcutaneous monitors. If a calibration (regression) line comparing the *in vivo* and *in vitro* observations is available, discrimination interval analysis can help one select either inverse estimation, if the inverse estimates are highly accurate, or trend following, if the inverse estimates are not highly accurate (Figs. 27.20B–D).[389a] Discrimination intervals for the indirect variable, transcutaneous p_{CO_2} (TC p_{CO_2}), which represents a complex transformation of intravascular p_{CO_2}, show that the primary value of TC p_{CO_2} lies not in providing accurate inverse estimates of arterial p_{CO_2}, but instead, in tracking short-term clinical trends. Therefore, this type of statistical analysis can facilitate the objective assessment of the reliability of *in vivo* monitoring data, as well as interpretation and clinical use.

The method proposed by Bland and Altman[375] is increasingly becoming a standard methodology for assessing agreement between monitors and laboratory analyzers. For a blood chemistry monitor, this approach involves the following steps: (1) decide on an acceptable level of agreement between monitoring and *in vitro* testing that will support the conclusion that for the desired application, monitoring can replace *in vitro* testing; (2) obtain a large series of simultaneous paired measurements covering the physiologic range of the target analytes; (3) plot the average of the two measurement techniques versus the difference in the measurements; and (4) add lines representing the mean difference and plus or minus two standard deviations on either side of the mean difference. Figure 27.21 shows a diagram of a Bland–Altman-style analysis. The mean difference ±2 standard deviations is termed the "limits of agreement." Assuming that the differences in the measurements are normally distributed, 95% of the data points will lie within this range. If the limits of agreement fall within the acceptable level of agreement, then the monitor could, according to this method, be judged an acceptable replacement for *in vitro* testing. Additional analyses also can be performed to assess the precision of estimated limits of agreement, systematic bias, and repeatability.[375]

What are acceptable levels of agreement? One approach is to use the standards published by the College of American Pathologists (CAP) and the Health Care Financing Administration (HCFA). These organizations have established proficiency testing programs to assure that the performance of an individual laboratory matches that of peer groups. Target values are established by determining the mean results for samples analyzed by all laboratories. Table 27.8

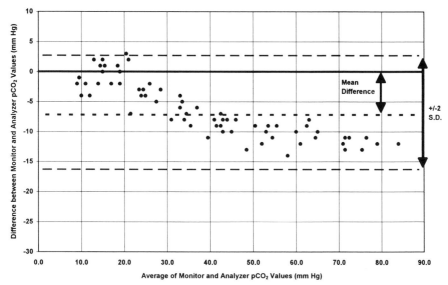

Figure 27.21. Bland–Altman method for assessing agreement between an *ex vivo* monitor (*m*) and an *in vitro* analyzer (*a*). Paired observations (m_i, a_i), consisting of p_{CO_2} from an *ex vivo* monitor and p_{CO_2} from an *in vitro* analyzer, are plotted as a single point where the *x* value is the average [$(m_i + a_i)/2$], and the *y* value is the difference ($m_i - a_i$). If all points fell on the horizontal line, $y = 0$, there would be no difference (bias) between the monitor and analyzer. In this example, the mean difference is −7 mm Hg, and the limits of agreement are +3 mm Hg and −16 mm Hg (±2 standard deviations). The plot also shows that as p_{CO_2} increases, the *ex vivo* monitor reports lower values relative to the analyzer and that the bias is nonlinear.

shows an example of the HCFA standards for pH, p_{CO_2} and p_{O_2}.[380] These values apply only to a group of comparable laboratory analyzers. For blood gas monitors, it is suggested that the minimum acceptable level of performance should be the bias and precision at least equivalent to that clearly demonstrated in a prospective multicenter study.[115] For other types of blood chemistry monitors, the desired agreement with laboratory analyzers will vary with the analyte being measured and the intended application. For example, ambulatory glucose monitors generate trend information that is more important than absolute agreement with laboratory analyzer values. The goals are to allow the patient to maintain their own glucose levels within a fairly wide target range and to provide an alert if they rise above or fall below that range. For this application, meeting the HCFA standard of ±10% of the peer group target glucose values across the full measurement range of the monitor may not be necessary to fulfill the clinical goals.[361]

Monitoring also presents several quality control challenges. Current quality-control methods for *in vitro* testing are designed to detect persistent errors found with batch analyzers, versus the singular or random failure events of

TABLE 27.8. Healthcare Financing Administration Proficiency Testing Standards for Blood Gases and pH[a]

Analyte	Criteria for Acceptable Performance
p_{O_2}	Target value ±3 standard deviations
p_{CO_2}	Target value ±5 mm Hg or $\pm8\%$ (whichever is greater)
pH	Target value ±0.04

[a]*Notes*

1. Satisfactory performance requires that a minimum of 80% of the results for each analyte in each testing event are within the specified limits.
2. For p_{O_2}, a given result must be within three standard deviations of the target value as established by the mean and standard deviation from referee laboratories testing common samples.
3. From the Clinical Laboratory Improvement Amendments of 1988.[379,380]

disposable sensors for which size of the population under review is only one. This is further complicated by the need to maintain sensor sterility with most monitoring systems. For example, it does not make sense to waste a $300 disposable *in vivo* blood gas sensor by testing it with three levels of conventional control solutions in the laboratory. Not only is this costly since the sensor is rendered nonsterile in the process and therefore cannot be used on a patient, but it provides essentially no information on the performance of the sensor that actually will be used. To address this issue, some monitoring systems provide a means of checking the performance of the electronics and software at several signal levels through use of a custom test fixture. Testing can be scheduled at periodic intervals to assure that the system, exclusive of the sensor, is performing within specifications. In addition, monitors typically conduct a number of quality checks on the sensors themselves during initial calibration and use.

Automatic recalibration during use also can improve the quality of measurements. However, a significant issue remains—if the performance of a sensor changes during use in a way that cannot be detected by software or hardware checks, the only way to know for certain is to verify its output against a simultaneous *in vitro* measurement or to measure controls. As discussed earlier, *in vitro* measurements have their own sources of error, so comparisons must be conducted carefully to avoid incorrect conclusions regarding monitor performance. Use of controls requires either (1) sterile, nontoxic, and nonpyrogenic control solutions with a provision in the monitor's design that allows taking the sensor off line during use for aseptic testing or (2) a system design that does not require sensor sterility (e.g., an *ex vivo* monitor where the blood sample is not returned to the patient). How often it will be necessary to verify the performance of a monitor during use will depend on historical reliability and manufacturer recommendations. Besides results from multicenter studies and institutional quality control records of simultaneous measurements obtained with reference analyzers during use, an additional method for assessing historical performance is to conduct a post-use audit on a percentage of sensors with *in vitro* controls.

27.4.5. Technical Challenges of Monitoring

There are many applications for which blood chemistry monitoring is of potential clinical value, yet despite years of effort, there are very few commercial systems available.[76] The primary reason for this lies in the numerous technical challenges (Table 27.9) to the development of sensor systems that meet the clinical requirements discussed earlier.

27.4.5.1. COMPATIBILITY WITH BLOOD AND OTHER BODY FLUIDS.

Compatibility of sensor surfaces with blood or other body fluids has been one of the most difficult challenges, particularly with *in vivo* sensors. Exposure to blood or extracellular fluid may result in the buildup of biological deposits on sensor surfaces and interference with the performance of the sensor membranes.[438] For example, deposits of protein have been thought to directly alter local pH, thus affecting the accuracy of both pH and p_{CO_2} measurements.[191] More recently, thrombus formation is believed to play a more significant role in affecting *in vivo* performance of blood gas and pH sensors.[471] Protein adsorption to the sensor is followed by the adherence of activated platelets, the formation of fibrin and ultimately, the deposition of a thrombus layer containing respiring blood cells over the entire sensor surface. This metabolically active layer changes the local environment around the sensor, causing it to report decreasing p_{O_2}, increasing p_{CO_2}, and decreasing pH over time relative to comparative *in vitro* measurements. This creates the "down–up–down" pattern,

---

TABLE 27.9. Major Technical Challenges—Automated Biochemical Monitoring

Microfabrication, reproducibility of sensor manufacturing, and practical shelflife

Size constraint by the inner diameter of the artery (or other vessel) with *in vivo* sensors

Impact of sterilization processes on sensor materials and performance

Biocompatability with blood and other body fluids

Avoidance of inflammatory response and fibrous encapsulation

Insignificant permeability to biofluids *in vivo* with minimum error from physical changes

Suitable for patients of different age and physical size (e.g., prematures, infants, and adults)

Not affected by changes in patient milieu (e.g., hyperlipidemia, hyperproteinemia, or hyperviscosity)

Local site problems (wall effect, positional lines, flush solution mixing with blood, flow-by, blood pressure waveform, vasospasm, pooling, hematoma, thrombosis, embolus, perforation, and infection)

Electrical noise, interference, and drift with electrochemical sensors

Calibration and stability of accuracy over time (e.g., 72 h) or between *in vivo* calibrations

Consistent and fast response time (i.e., short lag) for measurements *in vivo*

Manufacturing cost of disposable sensors for single patient use *in vivo* or *ex vivo*

referred to as the "DUD" effect.[444] Efforts to address this issue have included changing the sensor shape, modifying the chemical and physical surface properties of sensor materials, and using antithrombogenic coatings such as covalently bonded heparin or albumin.[438,471,521] Recent reports indicate that the blood compatibility problem may have been addressed with a recently introduced *in vivo* blood gas monitor.[405,509,510] However, variability in the thrombogenic response of individual patients to a foreign body means that local perturbations may still represent potential sources of error in clinical interpretation.

27.4.5.2. ACCESS SITE PROBLEMS.   Another major issue that affects the performance of invasive monitors is access site problems. These also can change the local environment around *in vivo* sensors or in the case of *ex vivo* systems, the local conditions where the sample is being withdrawn. One of the more frequently reported examples of this is the "wall effect" associated with *in vivo* blood gas and pH sensors.[465] In this case, the sensor surface is unintentionally pressed up against the wall of the artery and measures the pH, p_{CO_2}, and p_{O_2} at the surface of the endothelial cells instead of the blood. Efforts to address this issue have included modification of the sensor shape and the location of the sensor surfaces to minimize contact with the vessel wall, and flexibility in allowing the sensor to be rotated for optimal positioning within the artery.[521] Other site problems are those typically encountered with intravascular or subcutaneous infusion systems, including positional lines, vasopasm, vessel perforation, infiltration, local hematoma, and infection. These can cause changes in the ambient conditions at the access site, such as pooling of blood, mixing of blood and flush solutions, or changes related to bacterial metabolism. Although severe problems have been reported infrequently, close attention to site management and hygiene clearly are important for both *in vivo* and *ex vivo* monitoring systems. Site problems should be considered with any suspect readings.

27.4.5.3. CALIBRATION AND ACCURACY OVER TIME.   Long-term calibration stability (> 72 h) has been another major technical obstacle. Most monitoring systems currently involve an initial two-point calibration prior to attachment to the patient. As discussed earlier, electrochemical sensors are prone to drift over time. Although fiber optic and fiber optic chemical sensors are theoretically more stable, without periodic recalibration or verification of accuracy, there is no way to be certain that drift has not occurred or that erroneous measurements are not being reported. As a result, both *ex vivo* and *in vivo* systems involve some type of periodic recalibration. Although ideally this should be a two-point recalibration, most commercial systems provide for only one-point recalibrations. One-point calibrations can correct for either a change in sensor offset or change in slope, but not both. This implies an additional design constraint, in that the component of sensor output that is not being recalibrated, either offset or slope, must be stable enough to maintain accurate measurements for the duration of sensor use.

For some *ex vivo* systems, it is possible to use external or infusible solutions for recalibration, analogous to calibration methods employed with *in vitro* analyzers. In this way, recalibration can be conducted automatically. With current *in vivo* monitor designs, however, the only feasible approach is manual *in vivo* recalibration. This indirect method involves drawing a blood sample, measuring analytes with a conventional *in vitro* analyzer, and entering the time and values into the *in vivo* monitor. The monitor then automatically adjusts the reporting of subsequent measurements based on any differences between calculated values and the *in vivo* recalibration. If the frequency of *in vivo* recalibrations, which require operator labor and an *in vitro* analyzer, are too high, this can offset the benefits of using a monitor. Potentially more serious, however, is that if the *in vitro* measurement used to conduct the *in vivo* recalibration has significant error itself, this error may be propagated throughout the subsequent *in vivo* measurements until the next recalibration. In addition, if the differences between the sensor output and the *in vitro* measurement are due to local site conditions around the sensor and not actual sensor drift, *in vivo* recalibration may correct for apparent sensor error at the current analyte levels, but introduce additional error if the analyte levels subsequently change.

27.4.5.4. NOISE. With electrochemical sensors, discrimination of the sensor signals from electrical noise is another significant challenge. With *in vivo* systems and with *ex vivo* systems where the sensors are in a tube set connected directly to the patient, electrical noise from wiring, other bedside equipment, and the patient can all interfere with the low amplitude signals coming from the sensors. In such systems, electrical isolation generally is not possible or practical, so some effective means of noise reduction or signal discrimination must be designed into the monitor's electronics.

27.4.5.5. SENSOR SIZE. Sensor size has been another technical hurdle, primarily in the development of *in vivo* sensors. With intravascular blood gas and pH sensors, for example, the sensor probe must typically fit through a 20-gauge radial artery catheter, allow withdrawal of blood samples and infusion of flush solution, and not adversely affect signal fidelity from the continuous arterial pressure monitor. Since it is desirable to have the pH, p_{CO_2}, and p_{O_2} sensors in a single sensor unit, this requires three chemical sensors, three to six or more optic fibers or wires, a thermocouple for temperature correction, and a smooth external nonthrombogenic surface layer, all included in a probe having an outer diameter of <0.55 mm.[471] Adding additional sensors such as potassium or sodium to the same probe presents an even greater difficulty. For special applications, such as *in vivo* subcutaneous glucose sensors, the sensor must be small enough to allow easy insertion through the skin. For bioactive probes, the biosensor and conduit also must be cleverly configured as part of the endoscope, thin-needle biopsy, or other medical apparatus.

27.4.5.6. STERILIZATION. Sterilization has been a major obstacle to the development of *in vivo* monitoring systems and those *ex vivo* systems that return

TABLE 27.10. Invasive Blood Chemistry Monitors Currently Available and Under Development

Company	Model	Monitor Type	Status	Measurements
Abbott Critical Care Systems Mountain View, CA	Oximetrix/Opticath	*In vivo* Vascular	Commercial	O_2 Saturation
AVL Medical Instruments, AG Graz, Austria	G-Box and GI-Box	*Ex vivo* Open Perfusion	Development	Glucose
Baxter Edwards Critical-Care Irvine, CA	Vigilance/CCOmbo (SAT-2)	*In vivo* Vascular	Commercial	O_2 Saturation
CDI-3M Health Care Irvine, CA	CDI 300, 400	*Ex vivo* Flow Through	Commercial	pH, p_{CO_2}, p_{O_2}
	CDI 2000	*Ex vivo* Withdraw/Reinfuse	Development (on hold)	pH, p_{CO_2}, p_{O_2}
Institute for Diabetes Technology Ulm, Germany	Glucosensor Unitec Ulm	*Ex vivo* Withdraw/Discard	Commercial	Glucose
LightSense Laguna Hills, CA	(undetermined)	*In vivo* Vascular	Development	pH, p_{CO_2}, p_{O_2}
Mallinckrodt Sensor Systems, Inc. Ann Arbor, MI	GEM 6 Plus	*Ex vivo* Withdraw/Discard	Commercial	pH, p_{CO_2}, p_{O_2}, K^+, Ca^{2+}, Hct,
MiniMed Technologies Sylmar, CA	(undetermined)	*In vivo* Subcutaneous	Development	Glucose
Optex Biomedical, Inc. The Woodlands, TX	BioSentry	*In vivo* Vascular	Discontinued	pH, p_{CO_2}, p_{O_2}
Optical Sensors, Inc. Minneapolis, MN	SensiCath	*Ex vivo* Withdraw/Reinfuse	Development	pH, p_{CO_2}, p_{O_2}
Pfizer Biomedical Sensors Malvern, PA	Paratrend 7	*In vivo* Vascular	Commercial	pH, p_{CO_2}, p_{O_2}
Sintong Chemical Industries, Ltd. Taoyuan, Taiwan	Track-Bio	*Ex vivo* Withdraw/Discard	Development	UN
	Track-Ely	*Ex vivo* Withdraw/Discard	Development	K^+, Na^+, Ca^{2+}, Cl^-
UniFET Corporation La Jolla, CA	(undetermined)	*Ex vivo* Withdraw/Discard	Discontinued	UN, pH
VIA Medical San Diego, CA	VIA 1-01 (adult, neonatal, and glucose versions)	*Ex vivo* Withdraw/Reinfuse	Development	pH, p_{CO_2}, p_{O_2}, Na^+, K^+, Ca^{2+}, Hct, Glucose

Footnotes:
1. References 410, 411, 436, 448, 481, 486, & 515
2. References 414, 445, 466, & 502.
3. References 435, 463, 479, & 491.

Sensor Technology	Measurement Cycle Time	Initial *In Vitro* Calibration	Calibration During Use	Display	Printer	RS-232 Port	References
Fiber Optic	Continuous	1-point	In vivo (paired *in vitro* sample)	Num/Graph	Y	Y	Note 1
Electrochem. (enzyme)	Continuous	2-point	2-point	Num	N	N	282, 338
Fiber Optic	Continuous	1-point	In vivo (paired *in vitro* sample)	Num/Graph	Y	Y	410, 515
FibOp. Chem.	Continuous	2-point	In vivo (paired *in vitro* sample)	Num	Y	Y	Note 2
FibOp. Chem	3 min	2-point	In vivo (paired *in vitro* sample)	Num	Y	Y	Note 3
Electrochem. (enzyme)	Continuous	2-point	In vivo (paired *in vitro* sample)	Num	N	Y	234
FibOp. Chem	Continuous	2-point	In vivo (paired *in vitro* sample)	Num/Graph	Y	Y	None Listed
Electrochem.	6 min	2-point	2-point	Num	Y	Y	413, 478, 482
Electrochem. (enzyme)	Continuous	(undetermined)	In vivo (paired *in vitro* sample)	Num	N	Y	None Listed
FibOp. Chem.	Continuous	2-point	In vivo (paired *in vitro* sample)	Num/Graph	Y	Y	496, 498, 521
FibOp. Chem.	3 min	2-point	In vivo (paired *in vitro* sample)	Num/Graph	Y	Y	None Listed
FibOp. Chem / Electrochem.	Continuous	3-point / 2-point	In vivo (paired *in vitro* sample)	Num/Graph	Y	Y	405, 509, 510
Electrochem.	5 min	2-point	2-point	Num	Y	?	None listed
Electrochem.	5 min	2-point	2-point	Num	Y	?	None listed
Electrochem.	5 min	2-point	2-point	Num	Y	Y	None listed
Electrochem. / Electrochem. (enzyme)	5–10 min	2-point	1-point	Num	Y	Y	251, 499, 500, 516

blood to the patient. Heat, gamma radiation, and ethylene oxide gas, the traditional techniques for sterilization of medical devices, all can adversely affect the integrity, material properties, and consequent performance of chemical sensors.[438] *In vitro* systems typically do not require sensor sterilization. Hence, sterilization is a new constraint for monitoring systems, and one which has entailed major design effort.

27.4.5.7. COST.   Finally, manufacturing cost is an important consideration in the commercialization of both *in vivo* and *ex vivo* monitoring systems. Unlike many *in vitro* systems, where electrochemical or optical sensors can last for days or months and be used with many different patients, virtually all monitoring systems developed to date involve disposable sensors for single-patient use. The challenge of cost-effective initial sensor design and continued cost reduction over time is one that will remain an overriding factor for all commercial monitoring systems.

27.4.5.8. THE ONGOING CHALLENGE.   Given the magnitude of the technical challenges in the development of invasive blood chemistry monitoring systems, it is not surprising that there have been many unsuccessful attempts to produce commercial products. During the past 5 years several companies canceled their monitoring development projects. The majority were for *in vivo* blood gas or glucose systems. These companies include Abbott Laboratories, CR Bard, Baxter International, Becton Dickinson, BOC Group, Eli Lilly & Co., Medtronic Inc., Nellcor, Optex, Otto Sensors, Puritan-Bennett, Siemens, and Viggo Spectramed—a virtual "who's who" of the largest medical device companies in the world.[72,76] Most of the projects were canceled because of one or more of the technical challenges discussed above. For example, high initial sensor costs, limited early market acceptance (due to lack of cost-effectiveness studies), and compliance problems with the Food and Drug Administration played a role in hastening the exit of Puritan-Bennett, the first company to commercialize an *in vivo* blood gas monitor and the first to discontinue production.[76] Others, including 3M/CDI and Optical Sensors, Inc., have switched their development focus from *in vivo* to *ex vivo* systems. Despite the difficulties, however, several commercial products were introduced and are currently available, and a number are still under development. Table 27.10 provides a summary of the features and operating characteristics of current monitoring systems. The far-right column lists references where investigators have studied the systems. *Ex vivo* and *in vivo* monitors are reviewed briefly in the following sections.

27.5. SURVEY OF *EX VIVO* MONITORING SYSTEMS

27.5.1. Design Philosophy and Rationale

To some degree *ex vivo* monitors all isolate their sensors from the body. There are several reasons why this has been important in the development of monitoring systems (Table 27.11). For example, it allows much better control of the interface between the sensor and the body fluid being measured. If necessary, sample temperature can be regulated directly, rather than measured and compensated for by temperature correction algorithms.[169a] Duration and frequency of sensor surface exposure to blood or other body fluids can be controlled. Post-measurement flushing of the sensors is possible with some approaches, thereby reducing the likelihood of changes in sensor performance over time due to the buildup of proteins, blood clots, or living cells. There also are no rigorous limitations on sensor size as are imposed on *in vivo* probes. With external sensors it is possible to devise methodologies for automatic one- and two-point recalibrations to either validate or correct for changes in sensor performance during monitoring. Several different approaches to *ex vivo* monitoring have been developed and reported in the literature, including (1) withdrawal, measurement, and disposal of blood; (2) placement of sensors directly in an extracorporeal loop; (3) withdrawal, measurement, and reinfusion of blood; (4) microdialysis of extracellular fluid and measurement of the dialysate; and (5) open-tissue perfusion with measurement of the incompletely equilibrated perfusate. Each of these approaches is discussed below.

27.5.2. Withdrawal, Measurement, and Disposal of Blood

This method can be accomplished by withdrawing blood directly from a vascular access device or from an extracorporeal loop through which blood is flowing (e.g., a heart–lung machine). Blood can be withdrawn continuously, passed over the sensors, and pumped to a waste reservoir. Alternately, blood can be withdrawn in discrete samples, held over the sensors long enough for analysis, and then pumped to a waste reservoir. There are several advantages to withdrawing, measuring, and disposing of blood or dialysate when designing an automated monitor. A key element is that the sensors can be directly recalibrated at periodic intervals during use, either manually or automatically. This can be accomplished by interrupting measurements to pass solutions over the sensors for either one- or two-point calibration, or for other quality control checks. The calibration solutions can be relatively unrestricted, as they are not infused into the patient. In addition, the sensors need not be sterile. This eliminates a significant technical challenge and makes it possible to design systems that use the same sensors on successive patients. The major disadvantage of this method is

---

TABLE 27.11. Technical Advantages of *Ex Vivo* Monitoring

Relaxed constraints on sensor sizes, shapes, and designs
Temperature control rather than temperature correction
Better control of interface between sensor and blood or intravenous fluids
Fewer compatibility requirements of sensor surfaces for body fluids, particularly blood
Direct recalibration of external sensors and flexible calibration protocols
Design flexibility to interface with other technologies for combined or simultaneous
  operation

that the blood withdrawn for measurement is permanently lost from the patient or from the extracorporeal circulation system.

One of the first commercial automated blood chemistry monitoring systems, the Biostator (Miles Laboratories, Elkhart, IN), was an *ex vivo* monitor that used the continuous withdrawal, measurement, and disposal approach (Fig. 27.22). It was introduced in the late 1970s for continuous measurement of blood glucose. One configuration was capable of controlling glucose and insulin infusions to automatically regulate the patient's blood glucose level—a true closed-loop control system.[229] The Biostator used a custom dual-lumen intravenous catheter to withdraw venous blood continuously at 2 mL/h. The outer lumen was used to mix a heparin solution with the blood sample to prevent clotting as blood was drawn through the inner lumen to the analyzer, and to dilute the sample to 10 : 1. The sensor was a conventional glucose oxidase-based amperometric cell. The system incorporated a means of automatically performing one- and two-point calibrations on a periodic basis to maintain accuracy. Although the Biostator has been used extensively in research applications,[313] it did not adequately meet several of the key clinical requirements, including size, ease of use, and cost. It weighed close to 100 lb, required a full-time technician to operate, frequently had problems with clotting and occluded lines, and in 1979 cost between $45,000 and $60,000, depending on the configuration. A remarkable advance for its time, the Biostator unfortunately was not a commercial success and did not receive widespread acceptance in general clinical practice. Production stopped in the 1980s with approximately 500 systems in use. It did, however, make possible significant advances in the understanding of diabetes and the regulation of glucose levels.[313] There have been other development efforts to produce continuous withdrawal systems similar to the Biostator (e.g., by the Institute for Diabetes Technology, Ulm, Germany; Gambro Analysis Systems Division, Lund, Sweden; Esaote Biomedica, Toscana, Italy; and Nikkiso Co. Ltd, Tokyo, Japan). As of this date, only the Institute for Diabetes Technology's instrument is in limited clinical use.[234]

A commercial monitor based on withdrawal of discrete blood samples, measurement, and disposal of the blood is the GEM-6 Plus (Mallinckrodt Sensor Systems, Inc., Ann Arbor, MI). It is used as a monitor on the extracorporeal circuit during cardiopulmonary bypass and as an *in vitro* analyzer at other times. While attached to the extracorporeal circuit, the GEM-6 Plus can measure pH, p_{CO_2}, p_{O_2}, potassium, ionized calcium, and hematocrit on both the arterial and venous lines. Sampling can be performed either automatically as often as six arterial/venous pairs or 10 single arterial and/or venous samples per hour, or on demand by the press of a key. The 2-mL blood sample is drawn into the monitor through a one-way line, analyzed, and then flushed with a rinse solution into a waste reservoir in the disposable sensor cartridge. Results are available approximately 2.5 min after initiation of a measurement cycle (5 min for an arterial/venous pair) and are displayed numerically and printed with the monitor's integrated printer. The disposable cartridge contains conventional electrochemical sensors and all the calibration solution required for 50 samples or up

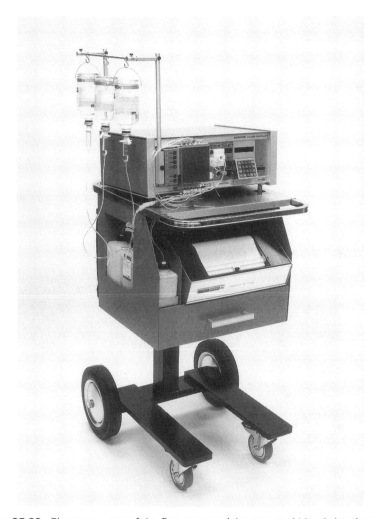

Figure 27.22. Biostator—one of the first commercial automated blood chemistry moni-tors. This transportable unit measured blood glucose by continuously withdrawing blood, passing it over an enzyme-based amperometric sensor, and discarding the blood into a waste container. In addition to monitoring, one Biostator configuration allowed the automated control of insulin delivery. (Courtesy of Miles Laboratories, Diagnostics Division.)

to 8 h of continuous use. There also is a standby mode of up to 28 h. This allows a cartridge life of 36 h and the possibility of using the same cartridge on more than one patient. Cross-contamination is not possible, since the sterile dispos-able tube set is discarded after each patient, and all blood and rinse solution is routed into the disposable cartridge. Sensor equilibration time at startup is 45 min. The system conducts an automatic two-point calibration initially and every hour during use. Both *in vitro* testing and clinical studies have found the GEM-6 Plus to be comparable to laboratory analyzers for blood gases, pH, and electrolytes, with hematocrit measurements 2–5% above *in vitro* laboratory values in patients with low pre-operative sodium levels or in patients who receive large amounts of albumin.[413,478,482]

Two companies currently are developing *ex vivo* monitoring systems for attachment to the extracorporeal loop of hemodialysis machines for automatic measurement of the dialysate. UniFET Corporation (La Jolla, CA) is developing a system to measure blood urea nitrogen (UN) and pH. Sintong Chemical Industries, Ltd (Taoyuan, Taiwan) is developing a system to measure UN as well as potassium, sodium, ionized calcium, and chloride. Both monitors withdraw, analyze, and discard a small volume of dialysate on an intermittent basis, with periodic interruptions for automatic two-point calibration.

27.5.3. Flow-Through Sensors in the Extracorporeal Loop

A second major approach to *ex vivo* monitoring is the placement of sensors directly in an extracorporeal blood loop, thereby providing for continuous measurement of analytes. A commercially successful product using this method for the measurement of p_{O_2}, p_{CO_2}, and pH in both the arterial and venous blood loops of heart–lung machines is the CDI 400 (CDI 3M Health Care, Irvine, CA) (Fig. 27.23). The sensors (Fig. 27.24) are optodes, based on the fluorescence intensity method. They undergo a 15–20 min automatic two-point calibration in a tonometered buffer solution prior to placement in the blood loop, after which the system provides continuous measurements of blood gases and pH during cardiopulmonary bypass. Results are displayed continuously on the monitor and also are available via an integrated printer and an RS-232 port. The sensor module measures blood temperature at the sensors, so that measurements can be corrected to 37°C.

There are several critical issues with this approach. Unlike the biosensors in a system where blood is withdrawn, analyzed, and discarded, the sensors used in an extracorporeal loop must be sterile or in some way be isolated from the blood by a sterile barrier. The CDI 400, for example, separates the sensors from the blood with a very thin sterile gas-permeable membrane. This eliminates the design constraint of sterility on the sensors themselves. The sensors also must be compatible with blood, although this requirement is less important than with *in vivo* sensors. The duration of use for flow-through extracorporeal sensors is very short, typically 3–6 h for a heart bypass procedure. Additionally, the patient is systemically heparinized to prevent thrombus formation in the extracorporeal circuit. These conditions significantly reduce the likelihood that buildup of protein, clots, or living cells on sensor surfaces will affect performance. Sensor stability also is an issue. Methods for automatic recalibration of the sensors after attachment to the blood loop have not been developed. *In vivo* recalibration can be accomplished by drawing a discrete blood sample from the loop, measuring it on a conventional blood gas analyzer, and entering the time and values into

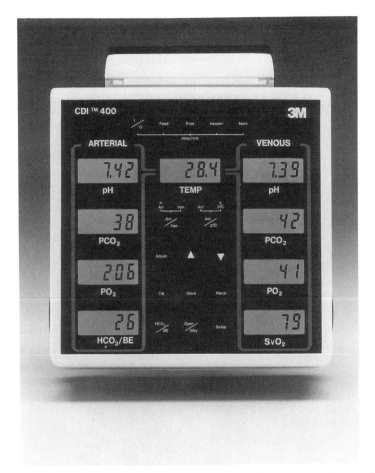

Figure 27.23. CDI 400 *ex vivo* monitor. The monitor acquires data simultaneously from two sets of extracorporeal flow-through sensors, one in the arterial path and one in the venous path of the cardiopulmonary bypass system. The sensors are shown in Figure 27.24. (Courtesy of CDI 3M Health Care.)

the monitor. As discussed earlier, however, this method potentially introduces into the monitor's subsequent output any error that might have been associated with the *in vitro* sample.

Performance studies for extracorporeal systems have in general shown good agreement with conventional blood gas analyzers.[62,445,466,502] Clinicians have found that the systems are useful in guiding the perfusionist with crucial trend information, although some authors conclude that because of discrepancies between monitor and laboratory values, a reference blood gas analyzer still is required.[414,466,502] Air bubbles in the sensor module, temperature-correction methodology, timing of *in vitro* samples relative to sensor response time during

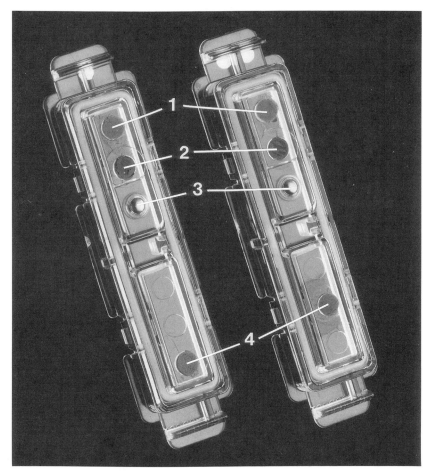

Figure 27.24. CDI 400 disposable *ex vivo* sensor chambers. The arterial unit is on the left, and the venous unit is on the right. Measurements include (1) p_{CO_2}, (2) pH, (3) temperature, and (4) p_{O_2}. Dimensions are approximately 1 × 5 in. (Courtesy of CDI 3M Health Care.)

rapid changes in patient status, and errors in the *in vitro* comparison samples have all been possible factors contributing to the observed discrepancies.[502] In view of these operating difficulties, the applicability of flow-through extracorporeal sensors is likely to remain limited. For bypass surgery, additional sensors could be added to current systems to provide a more complete cluster of blood chemistries that includes sodium, potassium, ionized calcium, ionized magnesium, lactate, hematocrit, and glucose. Nonetheless, these systems probably will not be used outside of bypass surgery or hemodialysis,[62,67] since implementation of an extracorporeal loop involves extra costs and risks that are unlikely to be outweighed by the potential benefits of automated monitoring. These include setup costs, intensive clinical management, systemic heparinization, and increases in complications from bleeding.[173]

27.5.4. Withdrawal and Reinfusion of Blood

A third major approach to *ex vivo* monitoring involves withdrawal of blood to sensors located in a tubing set, analysis, and reinfusion of the blood. Several commercial systems are currently under development for the measurement of one or a combination of blood gases (p_{O_2}, p_{CO_2}), pH, electrolytes (Na$^+$, K$^+$, Ca^{2+}), hematocrit and glucose.[251,435,491,499,500,516] The challenges facing *ex vivo* monitors that withdraw and reinfuse blood are similar to those for the flow-through extracorporeal loop systems—the sensors must be sterile and compatible with blood. The constraint of blood compatibility, however, is relaxed considerably compared to *in vivo* sensors, since the *ex vivo* sensor surfaces are in contact with blood for only a short period of time during each measurement cycle. Following sampling, they are flushed continuously with an aqueous electrolyte solution containing a small amount of heparin, typically 1 unit/mL, and remain in contact with that solution until the next sample. This decreases the likelihood that buildup of protein, clots, or living cells on sensor surfaces will affect performance during extended use. The major limitation of this approach is that measurements are not continuous, although the assumption that intermittent monitors are clinically less desirable than continuous monitors has been questioned.[494]

The VIA Monitor Model 1-01 (VIA Medical, San Diego, CA) is being developed in two configurations, one for the measurement of blood gases, electrolytes, and hematocrit, and one for the measurement of glucose (Fig. 27.25). Early clinical reports with limited numbers of patients show promising results.[251,499,500,516] The monitor is set up like a conventional intravenous infusion pump. The sensor array is integrated into the tubing set and located just external to the patient's vascular access site. An infusible calibration solution containing known analyte concentrations is pumped continuously over the sensors at a low rate to maintain site patency and to provide one-point calibrations with each sample. Sample cycles are initiated either automatically at preset intervals, or on demand by the press of a key. A sample cycle consists of the following steps: (1) the sensors are calibrated against the known values in the infusible calibration solution; (2) the monitor's pump reverses direction and draws a blood sample up the line and over the sensors, while a blood sensing algorithm ensures that undiluted blood is positioned correctly over the sensors and also allows for some variability in the internal volume of the tubing and catheter downstream from the sensor; (3) the blood sample is analyzed and for the blood gas, electrolyte, and hematocrit determinations, is also thermostated to 37°C; and (4) the results are displayed while the monitor's pump reverses direction again to flush the blood sample back into the patient. The disposable sensors in the VIA system are based on conventional electrochemical technologies (Fig. 27.26). The sensor array requires 15–20 min for equilibration prior to an initial two-point calibration. After

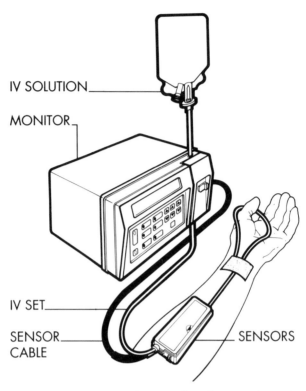

IV SOLUTION

MONITOR

IV SET

SENSOR
CABLE

SENSORS

Figure 27.25. VIA *ex vivo* blood chemistry monitor. At preset intervals or on demand, the monitor automatically withdraws blood over the sensors, analyzes it, and returns it to the patient via the intravascular line, thereby conserving patient blood volume. The intravenous (IV) solution serves as a calibration fluid for automatic one-point calibrations between each measurement cycle. The unit includes audible tones and diagnostic messages for alarms and advisories. (Courtesy of VIA Medical.)

attachment to the patient, one-point calibrations are automatically conducted prior to each measurement. The time from the initiation of the sample cycle to the completion of the analysis is approximately 1 min. Measurements can be repeated as often as every 5 min. Results are available on a numeric display, a paper printout, and over an RS-232 port. This approach involves flushing several milliliters of calibration solution into the patient with each sample. Hence, it is not suitable for neonates or other patients who cannot tolerate changes in intravascular volume. For these patients, a configuration is available that enables the clinician to manually shunt most of the calibration solution into a waste reservoir.

The CDI 2000 (CDI-3M Healthcare, Tustin, CA) was developed for the monitoring of p_{O_2}, p_{CO_2}, and pH. The sensor array is placed in the conventional arterial line tubing near the catheter (Fig. 27.27). Sampling is conducted manually by the following process: (1) a stopcock above the sensor array is turned off

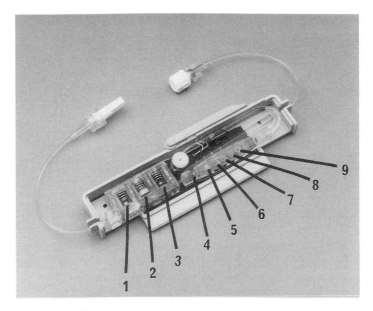

Figure 27.26. VIA critical-care sensor. Electrochemical measurements include (1) p_{CO_2}, (2) p_{O_2}, (6) K^+, (7) Ca^{2+}, (8) Na^+, and (9) pH; (3) is the reference electrode. Hematocrit is measured by conductance (4) and temperature with a thermistor (5). Measurement of glucose will be added later and also is available in a separate module. Measurement ranges are p_{CO_2}, 10–99 mm Hg; p_{O_2}, 10–600; K^+, 0.2–20 mmol/L; Ca^{2+}, 0.25–4.25 mmol/L; Na^+, 80–190 mmol/L; pH, 6.80–7.80; hematocrit, 10–75%; and glucose, 40–400 mg/dL. Dimensions are approximately 1 × 5 in. (Courtesy of VIA Medical.)

to the arterial line fluid source; (2) a syringe attached to the stopcock is used to draw a blood sample up the tubing and over the sensor array; (3) the stopcock is then turned back to the original position, allowing fluid flow to resume, and a key is pressed on the monitor to indicate that sampling is in progress; then (4) within 2 min the monitor displays the numeric measurement results and signals the clinician to manually flush the blood back to the patient. Results are printed and also available over an RS-232 port. The sensors in the CDI-2000 are based on fiber optic chemical sensor technology using the fluorescence intensity method. The sensor array first undergoes an automatic 20-min two-point calibration. After connection to the patient, the sensors require daily *in vivo* recalibrations. The *in vivo* calibration consists of a simultaneous blood sample drawn from a stopcock downstream from the sensor array during the manual measurement cycle. This sample is then analyzed *in vitro* on a conventional instrument and the results are entered into the monitor. A controlled study, involving *in vitro* testing with tonometered bovine blood and patient testing with normal volunteers in whom large changes in blood gas levels were induced, demonstrated performance comparable to conventional blood gas analyzers.[463] Several clinical studies, including a prospective multicenter trial,[491] have demonstrated good agree-

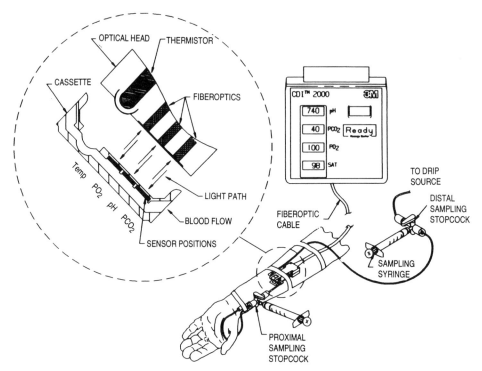

Figure 27.27. CDI 2000 *ex vivo* blood gas and pH monitor. The close-up shows the fiber optic chemical sensors, thermistor, and blood flow channel. The operator uses the distal sampling stopcock and syringe to draw blood over the sensors and then, presses a button on the monitor to start the analysis. After the analysis is complete, the monitor prompts the operator to reinfuse the blood. (Courtesy of CDI 3M Health Care.)

ment between this system and conventional *in vitro* analyzers for both radial artery[491] and pulmonary artery[435,479] blood gas measurements. The authors concluded that the CDI 2000 can be reliably utilized to guide therapy in critically ill patients with cardiopulmonary insufficiency,[435,479] and can replace the use of blood gas analyzers for intensive care unit patients with indwelling arterial catheters.[491]

27.5.5. Microdialysis

Microdialysis has been used for measuring amino acid and neurotransmitter concentrations in brain tissue[53,57] and extracellular glucose concentration in subcutaneous tissue.[50,58,60] Several research teams currently are developing *ex vivo* monitors based on this concept for the continuous measurement of extracellular glucose.[55,61,65] The principle involves placement of a microdialysis probe (Fig. 27.28) in the subcutaneous tissue, generally in the abdominal area, perfusing it continuously with an isoosmotic electrolyte solution, measuring the glucose level in the dialysate with a glucose oxidase-based amperometric sen-

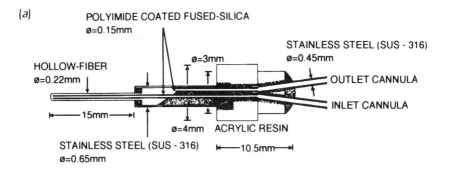

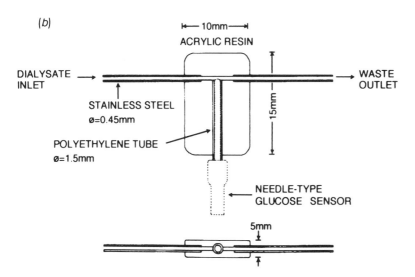

Figure 27.28. Schematic diagram of a microdialysis probe (*a*) and associated glucose sensor (*b*) for *ex vivo* monitoring of subcutaneous glucose levels. Perfusate is delivered to the tip of the hollow fiber probe via the inlet cannula. The dialysate returns via the outlet cannula, passes over the glucose sensor, and then flows to waste. (Courtesy of Yasuhiro Hashiguchi, M.D., Kumamoto University School of Medicine, Kumamoto, Japan.)

sor, and using that value to calculate extracellular glucose concentration. A variant of this method is to perfuse the microdialysis probe with a solution containing glucose oxidase. By measuring the change in oxygen level in the perfusate with an oxygen sensor, glucose concentration can be calculated.[205,330] Microdialysis allows sensors to be isolated from most components of the blood including all cells and recalibrated directly at periodic intervals during use. A key assumption of this method is that the rate of analyte recovery in the dialysate remains constant at a given perfusion rate. The adsorption of protein to the surface of the hollow-fiber membranes or the formation of protein plugs inside the hollow-fiber membrane may both contribute to reduced analyte recovery.

Day-to-day and intra- and interindividual variability in glucose recovery has been reported.[60,205] Local tissue changes, including blood flow and temperature, also can contribute to variable recovery.[262] Despite these potential problems, recent reports indicate that microdialysis systems can provide accurate glucose measurements,[61,65] in some cases up to several days between changes of the microdialysis probes.[55]

27.5.6. Open Perfusion

A novel approach to the continuous measurement of glucose concentration in subcutaneous tissue is open tissue perfusion with incomplete equilibration.[282,338] This method involves placing a double-lumen catheter (Fig. 27.29) in the subcutaneous tissue of the abdomen, pumping an isotonic nonconductive fluid containing no glucose through the inner lumen, and simultaneously pumping back a mixture of the infusate and extracellular fluid through the outer lumen. Partial equilibration between the infusate and extracellular fluid occurs along a series of 0.2-mm openings in the distal portion of the outer lumen of the catheter. The partially equilibrated fluid is then pumped over a sensor module containing glucose and electrical conductivity sensors. Glucose level in the recovered fluid is measured with glucose oxidase-based amperometric sensors. The percent equilibration of the recovered fluid is determined by conductivity. The actual extracellular glucose concentration is then calculated. In principle, if the conductivity of the recovered solution is 20% of the conductivity of the extracellular fluid, the measured glucose value would be multiplied by 5 to obtain the actual extracellular glucose concentration. In practice, a correction algorithm is used to assess the measurements obtained and arrive at the displayed glucose level. The assumption that the equilibration of ions and glucose takes place at the same rate along the catheter has been confirmed by human clinical testing.[282] However, using conductivity as the measure of equilibration also means that the calculated glucose concentration is potentially independent

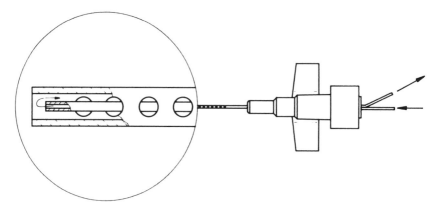

Figure 27.29. Subcutaneous double-lumen perfusion catheter for the system shown in Figure 27.30. (Courtesy of AVL List GMBH.)

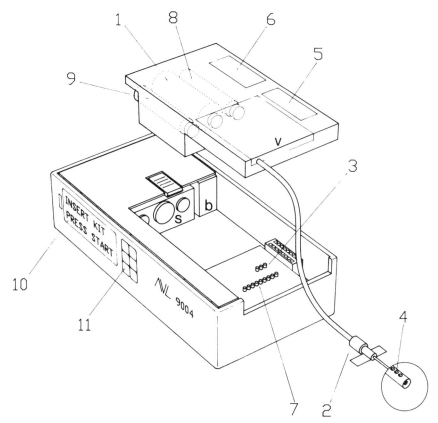

Figure 27.30. Open perfusion *ex vivo* monitor for the measurement of subcutaneous glucose levels and infusion of insulin. The system components are (1) perfusion fluid, (2) double-lumen catheter, (3) actuator for the peristaltic pump, (4) custom perfusion catheter (see Fig. 27.30), (5) measuring chamber, (6) waste, (7) actuator for the valves, (8) calibration fluid, (9) insulin (used for a closed-loop control system), (10) display, and (11) key pad. A valve unit (v) is in the top assembly. A battery pack (b) and the syringe drives (s) are in the lower one. (Courtesy of AVL List GMBH.)

of both fluid flow rate through the catheter and the equilibration rate, neither of which is true for the microdialysis approach.

Figure 27.30 shows the monitor currently under development at AVL List GMBH (Graz, Austria). It is portable and provides for periodic automatic two-point recalibrations. In addition, it contains two glucose sensors and four conductivity sensors for measurement redundancy and a thermistor for temperature correction. One version includes an insulin delivery system integrated with the monitor. The goal of this configuration is to provide automated regulation of subcutaneous insulin delivery based on an algorithm that considers both monitored glucose levels and individual patient sensitivity to insulin. Open perfusion depends on the assumption that the conductivity of extracellular fluid remains fairly constant. In some critical clinical conditions (e.g., heart surgery or burn patients), this may not be a valid assumption. However, open perfusion does represent an intriguing approach to the development of minimally invasive automated monitoring systems for any analyte where continuous measurement in the extracellular fluid would provide meaningful clinical information and adequate guidance for safe automated therapy.

27.6. SURVEY OF *IN VIVO* MONITORING SYSTEMS

27.6.1. Advantages and Hurdles

A major advantage of *in vivo* monitoring is the ability to generate essentially continuous information on the blood chemistry variables being measured. Invasive *in vivo* probes have sensors located directly in the body and therefore, in continual contact with the body fluid being analyzed. Although there may be a slight lag between the change in the target analyte level and its equilibration with the sensor, generally this is only 1 or 2 min. With current *ex vivo* systems, continuous measurement in blood is only possible with flow-through extracorporeal sensors or by means of continuous removal and disposal of blood. Neither approach is likely to receive clinical acceptance beyond certain narrow applications. Another potential advantage of *in vivo* systems is the ability to place the sensor directly in a specific location or target organ. As discussed in earlier sections, however, it is exactly because the sensors are placed directly in the body that *in vivo* monitors face the most difficult developmental hurdles. Two major systems approaches to *in vivo* monitoring—intravascular and subcutaneous—have been developed and reported in the literature. Intravascular systems have been confined primarily to the measurement of oxygen saturation, blood gases, and pH, while subcutaneous systems have focused almost exclusively on the measurement of glucose. Examples of each of these approaches are discussed below.

27.6.2. Intravascular Systems—Oxygen Saturation

The earliest *in vivo* blood chemistry monitoring technology involved the measurement of blood oxygen saturation by means of fiber optic catheters. Originally developed in the 1960s and 1970s,[424,430,455,503] oxygen saturation monitors were not successfully commercialized until the early 1980s.[432,456] A significant problem common to early systems was sensitivity to changes in hematocrit, blood flow velocity, and light reflected from the cells in blood vessel walls. This was due in part to reliance on two wavelength systems that allowed the calculation of only a single ratio between hemoglobin and oxyhemoglobin. Another difficulty involved the need to calibrate the sensors with one or more blood samples of known oxygen saturation prior to insertion into the patient.

The most widely adopted commercial system is the Oximetrix monitor (Abbott Critical Care Systems, Mountain View, CA), which measures cardiac output in addition to oxygen saturation. It consists of a monitor, an optical module, an external printer, several different configurations of arterial and pulmonary artery catheters with integrated fiber optic sensors, and an optical reference standard packaged with each catheter. Oxygen saturation levels are measured continuously, displayed in both numeric and graphical format, and printed on a strip chart. The optical module contains light-emitting diodes that transmit three wavelengths of light down one of the optic fibers. This optic fiber illuminates blood flowing past the catheter tip. The optical module also contains a photodetector that receives the light reflected back from a second optic fiber and converts the light intensity levels into electrical signals for analysis by the monitor. The use of three wavelengths of light allows two independent light ratios to be calculated. This approach helps avoid the limitations of the early two-wavelength systems and minimize errors related to changes in hematocrit, pulsatile flow, and noise from reflection of light off vessel walls. Calibration is accomplished with the optical reference standard, a small block that fits over the catheter tip and provides an absolute color standard for direct calibration prior to insertion of the catheter. This protocol simplifies the calibration process for the operator and avoids errors associated with calibration that uses *in vitro* blood samples. The system also supports *in vivo* recalibration if the sensor is left in place for more than 24 h.

One recent study reported unacceptable precision with the Oximetrix system compared to intermittently measured jugular bulb oxygen saturation.[481] In general, however, clinical reports have found the performance of the Oximetrix system both clinically acceptable and of clinical value.[411,448,486] The three-wavelength approach has been reported to show significantly less drift than a two-wavelength system,[436] although several recent studies indicate that a two-wavelength system (SAT-2, Baxter Edwards Critical Care, Irvine, CA) may provide comparable performance.[410,515]

27.6.3. Intravascular Systems—Blood Gas

With *in vivo* blood gas and pH monitors, all three sensors (p_{O_2}, p_{CO_2}, and pH) generally are located on or near the tip of a single probe that is inserted through a catheter, typically into the radial artery. The space between the sensor and the wall of the catheter must be large enough to allow a continuous flush solution to be infused in order to maintain line patency and to allow the withdrawal of blood samples for *in vitro* testing. The sensor also should not interfere with the measurement of arterial blood pressure through the catheter, either by blocking the signal or distorting the waveform. As discussed earlier in the chapter, there have been many unsuccessful attempts to commercialize continuous *in vivo* blood gas and pH monitors. A large body of literature has been published recently on clinical evaluations of *in vivo* systems,[206,405,412,416,433,439,440,442–444,
449,451,460,462,474–476,489,490,496,498,505,507,509,510,521] although most involved the Puri-

tan Bennett 3300 or other systems that are no longer available.[412,416, 433,439,440, 442,443,444,449,451,460,462,474–476,489,490,505,507] The commercial *in vivo* system currently available is the Paratrend 7 (Pfizer Biomedical Sensors, Malvern, PA). One other is under development (LightSense Corporation, Laguna Hills, CA). The BioSentry was discontinued recently. Initial clinical studies showed promising results,[496,498,521] although for some patients, the use of a 20-gauge radial artery catheter may have led to significant arterial waveform dampening on insertion of the optode.[496] With the exception of a fiber optic chemical sensor for p_{O_2}, the BioSentry is similar to the Paratrend 7, which we describe in detail next.

The Paratrend 7 (Fig. 27.31) provides continuous measurements of p_{O_2}, p_{CO_2}, pH, and temperature. The monitor also continuously calculates values for oxygen saturation, bicarbonate, and base excess and displays these parameters, with a user option of displaying the blood gases and pH in a graphical trend format (Fig. 27.32). The interface is flexible, allowing the clinician to adjust the scaling for each parameter, as well as vary the time window. Results also are available from an integrated printer or over an RS-232 port. The sensor probe (Fig. 27.33) is packaged in a disposable tonometer containing a sterile buffer solution. Prior to use, an automatic two-point calibration is conducted by bubbling gases of known concentration through the tonometer. After the 30-min calibration procedure, the sensor is inserted through a custom 20-gauge arterial catheter into the patient's radial artery. The sensor is connected to the monitor via a cable and a patient data module (see Fig. 27.31). The data module has nonvolatile memory. With the intravascular sensor in place, the data module can be disconnected from the monitor during patient transport and reconnected to the same or another monitor without loss of calibration and patient data. This is highly convenient, for although the monitor is mounted on a wheeled base, the system weighs approximately 95 lb. Every 12 h a one-point *in vivo* calibration is performed by drawing a paired blood sample, analyzing it with an *in vitro* analyzer, and entering the values into the monitor.

The sensor probe (Fig. 27.34) includes fiber optic chemical sensors for the measurement of p_{CO_2} and pH by the absorption method, an electrochemical Clark electrode for the measurement of p_{O_2}, and a thermocouple for the measurement of temperature. The manufacturer's published accuracy is p_{O_2}, ±5% < 120 mm Hg and ±10% ≥ 120 mm Hg; p_{CO_2}, ±3 mm Hg; pH, ±0.03; and temperature, ±0.2°C. Drift is p_{O_2}, < 1%/h; p_{CO_2}, < 1%/h; and pH, < 0.005/h. Response time is 0–90% in ≤ 180 s at 37°C. These specifications meet 95% confidence limits based on *in vitro* evaluations using tonometered solutions. The outer dimension of the sensor is less than 0.5 mm (Fig. 27.35). The entire surface has a covalently bonded bioactive surface treatment (Carmeda, Sweden) to reduce fibrin deposition and thrombus formation. Several clinical studies have demonstrated good agreement between the Paratrend 7 and *in vitro* analyzer values both intraoperatively[509] and in the intensive care unit.[405,510] Use during cardiac surgery and cardiopulmonary bypass has demonstrated that blood sampling was not impeded, fidelity of the arterial waveform was not

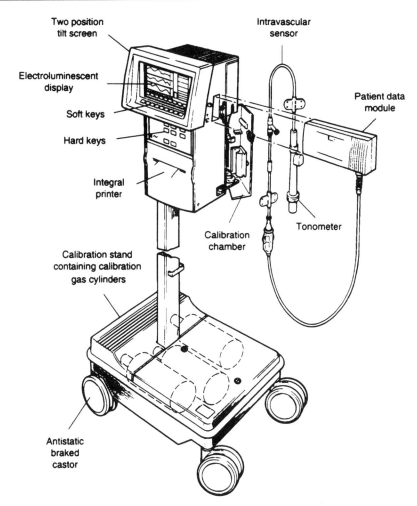

Two position
tilt screen

Intravascular
sensor

Electroluminescent
display

Patient data
module

Soft keys

Hard keys

Integral
printer

Calibration
chamber

Tonometer

Calibration stand
containing calibration
gas cylinders

Antistatic
braked
castor

Figure 27.31. Paratrend 7 biosensor system for *in vivo* intravascular monitoring. The patient data module allows temporary disconnection of the sensor from the monitor for easier transport with the patient. The module retains sensor calibration data and can be reconnected to the same or a different monitor. (Courtesy of Pfizer Biomedical Sensors.)

affected, and bias and precision were similar before, during, and after the bypass phase.[509] In the studies involving intensive care unit patients, the duration of sensor use was up to 5 or 6 days. The wall effect was not observed, no evidence of line thrombosis due to sensor placement occurred, and examination after sensor removal showed no observable buildup of organic material on the sensor surfaces.[510]

The challenges facing *in vivo* blood gas systems are the most demanding of any type of blood chemistry monitor and were discussed extensively in earlier sections. The key issues include (1) biocompatibility of sensors to withstand

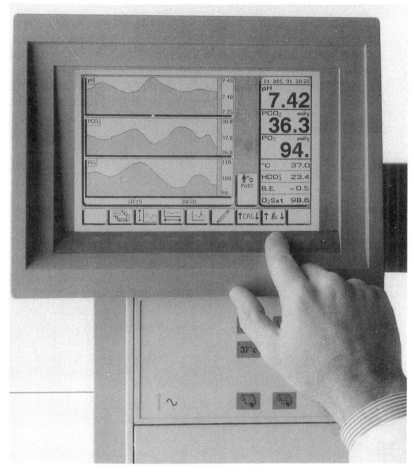

Figure 27.32. Graphical/numerical–user interface for the Paratrend 7 *in vivo* monitor. Scaling can be set individually for each measurement. The time interval for the graphical display of data is from 10 min to 24 h. Measurement ranges are p_{O_2}, 20–500 mm Hg; p_{CO_2}, 10–80 mm Hg; and pH, 6.80–7.80. (Courtesy of Pfizer Biomedical Sensors.)

continuous exposure to blood, (2) assurance that the sensors measure blood gas values in arterial blood rather than artifacts created locally, (3) microfabrication of sensors small enough to insert through appropriately sized catheters, (4) dependence on *in vivo* calibration, (5) the ability of the sensors to tolerate sterilization, and (6) high manufacturing costs. Adding additional sensors such as electrolytes and hematocrit to blood gas optodes, while at the same time maintaining size constraints, also represent significant technical and clinical hurdles. The key advantage of *in vivo* blood gas monitoring is the ability to obtain continuous information on pH, p_{CO_2}, and p_{O_2}, which for certain proce-

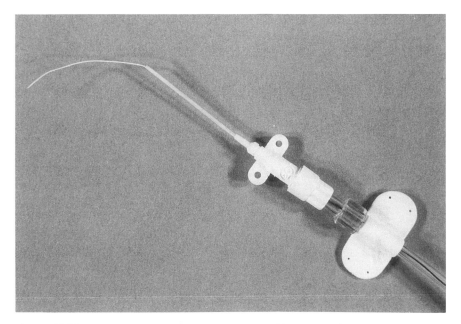

Figure 27.33. Paratrend 7 probe inserted through a 20-gauge radial artery catheter. The diameter of the probe at the end where the sensors are located is approximately 0.45 mm. (Courtesy of Pfizer Biomedical Sensors.)

dures (e.g., lung and liver transplants), may provide significant clinical value[440,476] and improve patient outcomes.

27.6.4. Subcutaneous Systems—Glucose

There have been many attempts to develop a reliable subcutaneous glucose sensor during the past decade.[206,233,257,258,270,275,284,298,302,304,306,314,316,325,333,334,348,349,355,356,366] A more recent attempt has been the development of noninvasive transcutaneous glucose monitors.[266,267] To date, however, there have been no successful commercial products based on the subcutaneous approach. In view of the difficulties encountered by placing the sensors directly in the subcutaneous tissue, several research teams that have been involved for many years in the development of *in vivo* glucose sensors have redirected their efforts to *ex vivo* microdialysis.[55,65] There is at least one company, however, that is actively developing a continuous glucose monitor based on an *in vivo* subcutaneous glucose sensor (MiniMed Technologies, Sylmar, CA). A major benefit of an *in vivo* glucose sensor is a relatively simple monitoring system without the need for pumps and calibration solutions required with *ex vivo* glucose monitors. Another benefit is the ability to generate continuous information on glucose levels, although this also is possible with *ex vivo* microdialysis and open perfusion. The design

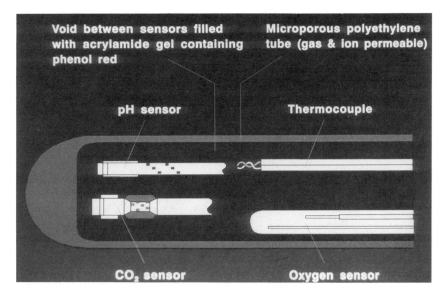

Figure 27.34. Schematic of the Paratrend 7 *in vivo* probe tip. The pH and p_{CO_2} sensors are fiber optic chemical sensors based on the absorption method. The p_{O_2} sensor is an electrochemical sensor based on a Clark oxygen electrode. The thermocouple measures local temperature in the tip. (Courtesy of Pfizer Biomedical Sensors.)

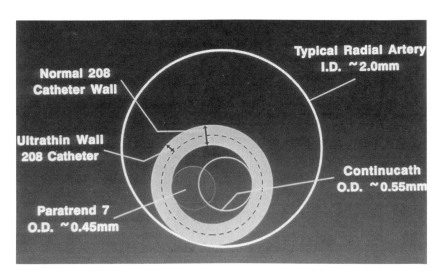

Figure 27.35. Cross-sectional schematic of the radial artery. The Paratrend 7 *in vivo* probe is small enough to allow blood to flow by it. This helps to avoid problems associated with local pertubations (see text and Table 27.9). (Courtesy of Pfizer Biomedical Sensors.)

principle for subcutaneous glucose monitors typically involves the fabrication of a glucose oxidase-based sensor on the tip of a needle or catheter small enough to be inserted easily through the skin, generally in the abdominal area. The sensor is sterilized during production and may or may not be calibrated *in vitro* prior to insertion into the subcutaneous tissue. After insertion, there is a settling or stabilization time of as long as 2–4 h,[270,321] after which a one or more point *in vivo* calibration is conducted using either an *in vitro* glucose analyzer or portable glucose meter.[270,321,353,356,366] *In vivo* calibrations are repeated on a periodic basis thereafter to correct for sensor drift. The sensor is replaced every 2–7 days. The obstacles to producing a reliable *in vivo* system, however, have yet to be overcome. We discuss these briefly next.

Fouling of the sensor membranes, lack of correlation between *in vitro* and *in vivo* calibrations, and changes in sensor performance over time all have been reported frequently throughout the literature on *in vivo* glucose sensors. The local subcutaneous environment around the sensor can affect measurements. There have been numerous conflicting reports on the relationship between extracellular glucose and blood glucose levels. These are reviewed in an elegant study by Schmidt et al.,[329] who recently demonstrated that extracellular glucose concentration is probably half that of blood glucose. Following insertion of the sensor, or at other times when capillaries around the sensor tip are ruptured (e.g., through bumping the insertion site), the small amount of extracellular fluid around the sensor is overwhelmed by blood, and the sensor measures blood glucose. After local capillary damage is resolved and normal extracellular glucose levels are restored, the sensor measures extracellular glucose. Since these values may differ by up to 50%, uncertainty could be introduced into normal sensor output, as well as during the *in vivo* calibration procedure. Another local site issue is the possibility of a variable amount of extracellular fluid around the sensor. This could influence both the rate of equilibration following changes in blood glucose levels, and the equilibrium value, since the sensor consumes glucose. Infection, the inflammatory response, and fibrous encapsulation at the site all could affect local glucose levels as well.

27.7. FUTURE PROSPECTS

The clinical success of *in vitro, ex vitro,* and *in vivo* biosensor systems position this technology at the center of an accelerating major trend in patient care. Although the development of *ex vivo* and *in vivo* systems has not been as fast or easy as initially projected, nonetheless, biosensors per se are a major factor in the paradigm shift to point-of-care testing. Now well established, *in vitro* point-of-care testing will increase rapidly in importance, utility, and versatility. On-site diagnosis decreases main laboratory test volume and diminishes the need for conventional specimen collection and transport. *In vitro* devices are now being integrated with other physiological patient monitoring systems. The role of the clinical laboratory has changed. The new collaborative consortium is a hybrid laboratory[92-98] shared with the clinical team. Emerging biosensor technologies reveal numerous new approaches[1-68,131-204] (e.g., DNA biosensors for cystic fibrosis[150a]). Therefore, *in vitro* test menus will expand, but with a premium on microsampling, compactness, portability, and one-step analysis. As biosensor technologies mature, economies of scale and competition will lower costs. Competition includes both commercial and medical competition, since managed care and capitation are transforming the criteria for inpatient care, particularly critical care. Hospitals will no longer automatically pay for an improvement in patient care unless that improvement is medically significant, attracts patients, or justifies the extra expense.[69-130]

Hospitals are concentrating critically ill patients in referral centers and when possible, managing others as outpatients. Rapid response and timeliness of decisions have taken on new meaning. Integrated healthcare systems create new demands that are satisfied by point of care testing. Critical care profiling,[90-93,117] when performed in a conventional main laboratory, no matter how efficient, is likely to be criticized as insufficient for critically ill patients. Test results age quickly, and errors due to time obsolescence are rarely considered in evaluating the performance of main laboratories. The immediacy of selecting the most important tests at the point of care while evaluating the patient, and then identifying critical alternatives in the differential diagnosis, as well as detecting sudden, unexpected, or rapid changes in the patient's metabolic condition are paramount to the clinician. *In vitro* testing using fast microanalysis at the point of care provides these advantages and will continue to be necessary in critical care whenever intravascular access for *ex vivo* and *in vivo* monitoring is not immediately available, not planned, or contraindicated. However, *in vitro* testing consumes blood and incurs costs with each set of tests performed. These inherent disadvantages discourage serial testing. They create medical and economic tradeoffs where *ex vivo* and *in vivo* monitoring have distinct advantages, especially during the initial stages of care when the patient is critically ill or during procedures like dialysis, where patient access is limited by time and equipment constraints.

Ex vivo systems are beneficial when they alleviate the need for serial *in vitro* tests, facilitate the temporal optimization of critical care, and help optimize diagnostic–therapeutic process.[97] Evidence indicates that *ex vivo* systems are clinically reliable (see references in Table 27.11). Since they eliminate unwanted sources of preanalytical error (e.g., handling, labeling, transport, delays, centrifugation, and splitting), *ex vivo* systems ultimately may prove to be more accurate than *in vitro* testing. The blood sample contacts the *ex vivo* biosensors briefly and then after measurement, returns to the patient with minimal or no loss. Hence, biocompatibility problems are diminished and blood volume is conserved. This obviates the expense and morbidity associated with transfusions. In the future, these systems will benefit from rapid expansion of test menus, nanofabrication of patient-portable units, and defined use in care paths and treatment algorithms. While most *ex vivo* systems generally do not provide continuous information, the intermittent measurements they do provide should improve the ability to discern trends before deleterious or catastrophic events occur. This will contract the therapeutic turnaround time. Therefore, integration with optimized treatment protocols, physiological information, and other bedside systems (including alarms, advisories, trends detectors, and telemetry) will be clinically beneficial.

Commercial development of *ex vivo* systems promises to be both creative and intense, given the large number of new devices and competitors (see Table 27.11). Implementation of *ex vivo* systems should be based on quantitative *proof* of clinical reliability, medical efficacy, and economic benefit.[115,116,494] Similar to what is emerging in managed care, a "report card" program of evaluation might be useful to help define appropriate clinical indications, cost-effective uses, and precautions in widely divergent groups of critically ill patients. Straightforward criteria for clinical adoption include evidence of better quality of care and major advantages over existing approaches at the same or lower cost. Now that academic medical center grants and research budgets are decreasing, industrial funding of outcomes research for these systems will become essential. The only data available on accuracy, bias, precision, drift, and complication rates are from relatively small clinical trials. Well-designed, prospective, multicenter studies targeting endpoint and intermediate outcomes (see Table 27.5) will be needed to determine the clinical reproducibility and critical niches of *ex vivo* systems, as well as *in vivo* systems. In the future it will become increasingly unlikely that these new monitoring technologies will be accepted without documentation of improved outcomes or lower costs.[116] A recent survey[503a] estimated an acceptable charge of $50–150 for continuous blood gas monitoring (approximately equal to the patient charge per blood gas analysis) and an acceptable daily charge of $250–750.

Current invasive *in vivo* systems, particularly for p_{O_2}, p_{CO_2}, and pH, have significantly improved since their initial introduction, but remain problematic.[512] For example, the performance of *in vivo* biosensor probes should not be degraded by sensor artifacts. Sensor biocompatibility, sensitivity, and stability are crucial. The physical form must match the measurement site. Approved sites generally include only the radial and femoral arteries. Variability in the local environment around the probe tip where the active sensors are located intravascularly has proved to be a much more difficult issue to address than originally envisioned. Thrombosis and thromboembolism represent additional inherent risks. Design, packaging, manufacturing constraints, and high costs per unit are major obstacles that impede the progress of *in vivo* biosensor systems and the expansion of their measurement capabilities. Probe insertion and maintenance consume physician and/or nurse time. Despite these challenges, there is growing evidence that invasive *in vivo* biosensor systems now achieve a level of performance that is clinically useful, for instance, to look for unexpected changes in cardiopulmonary homeostasis as early signs of problems that would have gone unnoticed until too late using routine *in vitro* testing. A recent report of a human closed-loop control system for oxygenation[408] is predictive of closed-loop regulation of biochemical variables and automated therapy (e.g., anesthesia, dialysis, and diabetes) in the future. New *in vivo* approaches (e.g., hematocrit,[467] lactate,[52,309,415,441,470,497,513] and urea[56]) and biosensors in bioactive *in vivo* probes (e.g., sensing endoscopes[406,407] and cancer probes[139a]) forecast exciting future prospects for *in vivo* biosensors.

Invasive *in vivo* systems (e.g., fiber optic sensors) have focused on the measurement of pH, p_{CO_2}, and p_{O_2}. Blood gases are some of the most frequently ordered tests in critical care. A recent survey[503a] showed that the patients most likely to benefit from use of continuous invasive *in vivo* monitoring are intensive care unit patients with acute respiratory failure, adult respiratory distress syndrome (ARDS), and systemic inflammatory reponse syndrome (SIRS), and surgery patients undergoing and recovering from cardiothoracic surgery, neurosurgical procedures, and organ transplantation. As an adjunct to conventional blood gas analysis, the clinical usefulness of transcutaneous p_{CO_2} and p_{O_2} monitoring illustrates how *noninvasive monitoring* can help vulnerable patients (e.g., tiny premature infants in a neonatal intensive care unit) to avoid *in vitro* tests and conserve precious blood volume. Eventually noninvasive monitoring (e.g., near-infrared spectroscopy; see Arnold[132]) should contribute many useful clinical solutions. Critically ill patients (and others) would benefit from the accelerated progress of noninvasive monitoring. Clinical progress has been slow or of limited scope (e.g., pulse oximetry). In general, monitoring, whether based on biosensors or other technologies, allows physicians to rapidly detect and treat metabolic changes, and then sort out the effectiveness of interventions by comparing cause and effect immediately and continuously. Once *ex vivo* and *in vivo* monitoring are accepted for general use, the enhancement in the *quality and timeliness* of the continuous information they provide is likely to improve patient outcomes and change medical practice in a profound way.

REFERENCES

Biosensor Development

1. Albantov AF, Levin AL: New functional possibilities for amperometric dissolved oxygen sensors. *Biosens Bioelectron* 9:515–526, 1994.
2. Altura BM, Altura BT: Characterization and studies of a new ion selective electrode for free extracellular magnesium ions in whole blood, plasma and serum. *Proc 14th Internal Symp Blood Gases and Electrolytes.* Chatham, MA, 1992, pp. 3–2.
3. Altura BT, Altura BM: Measurement of ionized magnesium in whole blood, plasma, and serum with a novel new ion selective electrode. *Proc American Society for Magnesium Research,* La Jolla, CA, 1991.
4. Altura BT, Dell Orfano K, Yeb Q, et al: A new ion selective electrode (ISE) for ionized magnesium (IMg^{2+}) in while blood (WB), plasma (PL) and serum (S). *Clin Chem* 37:948–949, 1991.
5. Altura BT, Shirey TL, Young CC, et al: A new method for the rapid determination of ionized Mg^{2+} in whole blood, serum and plasma. *Meth Find Exp Clin Pharmacol* 14:297–304, 1992.

6. Astles JR, Miller WG: Measurement of free phenytoin in blood with a self-contained-fiber optic immunosensor. *Anal Chem* 66:1675–1682, 1994.

7. Athey D, McNeil CJ, Bailey WR, Hager HJ: Homogeneous amperometric immunoassay for theophylline in whole blood. *Biosens Bioelectron* 8:415–420, 1993.

8. Chen Y, Tan TC: Selectivity enhancement of an immobilized apple power enzymatic sensor for dopamine. *Biosens Bioelectron* 9:401–410, 1994.

9. Cooper JC, Hämmerle M, Schuhmann, Schmidt HL: Selectivity of conducting polymer electrodes and their application in flow injection analysis of amino acids. *Biosens Bioelectron* 8:65–74, 1993.

10. Coulet PR, Blum LJ, Cautier SM: Luminescence optical biosensor oriented to clinical analysis. *In* Okuda K, ed: *Automation and New Technology in the Clinical Laboratory.* Oxford, UK: Blackwell Scientific Publications, 1988, pp. 239–244.

11. Crumbliss AL, Zhao J, Stonehuerner JG, O'Daly JP, Hendens RW: A carrageenan hydrogel stabilized colloidal gold multi-enzyme biosensor electrode utilizing immobilized horseradish peroxidase and cholesterol oxidase/cholesterol esterase to detect cholesterol in serum and whole blood. *Biosens Bioelectron* 8:331–338, 1993.

12. Garguilo MG, Michael AC: Quantitation of choline in the extracellular fluid of brain tissue with amperometric microsensors. *Anal Chem* 66:2621–2629, 1994.

13. Gilmartin MA, Hart JP: Novel, reagentless, amperometric biosensor for uric acid based on a chemically modified screen-printed carbon electrode coated with cellulose acetate uricase. *Analyst* 119:833–840, 1994.

14. Hampson SJ, Notley RG, Fletcher JE, et al: Prostate specific antigen estimation with optical biosensor. *Lancet* 343:301–302, 1994.

15. Hlavay J, Haemmerli SD, Guilbault GG: Fibre-optic biosensor for hypoxanthine and xathine based on a chemiluminescence reaction. *Biosens Bioelectron* 9:189–195, 1994.

16. Kaku T, Karan HI, Okamoto Y: Amperometric glucose sensors based on immobilized glucose oxidase-polyquinone system. *Anal Chem* 66:1231–1235, 1994.

17. Konig B, Gratzel M: A novel immunosensor for herpes viruses. *Anal Chem* 66:341–344, 1994.

18. Kost GJ: Ionized magnesium: measurement and clinical indications. *American Association for Clinical Chemistry National Meeting Roundtable. Clin Chem* 38:1125, 1992.

19. Külpmann WR, Kallien T: Evaluation of an ion-selective electrode for the determination of "ionized magnesium." *Proc 14th Internatl Symp Blood Gases and Electrolytes.* Chatham, MA, 1992, P P-12.

20. Lee SJ, Scheper T, Buckmann AF: Application of a flow injection fibre optic biosensor for the analysis of different amino acids. *Biosens Bioelectron* 9:29–32, 1994.

21. Maj-Zurawska M, Lewenstam A: Fully automated potentiometric determination of ionized magnesium in blood serum. *Anal Chim Acta* 236:331–335, 1990.

22. Mani JC, Marchi V, Cucurou C: Effect of HIV-1 peptide presentation on the affinity constants of two monocloncal antibodies determined by BIAcore technology. *Mol Immunol* 31:439–444, 1994.

23. Marsoner HJ, Sachs C, Ritter CH, et al: Ionized magnesium measurement in blood. *Proc 14th Internatl Symp Blood Gases and Electrolytes.* Chatham, MA, 1991, P P-10.

24. Marsoner HJ, Spichiger U, Ritter CH, et al: Measurement of ionized magnesium with neutral carrier based ISE's. Progress and results with the AVL 988-4 ionized magnesium analyzer. *Proc 14th Internatl Symp Blood Gases and Electrolytes.* Chatham, MA, 1992, pp. 174–187.

25. McEnroe E, McKenna MJ, Diamond D, et al: Dependence of measured ionized calcium on protein concentration as measured by three ion-selective electrodes. *Ann Clin Biochem* 29:443–449, 1992.

26. Moulds JJ: Blood grouping using a galvanic immunoelectrode sensor. *Transfus Clin Biol* 1:129–133, 1994.

27. Nguyen AL, Luong JHT: Development of mediated amperometric biosensors for hypoxanthine, glucose and lactate: a new format. *Biosens Bioelectron* 8:421–432, 1993.

28. Nice E, Lackmann M, Smyth F, Fabri L, Burgess AW: Synergies between micro-preparative high-performance liquid chromatography and an instrumental optical biosensor. *J Chromatogr A* 660:169–185, 1994.

29. Palmisano F, Centonze D, Zambonin PG: An in situ electrosynthesized amperometric biosensor based on lactate oxidase immobilized in a poly-o-phenylenediamine film: determination of lactate in serum by flow injection analysis. *Biosens Bioelectron* 9:471–479, 1994.

30. Pandey PC, Pandey V, Mehta S: An amperometric enzyme electrode for lactate based on graphite paste modified with tetracyanoquinodimethane. *Biosens Bioelectron* 9:365–372, 1994.

31. Payne RB, Buckley BM, Rawson KM: Protein interference with ion-selective electrode measurement depends on reference electrode composition and design. *Ann Clin Biochem* 28:68–72, 1991.

32. Pereiro Garcia R, Alava Moreno F, Diaz Garcia ME, Sanz-Medel A, Narayanaswamy R: Serum analysis for potassium ions using a fibre optic sensor. *Clin Chim Acta* 207:31–40, 1992.

33. Post PL, Trybus KM, Taylor DL: A genetically engineered, protein-based optical biosensor of myosin II regulatory light chain phosphorylation. *J Biol Chem* 269:12880–12887, 1994.

34. Rehak M, Snejdarkova M, Otto M: Application of biotin-streptavidin technology in developing a xanthine biosensor based on a self-assembled phospholipid membrane. *Biosens Bioelectron* 9:337–341, 1994.

35. Rio CS, Kato Y, Sonomoto K: Amperometric flow-injection analysis of creatinine based on immobilized creatinine deiminase, leucine dehydrogenase and L-amino acid oxidase. *Biosens Bioelectron* 9:429–437, 1994.

36. Rouilly M, Rusterholz B, Spichiger UE, et al: Neutral ionophore-based selective electrode for assaying the activity of magnesium in undiluted blood serum. *Clin Chem* 36:466–469, 1990.

37. Sachs C, Levillain P: The real cause of discrepancy between plasma sodium results obtained by ISE and "dilution" techniques: an error in the dilution factor. *AACC Electrolyte/Blood Gas Div Newsl* 9:2–4, 1994.

38. Sansubrino A, Mascini M: Development of optical fibre sensors for ammonia, urea, urease and IgG. *Biosens Bioelectron* 9:207–216, 1994.

39. Sena SF, Bowers Jr GN: Measurements of ionized calcium in biological fluids:ion-selective electrode methods. *Meth Enz* 158:320–334, 1988.

40. Shakhsher Z, Seitz WR, Legg KD: Single fiberoptic pH sensor based on changes in reflection accompanying polymer swelling. *Anal Chem* 66:1731–1735, 1994.

41. Suri CR, Raje M, Mishra CG: Determination of immunoglobulin M concentration by piezoelectric crystal immunobiosensor coated with protamine. *Biosens Bioelectron* 9:325–332,535–542, 1994.

42. Vreman HJ, Stevenson DK, Oh W, et al: Semiportable electrochemical instrument for determining carbon monoxide in breath. *Clin Chem* 40:1927–1933, 1994.

43. Watts HJ, Lowe CR, Pollard-Knight DV: Optical biosensor for monitoring microbial cells. *Anal Chem* 66:2465–2470, 1994.

44. Williams RA, Blanch HW: Covalent immobilization of protein monolayers for biosensor applications. *Biosens Bioelectron* 9:159–167, 1994.

45. Wolfbeis OS, Li H: Fluorescence optical urea biosensor with an ammonium optrode as transducer. *Biosens Bioelectron* 8:161–166, 1993.

46. Wolthuis R, McCrae D, Saaski E, Hartl J, Mitchell G: Development of a medical fiberoptic pH sensor based on optical absorption. *IEEE Trans on Biomed Eng* 39:531–537, 1992.

47. Wu AHB, Wong SS, Johnson KG, et al: Evaluation of the triage system for emergency drugs-of-abuse testing in urine. *J Anal Toxicol* 17:241–245, 1993.

48. Xie B, Harborn U, Medclenburg M: Danielsson B: Urea and lactate determined in 1-microL whole-blood samples with a miniaturized thermal biosensor. *Clin Chem* 40:2282–2287, 1994.

49. Yang VC, Ma SC, Liu D, Brown RB, Meyerhoff ME: A novel electrochemical heparin sensor. *ASAIO Journal* 39:M195–M201, 1993.

Dialysis Systems

50. Bolinder J, Hagstrom E, Ungerstedt U, Arner P: Microdialysis of subcutaneous adipose tissue *in vivo* for continuous glucose monitoring in man. *Scan J Lab Invest* 49:465–474, 1989.

51. Bolinder J, Ungerstedt U, Arner P: Microdialysis measurement of the absolute glucose concentration in subcutaneous adipose tissue allowing glucose monitoring in diabetic patients. *Diabetologia* 35:1177–1180, 1992.

52. DeBoer J, Korf J, Plijter-Groendijk H: In vivo monitoring of lactate and glucose with microdialysis and enzyme reactors in intensive care medicine. *Internatl J Artif Organs* 17:163–170, 1994.

53. Delgado JM, DeFeudis FV, Roth RH, Ryugo DK, Mitruka BK: Dialytrode for long term intracerebral perfusion in awake monkeys. *Arch Internatl Pharmacodyn* 198:9–21, 1972.

54. Gotch F, Evans M, Metzner K, Westphal D, Polaschegg H: An on-line monitor of dialyzer Na and K flux in hemodialysis. *ASAIO Trans* 36:M359–M361, 1990.

55. Hashiguchi Y, Sakakida M, Nishida K, Uemura T, Kajiwara KI, Shichiri M: Development of a miniaturized glucose monitoring system by combining a needle-type

glucose sensor with microdialysis sampling method. *Diabetes Care* 17:387–396, 1994.

56. Jacobs P, Suls J, Sansen W, Hombrouckx R: A disposable urea sensor for continuous monitoring of hemodialysis efficiency. *ASAIO J* 39:M353–M358, 1993.

57. Johnson RD, Justice JB: Model studies for brain dialysis. *Brain Res Bull* 10:567–571, 1983.

58. Lonnroth P, Jansson PA, Smith U: A microdialysis method allowing characterization of intercellular water space in humans. *Am J Physiol* 253:E228–231, 1987.

59. Meyerhoff C, Bischof F, Mennel FJ, Sternberg F, Pfeiffer EF: Use of the microdialysis technique in the monitoring of subcutaneous tissue glucose concentration. *Internatl J Artif Organs* 16:268–275, 1993.

60. Meyerhoff C, Bischof F, Sternberg F, Zier H, Pfeiffer EF: On line continuous monitoring of subcutaneous tissue glucose in men by combining portable glucosensor with microdialysis. *Diabetologia* 35:1087–1092, 1992.

61. Moscone D, Mascini M: Microdialysis and glucose biosensor for *in vivo* monitoring. *Ann Biol Clin* (Paris) 50:323–327, 1992.

62. Nielsen G, Bredahl C, Nielsen C: Continuous blood gas monitoring in haemodialysis using an electrode inserted in the extracorporeal dialysis circulation. *Scand J Clin Lab Invest* 53:197–200, 1993.

63. Palmissano F, Centonze D, Guerrieri A, Zambonin PG: An interference-free biosensor based on glucose oxidase electrochemically immobilized in a non-conducting poly(pyrrole) film for continuous subcutaneous monitoring of glucose through microdialysis sampling. *Biosens Bioelectron* 8:393–400, 1993.

64. Persson L, Hillered L: Chemical monitoring of neurosurgical intensive care patients using intracerebral microdialysis. *J Neurosurg* 76:72–80, 1992.

65. Pfeiffer EF, Meyerhoff C, Mennel FJ, Sternberg F, Bischof F: Presentation of the "Ulm Zuckeruhr" system in diabetes care: implantable microdialysis probe, glucosensor and telemetrically operated sugar watch for on-line s.c. glucose monitoring over 48 hours in men. *Endocrine Soc Annu Mtg Abstr* 350:601C, 1994.

66. Schindler JG, Schindler MM, Herna K, et al: Urea sensor for the continuous ammonium-selective enzymatic process control of the artificial kidney. *Eur J Clin Chem Clin Biochem* 32:145–152, 1994.

67. Schindler JG, Schindler MM, Herna K, Reisinger E, et al: Ion-selective electroanalyzer with tubular solid contact flow-through sensors for continuous bio-electrochemically controlled hemodialysis of K^+, Na^+, Ca^{++}, Cl^-, and pH. *Biomedizinishe Technik* 36:271–284, 1991. (In German.)

68. Stjernstrom H, Karlsson T, Ungerstedt U, Hillered, L: Chemical monitoring of intensive care patients using intravenous microdialysis. *Intensive Care Med* 19:423–428, 1993.

Economics and Strategies

69. Bauer S: A blood gas network: using blood gas and electrolyte analyzers at the point of care. *Med Lab Observ* 26(9S):2–9, 1994.

70. Bishop MS, Husain I, Aldred M, Kost GJ: Multisite point-of-care potassium testing for patient-focused care. *Arch Pathol Lab Med* 118:797–800, 1994.

71. *Blood Gas Monitoring: Economic Assessment and Market Strategies.* Washington, DC: The Lash Group, 1992.

72. Blood gas technology. *MedPRO Month* 31–32, Feb 1994.

73. Coalition for Critical Care Excellence: *ICU Cost Reduction: Practical Suggestions and Future Considerations.* Anaheim, CA: Society of Critical Care Medicine; 1994.

74. *Control Destiny: Control Cost.* Society of Critical Care Medicine 24th Educational and Scientific Symposium. Video produced by Abbott Critical Care Systems, Chesterfield, MI, 1995.

75. *Cost Benefit Analysis of the GEM Premier Blood Gas and Electrolyte Analyzer.* Salt Lake City, UT: The International Healthcare Consulting Group, 1994.

76. Diller W: Corporate strategies: Puritan-Bennett's Gamble. *In Vivo* 33–37, May 1994.

77. Elevitch FR: Multimedia communications networks: patient care through interactive point-of-care testing. *Clin Lab Med* 14:559–568, 1994.

78. Felder RA: Robotic automation of near-patient testing. In: Kost GJ, ed: *Handbook of Clinical Automation, Robotics, and Optimization.* New York: John Wiley and Sons, Inc., 1996:Chapter 24.

79. Frankel HL, Rozycki GS, Ochsner MG, et al: Minimizing admission laboratory testing in trauma patients: use of a microanalyzer. *J Trauma* 37:728–736, 1994.

80. Friedman BA, Mitchell W: Integrating information from decentralized laboratory testing sites: the creation of a value-added network. *Am J Clin Pathol* 99:637–642, 1993.

81. Gafni A, Birch S: Guidelines for the adoption of new technologies: a prescription for uncontrolled growth in expenditures and how to avoid the problem. *Can Med Assoc J* 148:913–917, 1993.

82. Ginsberg BH: An overview of minimally invasive technologies. *Clin Chem* 38:1596–1600, 1992. [Published erratum *Clin Chem* 38:2360, 1992.]

83. Greendyke RM: Cost analysis: bedside glucose testing. *Am J Clin Pathol* 97:106–107, 1992.

84. Herr DM, Newton NC, Santrach PJ, Hankins DG, Burritt MF: Airborne and rescue point-of-care testing. *Pathol Patterns, Am J Clin Pathol* 104:S54–S58, 1995.

85. Hortin GL, Utz C, Gibson C: Managing information from bedside testing. *Med Lab Observ* 27:28–32, 1995.

86. *International Classification of Clinical Services Database.* Ann Arbor, MI: Healthcare Knowledge Resources, 1991, Table 1.B.

87. Jacobs E: Information integration for point-of-care and satellite testing. In: Kost GJ, ed. *Handbook of Clinical Automation, Robotics, and Optimization.* New York: John Wiley and Sons, Inc.; 1996:Chapter 25.

88. Keffer JH: *Economic Aspects of Decentralized Testing.* Washington, DC: American Association for Clinical Chemistry Teleconference, Nov 15, 1994.

89. Keffer JH: The economic aspects of new delivery options for diagnostic testing. In: Kost GJ, ed. *Handbook of Clinical Automation, Robotics, and Optimization.* New York: John Wiley and Sons, Inc.; 1996:Chapter 23.

90. Kost GJ: Role of new whole blood analytical techniques in critical care. *Clin Chem* 35:1232–1233, 1989.

91. Kost GJ, Shirey TL: New whole-blood testing for laboratory support of critical care at cardiac transplant centers and U.S. hospitals. *Arch Pathol Lab Med* 114:864–868, 1990.

92. Kost GJ: The hybrid laboratory: shifting the focus to the point of care. *Med Lab Observ* 24(9S):17–28, 1992.

93. Kost GJ: The hybrid laboratory: the clinical laboratory of the 1990s is a synthesis of the old and the new. *Arch Pathol Lab Med* 116:1002–1003, 1992.

94. Kost GJ, Lathrop JP: Designing hybrid laboratories, performance maps, and quality paths for patient-focused care. *Med Lab Observ* 25(9S):16–26, 1993.

95. Kost GJ: Point-of-care testing: patient focusing for the future. *In* Howanitz PJ, McBride JH, eds: *Professional Practice in Clinical Chemistry: A Review.* Washington, DC: American Association for Clinical Chemistry Press, 1994, pp. 443–454.

96. Kost GJ: The future is now! Patient-centered testing result of automation, robotics. *ADVANCE Med Lab Prof* April:10–11, 18, 1994.

97. Kost GJ: Point-of-Care Testing ⇒ The Hybrid Laboratory ⇒ Knowledge Optimization. In: Kost GJ, ed. *Handbook of Clinical Automation, Robotics, and Optimization.* New York: John Wiley and Sons, Inc.; 1996:Chapter 28.

98. Kost GJ, Hague C: The current and future status of critical care testing and patient monitoring. *Pathol Patterns, Am J Clin Pathol* 104:S2–S18, 1995.

99. *Laboratory Services Review: Report to the Ministry of Health.* Ontario, Canada: Queen's Printer (Catalog No. 2227248), 1994.

100. Lash Group: *Blood Gas Monitoring—Economic Assessment and Market Strategies.* Washington, DC: The Lash Group, 1992.

101. Laupacis A, Feeny D, Detshy AS, Tugwell PX: How attractive does a new technology have to be to warrant adoption and utilization? Tentative guidelines for using clinical and economic evaluation. *Can Med Assoc J* 146:473–481, 1992.

102. Lee-Lewandrowski E, Laposata M, Eschenbach K, et al: Utilization and cost analysis of bedside capillary glucose testing in a large teaching hospital: implications for managing point of care testing. *Am J Med* 97:222–230, 1994.

103. May ME: Cost analysis of bedside glucose testing. [Comment, letter.] *Am J Clin Pathol* 98:383–384, 1992.

104. McIntire T: Cost analysis of bedside glucose testing. *Am J Clin Pathol* 98:383–384, 1992.

105. Misiano DR, Meyerhoff ME, Collison ME: Current and future directions in the technology relating to bedside testing of critically ill patients. *Chest* 97:204S–214S, 1990.

106. National Committee for Clinical Laboratory Standards: *Cost Accounting in the Clinical Laboratory: Proposed Guideline.* Villanova, PA: NCCLS, 1990, Publication GP11-P.

107. Naylor CD, Williams JI, Basinski A, Goel V: Technology assessment and cost-effectiveness analysis: misguided guidelines? *Can Med Assoc J* 148:921–924, 1993.

108. Nosanchuk JS, Keefner R: Cost analysis of point-of-care laboratory testing in a community hospital. *Am J Clin Pathol* 103:240–243, 1995.

109. Castro HJ, Oropello JM, Halpern NA: Point-of-care testing in the intensive care unit. The intensive care physician's perspective. *Pathology Patterns, Am J Clin Pathol* 104:S95–S99, 1995.

110. Owen VM: Market requirements for advanced biosensors in healthcare. *Biosens Bioelectron* 9:xxix–xxxv, 1994.

111. Popper C: Using cost-effectiveness analysis to weigh testing decisions. *Med Lab Observ* 24(9S):29–35, 1992.

112. Report: Medical, economic, and regulatory issues affecting point-of-care-testing. Na-

tional Academy of Clinical Biochemistry, May 6–7, 1994, Philadelphia, PA. *MDDI Gray Sheet,* May 23, 1994.

113. Roberts DE, Bell DD, Ostryniuk T, et al: Eliminating needless testing in intensive care—an information-based team management approach. *Crit Care Med* 21:1452–1458, 1993.

114. Roizen MF, Schreider B, Austin W, Carter C, Polk S: Pulse oximetry, capnography, and blood gas measurements: reducing cost and improving the quality of care with technology. *J Clin Monit* 9:237–240, 1993.

115. Shapiro BA: Evaluation of blood gas monitors: performance criteria, clinical impact, and cost/benefit. *Crit Care Med* 22:546–548, 1994.

116. Shapiro BA: Clinical and economic performance criteria for intraarterial and extraarterial blood gas monitors, with comparison with *in vitro* testing. *Pathol Patterns, Am J Clin Pathol* 104:S100–S106, 1995.

117. Shirey TL: Critical care profiling for informed treatment of severely ill patients. *Pathol Patterns, Am J Clin Pathol* 104:S79–S87, 1995.

117a. Sibbald WJ, Eberhard JA, Inman KJ, Sprug CL: New technologies, critical care, and economic realities. *Crit Care Med* 21:1777–1780, 1993.

118. Simpson KN, LaVallee RL, Halpern MT, et al: *The Economic and Clinical Efficiency of Point-of-Care Testing for Critically Ill Patients: GEM Premier versus Usual Laboratory Testing Procedures* (Executive Summary). Ann Arbor, Michigan: Mallinckrodt Sensor Systems, 1994.

119. Smith I. The economics of pulse oximetry. *J Resp Care Pract* 8:73–79, 1995.

120. Statland BE, Brzys K: Evaluating STAT testing alternatives by calculating annual laboratory costs. *Chest* 97:198S–203S, 1990.

121. Steiner JW, Root JM, Buck E: Lab networks: models of regional cooperation. *Med Lab Observ* 26:38–42, 1994.

122. Steiner JW, Root JM, Buck E: Lab regionalization: structural options for the age of managed competition. *Med Lab Observ* 26:48–51, 1994.

123. Steiner JW, Root JM, Buck E: The regionalization of laboratory services. *Med Lab Observ* 26:22–29, 1994.

124. Steiner J: *A Conceptual Framework for a Province-Wide Laboratory Services Delivery System.* Ontario, Canada: Chi Laboratory Systems, Inc., 1994.

125. Udvarhelyi IS, Colditz GA, Epstein AM: Cost-effectiveness and cost-benefit analyses in the medical literature. *Ann Intern Med* 116:238–244, 1992.

126. Weinstein MC, Stason WB: Foundations of cost-effectiveness analysis for health and medical practices. *N Eng J Med* 296:716–721, 1977.

127. White DL: Defining and measuring outcomes in laboratory medicine: focus of the 1994 clinical chemistry forum. *Clin Chem News* 20:2, 1994.

128. Winkelman JW, Wybenga DR: Quantification of medical and operational factors determining central versus satellite laboratory testing of blood gases. *Am J Clin Pathol* 102:7–10, 1994.

129. Zaloga GP: Evaluation of bedside testing options for the critical care unit. *Chest* 97(5):185S–190S, 1990.

130. Zaloga GP: The ideal critical care profile. *Proc Society of Critical Care Medicine Educational and Scientific Symposium.* Audio Recording. Palm Desert, CA: Convention Cassettes Unlimited, 24:8, 1995.

Emerging Technologies

131. Anderson GP, Golden P, Ligler FS: An evanescent wave biosensor. Part I: Fluorescent signal acquisition from step-etched fiber optic probes. *IEEE Trans Biomed Eng* 41:578–584, 1994.

132. Arnold MA: New developments and clinical impact of noninvasive monitoring. In: Kost GJ, ed. *Handbook of Clinical Automation, Robotics, and Optimization*. New York: John Wiley and Sons, Inc.; 1996:Chapter 26.

133. Arquint P, Koudelka-Hep M, van der Schoot BH, van der Wal P, de Rooij NF: Micro-machined analyzers on a silicon chip. *Clin Chem* 40:1805–1809, 1994.

134. Bluestein BI, Craig M, Slovacek R, et al: Evanescent wave immunosensors for clinical diagnostics. *In* Wise DL, Wingard LB, eds: *Biosensors with Fiberoptics*. Clifton, NJ: Humana Press, 1991, pp. 181–223.

135. Bos JA, Schelter W, Gumbrecht W, et al: Development of a micro transmission cell for in vivo measurement of SaO_2 and Hb. *Adv Exper Med Biol* 277:47–52, 1990.

136. Coulet PR, Blum LJ: Luminescence in biosensor design. *In* Wise DL, Wingard LB, eds: *Biosensors with Fiberoptics*. Clifton, NJ: Humana Press, 1991, pp. 293–324.

137. Daunert S, Bachas LG, Ashcom GS, Meyerhoff ME: Continuous on-line monitoring of biomolecules based on automated homogenous enzyme-linked competitive binding assays. *Anal Chem* 62:314–318, 1990.

138. De Vries EFA, Schasfoort RBM, Van der Plas J: Nucleic acid detection with surface plasmon resonance using cationic latex. *Biosens Bioelectron* 9:509–514, 1994.

139. Eisele S, Ammon HPT, Kindervater R, Gröbe A, Gospel W: Optimized biosensor for whole blood measurements using a new cellulose based membrane. *Biosens Bioelectron* 9:119–124, 1994.

139a. Frank CJ, Redd DC, Ganster TS, McCreery RL: Characterization of human breast biopsy specimens with near-IR Raman spectroscopy. *Anal Chem* 66:319–326, 1994.

140. Fu B, Bakker E, Yun JH, Yang VC, Meyerhoff ME: Response mechanism of polymer membrane-based potentiometric polyion sensors. *Anal Chem* 66:2250–2259, 1994.

141. Golden JP, Anderson GP, Rabbany SY, Ligler FS: An evanescent wave biosensor. Part II: Fluorescent signal acquisition from tapered fiber optic probes. *IEEE Trans Biomed Eng* 41:585–591, 1994.

142. Hall JW, Pollard A: Near-infrared spectrophotometry: a new dimension in clinical chemistry. *Clin Chem* 38:1623–1631, 1992.

143. Heideman RG, Kooyman RP, Greve J: Immunoreactivity of adsorbed anti human chorionic gonadotropin studied with an optical waveguide interferometric sensor. *Biosens Bioelectron* 9:33–43, 1994.

144. Haugland RP: Fluorescent labels. *In* Wise DL, Wingard LB, eds: *Biosensors with Fiberoptics*. Clifton, NJ: Humana Press, 85–110, 1991.

145. Jobst G, Urban G, Jachimowicz A, et al: Thin-film Clark-type oxygen sensor based on novel polymer membrane systems for in vivo and biosensor applications. *Biosens Bioelectron* 8:123–128, 1993.

146. Kricka LJ, Wilding P: Micromechanics and nanotechnology. In: Kost GJ, ed. *Handbook of Clinical Automation, Robotics, and Optimization*. New York: John Wiley and Sons, Inc.; 1996:Chapter 3.

147. Kumar P, Colston JT, Chambers JP, Rael ED, Valdes JJ: Detection of botulinum toxin using an evanescent wave immunosensor. *Biosens Bioelectron* 9:57–63, 1994.

148. Lackie SJ, Glass TR, Block MJ: Instrumentation for cylindrical waveguide evanescent fluorosensors. *In* Wise DL, Wingard LB, eds: *Biosensors with Fiberoptics.* Clifton, NJ: Humana Press, 1991, pp. 225–251.

149. Love WF, Button LJ, Slovacek RE: Optical characteristics of fiber optic evanescent wave sensors. Theory and experiment. *In* Wise DL, Wingard LB, eds: *Biosensors with Fiberoptics.* Clifton, NJ: Humana Press, 1991, pp. 139–180.

150. McDonald JA: Micromachining biosensors. *Biosens Bioelectron* 9:xvii–xx, 1994.

150a. Millan KM, Saraullo A, Mikkelsen SR: Voltametric DNA biosensor for systic fibrosis based on a modified carbon paste electrode. *Anal Chem* 66:2943–2948, 1994.

151. Mills A, Chang Q, McMurray N: Equilibrium studies on colorimetric plastic film sensors for carbon dioxide. *Anal Chem* 64:1383–1389, 1992.

152. Murphy AP, Rolfe P: Intravascular oxygen sensor with polyetherurethane membrane; in vitro performance. *Med Biol Eng Comput* 30:121–122, 1992.

153. Natsume T, Koide T, Yokota S, Hirayoshi K, Nagata K: Interactions between collagen-binding stress protein HSP47 and collagen. Analysis of kinetic parameters by surface plasmon resonance biosensor. *JAMA* 269:31224–31228, 1994.

153a. Nishizawa M, Menon VP, Martin CR: Metal nanotubule membranes with electro-chemically switchable ion-transport selectivity. *Science* 268:700–702, 1995.

154. Place JF, Sutherland RM, Riley A, Mangan C: Immunoassay kinetics at continuous surfaces. *In* Wise DL, Wingard LB, eds: *Biosensors with Fiberoptics.* Clifton, NJ: Humana Press, 1991, pp. 253–291.

155. Severs AH, Schasfoort RBM, Salden MHL: An immunosensor for syphilis screening based on surface plasmon resonance. *Biosens Bioelectron* 8:185–190, 1993.

156. Shinohara Y, Kim F, Shimizu M, Goto M, Tosu M, Hasegawa Y: Kinetic measurement of the interaction between an oligosaccharide and lectins by a biosensor based on surface plasmon resonance. *Eur J Biochem* 223:189–194, 1994.

157. Shoji S, Esashi M: Microfabrication and microsensors. *Appl Biochem Biotech* 41:21–34, 1993.

158. Shul'ga AA, Soldatkin AP, El'skaya AV, Dzyadevich SV, Patskovsky SV, Strikha VI: Thin-film conductometric biosensors for glucose and urea determination. *Biosens Bioelectron* 9:217–223, 1994.

159. Smith RL, Collins SD: Micromachined packaging for chemical microsensors. *IEEE Trans Elec Dev* 35:787–792, 1988.

160. Smith RL, Scott DC: An integrated sensor for electrochemical measurements. *IEEE Trans Biomed Eng* BME-33:83–90, 1986.

161. Striebel C, Brecht A, Gauglitz G: Characterization of biomembranes by spectral ellipsometry, surface plasmon resonance and interferometry with regard to biosensor application. *Biosens Bioelectron* 9:139–146, 1994.

162. Takano E, Hatanaka M, Haki M: Real-time-analysis of the calcium-dependent interaction between calmodulin and a synthetic oligopeptide of calcineurin by a surface plasmon resonance biosensor. *FEBS Lett* 352:247–250, 1994.

163. Thompson JM: Performance evaluation if ISFETs and other ISE sensors for whole blood ion assay. *Med Biol Engr Comput* 28:B29–B33, 1990.

164. Thompson RB, Ligler FS: Chemistry and technology of evanescent wave biosensors. *In* Wise DL, Wingard LB, eds: *Biosensors with Fiberoptics.* Clifton, NJ: Humana Press, 1991, pp. 111–138.

165. Van Kerkhof JC, Bergveld P, Schasfoort RBM: Development of an ISFET based heparin sensor using the ion-step measuring method. *Biosens Bioelectron* 8:463–472, 1993.

166. Wilding P, Pfahler J, Bau HH, Zemei JN, Kricka LJ: Manipulation and flow of biological fluids in straight channels micromachined in silicon. *Clin Chem* 40:43–47, 1994.

General Biosensors

167. Aizawa M: Biosensors: principles and applications. *In* Okuda K, ed: *Automation and New Technology in the Clinical Laboratory.* Oxford, UK: Blackwell Scientific Publications, 1988, pp. 233–238.

168. Albery WJ: Molecular recognition and molecular sensors. *Ciba Foundation Symp* 158:55–72,92–97, 1991.

169. Arnold MA: Motivation for developing optical sensors for blood electrolyte measurements. *Clin Chem* 37:1319–1320, 1991.

169a. Ashwood ER, Kost G, Kenny M: Temperature correction of blood-gas and pH measurements. *Clin Chem* 29:1871–1885, 1983.

170. Bilitewski U: Mass production of biosensors. *Anal Chem* 65:525A–533A, 1993.

171. Byfield M, Abuknesha RA: Review. Biochemical aspects of biosensors. *Biosens Bioelectron* 9:373–399, 1994.

172. Camara C, Moreno MC, Orellana G: Chemical sensing with fiberoptic devices. *In* Wise DL, Wingard, LB, eds: *Biosensors with Fiberoptics.* Clifton, NJ: Humana Press, 1991, pp 29–84.

172a. Claremont DJ: Biosensors: Clinical requirements and scientific promise. *J Med Eng Technol* 11:51–56, 1987.

173. Collison ME, Meyerhoff ME: Chemical sensors for bedside monitoring of critically ill patients. *Biochimica Clinica* 14(12):1288–1296, 1990; *Anal Chem* 62:425A–437A, 1990.

174. Durst RA, Siggaard-Anderson O: Electrochemistry. *In* Burtis CA, Ashwood ER, eds: *Clinical Chemistry.* Philadelphia: Saunders, 1994, pp. 159–183.

175. Eberhart RC, Weigelt JA: New chemical sensing techniques for critical care medicine. *In* Shoemaker WC, Ayres S, Grenvik A, Holbrook PR, Thompson, WL, eds: *Textbook of Critical Care.* Philadelphia: Saunders, 1989, pp. 223–230.

176. Gottlieb A: The optical measurement of blood gases—approaches, problems, and trends. *Fiber Opt Med Fluor Sensors Appl* 1648:4–11, 1992.

177. Henry JB: The impact of biosensors on the clinical laboratory. *MLO (Med Lab Observ)* 22:32–35, 1990.

178. Hodinar A: Biosensors in the clinical chemistry laboratory and in clinical medicine. *Cas Lek Cesk* 133:359–362, 1994.

179. Hunter KWW: Technological advances in bedside monitoring: biosensors. *Arch Pathol Lab Med* 111:633–636, 1987.

180. Janata J, Josowicz M, DeVaney DM: Chemical sensors. *Anal Chem* 66:207R–228R, 1994.

181. Kiel JL: The ultimate biosensor. *Aviat Space Environ Med* 65:A121–A124, 1994.

182. Kyes K: The future of blood gases: Analysis & monitoring. *J Resp Care Pract* 6:17–24, 1993.

183. McNeil C: Biosensors in clinical biochemistry—where to now? *Biosens. Bioelectron* 7/8:i–iii, 1993.

184. Monroe D: Potentiometric (bioselective electrodes) assay systems: utility and limitations. *Crit Rev Clin Lab Sci* 27:109–158, 1989.

185. Motta N, Guadalupe AR: Activated carbon paste electrodes for biosensors. *Anal Chem* 66:566–571, 1994.

186. Newman JD, Turner APF: Biosensors: the analyst's dream? *Chem Industr* 374–378, May 16, 1994.

187. Oesch U, Ammann D, Simon W: Ion selective membrane electrodes for clinical use. *Clin Chem* 32:1448–1459, 1986.

188. Optiz N, Lubbers DW: Theory and development of fluorescence-based optochemical oxygen sensors: oxygen optodes. *Internatl Anesthesiol Clin* 25:177–197, 1987.

189. Owen VM: Optical sensors in medicine. *Biosens Bioelectron* 9:xv–vi, 1994.

190. Peterson JL, Vurek GG: Fiber-optic sensors for biomedical applications. *Science* 224:123–127, 1984.

191. Regnault WF, Picciolo GL: Review of medical biosensors and associated materials problems. *J Biomed Nater Res: Appl Biomater* 21:163–180, 1987.

192. Robinson GA: Optical immunosensing systems—are they meeting market needs? *Biosens Bioelectron* 8:xxxvii–xxxx, 1993.

193. Rosen S: Biosensors: where do we go from here. *MLO* 27:24–29, 1995.

194. Scheper T, Müller C, Anders KD, et al: Optical sensors for biotechnological applications. *Biosens Bioelectron* 9:73–83, 1994.

195. Schultze JS: Biosensors. *Sci Am* 265:64–69, 1991.

196. Sethi RS: Transducer aspects of biosensors. *Biosens Bioelectron* 9:243–264, 1994.

197. Toffaletti J: Physiology and regulation: Ionized calcium, magnesium, and lactate measurements in critical care settings. Pathology Patterns. *Am J Clin Pathol* 104:S88–S94, 1995.

198. Walford S, Alberti KG: Biochemical self-monitoring: promise, practice and problems. *Contemp Issues Clin Biochem* 2:200–213, 1985.

199. Wang J, Naser N, Lopez D: Organic-phase biosensing of secondary alcohols with a Ta. brockii alcohol dehydrogenase electrode. *Biosens Bioelectron* 9:225–230, 1994.

200. Weetall HH: The biosensor technology program at the National Institute of Standards and Technology (NIST). *Biosens Bioelectron* 8:xii–xiii, 1993.

201. Widdowson G: Electrode technology in clinical chemistry today and tomorrow. *Lab Med* 19:483–489, 1988.

202. Wingard LB, Ferrance JP: Concepts, biological components, and scope of biosensors. *In* Wise DL, Wingard LB, eds: *Biosensors with Fiberoptics*. Clifton, NJ: Humana Press, 1991, pp. 1–27.

203. Wise DL, Wingard LB: Biosensors with Fiberoptics. Clifton, NJ: Humana Press, 1991.

204. Woo J, Henry JB: The advance of technology as a prelude to the laboratory of the twenty-first century. *Clin Lab Med* 14:459–472, 1994.

Glucose

205. Aalders AL, Schmidt FJ, Schoonen AJM, Broek IR, et al: Development of a wearable glucose sensor: studies in healthy volunteers and in diabetic patients. *Internatl J Artif Organs.* 14:102–108, 1991.

206. Abel P, Muller A, Fischer U: Experience with an implantable glucose sensor as a prerequisite of an artificial beta cell. *Biomed Biochim Acta* 43:577–584, 1984.

207. Aldhous P: Race quickens for non-stick blood monitoring technology. *Science* 258:892–893, 1992.

208. Allen BT, DeLong ER, Feussner JR: Impact of glucose self-monitoring on non-insulin-treated patients with type II diabetes mellitus. Randomized controlled trial comparing blood and urine testing. *Diabetes Care* 13:1044–1050, 1990.

209. Allen KR, Hamilton A, Bodansky J: Comparison of a new extra-laboratory reference method. *clin Chem News* 19:16, Jan 1993.

210. American Diabetes Association: Bedside blood glucose monitoring in hospitals. *Diabetes Care* 9:89, 1986.

211. American Diabetes Association: Consensus statement on self-monitoring of blood glucose. *Diabetes Care* 10:95–99, 1987.

212. American Diabetes Association: Self-monitoring of blood glucose. *Diabetes Care* 17:81–86, 1994.

213. Arnold MA: Can blood glucose be measured noninvasively by NIR spectroscopy? *Proc 14th Internatl Symp Blood Gases and Electrolytes,* Chatham, MA, 1992, pp. 3–6.

214. Ash SR, Poulos JT, Rainier JB, Zopp WE, Janle E, Kissinger PT: Subcutaneous capillary filtrate collector for measurement of blood glucose. *ASAIO* 38:M416–M420, 1992.

215. Ashworth L, Gibb I, Alberti KGMM: HemoCue: evaluation of a portable photometric system for determining glucose in whole blood. *Clin Chem* 38:1479–1482, 1992.

216. Atkin SH, Dasmahapatra A, Jaker MA, Chorost MI, Reddy S: Fingerstick glucose determination in shock. *Ann Intern Med* 114:1020–1024, 1991.

217. Atsushi S, Kimura J, Shionoya K, Kuriyama T: Continuous non-diluted serum sample measurements with an ISFET glucose sensor. *Biosens Bioelectron* 8:149–154, 1993.

218. Bachner P, Howanitz PJ, Jones BA: Bedside monitoring of glucose: Is better "bad"? [letter]. *Arch Pathol Lab Med* 118:594, 1994.

219. Baer DM, Petersen J, Belsey RE, Eyberg R: Bedside testing. Part 3. Quality management of bedside glucose testing. *MLO* 25:46–52, 1993.

220. Baer DM, Petersen J, Belsey RE, Eyberg R: Quality managemenet of bedside glucose teseting. *MLO* 25:46–58, 1993.

221. Ballerstädt R, Ehwald R: Suitability of aqueous dispersions of dextran and Concanavilin A for glucose sensing in different variants of the affinity sensor. *Biosens Bioelectron* 9:557–568, 1994.

222. Barr JT, Betschart J, Bracey A, et al: *Ancillary (Bedside) Blood Glucose Testing in Acute and Chronic Care Facilities.* Villanova, PA: National Committee for Clinical Laboratory Standards, Document C30-A, 1994.

223. Barreau P, Buttery JE: Effect of hematocrit concentration on blood glucose value determined on Glucometer II. *Diabetes Care* 11:116–118, 1988.

224. Barreau PB, Buttery JE: The effects of haematocrit value on the determination of glucose levels by reagent-strip methods. *Med J Austral* 147:286–288, 147.

225. Bataillard P, Steffgen E, Haemmerli S, Manz A, Widmer HM: An integrated silicon thermopile as biosensor for the thermal monitoring of glucose, urea and penicillin. *Biosens Bioelectron* 8:80–90, 1993.

226. Belsey R, Morrison JI, Whitlow KJ, et al: Managing bedside glucose testing in the hospital. *JAMA* 258:1634–1638, 1987.

227. Bernbaum M, Albert SG, McGinnis J, et al: Laboratory assessment of glucose meters does not predict reliability of clinical performance. *Lab Med* 25:32–34, 1994.

228. Beu DS: Hazards of inaccurate readings obtained by self-monitoring of blood glucose. [letter]. *Diabetes Care* 13:1131–1132, 1990.

229. Beyer J, Wolf, E, Cordes U, Hassinger W: The artificial beta cell (Biostator) in the adjustment of instable diabetics—results after 20 months. *Horm Metab Res* 8:127–131, 1979.

230. Bindra DS, Zhang Y, Wilson GS, et al: Design and in vitro studies of a needle-type glucose sensor for subcutaneous monitoring. *Anal Chem* 63:1692–1696, 1991.

231. Blood glucose monitoring in the emergency department. *J Emerg Nurs* 20:315–317, 1994.

232. Bolinder J, Frid A: Ultrasonic measurements of forearm subcutaneous adipose tissue thickness suitable for monitoring of subcutaneous glucose concentrations? [letter]. *Diabetes Care* 12:305–306, 1989.

233. Bruckel J, Kerner W, Zier H, et al: *In vivo* measurement of subcutaneous glucose concentrations with an enzymatic glucose sensor and a wick method. *Klin Wochenschr* 67:491–495, 1989.

234. Bruckel J, Zier H, Kerner W, Pfeiffer EF: Progress in practical endocrinology. The Glucosensor Unitec Ulm—a portable monitor for continuous blood glucose measurement. *Horm Metab Res* 22:382–384, 1990.

235. Burrin JM, Alberti KGMM: What is blood glucose: can it be measured. *Diabetic Med* 7:199–206, 1990.

236. Butler LA, Karp T, McCance KL, Ward RM: Neonatal glucose determinations obtained from an umbilical artery catheter: evaluation for accuracy using an in vitro model. *Neonatal Network* 12:31–35, 1993.

237. Campanella L, Mazzei F, Tomassetti M: Biosensor for direct determination of glucose and lactate in undiluted biological fluids. *Biosens Bioelectron* 8:307–314, 1993.

238. Campbell EM, Redman S, Dunkley PR, Moffitt PS: The use of portable blood glucose monitors by trained lay operators. *Med J Austra* 157:446–448, 1992.

239. Campbell LV, Ashwell SM, Borkman M, Chisholm DJ: White coat hyperglycaemia: disparity between diabetes clinic and home blood glucose concentrations. *Br Med J* 305:1194–1196, 1992.

240. Castellini MA, Castellini JM: Influence of hematocrit on whole blood glucose levels: new evidence from marine mammals. *Am J Physiol* 256:R1220–R1224, 1989.

241. Chabert MF, Verger P, Louis-Sylvestre J: A method for long-term and accurate measurement and recording of the blood glucose level in man. *Physiol Behav* 49:827–830, 1991.

242. Chen PT, Chen SS: Redox electrode for monitoring oxidase-catalyzed reactions. *Clin Chim Acta* 193:187–192, 1990.

243. Chun TY, Hirose M, Sawa T, et al: The effect of the partial pressure of oxygen on blood glucose concentration examined using glucose oxidase with ferricyan ion. *Anesth Analg* 79:993–997, 1994.

244. Colagiuri R, Colagiuri S, Jones S, Moses RG: The quality of self-monitoring of blood glucose. *Diabetic Med* 7:800–804, 1990.

245. Considine JM, Law T: Glucometers: accuracy and precision. Part II. Selection of a blood glucose monitor for standard hospital use. *J Ped Nurs* 8:193–196, 1993.

246. Csoregi E, Quinn CP, Schmidtke DW, et al: Design, characterization, and one-point in vivo calibration of a subcutaneously implanted glucose electrode. *Anal Chem* 66:3131–3138, 1994.

246a. Csoregi E, Schmidtke DW, Heller A: Design and optimization of a selective subcutaneous implantable glucose electrode based on "wired" glucose oxidase. *Anal Chem* 67:1240–1244, 1995.

247. De Boer J, Baarsma R, Okken A, Plijter-Groendijk H, Korf J: Applications of transcutaneous microdialysis and continuous flow analysis for on-line glucose monitoring in newborn infants. *J Lab Clin Med* 124:210–217, 1994.

248. De Boer J, Plijter-Groendijk H, Korf J: Microdialysis probe for transcutaneous monitoring of ethanol and glucose in humans. *J Appl Physiol* 75:2825–2830, 1993.

249. Degroote NE, Pieper B: Blood glucose monitoring at triage. *J Emerg Nurs* 41:55–58, 1993.

250. Diabetes Control and Complications Trial Research Group: The effect of intensive treatment of diabetes on the development and progression of long-term complications in insulin-dependent diabetes mellitus. *N Engl J Med* 329:977–986, 1993.

251. Edelman SV, Baloga J: Preliminary evaluation of a novel real-time blood glucose monitor. *Am Diab Assoc Scientific Sessions,* June 1994.

252. Fogh-Anderson N, Wimberley PD, Thode J, Siggaard-Andersen O: Direct reading glucose electrodes detect the molality of glucose in plasma and whole blood. *Clin Chim Acta* 189:33–38, 1990.

253. Frishman D, Ardito DM, Graham SM: Performance of glucose monitors. *Lab Med* 23:179–184, 1992.

254. Furbee JW Jr, Kuwant T, Kelly RS: Fractured carbon fiber-based biosensor for glucose. *Anal Chem* 66:1575–1577, 1994.

255. Genter PM, Ipp E: Accuracy of plasma glucose measurements in the hypoglycemic range. *Diabetes Care* 17:595–598, 1994.

256. Ghindilis Al, Kurochkin IN: Glucose potentiometric electrodes based on mediatorless bioelectrocatalysis. A new approach. *Biosens Bioelectron* 9:353–359, 1994.

257. Gilligan BJ, Shults MC, Rhodes RK, Updike SJ: Evaluatoin of a subcutaneous glucose sensor out to 3 months in a dog model. *Diabetes Care* 17:882–887, 1994.

258. Gough DA, Armour JC, Lucisano JY, McKean BD: Short term *in vivo* operation of a glucose sensor. *Trans Am Soc Artif Intern Organs* 32:148–150, 1986.

259. Gough JE, Jones JL, Garrison HG: Fingerstick detection of hypoglycemia can prevent dangerous doses of dextrose. *NC Med J* 53:466–467, 1992.

260. Greenough KR, Skillen AW, McNeil CJ: Potential glucose sensor for perioperative blood lucose control in diabetes mellitus. *Biosens Bioelectron* 9:23–28, 1994.

261. Greyson J: Quality control in patient self-monitoring of blood glucose. *Diabetes Care* 16:1306–1308, 1993.

262. Hagstrom E, Arner P, Engfeldt P, Rossner S, Bolinder J: *In vivo* subcutaneous adipose tissue glucose kinetics after glucose ingestion in obesity and fasting. *Scand J Clin Lab Invest* 50:129–136, 1990.

263. Halloran SP: Influence of blood oxygen tension on dipstick glucose determinations. *Clin Chem* 35:1268–1269, 1989.

264. Havlin CE, Parvin CA, Cryer PE: The accuracy of blood glucose monitoring devices. *Clin Diabetes* 92–93, Nov/Dec 1991.

264a. Heise HM, Marbach R, Koschinsky T, Gries FA: Noninvasive blood glucose sensors based on near-infrared spectroscopy. *Artificial Organs* 18:439–447, 1994.

264b. Heise HM, Marbach R, Janatsch G, Kruse-Jarres JD: Multivariate determination of glucose in whole blood by attenuated total reflection infrared spectroscopy. *Anal Chem* 61:2009–2015, 1989.

265. Ingram-Main R, Kiechle FL: Implementing a successful bedside glucose program. *MLO* 25:25–28, 1993.

266. Ito N, Kayashima S, Kimura J, et al: Development of a transcutaneous blood-constituent monitoring method using a suction effusion fluid collection technique and an ion-sensitive field-effect transistor glucose sensor. *Med Biol Eng Comput* 32:242–246, 1994.

267. Ito N, Saito A, Kuriyama T, et al: Development of a non-invasive transcutaneous blood glucose monitoring method using an ISFET biosensor. *Front Med Biol Eng* 4:35–45, 1992.

268. Jacobs E: The influence of hematocrit, uremia and hemodialysis on whole blood glucose analysis. *Lab Med.* 24:295–300, 1995.

269. James K, MacPhail G, Davis R: Evolving issues related to bedside glucose testing. *MLO* 22:31–36, 1990.

270. Johnson KW, Mastrototaro JJ, Howey DC, et al: *In vivo* evaluation of an electro-enzymatic glucose sensor implanted in subcutaneous tissue. *Biosens Bioelectron* 7:709–714, 1992.

271. Jones BA, Bachner P, Howanitz PJ: Bedside glucose monitoring: A College of American Pathologists Q-Probes study of the program characteristics and performance in 605 institutions. *Arch Pathol Lab Med* 117:1080–1087, 1993.

272. Jones BA: Testing at the patient's bedside. *Clinics Lab Med* 14:473–492, 1994.

273. Jurf JB, Outlaw EG: Designing and implementing a comprehensive quality assurance program for bedside glucose testing. *Diabetes Educ* 19:105–108, 1993.

274. Kaplan M, Blondheim O, Alon I, Eylath U, Trestian S, Eidelman AI: Screening for hypoglycemia with plasma in neonatal blood of high hematocrit value. *Crit Care Med* 17:279–282, 1989.

275. Kerner W, Kiwit M, Linke B, Keck FS, Zier H, Pfeiffer E: The function of a hydrogen peroxide-detecting electroenzymatic glucose electrode is markedly impaired in human subcutaneous tissue and plasma. *Biosens Bioelectron* 8:473–482, 1993.

276. Kiechle FL, Ingram-Main R: Bedside testing: beyond glucose. *MLO* 25:65–68, 1993.

277. Kiechle F, Ingram R, Karcher R, et al: Transfer of glucose measurements outside the laboratory. *Lab Med* 21:504–511, 1990.

278. Kimura J: Noninvasive blood glucose concentration monitoring method with suction effusion fluid by IFSET biosensor. *Appl Biochem Biotechnol* 41:55–58, 1993.

279. Kinghorn HA: Quality control measures in glucose monitoring [letter]. *Diabetes Care* 15:1824, 1992.

280. Kishimoto M, Kawamori R, Kubota M, et al: Clinical usefulness of a non-wiping type glucose meter in diabetic patients. *Diabetes Res Clin Pract* 20:47–50, 1993.

281. Kisner HJ: Glucose monitoring—from fingersticks to Star Trek. *Clin Lab Management Rev* 7:336–338, 1993.

282. Kontschieder H, Ritter C, Grubler R, et al: On-line monitoring of subcutaneous tissue glucose concentration for glucose control in diabetic patients. *7th European*

Congress on Intensive Care Medicine, Innsbruck, Austria. Poster presentation. June 1994.

283. Kost GJ, Wiese DA, Bowen TP: New whole blood methods and instruments: glucose measurement and test menus for critical care. *J Internatl Fed Clin Chem* 3:160–172, 1991.

284. Koudelka M, Rohner-Jeanrenaud F, Terrettaz J, et al: In-vivo behavior of hypodermically implanted microfabricated glucose sensors. *Biosens Bioelectron* 6:31–36, 1991.

285. Kreitzer MJ, Marko M, Nettles A: Implementation of a quality improvement program for a bedside blood glucose testing system: a collaborative endeavor. *J Nurs Care Qual* Suppl:1–11, 1992.

286. Kucler MA, Goormastic M, Hoogwerf BJ: Influence of frequency, time interval from initial instruction, and method of instruction on performance competency for blood glucose monitoring. *Diabetes Care* 13:488–491, 1990.

287. Kulys J, Hansen HE: Carbon-paste biosensors array for long-term glucose measurement. *Biosens Bioelectron* 9:491–500, 1994.

288. Lager W, von Lucadou I, Nischik, et al: Electrocatalytic glucose sensor for long-term in vivo use. *Internatl J Artif Organs* 17:183–188, 1994.

289. Lager W, von Lucadou I, Preidel W, Ruprecht L, Saeger S: Electrocatalytic glucose sensor. *Med Biol Eng Comput* 32:247–252, 1994.

290. Lawrence PA, Dowe MC, Perry EK, Strong S, Samsa GP: Accuracy of nurses in performing capillary blood glucose monitoring. *Diabetes Care* 12:298–301, 1989.

291. Letellier G: Biochemical diagnosis and monitoring of diabetes: a laboratory perspective for the nineties. *Clin Biochem* 26:320–323, 1993.

292. Lewandrowski K, Cheek R, Nathan DM, et al: Implementation of capillary blood glucose monitoring in a teaching hospital and determination of program requirements to maintain quality testing. *Am J Med* 93:419–426, 1992.

293. Lin HC, Maguire C, Oh W, Cowett R: Clinical and laboratory observations: accuracy and reliability of glucose reflectance meters in the high-risk neonate. *J Ped* 115:990–1000, 1989.

294. Linke B, Kener W, Kiwit M, Pishko M, Heller A: Amperometric biosensor for in vivo glucose sensing based on glucose oxidase immobilized in a redox hydrogel. *Biosens Bioelectron* 9:151–158, 1994.

295. Luxton GC: Diabetes monitoring with out-of-laboratory tests. *Clin Biochem* 26:19–20, 1993.

296. Male KB, Luong JHT: Improvement of the selectivity of an FIA amperometric biosensor system for glucose. *Biosens Bioelectron* 8:239–248, 1993.

296a. Maley TC, D'Orazio P: Biosensors for blood glucose: A new question of what is measured and what should be reported. *Clin Chem News.* 1995;21(1):12–13.

297. Marcinkeviciene J, Kulys J: Bienzyme strip-type glucose sensor. *Biosens Bioelectron* 8:209–212, 1993.

297a. Maser RE, Butler MA, DeCherney GS: Use of arterial blood with bedside glucose reflectance meters in an intensive care unit: Are they accurate? *Crit Care Med* 22:595–599, 1994.

298. Matthews DR, Bown E, Bech TW, et al: An amperometric needle-type glucose sensor tested in rats and man. *Diabetic Med* 5:248–252, 1988.

299. Meehan CD, Silvestri A, Street ED: Improving blood glucose monitoring in a hospital setting using the PDCA approach. Plan, do, check, act cycle. *J Nurs Care Qual* 7:56–63, 1993.

299a. Mendelson Y, Clermont AC, Peura RA, et al: Blood glucose measurement by multiple attenuated total reflection and infrared absorption. *IEEE Trans Biomed Engr* 37:458–465, 1990.

300. Meters for measuring blood glucose at home. *Drug Ther Bull* 31:30–32, 1993.

301. Mizutani F, Yabuki S: Flow injection analysis for glucose using an amperometric enzyme electrode based on lipid-modified glucose oxidase as the detector. *Biosens Bioelectron* 9:411–414, 1994.

302. Moatti-Sirat D, Capron F, Poitout V, et al: Towards continuous glucose monitoring: *in vivo* evaluation of a miniaturized glucose sensor implanted for several days in rat subcutaneous tissue. *Diabetologia* 35:224–230, 1992.

303. Moatti-Sirat D, Poitout V, Thome V, et al: Reduction of acetaminophen interference in glucose sensors by a composite Nafion membrane: demonstration in rats and man. *Diabetologia* 37:610–616, 1994.

304. Moatti-Sirat D, Velho G, Reach G: Evaluating *in vitro* and *in vivo* the interference of ascorbate and acetaminophen on glucose detection by a needle-type glucose sensor. *Biosens Bioelectron* 7:345–352, 1992.

305. Moberg E, Lundblad S, Lins PE, Adamson U: How accurate are home blood-glucose meters with special respect to the low glycemic range? *Diabetes Res Clin Prac* 19:239–243, 1993.

306. Moussy F, Harrison DJ, Rajotte RV: A miniaturized Nafion-based glucose sensor: *in vitro* and *in vivo* evaluation in dogs. *Internatl J Artif Organs* 17:88–94, 1994.

307. Nichols JH, Howard C, Loman K, et al: Laboratory and bedside evaluation of portable glucose meters. *Am J Clin Pathol* 103:244–251, 1995.

308. Page SR, Peacock I: Blood glucose monitoring: Does technology help? *Diabetic Med* 10:793–801, 1993.

309. Palleschi G, Mascini M, Bernardi L, Zeppilli P: Lactate and glucose electrochemical biosensors for the evaluation of the aerobic and anaerobic threshold in runners. *Med Biol Eng Comput* 28:B25–B28, 1990.

310. Pandey PC, Glazier S, Weetall HH: An amperometric flow-injection analysis biosensor for glucose based on graphite paste modified with tetracyanoquinodimethane. *Anal Biochem* 214:233–237, 1993.

311. Patrick AW, Gill GV, MacFarlane IA, Cullen A, Power E, Wallymahmed M: Home glucose monitoring in type 2 diabetes: is it a waste of time? *Diabetic Med* 11:62–65, 1994.

312. Peterson KA, Peterson AM, Corbett V, Tongen S, Guzman M, Mazze R: Comparison of home glucose monitoring with the oral glucose tolerance test to detect gestational glucose intolerance. *J Fam Pract* 39:558–563, 1994.

313. Pfeiffer EF: On the way to the automated (blood) glucose regulation in diabetes: the dark past, the grey present and the rosy future. *Diabetologia* 30:51–65, 1987.

314. Pfeiffer EF: The glucose sensor: the missing link in diabetes therapy. *Hormone Metabol Res* 24:154–164, 1990.

315. Phillipou G, Farrant RK, Phillips PJ: Computer based quality assessment of hospital capillary blood glucose monitoring. *Diabetic Med* 7:234–237, 1990.

316. Pickup JC, Shaw GW, Claremont DJ: *In vivo* molecular sensing in diabetes mellitus: an implantable glucose sensor with direct electron transfer. *Diabetologia* 32:213–217, 1989.

317. Poitout V, Moatti-Sirat D, Reach G, Zhang Y, Wilson GS, Lemonnier F, Klein JC: A glucose monitoring system for on line estimation in man of blood glucose concentration using a miniaturized glucose sensor implanted in the subcutaneous tissue and a wearable control unit. *Diabetologia* 36:658–663, 1993.

318. Proposed strategies for reducing user error in capillary blood glucose monitoring. The National Steering Committee for Quality Assurance in Capillary Blood Glucose Monitoring. *Diabetes Care* 16:493–498, 1993.

319. Rainey PM, Jatlow P: Monitoring blood glucose meters. *Am J Clin Pathol* 103:125–126, 1995.

320. Rao G, Glikfeld P, Guy RH: Reverse iontophoresis: development of a noninvasive approach for glucose monitoring. *Pharmaceutical Res* 10:1751–1755, 1993.

321. Reach G, Wilson GS: Can continuous glucose monitoring be used for the treatment of diabetes? *Analyt Chem* 64:381A–386A, 1992.

322. Reynolds ER, Yacynych AM: Direct sensing platinum ultramicrobiosensors for glucose. *Biosens Bioelectron* 9:283–293, 1994.

323. Rhodes RK, Shults MC, Updike SJ: Prediction of pocket-portable and implantable glucose enzyme electrode performance from combined species permeability and digtal stimulation analysis. *Anal Chem* 66:1520–1529, 1994.

324. Robinson MR, Eaton RP, Haaland DM, et al: Noninvasive glucose monitoring in diabetic patients: a preliminary evaluation. *Clin Chem* 38:1618–1622, 1992.

325. Robinson RJ, McDonald SD: Glucose-sensitive membrane and infrared absorption spectroscopy for potential use as an implantable glucose sensor. *ASAIO J* 38:M458–M462, 1992.

326. Rosenthal RD, Paynter LN: Investigation of non-invasive measurement of blood glucose. *Proc Internatl Diabetes Federation Congress,* 1991, pp. 1–6.

327. Ross D, Heinemann L, Chantelau EA: Short-term evaluation of an electro-chemical system (ExacTech) for blood glucose monitoring. *Diabetes Res Clin Pract* 10:281–285, 1990.

328. Schmidt FJ, Aalders AL, Schoonen AJM, Doorenbos H: Calibration of a wearable glucose sensor. *Internatl J Artif Organs* 15:55–61, 1992.

329. Schmidt FJ, Sluiter WJ, Schoonen AJM: Glucose concentration in subcutaneous extracellular space. *Diabetes Care* 16:695–700, 1993.

330. Schoonen AJM, Schmidt FJ, Hasper H, et al: Development of a potentially wearable glucose sensor for patients with diabetes mellitus: design and *in vitro* evaluation. *Biosens Bioelectron* 5:37–46, 1990.

331. Shaffar BP, Wolfbeis OS: A fast responding fibre optic glucose biosensor based on an oxygen optrode. *Biosens Bioelectron* 5:137–148, 1990.

332. Sharp S: Blood glucose monitoring in the intensive care unit. *Br J Nurs* 10:209–214, 1993.

333. Shaw GW, Claremont DJ, Pickup JC: *In vitro* testing of a simply constructed, highly stable glucose sensor suitable for implantation in diabetic patients. *Biosens Bioelectron* 6:401–406, 1991.

334. Shichiri M, Asakawa N, Yamasaki Y, et al: Telemetry glucose monitoring device with needle type glucose sensor: a useful tool for blood glucose monitoring in diabetic individuals. *Diabetes Care* 9:298–301, 1986.

335. Shtelzer S, Braun S: An optical biosensor based upon glucose oxidase immobilized in sol-gel silicate matrix. *Biotechnol Appl Biochem* 19:293–305, 1994.

336. Shults MC, Rhodes RK, Updike SJ, Gilligan BJ, Reining WN: A telemetry-instrumentation system for monitoring multiple subcutaneously implanted glucose sensors. *IEEE Trans Biomed Eng* 41:937–942, 1994.

337. Sidebottom RA, Williams PR, Kanarek KS: Glucose determination in plasma and serum: potential error related to increased hematocrit. *Clin Chem* 28:190–192, 1982.

338. Skrabal F, Kontschieder H, Kotanko P, et al: A portable insulin pump with continuous measurements of subcutaneous tissue glucose using open tissue perfusion. *Diabetes* 42:249A, 1993.

339. Snorgaard O, Binder C: Monitoring of blood glucose concentration in subjects with hypoglycaemic symptoms during everyday life. *Br Med J* 300:16–18, 1990.

340. Speicher CE: The bottom line. Can portable blood glucose monitoring improve the outcomes of diabetic patients? *Am J Clin Pathol* 95:112–116, 1991.

341. Sridhar GR: Portable blood glucose monitoring devices [letter]. *J Assoc Physicians India* 40:642, 1992.

342. Sternberg F, Meyerhoff C, Mehnel FJ, Bischof F, Mayer H, Pfeiffer EF: Comments on subcutaneous glucose monitoring. *Diabetologia* 37:540–542, 1994.

342a. Sylvain HF, Pokorny SM, English SM, et al: Accuracy of fingerstick glucose values in shock patients. *Am J Crit Care* 4:44–48, 1995.

343. Tate PF, Clements CA, Walters JE: Accuracy of home blood glucose monitors. *Diabetes Care* 15:536–538, 1992.

344. Tattersall R: Self monitoring of blood glucose concentrations by non-insulin dependent diabetic patients. *Br Med J* 305:1171–1172, 1992.

345. Taylor HM, Mujoomdar A: Bedside testing of the blood glucose level in neonates: What to use? [letter]. *Can Med Assoc J* 142:802, 1990.

346. Ting C, Nanji AA: Evaluation of the quality of bedside monitoring of the blood glucose level in a teaching hospital. *Can Med Assoc J* 138:23–26, 1988.

347. Trovati M, Burzacca S, Mularoni E, et al: Occurrence of low blood glucose concentrations during the afternoon in type 2 (non-insulin-dependent) diabetic patients on oral hypoglycaemic agents: importance of blood glucose monitoring. *Diabetologia* 34:662–667, 1991.

348. Turner RFB, Harrison DJ, Rajotte RV, Baltes HP: A biocompatible enzyme electrode for continuous *in vivo* glucose monitoring in whole blood. *Sensors Actuators B (Chemical)* B1:561–564, 1990.

349. Updike J, Shults MC, Rhodes RK, Gilligan BJ, Luebow JO, von Heimburg D: Enzymatic glucose sensors. Improved long-term performance *in vitro* and *in vivo*. *ASAIOI J* 40:157–163, 1994.

350. Vadasdi E, Jacobs E: HemoCue β-glucose photometer evaluated for use in a neonatal intensive care unit. *Clin Chem* 39:2329–2332, 1993.

351. Vaidya R, Wilkins E: Use of charged membranes to control interference by chemicals in a glucose biosensor. *Med Eng Phys* 16:416–421, 1994.

352. Vallera DA, Bissel MG, Barron W: Accuracy of portable blood glucose monitoring. Effect of glucose level and prandial state. *Am J Clin Pathol* 95:247–252, 1991.

353. Velho G, Froguel P, Thevenot DR, Reach G: Strategies for calibrating a subcutaneous glucose sensor. *Biomed Biochim Acta* 48:957–964, 1989.

354. von Woedtke T, Fischer U, Abel P: Glucose oxidase electrodes: effect of hydrogen peroxide on enzyme activity? *Biosens Bioelectron* 9:65–71, 1994.

355. von Woedtke T, Fischer U, Brunstein E, et al: Implantable glucose sensors: comparison between *in vitro* and *in vivo* kinetics. *Internatl J Artif Organs* 14:473–481, 1991.

356. von Woedtke T, Rebrin K, Fischer U, et al: *In situ* calibration of implanted electrochemical glucose sensors. *Biomed Biochim Acta* 48:943–952, 1989.

357. Walker EA: Quality assurance for blood glucose monitoring. The balance of feasibility and standards. *Nurs Clin N Am* 28:61–70, 1993.

358. Walker EA: The clinical utility of capillary blood glucose monitoring in the 1990s. *Connecticut Med* 55:637–640, 1991.

359. Walker EA, Paduano DJ, Shamoon H: Quality assurance for blood glucose monitoring in health-care facilities. *Diabetes Care* 14:1043–1049, 1991.

360. Wandrup J, Vadstrup S: Amperometric determinations of glucose in whole blood by the YSI 23AM analyzer. *Clin Chem* 36:1260–1261, 1990.

361. Watts NB: Bedside monitoring of blood glucose in hospitals: Speed vs precision and accuracy. *Arch Pathol Lab Med* 117:1078–1079, 1993.

362. Weiss SL, Cembrowski GS, Mazze RS: Patient and physician analytic goals for self-monitoring blood glucose instruments. *Am J Clin Pathol* 102:611–615, 1994.

363. Whalen F: An outreach program for home glucose monitoring. *MLO* 26:44–46, 1994.

364. Wiener K: An assessment of the effect of haematocrit on the HemoCue blood glucose analyser. *Ann Clin Biochem* 30:90–93, 1993.

365. Wiese DA, Bowen TP, Kost GJ: Enzyme electrode for glucose measurement in whole blood with a critical care profiling instrument. *Clin Chem* 35:1098, 1989.

366. Wilson GS, Zhang Y, Reach G, et al: Progress toward the development of an implantable sensor for glucose. *Clin Chem* 38:1613–1617, 1992.

367. Wimberley PD, Burnett RW, Covington AK, et al: Guidelines for transcutaneous PO_2 and PCO_2 measurement. *J Internatl Fed Clin Chem* 2:128–135, 1990.

368. Winkelman JW, Wybenga DR, Tanasivevic MJ: The fiscal consequences of central vs distributed testing of glucose. *Clin Chem* 40:1628–1630, 1994.

369. Zhang Y, Hu Y, Wilson GS, Moatti-Sirat D, Poitout V, Reach G: Elimination of the acetaminophen interference in an implantable glucose sensor. *Anal Chem* 66:1183–1188, 1994.

370. Zhu J, Tian C, Wu W, et al: Fabrication and characterization of glucose sensors based on a microarray H_2O_2 electrode. *Biosens Bioelectron* 9:295–300, 1994.

371. Zier H, Kerner W, Bruckel J, Pfeiffer EF: "Glucosensor Unitec Ulm." A portable, continuously measuring glucose sensor and monitor. *Biomedizinische Technik* 35:2–4, 1990.

Guidelines, Accreditation, and Quality

372. Barker SJ, Hyatt J, Shah NK, Kao YJ: The effect of sensor malpositioning on pulse oximeter accuracy during hypoxemia. *Anesthesia* 79:248–254, 1993.

373. Belanger AC: Point-of-care testing: The JCAHO perspective. *MLO* 26:46–49, 1994.

374. Biswas CK, Ramos JM, Agroyannis B, et al: Blood gas analysis: effect of air bubbles in syringe and delay in estimation. *Br Med J* 284:923–927, 1982.

375. Bland JM, Altman DG: Statistical methods for assessing agreement between two methods of clinical measurement. *Lancet* 1:307–310, 1986.

376. Boink ABTJ, Buckley BM, Christiansen TF, et al: IFCC recommendation on sampling, transport and storage for the determination of the concentration of ionized calcium in whole blood, plasma, and serum. *Ann Biol Clin* 49:434–438, 1991; *Clin Chim Acta* 202:S13–S22, 1991; *Eur J Clin Chem Clin Biochem* 29:767–772, 1991; *J Internatl Fed Clin Chem* 4:147–152, 1992.

377. Burnett RW, Covington AK, Fogh-Andersen N, et al: Recommendations on whole blood sampling, transport, and storage for simultaneous determination of pH, blood gases, and electrolytes. International Federation of Clinical Chemistry Scientific Division. *J Internatl Fed Clin Chem* 6:115–120, 1994.

378. Clausen JL, Murray KM: Clinical applications of arterial blood gases: How much accuracy do we need? *J Med Tech* 2:19–32, 1985.

379. Clinical Laboratory Improvement Amendments of 1988; Final Rule. *Federal Register.* 57(40):7008, 1992.

380. Clinical Laboratory Improvement Amendments of 1988; Final Rule. *Federal Register.* 57(40):7158, 1992.

381. Ehrmeyer SS, Laessig RH: Regulatory requirements (CLIA '88, JCAHO, CAP) for decentralized testing. *Pathol Patterns, Am J Clin Pathol* 104:S40–S49, 1995.

382. Eichorn J, Moran R, Cormier A: Blood gas pre-analytical considerations: specimen collection, calibration and control. *National Committee for Clinical Laboratory Standards* (NCCLS) Publication C-27, Villanova, PA, 1985.

383. Goldsmith BM, Travers EM, Bakes-Martin R, et al: *Point-of-Care in Vitro Diagnostic (IVD) Testing.* Villanova, Pennsylvania: National Committee for Clinical Laboratory Standards, Document AST2. (Proposed version, 1994; approved version, 1995.)

384. Graham GA, Bergkuist C, Cormier AD, et al: *Ionized Calcium Determinations: Precollection Variables, Specimen Choice, Collection, and Handling.* Villanova, Pennsylvania: National Committee for Clinical Laboratory Standards, Document C31, 1993.

385. Hamlin WB: Regulatory and accreditation implications of alternate-site laboratory testing. *Clin Lab Med* 14:605–662, 1994.

386. Handorf CR: Quality control and quality management of alternate-site testing. *Clin Lab Med* 14:539–558, 1994.

387. Herring K, McLellan W, Plaut D: QC and new technology: Do the old rules still apply? 25(9S):7–15, 1993.

388. Jacobs E: Total quality management and point-of-care testing. *MLO* 25(9S):2–6, 1993.

389. JCAHO: HAP (Hospital Accreditation Program) scoring guidelines: Decentralized laboratory testing standards. *Joint Commission Perspectives* 10:A15–A17, Jan/Feb 1990.

389a. Kost GJ: Discrimination and other statistical intervals for the interpretation of *in vivo* patient monitoring data. *Statistics Med* 5:347–354, 1986.

390. Kost GJ, Evans BD, Biltz JH, et al: Pattern recognition ("fingerprinting") for continuous quality improvement of point-of-care whole blood testing. *Proc Oak Ridge Conf Advanced Analytical Concepts for the Clinical Laboratory* No. 20, 1992.

390a. Kost GJ, Inn M, Johnson T: Regression workstation for clinical chemistry method evaluation. *Clin Chem* 39:1547–1548, 1993.

391. Kost GJ: Guidelines for point-of-care testing. *Proc Society of Critical Care Medicine Educational and Scientific Symposium.* 24:8, 1995; audio recording. Palm Desert, CA: Convention Cassettes Unlimited.

391a. Kost GJ: Guidelines for point-of-care testing: Improving patient outcomes. *Pathol Patterns (Am J Clin Pathol)* 104:S111–S127, 1995.

392. La Manta KR, O'Connor T, Barash PG: Comparing methods of measurement: an alternative approach. *J Anesth* 72:781–783, 1990.

393. Moran RF, Bergkuist C, Graham GA, Misiano DR, O'Connell KO, Sena SF: *Considerations in the Simultaneous Measurement of Blood Gases, Electrolytes, and Related Analytes in Whole Blood.* Villanova, Pennsylvania: National Committee for Clinical Laboratory Standards, Document C32, 1993.

394. Nani AA, Poon R, Hinberg I: Decentralized clinical chemistry testing: quality of results obtained by residents and interns in an acute care setting. *J Intern Care Med* 3:272–277, 1988.

395. Nanji AA, Poon R, Hinberg I: Quality of laboratory test results obtained by nontechnical personnel in a decentralized setting. *Am J Clin Pathol* 89:797–801, 1988.

396. Nickel K: *Emergency Regulations for Point-of-Care Testing.* Lab Field Services, Dept Health Services, State of California, 2151 Berkeley Way, Berkeley, CA 94704, Dec 27, 1994.

397. Pickup JC, Alcock S: Clinicians' requirements for chemical sensors for *in vivo* monitoring: a multinational survey. *Biosens Bioelectron* 6:639–646, 1991.

398. Pikul FJ: CLIA and point-of-care testing. *MLO* 25(9S):42–47, 1993.

399. Sasse SA, Chen PA, Mahutte CK: Variability of arterial blood gas values over time in stable medical ICU patients. *Chest* 106:187–193, 1994.

400. Shapiro BA: Quality improvement standards for intensive care unit monitors: we must be informed and involved. *Crit Care Med* 20:1629–1630, 1992.

401. Thorson SH, Marini JJ, Pierson DJ, et al: Variability of arterial blood gas values in stable patients in the ICU. *Chest* 84:14–18, 1983.

402. Van Woerkens EC, Trouwborst A, Tenbrinck R: Accuracy of a mixed venous saturation catheter during acutely induced changes in hematocrit in humans. *Crit Care Med* 19:1025–1029, 1991.

403. Vanderlinde RE, Goodwin J, Koch D, et al: *Guidelines for Providing Quality Stat Laboratory Services.* Washington, DC: American Association for Clinical Chemistry Press, 1987.

404. Winckers EK, Teunissen AJ, Van den Camp RA, et al: A comparative study of the electrode systems of three pH and blood gas apparatus. *J Clin Chem Biochem* 16:175–185, 1978.

In Vitro, Ex Vivo and In Vivo Systems

405. Abraham E, Gallagher TJ, and Fink S: Clinical evaluation of a multiparameter intraarterial blood gas sensor. *Crit Care Med* 22:A60, 1994.

406. Alcock J: Advances in the use of in-vivo sensors. *Biosens Bioelectron* 7:243–254, 1992.

407. Alcock SJ, Karayannis M, Turner APF: The design and development of new chemical sensors for *in vivo* monitoring. *Biosens Bioelectron* 6:647–652, 1991.

408. Anderson JR, East TD, Coombs J, et al: Clinical trial of a non-linear closed-loop controller for oxygenation during ARDS. *Crit Care Med* 22:A188, 1994.

409. Arnold WP: Perioperative biochemical monitors. *In* Lake CL, ed: *Clinical Monitoring for Anesthesia and Critical Care*. Philadelphia: Saunders, 1994, pp. 539–560.

410. Auger WR, Hoyt DB, Wayne F, et al: Continuous cardiac output/mixed venous O_2 monitoring system—a comparative evaluation in critically ill patients. *Crit Care Med* 22:A190, 1994.

411. Baele PL, McMichan JC, Marsh HM, et al: Continuous monitoring of mixed venous oxygen saturation in critically ill patients. *Anesth Analg* 61:513–517, 1982.

412. Barrera R, Loiacono J, Groeger JS, Carlon GC: Evaluaton of an intra-arterial blood gas monitor in mechanically ventilated patients. *Anesthesia* 81(3A):A615, 1994.

413. Bashein G, Greydanus WK, Kenny MA: Evaluation of a blood gas and chemistry monitor for use during surgery. *Anesthesia* 70:123–127, 1989.

414. Bashein G, Pino JA, Nessly ML, Kenny MA, et al: Clinical assessment of a flow-through fluorometric blood gas monitor. *J Clin Monit* 4:195–203, 1988.

415. Battersby CM, Vadgama P: A lactate needle enzyme electrode for whole blood measurement. *Diab Nutr Metab* 1:43–48, 1988.

416. Bearden E, Lopez, JA, Solis RT: Evaluation of a continuous intra-arterial blood gas sensor in critically ill patients. *Crit Care Med* 22:A25, 1994.

417. Boycks E, Michaels S, Weil MH, Shubin H, Marbach EP: Continuous-flow measurement of lactate in blood: a technique adapted for use in the emergency room. *Clin Chem* 21:113–118, 1975.

418. Bratanow N, Polk K, Bland R, et al: Continuous polarographic monitoring of intra-arterial oxygen in the perioperative period. *Crit Care Med* 13:859–860, 1985.

419. Bucholz F, Buschmann N: A fibre-optical sensor for the determination of sodium with a reversible response. *Sensors Actuators B* 9:41–47, 1992.

420. Chicoine RE, Gettinger A, Polito F, Fairweather RB: Reproducibility of laboratory results from a whole-blood analyzer in the ICU: effect of Sample Size. *Crit Care Med* 22:A29, 1995.

421. *Ciba-Corning 800 Series Operator Manual*. Ciba-Corning Diagnostics, Medfield, MA. *NOVA Biomedical Stat Profile Series Operator Manual*. NOVA Biomedical, Waltham, MA. Other whole-blood analyzer operator manuals.

422. Clark CL, O'Brien J, McCulloch J, et al: Early clinical experience with Gas-STAT. *J Extra-Corporeal Technol* 18:185–189, 1986.

423. Clark LC: Monitor and control of blood and tissue oxygen tensions. *Trans Am Soc Artif Intern Organs* 2:41–45, 1956.

424. Cole JS, Martin WE, Cheung PW, Johnson CC: Clinical studies with a solid state fiberoptic oximeter. *Am J Cardiol* 29:383–388, 1972.

425. Collison ME, Aebli GV, Petty J, Meyerhoff ME: Potentiometric combination ion/carbon dioxide sensors for in vitro and in vivo blood measurements. *Anal Chem* 61:2365–2372, 1989.

426. Coughlan ME, Alcock SJ: Chemical sensors for in vivo monitoring: packaging, biocompatibility, stability. *Biosens Bioelectron* 6:87–91, 1991.

427. Crespi F: In vivo voltammetry with micro-biosensors for analysis of neurotransmitter release and metabolism. *J Neurosci Meth* 34:53–65, 1990.

428. Dechert RE, Arnoldi D, Giacherio D, Bartlett, R: Evaluation of the GEM-Premier combined blood gas and electrolyte analyzer for point-of-care (POC) testing. *Crit Care Med Sci Poster Session* 22:A24, 1994.

429. Divers S: Advances in intra-arterial blood gas sesors. *Proc 14th Internatl Symp Blood Gases and Electrolytes,* Chatham, MA, 1992, pp. 4–2.

430. Enson Y, Briscoe WA, Polanyi ML, et al: *In vivo* studies with an intravascular and intracardiac reflection oximeter. *J Appl Physiol* 17:552–558, 1962.

431. Erickson KA, Wilding P: Evaluaton of a novel point-of-care system, the i-STAT portable clinical analyzer. *Clin Chem* 39:283–287, 1993.

432. Fahey PJ, Harris K, Vanderwarf C: Clinical experience with continuous monitoring of mixed venous oxygen saturation in respiratory failure. *Chest* 86:748–752, 1984.

433. Fennema M, van Krugten RJ, de Boer HJ, Prakash O, Erdman W: Continuous intra-arterial pO_2 monitoring during thoracic surgery. *Adv Exper Med Biol* 316:75–83, 1992.

434. Fogt EJ: Continuous ex vivo and in vivo monitoring with chemical sensors. *Clin Chem* 36:1573–1580, 1990.

435. Franklin M, Peruzzi W, Shapiro B: Evaluation of a rapid, intermittent on-demand bedside blood gas monitor on pulmonary artery blood. *Crit Care Med* 22:A23, 1994.

436. Gettinger A, DeTraglia MC, Glass DD: *In vivo* comparison of two mixed venous saturation catheters. *Anesthesia* 66:373–375, 1987.

437. Gong AK: Near-patient measurements of methemoglobin, oxygen saturation, and total hemoglobin: evaluation of a new instrument for adult and neonatal intensive care. *Crit Care Med* 23:193–201, 1995.

438. Gottlieb A, Divers S, Hui HK: *In vivo* applications of fiberoptic chemical sensors. *In* Wise DL, Wingard LB, eds: *Biosensors with Fiberoptics.* Clifton, NJ: Humana Press, 1991, pp. 325–367.

439. Greenblott GB, Tremper KK, Barker S, Gershultz S, Gehrich JL: Continuous blood gas monitoring with an intraarterial optode during one-lung anesthesia. *J Cardiothor Vasc Anesth* 5:365–367, 1991.

440. Groh J, Haller M, Kilger E, et al: Continuous blood gas monitoring during lung transplantation. *Anesthesiology* 81(3A):A617, 1994.

441. Hakanson H, Kyrolainen M, Mattiasson B: Portable system for continiuous ex vivo measurements of lactate. *Biosens Bioelectron* 8:213–218, 1993.

442. Halbert SA: Intravascular monitoring: problems and promise. *Clin Chem* 36:1581–1584, 1990.

443. Haller M, Kilger E, Briegel J, Forest H, Peter K: Continuous intra-arterial blood gas and pH monitoring in critically ill patients with severe respiratory failure: a prospective, criterion standard study. *Crit Care Med* 22:580–587, 1994.

444. Hansmann DR, Gehrich JL: Practial perspectives on the in-vitro and in-vivo evaluation of a fiber optic blood gas sensor. Optical Fibers in Medicine III; *Proc Soc Photo-Optical Instrumentation Engineers (SPIE)* 906:4–10, 1988.

445. Harloff M: Continuous blood gas monitoring using the CDI System 300. *J Extra-Corporeal Technol* 23:27–30, 1992.

446. Jacobs E, Nowakowski M, Colman N: Performance of Gem Premier blood gas/electrolyte analyzer evaluated. *Clin Chem* 39:1890–1893, 1993.

447. Jacobs E, Vadasdi E, Sarkozi L, Colman N: Analytical evaluation of i-STAT portable clinical analyzer and use by nonlaboratory health-care professionals. *Clin Chem* 39:1069–1074, 1993.

447a. Janle EM, Kissinger PT: Implanted sensors for glucose monitoring: a status report. *Clin Chem News* 21:10–11, 1995.

448. Jaquith SM: The Oximetrix Opticath: What is it and how can it facilitate nursing management of the critically ill patient? *Crit Care Nurs* 4:1–4, 1984.

449. Johnson FW, Burns DM, Kinninger KK, et al: Clinical evaluation of continuous intra-arterial blood gas monitor in hypoxic, hypercapnic and hypocapnic patients. *Crit Care Med* 22:A190, 1994.

450. Katayama M, Murray GC, Uchida T, et al: Intra-arterial continuous PO_2 monitoring by an ultra-fine microelectrode. *Crit Care Med* 15:A357, 1987.

451. Kilger E, Haller M, Briegel J, et al: Long term evaluation of a continuous intra-arterial blood gas monitor in critically ill patients. *Anesthesia* 81(3A):A613, 1994.

452. Kisner HJ: Talking about Technology. Mallinckrodt sensor systems GEM Premier. *Clin Lab Management Rev* 363–367, July/Aug 1994.

453. Kisner HJ: Talking about technology. i-STAT point-of-care blood analyzing system. *Clin Lab Management Rev* 454–457, Sept/Oct 1993.

454. Kost GJ: New whole blood analyzers and their impact on cardiac and critical care. *Crit Rev Clin Lab Sci* 30:153–202, 1993.

455. Krauss XH, Verdouw PD, Hugenholtz PG, Nauta J: On-line monitoring of mixed venous oxygen saturation after cardiothoracic surgery. *Thorax* 30:636–643, 1975.

456. Krouskop RW, Cabatu EE, Chelliah BP, et al: Accuracy and clinical utility of an oxygen saturation catheter. *Crit Care Med* 11:744–749, 1983.

457. Lake CL: Monitoring: history and philosophy. *In* Lake CL, ed: *Clinical Monitoring for Anesthesia and Critical Care.* Philadelphia: Saunders, 1994, pp. 2–10.

458. Larsson CP, Vender J, Seiver A: Multisite evaluation of a continuous intraarterial blood gas monitoring system. *Anesthesia* 81:543–552, 1994.

459. Larsson CP: Clinical experience with an intra-arterial blood gas monitor. *Proc 14th Internatl Symp Blood Gases and Electrolytes,* Chatham, MA, 1992, p. 4-3.

460. Lemus JF, Kearney T, Margulies DR, et al: Continuous intra-arterial oxygen monitoring: accuracy and reliability in the surgical intensive care unit. *Am Surgeon* 58:740–742, 1992.

461. Lübbers DW, Opitz N: Die pCO_2-/pO_2-Optode: eine neue pCO_2-bzw. pO_2-Messonde zur Messung des pCO_2 oder pO_2 von Gasen und Flüssigkeiten. *Z. Naturforsch* 30c:532–533, 1975.

462. Lumsden T, Marshall WR, Divers GA, Riccitelli SD: The PB3300 intraarterial blood gas monitoring system. *J Clin Monit* 10:59–66, 1994.

462a. Mahutte CK: Continuous intra-arterial blood gas monitoring. *Intensive Care Med* 20:85–86, 1994.

463. Mahutte CK, Holody M, Maxwell TP, Chen PA, Sasse SA: Development of a patient-dedicated, on-demand, blood gas monitor. *Am J Resp Crit Care Med* 149:852–859, 1994.

464. Mahutte CK, Sasse SA, Chen PA, Holody M: Performance of a patient dedicated, on-demand blood gas monitor in medical ICU patients. *Am J Resp Crit Care Med* 150:865–869, 1994.

465. Mahutte CK, Sassoon SH, Muro JR, et al: Progress in the development of a fluorescent intravascular blood gas system in man. *J Clin Monit* 6:147–157, 1990.

466. Mark JB, FitzGerald D, Fenton T, et al: Continuous arterial and venous blood gas monitoring during cardiopulmonary bypass. *J Thor Cardiovasc Surg* 102:431–439, 1991.

467. Mendelson Y, Galvin JJ, Wang Y: In-vitro evaluation of a dual oxygen saturation/hematocrit intravascular fiberoptic catheter. *Biomed Instrum Tech* 24:199–206, 1990.

468. Mendelson Y: Pulse oximetry: theory and applications for noninvasive monitoring. *Clin Chem* 38:1601–1607, 1992.

469. Metzler H: Continuous measurement of hepatic vein oxygen saturation with a new catheter. *Intensive Care Med* 18:131, 1992.

470. Meyerhoff C, Bischof F, Mennel FJ, Sternberg F, Bican F, Pfeiffer EF: On line continuous monitoring of blood lactate in men by a wearable device based upon an enzymatic amperometric lactate sensor. *Biosens Bioelectron* 8:409–414, 1993.

471. Meyerhoff ME: *In vivo* blood-gas and electrolyte sensors: progress and challenges. *Trends Analyt Chem* 12:257–266, 1993.

472. Meyerhoff ME: In vivo ion and gas sensors: progress and challenges. *Clin Chem* 38:925–926, 1992.

473. Meyerhoff ME: New in vitro analytical approaches for clinical chemistry measurements in critical care. *Clin Chem* 36:1567–1572, 1990.

474. Miller WW, Gehrich JL, Hansmann DR, Yafuso M: Continuous *in vivo* monitoring of blood gases. *Lab Med* 19:629–635, 1988.

475. Miller WW, Yafuso M, Yan CF, et al: Performance of an in-vivo, continuous blood-gas monitor with disposable probe. *Clin Chem* 33:1538–1542, 1987.

475a. Moussy F, Harrison J, O'Brien DW, et al: Performance of subcutaneously implanted needle-type glucose sensors employing a novel trilayer coating. *Anal Chem* 65:2072–2077, 1993.

476. Nakatsuka M, Posner M, Fisher R, et al: Validity of the continuous intra-arterial blood gas monitoring system during liver transplantation. *Anesthesia* 81(3A):A614, 1994.

477. Nicolson SC, Jobes DR, Steven JM, et al: Evaluation of a user-operated patient-side blood gas and chemistry monitor in children undergoing cardiac surgery. *J Cardiothor Anesth* 3:741–744, 1989.

478. Parault B: Technique for improved patient care: initial experience with the GEM-6. *J Extra-Corporeal Technol* 20:47–52, 1988.

479. Peruzzi WT, Franklin ML, Shapiro BA, Moen SG: Comparison of conventional blood gas analysis and an on-demand bedside blood gas monitor in the determination of mixed venous blood gas values. *Anesthesia* 81(3A):A620, 1994.

480. Pickup JC, Alcock S: Clinicians' requirements for chemical sensors for in vivo monitoring: a multinational survey. *Biosens Bioelectron* 6:639–648, 1991.

481. Reich DL, Vela-Cantos F, Silvay G: What is the accuracy and precision of continuous

jugular bulb oxyhemoglobin saturation monitoring using a fiberoptic catheter? *Soc Cardiovascular Anesthesiologists Scientific Papers* 257, 1993.

482. Riley J, Burgess B, Crowley J, Soronen S: *In vitro* measurement of the accuracy of a new patient side blood gas, pH, hematocrit and electrolyte monitor. *J Extra-Corporeal Technol* 19:322–327, 1987.

483. Rolfe P: *In vivo* chemical sensors for intensive-care monitoring. *Med Biol Eng Comput* 28:B34–B47, 1990.

484. Rubsamen DS: Continuous blood gas monitoring during cardiopulmonary bypass—how soon will it be the standard of care? *J Cardiothor Anesth* 4:1–4, 1990.

485. Sainato D: NASA tests point-of-care system on space shuttle. *Clin Chem News* 20:36, 1994.

485a. Schembri CT, Ostoich V, Lingane PJ, Burd TC, Buhl SN: Portable simultaneous multiple analyte whole-blood analyzer for point-of-care testing. *Clin Chem* 38:1665–1670, 1992.

486. Schmidt CR, Starr NJ: Evaluation of a continuous SvO2 monitoring system. *Anesthesia* 55:A125, 1981.

487. Seifert GP, Moore AA, Graves KL, Lahtinen SP: In vivo and in vitro studies of a chronic oxygen saturation sensor. *Pacing Clin Electrophysiol* 14:1514–1527, 1991.

488. Severinghaus JW, Bradley AF: Electrodes for blood pO_2 and pCO_2 determinations. *J Appl Physiol* 13:515–520, 1958.

489. Sha M, Katagiri J, Ohmura A, et al: Comparison of continuous blood gas monitoring and end-tidal carbon dioxide tension after CO_2 injection. *Anesthesia* 81(3A):A341, 1994.

490. Shapiro BA, Cane RD, Chomka CM, Bandala LE, Peruzzi WT: Preliminary evaluation of an intra-arterial blood gas system in dogs and humans. *Crit Care Med* 17:455–60, 1989.

491. Shapiro BA, Mahutte CK, Cane RD, Gilmour IJ: Clinical performance of a blood gas monitor: a prospective, multicenter trial. *Crit Care Med* 21:487–494, 1993.

492. Shapiro BA, Perruzi WTP, Templin R: Blood gas analyzers. In *Clinical Applications of Blood Gases,* 5th ed. St. Louis: Mosby-Year Book, 1994.

493. Shapiro BA: *In vivo* monitoring of arterial blood gases and pH. *Resp Care* 37:165–169, 1992.

494. Shapiro BA: Blood gas monitors: justifiable enthusiasm with a note of caution. *Am J Resp Crit Care Med* 149:850–851, 1994.

495. Shapiro BA: pH and blood gas measurements: discerning innovation from sophistication. *Crit Care Med* 17:966, 1989.

496. Shenaq SA, Zimmerman JL, Curling PE: Evaluation of a continuous intra-arterial blood gas monitor in cardiothoracic surgery. *Anesthesia* 81(3A):A616, 1994.

497. Shimojo N, Fujino K, Kitahashi S, et al: Lactate analyzer with continuous blood sampling for monitoring blood lactate during physical exercise. *Clin Chem* 37:1978–1980, 1991.

498. Smith BE, King PH, Schlain L: Clinical evaluation—continuous real-time intra-arterial blood gas monitoring during anesthesia and surgery by fiber optic sensor. *Internatl J Clin Monit Comput* 9:45–52, 1992.

499. Smith M, Gunning KE, Hayman G, Kinck JR: Evaluation of the VIA Medical Corporation VIA 1-01 electrolyte and pH analyzer. *Anesthesia* 79:3A, 1993.

500. Smith ML, Smith NT, Nesseler ES: In-line measurement of electrolytes, glucose, and blood gases. *Internatl Anesth Clin* 31:159–180, 1993.

501. Strickland RA, Hill TR, Zaloga GP: Bedside analysis of arterial blood gases and electrolytes during and after cardiac surgery. *J Clin Anesth* 1:248–252, 1989.

502. Svenmarker S, Lindholm R, Haggmark S, Jansson E, Benze S: Clinical evaluation of the CDI™ System 400 blood gas monitor. *Perfusion* 9:71–76, 1994.

503. Taylor JB, Lown B, Polany M: *In vivo* monitoring with a fiberoptic catheter. *JAMA* 221:667–673, 1972.

503a. *Technology Report: Continuous In Vivo Arterial Blood Gas Monitor Systems.* Oak Brook, IL: University Hospital Consortium, 1994.

503b. Technology subcommittee of the working group on critical care, Ontario Ministry of Health: Noninvasive blood gas monitoring. A review for use in the adult critical care unit. *Can Med Assoc J* 146:703–721, 1992.

504. Telting-Diaz M, Collison ME, Meyerhof ME: Simplified dual-lumen catheter design for simultaneous potentiometric monitoring of carbon dioxide and pH. *Anal Chem* 66:546–583, 1994.

505. Tortella BJ: Continuous arterial blood gas/pH/base excess monitoring: a new modality in critical care. *Crit Care Med* 22:A29, 1994.

506. Travers E, Wolke JC, Johnson, et al: Changing the way lab medicine is practiced at the point of care. *MLO* 26:33–40, 1994.

507. Uchida T, Makita K, Tsunoda Y, Toyooka H, Amaha K: Clinical assessment of a continuous intra-arterial blood gas monitoring system. *Canadian J Anaesth* 41:64–70, 1994.

508. Vender J, Gilbert H, Kehoe T: Evaluation of a new point-of-care blood gas monior. *Crit Care Med* 22:A24, 1994.

509. Venkatesh B, Clutton-Brock TH, Hendry SP: Intraoperative use of the Paratrend 7 intravascular blood gas sensor. *Crit Care Med* 22:A21, 1994.

510. Venkatesh B, Clutton-Brock TH, Hendry SP: A multiparameter sensor for continuous intra-arterial blood gas monitoring: a prospective evaluation. *Crit Care Med* 22:588–594, 1994.

511. Vurek GG: Intravascular fiber optic blood gas sensing: lessons from mixed venous oximetry. *Proc 14th Internatl Symp Blood Gases and Electrolytes,* Chatham, MA, 1992, p. 4-1.

512. Wahr JA, Tremper KK: Emerging technologies: Continuous intravascular blood gas monitoring. *J Cardiothor Vasc Anesth* 8:342–353, 1994.

513. Waite RI, Waite LR, Lim SP, Spieker C: A catheter-based enzyme-coupled electrode for measurement of lactate. *Biomed Instrum Technol* 25:461–464, 1991.

514. Walt DR: Fiber-optic sensors for continuous clinical monitoring. *Proc IEEE.* 80:903–911, 1992.

515. Wilmoth G, Nguyen D, Bongard F: Simultaneous in-vivo comparison of 2- vs 3-wavelength mixed venous oximetry catheters with varying hemoglobin concentrations. *Anesthesia* 81(3A):A619, 1994.

516. Wong DK, Jordan WS: Microprocessor-based near real-time bedside blood chemistry monitor. *Internatl J Clin Monit Comput* 9:95–102, 1992.

517. Wong RJ, Mahoney JJ, Harvey JA, Van Kessel AL: StatPal® II pH and blood gas analysis system evaluated. *Clin Chem* 40:124–129, 1994.

518. Woo J, McCabe JB, Chauncey D, Schug T, Henry JB: The evaluation of a portable clinical analyzer in the emergency department. *Am J Clin Pathol* 100:599–605, 1993.

519. Zaloga GP, Dudas L, Roberts P, Bortenschlager L, Black K, Prielipp R: Near-patient blood gas and electrolyte analyses are accurate when performed by non-laboratory-trained individuals. *J Clin Monit* 9:341–346, 1993.

520. Zaloga GP, Santamauro J, Roberts P, Klase E, Black K: Hand-held blood gas analyzer is accurate in the critical care setting. *Crit Care Med* 22:A26, 1994.

521. Zimmerman JL, Dellinger RP: Initial evaluation of a new intra-arterial blood gas system in humans. *Crit Care Med* 21:495–500, 1993.

Medical

522. Abbott N, Walrath JM, Scanlon-Trump E: Infection related to physiologic monitoring: venous and arterial catheters. *Heart Lung* 12:28–34, 1983.

523. Blanchette VS, Hume HA, Levy GJ, Luban NL, Strauss RG: Guidelines for auditing pediatric blood transfusion practices. *Am J Dis Child* 145:787–796, 1991.

524. Blanchette VS, Zipursky A: Assessment of anemia in newborn infants. *Clin Perinatol* 11:489–510, 1984.

525. Chernow B, Salem M, Sacey J: Blood conservation—a critical care imperative. *Crit Care Med* 19:313–314, 1991.

526. Chernow B: Blood conservation in critical care—the evidence accumulates. *Crit Care Med* 21:481–482, 1993.

527. Crow S, Conrad SA, Chaney-Rowell C, King JW: Microbial contamination of arterial infusions used for hemodynamic monitoring: a randomized trial of contamination with sampling through conventional stopcocks versus a novel closed system. *Infection Control Hosp Epidemiol* 10:557–561, 1989.

528. Fanaroff AA, Martin RJ, Merkatz IR: *Behrman's Neonatal-Perinatal Medicine: Diseases of the Fetus and Infant,* 8th ed. St Louis, MO: Mosby, 1983, p. 1109.

529. Harvey D, Cooke RW, Levitt GA: *The Baby Under 1000 g.* Boston: Wright, 1989, p. 173.

530. Hashimoto F: Bleeding less for diagnostics. *JAMA* 248:171, 1982.

531. Kakaiya RM, Morrison FS, Rawson JE, Lotz LL, Martin JW: Pedi-Pack transfusion in a newborn intensive care unit. *Transfusion* 19:19–24, 1979.

532. Kost GJ: The challenges of ionized calcium: cardiovascular management and critical limits. *Arch Pathol Lab Med* 111:932–934, 1987.

533. Kost GJ: Critical limits for urgent clinical notification at US medical centers. *JAMA* 263:704–707, 1990.

534. Kost GJ: Critical limits for emergency clinician notification at United States children's hospitals. *Pediatrics* 88:597–603, 1991.

535. Kost GJ: Ionized calcium: cardiac significance, critical limits and clinical challenges. *Clin Chem* 38:926–927, 1992.

536. Kost GJ: Using critical limits to improve patient outcome. *MLO* 25:22–27, 1993.

537. Kost GJ: The significance of ionized calcium in cardiac and critical care: availability and critical limits at US medical centers and children's hospitals. *Arch Pathol Lab Med* 177:890–896, 1993.

538. Maier RF, Obladen MO, Scigalla P, et al: The effect of Epoetin Beta (recombinant human erythropoietin) on the need for transfusion in very-low-birth-weight infants. *N Engl J Med* 330:1173–1178, 1994.

539. Maukkassa FF, Rutledge R, Fakhry SM, et al: ABGs and arterial lines: the relationship to unnecessarily drawn arterial blood gas samples. *J Trauma* 30:1087–1095, 1991.

540. McMahon DJ, Carpenter RL: A comparison of conductivity-based hematocrit determinations with conventional laboratory methods in autologous blood transfusions. *Anesth Analg* 71:541–544, 1990.

541. Meyer J, Sive A, Jacobs P: Empiric red cell transfusion in asymptomatic preterm infants. *Acta Paediatrica* 82:30–34, 1993.

542. Nexo E, Christensen NC, Olesen H: Volume of blood removed for analytical purposes during hospitalization of low-birthweight infants. *Clin Chem* 27:759–761, 1981.

543. Peruzzi WT, Moen S, Lichtenthal P, Noskin G, Yungbluth M: Bacterial and fungal contamination of blood conservation devices in ICU patients. *Anesthesia* 81(Suppl): A582, 1994.

544. Peruzzi WT, Parker MA, Lichtenthal PR, Cochran-Zull C, Toth B, Blake M: A clinical evaluation of a blood conservation device in medical intensive care unit patients. *Crit Care Med* 21:501–506, 1993.

545. Polish LB, Shapiro CN, Bauer F, Klotz P, Ginier P, Roberto RR, Margolis HS, Alter MJ: Nosocomial transmission of hepatitis B virus associated with the use of a spring-loaded fingerstick device. *N Engl J Med* 326:721–725, 1992.

546. Preusser BA, Lash J, Stone KS, Winningham ML, Gonyon D, Nickel JT: Quantifying the minimum discard sample required for accurate arterial blood gases. *Nurs Res* 38:276–279, 1989.

547. Salem M, Chernow B, Burke R, et al: Bedside diagnostic testing: its accuracy, rapidity, and utility in blood conservation. *JAMA* 226:382–389, 1991.

548. Shinozaki T, Deane RS, Mazuzan JE: Bacterial contamination of arterial lines: a prospective study. *JAMA* 249:223, 1983.

549. Silver MJ, Jubran H, Stein S, McSweeney T, Jubran F: Evaluation of a new blood-conserving arterial line system for patients in intensive care units. *Crit Care Med* 21:507–511, 1993.

550. Skrabal F, Kleinhappl E, Kotanko P, Wiesspeiner G, Wach P, Marsoner H: A new device for continuous ambulatory 24-h fractionated blood sampling. *Biomedizinische Technik* 35:242–243, 1990.

551. Smoller BR, Kruskall MS: Phlebotomy for diagnostic laboratory tests in adults: pattern of use and effect on transfusion requirements. *N Engl J Med* 314:1233–1235, 1986.

552. Soong WJ, Hwang B: Contamination errors when sampling blood from an arterial line. *Clin Ped* 32:501–503, 1993.

552a. Stott RAW, Hortin GL, Wilhite TR, Miller SB, Smith CH, Landt M: Analytical artifacts in hematocrit measurements in whole-blood chemistry analyzers. *Clin Chem* 41:306–311, 1995.

553. Thorson SH, Pierson DJ, Hudson L: Variability of arterial blood gas values in stable patients in the ICU. *Chest* 84:14–18, 1983.

554. Ziai M, Clarke TA, Merritt TA: *Assessment of the Newborn—a Guide for the Practitioner.* Boston: Little, Brown, 1984, p. 358.

Surface Monitoring

555. Binder N, Atherton H, Thorkelsson T, Hoath SB: Measurement of transcutaneous carbon dioxide in low birth-weight infants during the first two weeks of life. *Am J Perinatol* 11:237–241, 1994.

556. Chow JL, Kost GJ, Kenny MA: Reliability of transcutaneous carbon dioxide monitoring in premature infants with chronic lung disease. *Singapore Med J* 27:489–495, 1986.

557. Hasibeder W, Haisjaukl M, Sparr H, et al: Factors influencing transcutaneous oxygen and carbon dioxide measurements in adult intensive care patients. *Intensive Care Med* 17:272–275, 1991.

558. Hoppenbrouwers T, Hodyman JE, Arakawa K, Durand M, Cabal LA: Transcutaneous oxygen and carbon dioxide during the first half year of life in premature and normal infants. *Ped Res* 31:73–79, 1992.

559. Kesten S, Chapman KR, Rebuck AS: Response characteristics of a dual transcutaneous oxygen/carbon dioxide monitoring system. *Chest* 99:1211–1215, 1991.

560. Kost GJ: Utilization of surface pH electrodes to establish a new relationship for muscle surface pH, venous pH, and arterial pH. *Proc San Diego Biomedical Symp* 16:25–33, 1977; *IEEE Trans Biomedical Engineering* 25:110, 1978.

561. Kost GJ: Muscle surface pH: Measurement technique and response to acidosis and alkalosis. *J Appl Physiol Resp Environ Exer Physiol* 52:85–90, 1982.

562. Kost GJ, Chow JL, Kenny M: Unpredictable fluctuations in transcutaneous pCO_2 from capillary blood gas determinations. *Clin Chem* 28:1514–1516, 1982.

563. Kost GJ: Surface pH responses of muscles of different fiber-type compositions to catecholamines. *J Appl Physiol Resp Environ Exer Physiol* 54:1667–1672, 1983.

564. Kost GJ, Chow JL, Kenny MA: Monitoring of transcutaneous carbon dioxide tension. *Am J Clin Pathol* 80:832–838, 1983.

565. Kost GJ, Chow JL, Kenny MA: Transcutaneous carbon dioxide for short-term monitoring of neonates. *Clin Chem* 29:1534–1536, 1983.

566. Kost GJ: Hypothesis relating catecholamine release to changes in electrode pH during fetal scalp monitoring. *Ob Gyn* 64:597, 1984.

567. Kost GJ: Surface pH of the medial gastrocnemius and soleus muscles during hemorrhagic shock and ischemia. *Surgery* 95:183–190, 1984.

568. Ravindranath T: Non-invasive monitoring in the pediatric ICU. Part II: Transcutaneous carbon dioxide monitoring ($PtcCO_2$). *Indian J Ped* 57:175–178, 1990.

569. Rennie M: Transcutaneous carbon dioxide monitoring. *Arch Dis Child* 65:345–346, 1990.

570. Rithalia SV, Farrow P, Doran BR: Comparison of transcutaneous oxygen and carbon dioxide monitors in normal adults and critically ill patients. *Intensive Crit Care Nurs* 8:40–46, 1992.

VI

OPTIMIZATION

CHAPTER

28

Point-of-Care Testing ⇒ The Hybrid Laboratory ⇒ Knowledge Optimization

GERALD J. KOST

CONTENTS

Handbook of Clinical Automation, Robotics, and Optimization, Edited by Gerald J. Kost with the collaboration of Judith Welsh.
ISBN 0-471-03179-8 © 1996 John Wiley & Sons, Inc.

28.1. GOAL, OBJECTIVES, AND RATIONALE

Our goal is to gather the pieces of a puzzle that, once assembled, will reveal a new paradigm—*knowledge optimization*. The fast-paced evolution—perhaps better termed, *revolution*—in medicine is generating more pieces of the puzzle than we can present here. However, point-of-care testing, its clinical frontier— the hybrid laboratory, and patient focusing are dynamic enablers of future change. Collectively, physicians must do more for patients, despite fewer resources and less time! How can this be done? One solution is to identify how these new paradigms allow us to optimize the use of time (temporal optimization) for the individual patient and help us optimize diagnostic and therapeutic actions (process optimization) in critical care—a good start, since this is expensive care where performance measures success for the critically ill patient and also determines the standard for accreditation, if not survival, in an increasingly competitive medical marketplace.

    Point-of-care testing should be evaluated from a broad perspective and must be both *economically sound* and *medically efficacious*. Point-of-care testing is a new and challenging field. How can we nourish its strengths? We will focus on three important medical objectives: (1) clinical integration, (2) synthesis of rapid diagnostic results, and (3) improvement in patient outcomes. Outcomes, of course, must include both medical and economic ones. Evidence is accumulating to help us piece together the puzzle, and that evidence points toward optimization—but what should we optimize? The answer proposed here is *knowledge*. The knowledge optimization concept is intuitive. It draws on experience, published evidence, and good judgment, and encourages us to center our attention on the patient in order to balance medical and economic objectives during this period of tumultuous change. A fundamental goal of knowledge optimization is to assure the collaborative practice of medicine and the maximum welfare of patients.

28.2. INTRODUCTION: THREE SYNERGISTIC PARADIGM SHIFTS

A *paradigm* is an accepted system of rules that promotes success by solving problems within defined boundaries. It serves as the springboard for professional traditions. In the past two decades, a dominant paradigm has been the main laboratory, usually located far from the patient and characterized by slow response times. A paradigm shift is a change to a new set of rules that occurs when the dominant paradigm becomes inefficient at solving problems and thus, less successful. The trigger for a paradigm shift is the sudden appearance of ideas and inventions that are not foreshadowed by trends. This redefines traditional practices and stimulates a new trend or dramatically alters the existing one. The more powerful the new paradigm, the more problems it will solve as innovation and implementation proceed over time. Occasionally, two or more new paradigms combine synergistically to create a period of rapid change, as we experience now with point-of-care testing and medicine in general.

28.2.1. Point-of-Care Testing—Hybridization

Critical medical needs stimulated a paradigm shift in diagnostic testing more than one decade ago. *Point-of-care testing* first became essential when rapid changes during liver transplant protocols demanded immediate knowledge of levels of ionized calcium,[1] the physiologically active form of calcium in blood.[2] It became clear that because the citrate from transfused blood bound calcium, total calcium levels could not be used for patient management during transplantation.[1] Direct biosensor-based measurements of ionized calcium were needed every few minutes for cardiac and therapeutic management. Whole blood analyzers placed adjacent to or in the operating room eliminated processing steps and centrifugation. The immediate availability of critically fast and physiologically relevant ionized calcium results during acute patient treatment was a key innovation in the paradigm shift (Fig. 28.1). These analyzers also provided medically accurate measurements of electrolytes in the presence of hyperlipidemia, hyperproteinemia, and hyperviscosity, which, with indirect measurement, cause pseudohyponatremia that sometimes leads to fatal treatment errors.[3-9] United States liver and heart transplant centers quickly shifted to the use of whole-blood analysis and became the vanguard of point-of-care testing, that is, *testing at the point of patient care, wherever that medical care is needed.*[10-12]

A national survey showed that whole-blood electrolyte testing increased several-fold between 1982[13] and 1989[14] (Fig. 28.2). The percentage of blood gas laboratories that performed chemistry tests more than doubled, and in cardiac

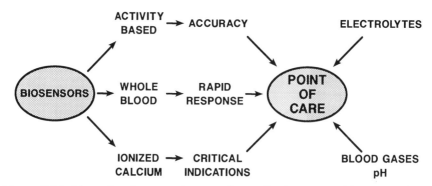

Figure 28.1. The point-of-care testing paradigm shift. Accurate activity-based biosensors enabled medically critical whole-blood tests like ionized calcium to be performed quickly at the point of care.[1,10,11] Next, innovation brought compact transportable and portable instruments that simultaneously measured ionized calcium, electrolytes, blood gases, pH, and hematocrit. Then, metabolites like glucose[69] and lactate[285] were added. The rapid response engendered clinician efficiency and enthusiasm, two of the most powerful forces perpetuating the paradigm shift. Now, biosensor and instrument technologies are maturing swiftly. This assures universal access to point-of-care testing wherever physicians, nurses, or patients need fast diagnostic test results. (Reproduced with permission from Ref. 22a.)

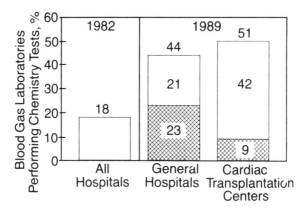

Figure 28.2. The national shift in diagnostic testing to the point of care. The percentage of blood gas laboratories that perform tests for potassium, sodium, free calcium, and/or glucose, in addition to tests for blood gases and pH has increased (see text). Historically, liver[1] and cardiac transplantation centers[14] satisfied critical needs for short therapeutic turnaround time by placing whole-blood analyzers at the point of care. Transplantation centers used satellite labs more than central labs (cross-hatched). Survey data were compared with a survey conducted in 1982 and published in 1984 by Hall and Shapiro.[13] (Reproduced with permission of *Archives of Pathology and Laboratory Medicine,* 1990;114:865–868. Copyright 1990, American Medical Association.)

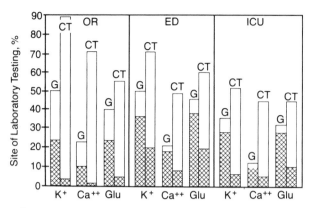

Figure 28.3. Sites of point-of-care testing. This graph compares the sites of laboratory testing for potassium, ionized calcium (Ca^{2+}), and glucose (Glu).[14] Clinical departments are the operating room (OR), emergency department (ED), and intensive care unit (ICU). Cardiac transplantation centers relied extensively on whole-blood instruments located at the point of care, particularly in the OR. (Reproduced with permission of *Archives of Pathology and Laboratory Medicine*, 1990;114:865–868. Copyright 1990, American Medical Association.)

transplant centers, nearly tripled. Figure 28.3, from the same survey, illustrates the clinical sites of potassium, ionized calcium, and glucose testing.[14] Critical testing shifted to the operating room, emergency department, and intensive care unit. Clinical departments controlled nearly two-thirds of testing sites during this phase of the initial expansion of point-of-care testing.[14] Subsequently, innovations in microchemistry, accompanied by miniaturization and microcomputerization, generated smaller, smarter, and faster whole-blood analyzers, in a progression analogous to the development of handheld calculators, personal computers, and personal digital assistants. The success of point-of-care testing can be attributed to the quality, immediacy, and significance of the integrated medical solutions it provides (Table 28.1). The extent to which these solutions motivate physicians, nurses, and patients to use point-of-care testing explains the popularity of this paradigm shift and its rapid upward trend.

The innovation of a *critical care profile* further minimized the response time for whole-blood analyses.[10–12,14] Fast therapeutic turnaround time (the time from test ordering to treatment[10–12,14–16]) of 2–5 min was necessary during liver transplantation.[1] Transplant procedures (and massive transfusions) demonstrated the significance of ionized calcium, the time value of diagnostic test results, and the efficacy of the critical care profile. Initially, the critical care profile combined whole-blood ionized calcium (Ca^{2+}) and electrolytes (K^+, Na^+, Cl^-) with blood gases (pO_2, pCO_2), pH, and hematocrit. Now biosensor-based whole-blood measurements in critical care clusters include ionized magnesium, glucose, lactate, urea nitrogen, creatinine, and CO_2 content.[17–19] Several

TABLE 28.1. Point-of-Care Testing (POCT) Paradigm—the Solutions Provided

Event	Phase	Solutions Provided
Biosensors (e.g., Ca^{2+}) and whole-blood analysis	Initial paradigm shift—invention of new whole blood analyzers	Accuracy, rapid response, and critical medical indications (see Fig. 28.1)—discovery of time/diagnosis/therapy patterns for Ca^{2+} and later, for other biochemical and metabolic variables
Critical care profile and test clusters; POCT in the OR, ED, and ICU; more critically ill patients; and the emergence of the hybrid laboratory	Expanding test menus, shifting the focus to the patient, and bridging of the disciplines	Fast therapeutic turnaround time, results synthesis, efficient analysis of diagnostic–therapeutic processes, new emphasis on the episode of care and patient outcomes, and collaborative model of laboratory medicine and critical care
Transportable, portable, and handheld instruments—microchemistry, miniaturization, and microcomputerization	Innovations and paradigm pioneers—branching of test menus and more user-friendly instruments	Blood conservation; full clinical integration; physician capture; clinical insights for key electrolytes, metabolites, and new tests (e.g., hemostasis and myocardial injury) in critical care pathophysiology and treatment; and new practice patterns
Nanofabrication, multisensor arrays, microfluidics, and personal testing devices (PTDs)	Rapid upward trend in the POCT paradigm shift—PTD diffusion	Universal accessibility; empowerment of the physician, nurse, and patient with immediate knowledge for diagnosis and treatment; and sorting out of the medical and economic value
Remote automated review systems, robotic workstations, and connection of *in vitro* devices to patient monitors	Automation and robotization of POCT and of PTD gateways to the electronic record	Systems and information integration, informatics efficiency, improved outcomes optimization linkages, and fulfillment of regulatory requirements
Ex vivo and *in vivo* biosensor systems	Transformation to the automated and/or continuous measurement of medical variables	Economization of redundant discrete samples, greater facilitation of temporal and process optimization, better detection of rapid changes, and linkages of continuous biochemical variables to physiological variables
Algorithmic, automated, feedback, and knowledge systems for patient diagnosis and therapy—the future	Synergy of POCT, patient-focused care, and knowledge optimization paradigm shifts	Automated care paths and protocols, artificial intelligence-facilitated criticality trajectory decisions, formal outcomes optimization, minimized length of stay, and cost-effectiveness through improved outcomes performance

(Reproduced with permission from Ref. 22a.)

other medically important critical care tests,[20] combined strategies,[20a] and novel approaches[21,22] are available, or soon will be. User-definable and patient-focused tests clusters[23–25] provide valuable indicators of vital functions. Profound shifts in the availability and speed of testing stimulated rising expectations of physicians, nurses,[25a] and patients. Figure 28.4 shows how biosensor-based ionized calcium testing increased in importance from 1982 to 1992.[26–28] Figure 28.5 emphasizes the importance of the immediate communication of critical results. *The availability of pivotal diagnostic information at the point of care allows clinicians to make evidence-based medical decisions and to immediately prioritize the treatment of patients—this has changed the clinician's "mind-set" forever!*

From 1990[15–16] to 1995,[29–34] the demand for point-of-care testing, especially glucose monitoring, increased rapidly. Recent surveys showed that from about 41–50%[34,35] to as high as 75%,[36] 77% (near-patient testing),[37,37a] 78%,[38] 83% (handheld testing),[37,37a] and 87%[39] of United States hospitals have point-of-care

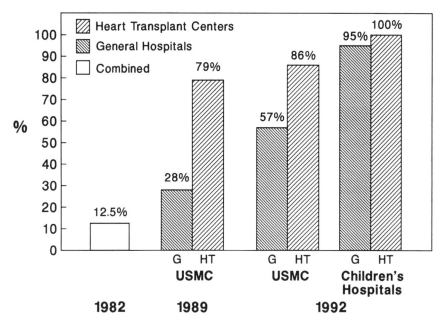

Figure 28.4 Ionized calcium—a driving force for point-of-care testing. The availability of ionized calcium testing has increased dramatically, particularly at heart transplant centers and children's hospitals. According to recommended guidelines,[17,17a,28] all hospitals caring for critically ill patients should provide rapid ionized calcium results. However, in 1992 a large percentage of United States general hospitals (43%) and some heart transplant centers (14%) still did not provide testing of ionized calcium levels in house. The percentages represent hospitals that performed ionized calcium testing in house. The 1992 survey[28] was compared to the previous surveys in 1989[14] and 1982.[13] (Reproduced with permission of the *Archives of Pathology and Laboratory Medicine*, 1993;117:890–896. Copyright 1993, American Medical Association.)

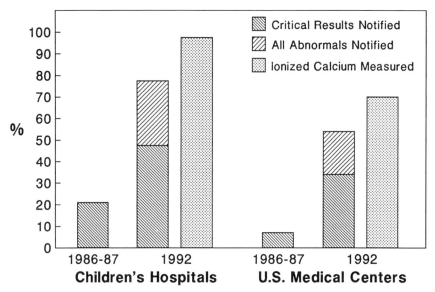

Figure 28.5. Emergency notification of ionized calcium critical results. Increasing numbers of institutions list ionized calcium critical limits or notify clinicians of all abnormal results. Of those institutions that perform ionized calcium measurement in house, 79% of children's hospitals and 77% of medical centers use a critical result emergency notification system or immediate communication. The 1986–87 survey addressed only critical limits; for historical trends in testing, please see Figure 28.4. (Reproduced with permission of the *Archives of Pathology and Laboratory Medicine,* 1993;117:890–896. Copyright 1993, American Medical Association.)

testing programs. In one survey,[36] 79% implemented point-of-care testing *with the main objective to improve patient care.* Projecting these survey results to two or three years from now, all United States hospitals will have point-of-care testing programs. Recently, the National Institute of Standards and Technology (NIST) organized a new program to promote biosensor technologies and to transfer these technologies to industry.[40] Fortunately, industry has embraced the point-of-care testing paradigm. There is an explosion in point-of-care technologies. Manufacturers are designing and introducing unique new *in vitro, ex vivo,* and *in vivo* systems[21,22]—future problem solvers in the point-of-care paradigm. Numerous new whole-blood biosensors,[22] nanofabrication,[41] thrombosis-hemostasis tests,[42–50] and new methods[51] are rapidly expanding test menus available at the point of care. Instruments for point-of-care testing soon will have extensive menus from which clinicians can select customized test clusters for near real-time diagnosis and therapy. The impact is far-reaching (e.g., more efficient use of blood products with rapid knowledge of hemostasis test results, or more cost-effective use of emergency room and coronary care facilities with rapid knowledge of myocardial injury markers). However, fulfilling the rising demand for point-of-care testing without restraint may not be economical. It is critical to maximize the value of the changes that are occurring. We will discuss recommended approaches to the economics of point-of-care testing later (see Section 28.4).

Point-of-care testing is becoming embedded in medical culture. In 1994 the Society of Critical Care Medicine established a multidisciplinary Point-of-Care Testing National Task Force to promote point-of-care testing, educate professionals in its use, and study its impact. In 1995 the University Hospital Consortium disseminated a technology report[37a] to help its approximately seventy members implement point-of-care testing effectively. Members previously reported that although operating costs were higher and information integration was harder, point-of-care testing was implemented because of priorities for rapid response, shortened length of stay, growth in admissions, and competition for patients.[37,38] Educational[52] and conference venues[53] focus on alternate site testing (primarily glucose meters) to help quality assure,[54-57] accredit, and regulate[58-60] these programs, and to address questions regarding the on-site accuracy, precision, and interpretability[29] of decentralized glucose testing.[61-79] Accreditation agencies (e.g., the College of American Pathologists) now inspect point-of-care testing (formerly called *alternate site testing*). These groups are balancing the expediency of testing logistics with the quality of the product.[79a,79b] Decentralized testing offers a challenging but exciting future, and one that must be tempered by preserving the quality of diagnostic testing and optimizing the use of increasingly scarce medical resources. *Personal testing devices* (PTDs) and soon, *automated testing machines* (ATMs!) will evolve much faster than regulatory oversight. Robotics[80,80a] and remote review[80b-80d] allow laboratory professionals to oversee several point-of-care testing sites, provide rapid response, sustain quality equivalent to the main laboratory, maintain accountability, preserve security, automatically enter patient results into the permanent electronic patient record, defray personnel and supplies expenses for relative cost-effectiveness, and improve outcomes. Simultaneously, regionalization[81-85] accelerates the restructuring and redistribution of diagnostic testing.

The clinical integration of whole-blood analyzers at the point of care created the *hybrid laboratory*.[24,25] Point-of-care testing, customized test clusters, minimized therapeutic turnaround time, optimized diagnostic–therapeutic strategies, and especially, *an emphasis on patient outcomes,* are the hallmarks of the hybrid laboratory. Current changes in medical and surgical practice continue to reward testing performed closer to the patient. The hybrid laboratory is quickly transforming diagnostic practices. Its practitioners are dynamically combining multidimensional technologies, quickly expanding test menus, efficiently integrating multiskilled "hybrid" professionals, and carefully satisfying clinical goals, while serving physicians and patients with a tighter focus and greater continuity that together facilitate clinical discovery. This trend toward *hybridization* is accelerating. As more professionals recognize its potential for solving integrated medical and economic problems[11,17-18,20,20a,35,86-105] when used in appropriate critical care settings, the significance and popularity of point-of-care testing will increase substantially. For example, a study of outcomes shows that point-of-care testing can result in earlier therapeutic intervention and more efficient use of emergency room resources.[95,100a] Ultimately, the objective of point-of-care testing is to improve outcomes.

28.2.2. Patient Focusing

Patient focusing directs resources efficiently to patient care.[106–108] In the 1980s, the innovation of the critical care profile facilitated the rapid acceptance of point-of-care testing because several tests were performed simultaneously and results were available immediately. For critically ill patients, immediate whole-blood analysis often is a strategic necessity.[1,2,10–12,14,17–18,20,20a,24,25] Acute changes in biochemical and physiological variables can indicate that a life-threatening condition exists. Expedient decisions improved the quality of cardiac, transplant, and critical care, and in the past decade, revealed the importance of *patient-focused testing,* that is, testing driven primarily by needs for efficient diagnosis, monitoring, and treatment, rather than by an overwhelmed conventional laboratory, a poorly designed hospital structure, or a dysfunctional bureaucracy.[107] The expansion of distributed modalities, such as *ex vivo* and *in vivo* monitoring, is broadening the scope of point-of-care technologies. These changes are fundamentally restructuring conventional clinical diagnostics for *patient-focused care.* Healthcare systems are investing heavily in patient-focused care, since this paradigm attracts patients, is competitive, and improves quality while reducing the overall costs of care through restructuring and reengineering.

Conventional methods of diagnostic testing suffer from unnecessary process steps, prolonged therapeutic turnaround times, and possibly clinically inaccurate results, in part, because the patient's medical status may change significantly by the time the physician receives test results that were ordered up to several hours earlier. Fortunately, technological advances in direct-reading biosensors and transportable microchemistry instruments have solved these problems and have enabled point-of-care testing to also become contemporary patient-focused testing. With no need for sample processing and centrifugation, whole-blood analysis is the fundamental key to rapid response.[11] An extremely rapid response of about 5 min is now a standard of care that clinicians expect.[14] *Ion-specific electrodes* (ISEs) allow accurate activity-based measurements to be performed simultaneously using less than 200 μL of whole blood. *Analyte-specific optical sensors* (ASOSs)[17] for whole-blood measurements are appearing on *in vitro, ex vivo,* and *in vivo* point-of-care systems.[22] *Substrate-specific electrodes*[69] (SSEs) provide measurements of metabolites. Hematocrit is measured with an *electrical conductance sensor* (ECS). Direct ISE, SSE, and ASOS, and ECS measurements conserve patient blood volume. This is especially advantageous in pediatric care, as illustrated by the popularity of ionized calcium testing at children's hospitals (see Fig. 28.4). Therefore, patient focusing is a powerful paradigm that works synergistically with point-of-care testing.

28.2.3. Knowledge Optimization

We are currently experiencing important and challenging multiple paradigm shifts[109,110] in medicine. Let us consider what these changes will produce. Dramatic economic and social forces continue to impel testing closer to the patient. Intensive care is expanding to serve increasing numbers of critically ill patients, including more elderly with complex multisystem diseases. At the same time, managed care is shrinking the population of patients without acute illnesses in most hospitals. Robotic, portable, and handheld instruments already allow point-of-care testing to be performed virtually anywhere it is medically indicated,[111]

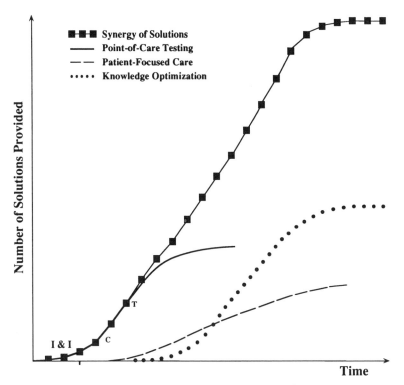

Figure 28.6. Knowledge optimization—a new paradigm shift? A paradigm shift arises when invention and innovation ("I & I") solve problems, at first slowly, but then rapidly. Medical criticality ("C") followed by intuitive adoption of point-of-care testing and technological explosion launched a major trend ("T"). Patient-focused care moves more slowly, since generally, remodeled or new structures are necessary for patient-focused care centers. Knowledge optimization generates problem solving through linkages, integration, synthesis, and optimization. The synergism of paradigm shifts accelerates the actual pace and tremendous force of the change that we experience. What appears extraordinary today will be ordinary tomorrow!

including emergency rescues.[112,112a] Hospitals are restructuring as semi-autonomous care centers, focusing on emergency diagnostic testing, and consolidating other testing into regional[81–85] laboratories. Point-of-care testing and patient focusing now are well established and widely accepted. Profound advances in the speed and availability of diagnostic information are transforming medical practices, the timelines for treatment, and the effectiveness of collaborative care. These new approaches should provide us with a clearer understanding of basic mechanisms and of integrated clinical pathophysiology. Clinical linkages, integration, results synthesis, and outcomes optimization are the essential "knowledge technologies" that will help us meet the challenges of the next decade.

Current trends suggest that in the future (1) the point-of-care testing paradigm will be universal, as well as pivotal to patient care, with 30 or 40 tests immediately available to the physician on one or two biosensor-based or microcassette-based instruments used during bedside patient evaluation; (2) the patient focusing paradigm will help physicians prioritize test clusters and re-value biochemical variables that are of greatest relevance for efficient patient triaging and critical care; and (3) the emergence of a new paradigm, *knowledge optimization,* will facilitate future problem solving by conceptually consolidating temporally dependent and process-related components that efficiently augment the efficacy of collaborative practice (Fig. 28.6). Technologically, it appears that point-of-care testing will evolve from discrete *in vitro* testing to semicontinuous *ex vivo* testing, and to invasive and noninvasive continuous *in vivo* monitoring.[21,22] These scientific and clinical advances, when used in appropriate combinations, will increase the speed, efficiency, and cost-effectiveness with which physicians engage and optimize *diagnostic–therapeutic processes.* Temporal optimization and diagnostic–therapeutic process optimization are components of knowledge optimization, a new knowledge structure[112b] that is constructed here to focus resources more effectively on improved patient outcomes, especially for the critically ill patient.

28.3. THEORETICAL FOUNDATIONS

28.3.1. Diagnostic–Therapeutic Processes

Critically ill patients enter a stream of diagnostic–therapeutic processes (Fig. 28.7). Optimization must simultaneously (1) identify an efficient trajectory, (2) reduce its duration, (3) eliminate process steps, and (4) decrease acuity and criticality. For a given diagnostic problem, generally, the number of major process steps is similar, although clinical courses vary in duration and criticality. Interventions yield regressive ("r"), neutral ("n"), or progressive ("p") changes. The synergistic paradigms (i.e., point-of-care testing—hybridization, patient-focused care, and knowledge optimization) eliminate or simplify diagnostic–therapeutic process steps more efficiently than do disunited approaches. Coalescence of discrete and stochastic observations into semicontinuous or continuous

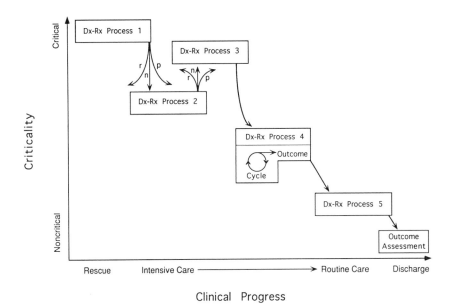

Figure 28.7. Diagnostic–therapeutic processes. The immediacy of point-of-care testing helps optimize the patient's clinical course by decreasing decision cycle times. Diagnostic–therapeutic ("Dx–Rx") processes evolve smoothly and quickly if diagnostic testing is open, flexible, and fast. Handheld, portable, and transportable instruments, as well as mobile carts, robotics, and remote review,[80–80d] provide diagnostic data quickly during critical care in the emergency department, operating room, and intensive care unit, and during rescues (field or airborne). Optimization is necessary in order to successfully complete several process steps each day and efficiently move through intermediate outcomes along the trajectory of decreasing patient criticality. (Rx means medical or surgical therapies.) (Reproduced with permission from Ref. 17a.)

ones can improve clinical performance by integrating diagnostic data needed for decisions. For example, a rising lactate level might trigger urgent patient evaluation that leads to the discovery of an unsuspected problem, followed by surgery and a transient increase in criticality (from process 2 to process 3), but ultimately, an advance (from process 3 to process 4) along an efficient and beneficial trajectory to recovery. Decreased decision cycle time for each process is crucial.

Diagnosis and therapy must be fast enough to prevent or rapidly reverse critical organ deterioration (e.g., the brain and heart). Point-of-care testing obviates time obsolescence of data, helps eliminate wasteful repetitive steps, contracts diagnostic–therapeutic cycles,[20] and speeds the identification of differential diagnoses and selection of a working hypothesis that points to an outcome target (in process 4, Fig. 28.7). Efficient therapeutic interventions then decrease the number of process steps, shorten the length of stay, and conserve resources. In the operating room, emergency department, or intensive care unit, the patient's criticality trajectory is largely data-driven. The change, rate of change, and quality of change in patient variables are important. Computer facilitation,[112C–155] information integration,[156–162] and decision analysis[163–170] can help streamline documentation, enhance insight, and identify medical trends. When the patient enters the phase of routine care (process 5), problems are more predictable and can be tracked more easily using care paths[170a] and documentation by exception (elements of patient-focused care—see below) to save time and expedite discharge. Therefore, the objectives of the analysis of diagnostic–therapeutic processes are to help diagnose and treat quickly and to effectively decrease patient criticality.

28.3.2. Axioms

Results[1,2,10–12,14,28,30–34,48,80,80a,80b,95,100a,101,108,111,112,112a,171–186] from investigators who studied rapid response or point-of-care testing support the principles posed here as fundamental axioms. For clarity, performance variables are limited to diagnostic efficiency (ε_d), therapeutic efficiency (ε_t), cluster effectiveness (e_c), response time (t_r), analysis time (t_a), and transit time (t_t). Cluster effectiveness refers to how well results from sets of necessary tests discriminate (rule in or rule out) differential diagnoses and change (start or stop) clinical therapies or actions. Morbidity and mortality decrease by clustering diagnostic tests shrewdly and receiving results rapidly to speed the analysis and execution of diagnostic–therapeutic processes. For discrete tests, t_t depends on the distance, x, of the measurement from the patient; t_a is instrument measurement (analysis) time; and t_r is equivalent to therapeutic turnaround time. For continuous monitors (*ex vivo* or *in vivo*, invasive or noninvasive), t_r approaches t_a. The equations illustrate relations among performance variables, and "*f*" is read as "*function of*".

- *Axiom 1. Patient outcome (Ω) depends fundamentally on optimization of decisions (D_i) and performance variables (P_{ij}) affected by the decisions (including financial ones); for the patient's successive critical care sites, i, the performance categories, j, and weightings, α and β:*

$$\Omega = \text{opt} \{ f_1 \, [\Sigma_i \, (\alpha_i D_i), \, \Sigma_{ij} \, (\beta_{ij} P_{ij}) \,]\}$$

- *Axiom 2. Morbidity and mortality (M) decrease as diagnostic and therapeutic efficiency increase:*

$$M = f_2 \, (\varepsilon_d, \, \varepsilon_t)$$

- *Axiom 3. Diagnostic efficiency increases as the cluster effectiveness of tests (or other diagnostic procedures) increases and response time decreases:*

$$\varepsilon_d = f_3 \, (e_c, \, t_r)$$

- *Axiom 4. For a critical care profile, optimum response time is achieved when the combination of analysis time and transit time (a function of the distance of the measurement from the patient) is minimized:*

$$t_r = \min \{ f_4 \, [t_a, \, t_t(x)] \}$$

The purpose of these axioms is to aid objectivity. Although most pertinent to critical care and patient-focused care, they apply broadly, and are particularly relevant when hybrid laboratory personnel are empowered to provide patient care and quality improvement directly. For example, financial decisions must be evaluated for their impact on performance variables and patient outcomes before excluding the use of whole-blood analyzers solely on the basis of startup expenses, in comparison to the currently lower marginal costs of tests performed by conventional methods. Thus, the axioms are rules for actional thought and a basis for blending strategic decisions by consensus, a process that is difficult to model analytically, and operational decision analysis, a process that can be aided by quantitative models (e.g., performance maps) of interrelated functional components.

28.3.3. Performance Maps and Quality Paths

Performance maps[106] are designed to integrate diagnostic testing and to facilitate performance improvement in critical care, patient-focused care centers, and point-of-care testing networks.[156–162] A sequence of activities *and* their performance indicators constitute a *quality path*. A network of quality paths constitutes a performance map, which graphically and quantitatively integrates interrelated activities (nodes), their durations, temporal sequences, and primary performance indicators (Table 28.2). Performance indicators emphasize quality drivers, controllable expenses, and clinical outcomes. Graphical visualization helps identify alternate levels of performance that the care team selects when analyzing diagnostic–therapeutic processes. Graphical visualization of the physical and temporal relationships among point-of-care, satellite, and main laboratory testing helps identify alternate routes for providing diagnostic testing, and hence, the relative levels of performance and speeds along high-priority quality paths (including critical paths). A performance map incorporates optimization, similar to the critical path method[187,188] (which also is used to design patient-focused care paths) and could be supported by influence diagrams, knowledge maps, and intelligent medical decision systems.[163,165]

Figure 28.8 illustrates a performance map for the support of emergency critical care. Performance indicators are assigned for each activity in the diagnostic support of cardiac resuscitation. Activity duration is indicated in minutes within the node. The number by the arrowhead is the cumulative time required by the slowest activities preceding. The "bottleneck route" (critical path) is the slowest route, determined by the critical path method, by starting at the last node, selecting the arrow showing the greatest elapsed time, and then continu-

TABLE 28.2. How to Design and Use a Performance Map

1. Define the key activities and their performance indicators (e.g., quality drivers and controllable expenses).
2. Estimate the durations of the activities, and if desired, include uncertainty in the time estimates.[187,188]
3. Formulate the arrow diagram by showing the precedence relationships and interrelationships of activities.
4. Determine the critical path using project management software (if available).
5. Identify and select the highest-priority quality paths based on patient focusing goals.
6. Find the fastest quality path and consider the relative tradeoffs of performance levels versus speed in terms of therapeutic turnaround time.
7. Select the current quality paths for action according to performance goals (grouping functions) and consensus criteria for optimization of patient outcomes.

Source: Modified from *MLO*[24,106] with permission.

ing backward to the first node. Quality path selection may vary depending on the stage of response, timing, and resolution. The care team prioritizes the speed of response in relation to resources available, test clusters, and impact on emergency care. Caregivers perform phlebotomy and are responsible for adequate volume, anticoagulation, specimen labeling, and other process steps. The bottleneck route goes through the main laboratory, where queuing, preanalytical, and postanalytical delays may degrade the integrity and medical usefulness of test results, unless, for example, transport, computer, priority, and urgent communication systems are in place. If whole-blood analysis is not available, handling, centrifugation, and splitting may increase the probability of specimen problems. This can result in specimen rejection, the need for redraw, and wasted effort. The uncertainty may generate anxiety, frustration, and possibly poor outcomes during periods of critical need.

Optimization of the quality path vector, **QP,** for a sequence of activities (nodes, i) depends on optimization of a grouping function (g) of activity-weighted (γ_i) performance indicators:

$$\text{opt} \{ \mathbf{QP} \} = \text{opt} \{ g [\gamma_i PI_{ij}, \delta_k PI_k] \}$$

Figure 28.8. Performance map for cardiac resuscitation. Optimizing a quality path depends on optimizing performance along that route. The therapeutic turnaround time (TTAT) is the time from the first to the last node in the performance map. Hence, TTAT depends on the route selected. The quality path using whole-blood analysis for point-of-care testing is the fastest route in this performance map. Use of a whole-blood analyzer,[11] wherever it is placed, is essential to expedite testing. The measurement cycle is ≤ 2 min, and results are available for synthesis in only 5–6 min, an emerging national standard of care.[11,17,17a] If centrifugation is required, the laboratory response time is an order of magnitude longer. Additional delays result if specimens must be transported to and processed by a the main laboratory. (Reprinted by permission from *MLO*.[106])

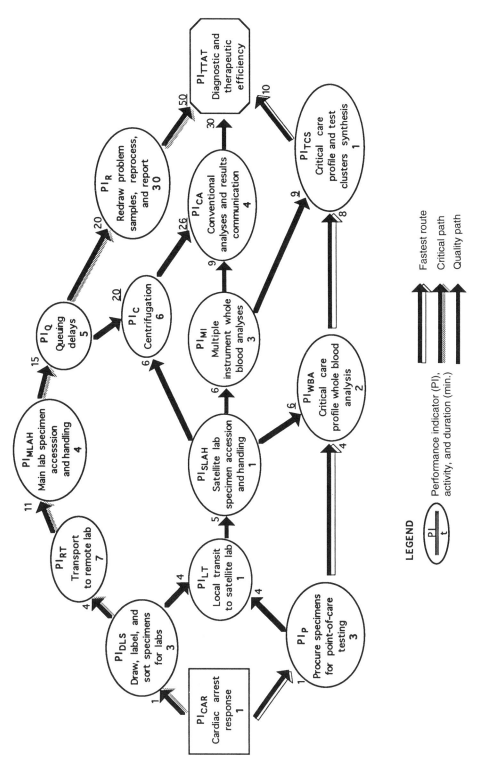

LEGEND

$\dfrac{PI}{t}$ — Performance indicator (PI), activity, and duration (min.)

Fastest route

Critical path

Quality path

PI$_{CAR}$ Cardiac arrest response **1**

PI$_P$ Procure specimens for point-of-care testing **3**

PI$_{DLS}$ Draw, label, and sort specimens for labs **3**

PI$_{LT}$ Local transit to satellite lab **1**

PI$_{RT}$ Transport to remote lab **7**

PI$_{MLAH}$ Main lab specimen accession and handling **4**

PI$_{SLAH}$ Satellite lab specimen accession and handling **1**

PI$_{WBA}$ Critical care profile whole blood analysis **2**

PI$_Q$ Queuing delays **5**

PI$_C$ Centrifugation **6**

PI$_{MI}$ Multiple instrument whole blood analyses **3**

PI$_{TCS}$ Critical care profile and test clusters synthesis **1**

PI$_R$ Redraw problem samples, reprocess, and report **30**

PI$_{CA}$ Conventional analyses and results communication **4**

PI$_{TTAT}$ Diagnostic and therapeutic efficiency

where the performance indicators may vary with time, $PI_{ij} = PI_{ij}(t)$, and $PI_k(t)$ are priority-weighted (δ_k) global performance indicators. Weightings (γ_i, δ_k) and the grouping function (g) should be defined by consensus according to goals and priorities established within the critical care unit or patient-focused care center and then, related to the institution as a whole by means of the global performance indicators. Performance indicators for the fastest route (Fig. 28.8) include the effectiveness of the response to cardiac arrest (PI_{CAR}); the efficiency of specimen procurement for point-of-care testing (PI_P); the integrated reliability, reproducibility, measurement cycle, and total error for whole-blood analysis (PI_{WBA}); critical care profile and test cluster synthesis (PI_{TCS}); and the therapeutic turnaround time (PI_{TTAT}). For this quality path (with only five activities):

$$\text{opt } \{ \textbf{QP} \} \approx \text{opt } \{ g\, [\, \gamma_1 PI_{CAR},\, \gamma_2 PI_P,\, \gamma_3 PI_{WBA},\, \gamma_4 PI_{TCS},\, \gamma_5 PI_{TTAT},\, \delta_1 PI_{PS},\, \delta_2 PI_{LE},$$
$$\delta_3 PI_{t_{1/2}},\, \delta_4 PI_C,\, \delta_5 PI_{LOS},\, \delta_6 PI_O\,]\}$$

Global performance indicators are included to reflect important distinctions in diagnostic–therapeutic processes: (1) the number and efficiency of the process steps (PI_{PS}); (2) the number of laboratory errors (PI_{LE}), including data communication, retrieval, and archiving errors; (3) the medically useful half-life of test results ($PI_{t_{1/2}}$); (4) the costs of diagnostic testing services (e.g., labor, supplies, and equipment) plus the costs of clinician time spent to order, locate, absorb, and integrate test results (PI_C); (5) the length of stay (PI_{LOS}); and (6) patient outcomes (PI_O), such as intubation, ventilation, morbidity, and mortality. Patient satisfaction can be assessed quantitatively by survey and is an important additional performance criterion.[38,106,107] Generally, performance indicators should be actionable. For example, reduction in the number of process steps, decreased laboratory errors, availability of test results before they obsolete medically (i.e., shift relative to time-varying patient changes[189,190]), elimination of transportation and personnel expenses, shortened length of stay, and better patient outcomes improve overall performance. Adjustments in activities can be made continuously as needs change. A primary quality principle is the continuous quality improvement in the performance of the multiskilled process group of practitioners, who work dynamically from the currently selected care path at the point of care.

Quality paths focus tightly on patient care. The quality path concept avoids the drawbacks of retrospective quality control by personnel not directly involved in patient care (Table 28.3). Conventional quality assurance emphasizes discrete measures of performance and retrospective statistical analyses. Ideally, software packages available for the critical path method will be enhanced, so that performance maps and quality paths can be monitored easily. Whole-blood analyzers are becoming more versatile. Eventually, testing systems could incorporate quality pattern recognition [FAST QC (*f*ingerprint *a*nalysis, *s*ystems *t*esting *q*uality control[191,192]], robotic automation,[80,80a] remote review,[80b–80d] and artificial intelligence to verify instrument operation, facilitate results interpretation, and pro-

TABLE 28.3. Benefits of Performance Maps and Quality Paths

1. Framework for the identification of patterns of diagnostic support of critical care and patient-focused care
2. Quantification of therapeutic turnaround time on quality paths, including the fastest and slowest (critical path)
3. Qualitative or quantitative analysis of performance indicators for key quality drivers and controllable expenses
4. Optimization of overall performance for high-priority quality paths
5. Comparison of the relative merits of each quality path and hence, of levels of diagnostic testing including point-of-care, satellite sites, and the main laboratory
6. Assessment of global performance indicators and of their changes with different quality paths and testing modalities
7. Proactive and dynamic adjustment in performance levels tailored to the fluxes in physician and patient needs
8. Objective quantitation of economic constraints and benefits in relation to performance levels
9. Ability to computerize for interactive assessments of critical paths, quality paths, and performance maps in relation to patient care paths
10. Potential for interfacing with knowledge maps and intelligent decision systems to assist professionals in making medical decisions

Source: Modified from *MLO*[24,106] with permission.

vide alerts, advisories, and clues for diagnosis. Quality paths and activity weightings may shift in parallel with clinical priorities, thereby altering global performance. Monitoring of practice parameters[193,194] helps identify important areas for continuous improvement. This approach is timely and useful in settings where the laboratory professional is a care team member who helps prioritize testing and balances the tradeoff between main laboratory versus point-of-care testing. A written protocol for quality paths is useful for describing how resources should be adjusted to match fluxes in patient census and criticality.

Laboratory professionals working in patient-focused care centers reported that the following performance indicators showed improvements:[106,108] (1) response time, (2) the number of process steps, (3) the frequency of laboratory errors, and (4) imprecision and inaccuracy. Specimen performance indicators included mislabeling, inadequate volume, clotting, contamination, and repeats. These must be monitored carefully, especially during the initial phases of a newly initiated point-of-care testing program. The diagnostic testing performance indicators that showed improvements beneficial to patients included (1) caregiver queuing (waiting for access to laboratory services); (2) follow-up tests, procedures, or actions taken immediately after the presentation of laboratory results; and (3) accelerated patient schedules (e.g., to surgery) that shortened the length of stay. Additional performance indicators that were useful were changes in the type, timing, or intensity of therapy, and in the medical or surgical strategy.

28.4. MACROECONOMICS AND MICROECONOMICS

28.4.1. Macroeconomic Perspective

Medical efficacy and economic benefits should be assessed together. Escalating healthcare costs, managed competition, capitation, an aging population, more critically ill patients, and national priorities demand a shift in focus and a reassessment of missions. Resource constraints call for collaborative economic efficiency.[35,86–105] The main laboratory can transfer expenses (e.g., phlebotomy, transport, labor, or reporting) to clinical sites where tests are performed, but this may or may not achieve global savings. Increasing scarcity of funds for staff and equipment necessitates careful deployment. Tradeoffs of accuracy and speed should be assessed carefully. Commercial competitors currently are introducing many new devices,[22] often birthed by venture capital and nursed to maturity by public stock offerings. As investors recoup startup costs and competition increases, point-of-care testing will become less expensive per test cluster, but the accessibility and increased volume of testing may still increase overall expenditures. Manufacturers must help by simultaneously improving quality and reducing the costs of equipment, consumables, and maintenance. If not, then utilization logically should target primarily high-priority critical care areas and critically ill patients. Multicenter studies are needed to determine how to efficiently hybridize and integrate the new technologies, but there is little research funding available for objective studies of new devices. *Ex vivo* and *in vivo* systems[22] can reduce the frequency of discrete samples, conserve blood, spare transfusions, improve the efficiency of medical decisions, and reduce risks of infection to patients and personnel, and additionally, may save money.[104] If, ultimately, these technologies reduce morbidity and mortality, or provide other important clinical benefits, they may be adopted, even if they are more costly than present practice. A solid understanding of the issues and common sense are important attributes for consensus decisions.[24,25] A macroscopic, that is, macroeconomic viewpoint is useful when establishing the overall direction of point-of-care testing and utilization of resources, without necessarily quantitating the fiscal impact of each alternative exactly in terms of cost per outcome.

28.4.2. Microeconomic Analysis (The "A-B-Cs")

For new or reengineered point-of-care testing programs, first define the mission, then, design *alternatives* (the "A") and determine *benefits* (the "B") versus *costs* (the "C").[195] In other words, establish clinical goals. Next, design care paths,[170a] testing modalities, and quality paths to satisfy these goals. Finally, balance tangible benefits (e.g., reduced length of stay) and intangible benefits (e.g., physician satisfaction) against *the marginal economic costs* associated with each different alternative to arrive at informed decisions and a strategic plan. Marginal economic costs are the additional expenditures needed to implement the alternative. Managed care is reducing main laboratory economies of scale.[37a] Undue emphasis on costs per test or per test cluster may "miss the forest for the trees." Factors such as physician time spent waiting for testing, finding results, calling if results are not found, identifying the specimen collection versus analysis times, remembering the pertinent history of each patient's clinical course at the time the orders were written, and reconstructing thoughts on an individual patient's diagnosis, should be figured into microeconomic analyses and studies of turnaround time, but are difficult to quantitate, generally are ignored, and rarely are included. The expansion of point-of-care testing has been and will continue to be justified, in part, by reducing these *value-added costs* to physicians and the care team in order to offset the added marginal economic costs of equipment, consumables, and space for point-of-care testing.[106]

28.4.3. Alternative Modalities

One should compare alternative modalities: (1) *in vivo* (invasive and noninvasive), *ex vivo,* or *in vitro* testing (see Kost and Hague[22]); (2) handheld, portable, or transportable (mobile) instruments; (3) rescue, bedside, satellite, or main laboratory sites; (4) patient, courier, or automated specimen transport; (5) personal testing devices, bedside analyzers, or remote automated review[80–80d] workstations; and (6) conventional, broadcast, or wireless resulting. Some investigators have compared modalities quantitatively. For example, whole-blood microanalyses in a resuscitation area may reduce the costs of testing and improve the efficiency of trauma care.[95] Remote review, which provides a rapid response of 3–5 min, can reduce nurse and messenger time, produce significant annual cost reduction, and improve patient outcomes.[80b,80d] In some cases, the use of handheld instruments can replace satellite laboratories.[195a] Other studies show that couriers and pneumatic-tube transport systems[101,101b,196–200] are useful. For instance, if blood gas[199] and glucose[101] testing are performed using computer-interfaced whole-blood analyzers located in a central laboratory that has fast specimen transport by pneumatic tube, priority specimen processing, and computerized results broadcasting, then the average turnaround time may be nearly comparable to that of a satellite laboratory serving the same area, and, if these support systems are already available and paid for, the marginal costs of centralized whole-blood analyses may be lower. However, the combination of testing modalities (*in vitro, ex vivo,* and *in vivo*[22]) still should be optimized for the level of patient criticality.

It is clear that *the fundamental key to minimizing response time is the use of whole-blood analysis,*[11] whether it is performed at the point of care, in a satellite laboratory, or in the main laboratory. Then, if a transport system or courier is fast enough to provide a state-of-the-art therapeutic turnaround time of about 5 min on the average, short delays in turnaround time of 1 or 2 min may be clinically unimportant. The acceptability of intermediate turnaround times depends on the analysis of medical and economic outcomes.[101,101b] Beware, however, of unpredictable long delays that occasionally may occur with transport systems. If the inflexibility of a fixed transport system delays testing, or if the situation is deemed critical, it is safer to perform testing directly at the point of care, since risk reduction has medical and economic value. An option is to use mobile laboratories[201] and mobile carts, which were introduced for monitoring over 15 years ago,[22] and first commercially manufactured for use with whole-blood analyzers in 1989. These are of value primarily when assisting emergency resuscitations, urgent procedures, and critical support of transplant or special surgical protocols. However, as point-of-care technologies mature, there will be less need to transport either specimens or instruments, since the devices will tend to become ubiquitous. Therefore, the clinical importance of a rapid response warrants careful analysis of competing modalities and their economic impact, including initial investments, amortization, retrofitting, and operating costs. Flexibility has distinct merit and economic value, which also should be considered.

28.4.4. Integrated Decisions

Use good judgment to design alternatives that best fit clinical goals and also are *economical on a relative or marginal basis.* Unless a single alternative is dominant, one can use formal sensitivity, cost-benefit, or cost-effectiveness analysis,[91,97,102] if desirable, affordable, and accessible. These approaches can be used to quantitatively compare point-of-care testing in different sites. To be effective, new technology must reduce the cost/benefit ratio. However, only about 7%[39] to 50%[38] of hospitals perform cost-effectiveness analysis prior to implementing point-of-care testing. Whole-blood microanalysis and fast test results can reduce "hidden" costs (e.g., duplicate tests, delayed treatment, iatogenic blood loss, or prolonged operating room time) or "downstream" costs (e.g., poor clinical outcomes).[37a,100] Therefore, a "cost-effectiveness judgment"[102] often is more practical. Be cautious! The least expensive alternative analyzed on the basis of main laboratory criteria may not be the best option from the perspective of the hospital. Point-of-care testing can help reduce turnaround time, shorten the length of stay, attract patients, and increase admissions.[37,38] Therefore, carefully select alternatives and prioritize them in collaboration with administrators and clinicians. The objective is to select alternatives that for the least expenditure, yield the greatest improvement in outcomes. Ideal alternatives are those that improve outcomes without any additional expenditure. A broad perspective is necessary to optimize the medical center, physician network, or healthcare system as an *integrated whole.* The hybrid laboratory concept, which we discuss next, can help integrate medical and economic decisions.

28.5. THE HYBRID LABORATORY

28.5.1. Goals

The fundamental goal of the *hybrid laboratory*[24,25] is to improve patient outcomes (prospects) by reducing morbidity and mortality (Table 28.4). The hybrid laboratory is dynamic, operating from a composite foundation of patient moni-

TABLE 28.4. The Hybrid Laboratory—Emergence and Definition

Conventional Laboratory (1980s)	Hybrid Laboratory (1990s)
Centralized	Patient-focused
Separate samples	Critical care profiles (test clusters)
Confusion	Whole-blood priority
Slow, high-volume panels	Fewer, more important tests faster
Data overload	Diagnostic synthesis
Laboratory turnaround time	Therapeutic turnaround time
Cost analysis by function	Cost-effectiveness from patient outcomes

Source: Modified from *MLO*[24,106] with permission.

tors, point-of-care testing, robotic workstations, and satellite laboratories, but integrated by interdisciplinary process teams, consistent technical performance, and continuous quality improvement. Access to equipment and testing is becoming cheaper and easier. Hybrid laboratory professionals are faced with the challenge of guiding the blossoming of point-of-care technologies, while meeting accreditation requirements, maintaining quality, recognizing fiscal realities, and planning sound collaborative care. Another goal is to provide a framework for rational decisions. A strictly centralized laboratory may worsen patient outcomes through confusion over test priorities, degradation of transit times, and excessive dwell time for analyses. Critical care testing must focus on the patient, respond to needs, and be site-specific. Point-of-care testing facilitates high-quality trend monitoring, faster treatment decisions, and patient and physician satisfaction. A critical care test cluster should target clinical priorities driven by diagnostic–therapeutic processes. With the benefit of integrated services and timely synthesis of results, physicians can optimize criticality trajectories and treatment protocols. The axioms (rules of actional thought) form the foundation of the hybrid laboratory and provide a theoretical basis for the synthesis of a wide spectrum of diagnostic modalities, from conventional laboratory functions to *in vitro* point-of-care testing and *in vivo* patient monitoring.

28.5.2. Applying the Axioms

Investigators[1,10,11,14,28,30–31,48,80,80a,80b,95,101,101b,108,111,112,112a,175,178,180,183,194,199] have demonstrated that whole-blood analysis facilitates availability of results and improves efficiency, and in some studies decreases morbidity. Whole-blood analysis also conserves patient blood volume,[111] eliminates multiple sampling for satellite and main laboratories, and reduces preanalytical errors due to centrifugation, splitting, and distribution of samples to several instruments. Generally, specimen transport time is a major factor slowing therapeutic turnaround time. For example, the immediate availability of test results should decrease mortality due to cardiac arrest.[202] The critical care profile improves cluster effectiveness (e_c) of tests by combining clinical indicators that pivot differential diagnoses and launch crucial therapies. For example, high-quality trend monitoring of K^+, Mg^{2+}, Ca^{2+}, Na^+, glucose, hematorcrit, pO_2, pCO_2, and pH is valuable to avoid arrhythmias during the restoration of cardiac function following cardiopulmonary bypass or cardiac arrest. Alternately, for a patient in renal failure, point-of-care results for Na^+, K^+, urea nitrogen, and creatinine might save a day of routine dialysis. In each example, whole-blood instruments (minimum t_a) close to patients or quickly accessible (minimum t_t) provide highly important tests faster (optimum t_r). Testing sites should create patient proximity, reduce transit time, or both, and also report results immediately to improve performance, increase diagnostic and therapeutic efficiency (ε_d, ε_t), decrease morbidity and mortality ($\mathcal{M}$), and thereby, improve patient outcome (Ω).

The strategic plan for the support of cardiac and critical care in the hybrid laboratory calls for one or two whole-blood analyzers in each testing zone or care center, plus two additional instruments, one available for emergencies, and one available for immediate replacement of any instrument with prolonged downtime. Availability of a fast transport system can reduce equipment duplication.[101,101b,199] This strategy provides local back-up, flexibility, continuity, and integrated cost-effectiveness. Portable instruments and mobile workstations should be used to provide testing for emergency resuscitation, transplantation, or special procedures. Personal testing devices (PTDs) and automated testing machines (ATMs) in different clinical centers should be overseen by a unified team, which also is responsible for education and credentials. A multidisciplinary hybrid staff can introduce point-of-care testing and expand quality paths to include new testing sites, according to consensus priorities and outcomes assessments. Laboratory professionals should contribute administrative, technical, and professional leadership to plan and coordinate these new activities, while embracing the collaborative care concept and exerting a broader span of control. Technical expertise is vital to the educational processes required for a successful point-of-care testing program. It is efficient and cost-effective to consolidate the management of proficiency testing and quality assurance, as well as instrument evaluation, purchase, backup, and maintenance. Continuous quality improvement and proficiency testing are essential for service and accreditation.

28.5.3. The Critical Care Profile and Test Clusters

Point-of-care test clusters should fulfill patient and physician goals. Historically, a key technical advance propelling the concept of a *critical care profile*[10–12,14] (a patient-focused[106] test cluster) was the simultaneous measurement of ionized calcium, potassium, sodium, chloride, pO_2, pCO_2, pH, and hematocrit in whole blood. Then, biosensors for glucose, lactate, ionized magnesium, urea nitrogen, and creatinine were added to whole-blood analyzers that supplied these in various test clusters for critical and cardiac care (see Kost and Hague[22] for test listings). CO_2 content (total CO_2) also now can be measured in whole blood. A total of 11 whole-blood measurements (and soon more) can be performed simultaneously. Expansion of the testing repertoire is clinically important since it conserves patient blood volume and avoids unnecessary transfusion and the attendant risks. Table 28.5 presents critical care profile tests in terms of vital functions and their *diagnostic pivots* or physiological indicators. Critical care profiles can be selected by considering their medical impact, by satisfying objectives established with clinical directors, and by monitoring performance variables and performance indicators. A benefit of the test cluster concept is selection of only those tests needed to accomplish the clinical goal. Extraneous tests add to costs directly through consumption of supplies and indirectly through obligatory evaluation of false indications of clinical problems.

Tests recently introduced add more breadth to the point-of-care amamentarium. For example, thrombosis and hemostasis tests[42–50] are useful to conserve transfused blood products in the operating room. Patient-focused tests, such as β-hydroxybutyrate for diabetes, rapid troponin and qualitative "spot" creatine kinase MB for myocardial injury, and toxicology screens for overdoses allow customization and site specificity. Tests requiring complex instrumentation (e.g., creatine kinase MB isoforms to assess myocardial injury) can help in assigning patients to observation or admission in order to improve the utilization of hospital inpatient resources. Evaluations of organ function (e.g., galactose clearance for hepatic function and D-xylose absorption for gastrointestinal function[20,203]) also are important in critical care.[175,178,180,194] The flexible and "open" (i.e., user-definable) selection of test clusters[23] enhances diagnostic efficiency, clinical effectiveness, and *physician capture* (see below). The immediate availability of results allow the physician to make and pursue evidence-based decisions before leaving the critical care area.[24,25] Timeliness and immediacy for accelerated medical decision making were documented by several investigators over one decade ago.[11] Now rapid response is cited as one of the most important advantages of point-of-care testing.[35–39]

The original critical care profile was designed with the philosophy, *"Fewer, more important tests faster!"* Increasingly, "time is money," and "faster is better," although this view is becoming tempered by the economic frugalities of managed care. Once a state-of-the-art therapeutic turnaround time of about five minutes is achieved, slight improvements in speed lose their medical relevance. Other factors then should be optimized. Hence, test menus should be selected to optimize diagnostic-therapeutic processes, care paths, treatment strategies, hospital utilization, and time itself. Consolidating the most frequently ordered rapid response tests in a critical care profile and specialty-oriented test clusters decreases the therapeutic turnaround time. Most states allow phlebotomy, testing, and other laboratory functions to be performed within the operating room, intensive care unit, emergency department, or patient-focused care center by appropriately cross-trained hybrid staff who can legally and competently do so.[17,17a] As instrument capabilities increase in the future, menus will encompass most urgent tests. Point-of-care approaches should integrate *in vitro* tests, *ex vivo* measurements, and *in vivo* monitoring[22] in optimized combinations that match patient criticality. For example, if a diagnostic–therapeutic process cycle warrants one or more blood gas determinations per hour, then *ex vivo* monitoring

TABLE 28.5. Critical Care Profile Tests

Vital Function	Diagnostic Pivots (Physiological Indicators)
Energy	Glucose[a] Hemoglobin[a] pO_2[a] O_2 saturation[a]
Conduction	Potassium[a] Sodium[a] Ionized magnesium[a] Ionized calcium[a]
Contraction	Ionized calcium[a] Ionized magnesium[a]
Perfusion	Lactate[a]
Acid–Base	pH[a] pCO_2[a] CO_2 content[a] End-tidal CO_2 tension Bicarbonate
Osmolality	Measured osmolality Calculated osmolality[6,11]
Hemostasis	Hematocrit[a] Prothrombin time (PT)[a] [INR] Partial thromboplastin time (PTT)[a] Activated PTT[a] Activated clotting time (ACT, ACT Plus[b])[a] Thrombin time[a] Platelets[a]
Homeostasis	Creatinine[a] Urea nitrogen[a] White blood cell count[a] Chloride[a] Inorganic phosphate

Source: Modified from *MLO*[24,106] with permission.

[a]Point-of-care whole-blood method available. For details of biosensor-based tests, please see Kost and Hague.[22]

[b]Used in cases of hypothermia, hemodilution, or antifibriolytic drugs (ITC, Edison, NJ).

General notes: Additional sets of point-of-care tests are discussed in the text and are found in references 17, 17a, 18, 20, 20a, 97, and 102. See reference 50 regarding tests for temporal optimization of thrombotic and anticoagulant therapy, such as the lysis onset time test for lytic state and the heparin management test for heparin levels (CDI, Raleigh, NC). INR = International Normalized Ratio.

(with blood replacement) and continuous *in vivo* monitoring are more cost-effective and less risky than repeated arterial sampling for discrete *in vitro* measurements that consume blood. Use of the critical care profile, patient-focused test clusters, and *ex vivo/in vivo* monitoring approaches are efficacious because they conserve blood, improve access to results, limit empirical therapy, speed diagnostic–therapeutic processes, and help physicians manage the patient in real time.

28.5.4. Critical Limits and Emergency Notification

Critical limits define the boundaries of the low and high life-threatening values of laboratory test results.[204-211] The primary objectives of an emergency notification system for critical results are to improve patient outcomes and to provide guidelines for the efficient use of resources. Critical limits should be patient-focused. Different types of critical limits include (1) continuous quantitative (e.g., glucose), (2) discrete quantitative (e.g., platelet count), (3) age-specific (newborn, child, and adult), (4) delta (sudden shift), and (5) temporal (first appearance). Critical limits reflect medical decision levels for emergency patient evaluation and ideally, pivotal points for critical therapy in diagnostic–therapeutic processes. Physicians adjust critical limits to balance their desire to know extremely abnormal test results with the need to treat life-threatening conditions. Because of limited resources and time constraints, this balance should be assessed carefully and continuously. Two national surveys established consensus critical limits.[204,206] A follow-up survey established critical limits for ionized calcium.[28] Critical limits are readily accessible in summary tables published elsewhere.[208-211] Please consult these references for listings of critical limits.

We will briefly consider how critical limits can be used in decisions regarding point-of-care testing. Critical results are test results that fall outside the low and high critical limits. Critical results arise frequently during medical emergencies and commonly in the operating room, intensive care unit, or emergency room. As portable and handheld instruments are used more to aid field rescues,[112,112a] critical results will be recognized earlier there as well. Glucose was the most commonly encountered test on critical limit lists at medical centers[204] and children's hospitals.[206] Hence, critical limit frequencies suggest priorities for urgent tests and can assist in the selection of effective point-of-care instruments and test clusters. One can estimate the instrument linear range that is required to span critical results from mean low and high critical limits (see Kost and Hague[22]). Linear ranges also should cover the extremes of quality control and proficiency testing. Accreditation agencies require clinical laboratories to establish lists of critical limits. These must be accompanied by formal notification policies that clearly delineate how clinicians are notified of emergency results and how the communication of critical results is documented. Point-of-care testing should be included in the policies. Critical results may belong to patients at other sites if specimens have been transported. Therefore, physicians at the other sites may need to be notified urgently. Critical limits and test clusters constitute one of the primary sets that make up the components of knowledge optimization (see below).

28.5.5. Hybridization

The objective of hybridization is to link time-dependent and process-related components of diagnostic testing for critical care. Hybridization guidelines encompass patient-focusing objectives, management and operations strategy, and laboratory medicine principles (Table 28.6). Hybridization of diagnostic testing draws on collaborative team skills, including vision, strong leadership, commitment, persistence, physician support, empowered staff, recognition of political barriers, assurance of quality, and fulfillment of accreditation requirements. Hybridization also calls for accountability, authority, responsibility, clear priorities, careful selection of sites for testing, continuous quality improvement, and awareness of state and federal laws. The efficiency of whole-blood analyzers is firmly established in critical care areas, such as, the operating room, emergency department, or intensive care unit.[11] However, the accessibility of point-of-care technologies currently outstrips parallel changes in operating approaches needed to optimize the use of decentralized testing outside of critical care areas. For example, instruments for decentralized testing should not be complex, since complexity degrades results.[211a] This development finds analogies in other industries where computerization and technical excellence eventually obsoleted the need for perpetual maintenance, repair, and oversight of instruments, and made universal access feasible. We should expect the same with decentralized testing, as instruments become simpler, more reliable, and easier to operate, and migrate to the point of care.

Hybridization helps match test clusters to critical care objectives, optimize care paths according to patient criticality, and blend point-of-care testing, staff, and sites through performance maps and quality paths. Critically ill patients with complex diagnostic–therapeutic processes require facilitated synthesis of diagnostic results. Providing fewer tests faster, a key concept of hybridization, helps improve therapeutic turnaround time, decision making, and patient outcomes in critical care. There is agreement that hospital infrastructure must support testing modalities in order to be successful. Historically, manufacturers were reluctant to design cheaper and smaller instruments scaled to the size and needs of point-of-care testing. However, several companies shifted emphasis to point-of-care diagnostics in lieu of other markets that were diminishing under tougher federal regulations and managed healthcare. For patient-focused care, typically each care center is designed for one specialty, such as orthopedics, oncology, surgery, cardiac care, general medicine, or an acute-care discipline such as critical care or trauma. Physicians and care teams design care paths to accommodate most routine care efficiently. Generally, a patient-focused care center requires a broader menu of approximately thirty tests that are appropriate for the medical or surgical specialty. Soon, we can expect that small handheld instruments will

TABLE 28.6. Hybridization Strategies

A. Clinical objectives
1. Customize objectives so that diagnostic-therapeutic processes drive different modalities of testing and speeds of response (not vice versa).
2. Involve physicians and care teams early and continuously.
3. Select test clusters to meet the clinical needs of the specialty and to improve quality path performance.
4. Provide integrated patient care according to the needs of the patients and their critically, as determined by a consensus of the care team.
5. Integrate planning carefully with the care paths (care plans) used by the physician specialists in order to decrease the time spent and the number of process steps.
6. Create ways to reduce non-value-added activities (e.g., scheduling, traveling, waiting, delaying, documenting, and repeating) in testing cycles, workflow, and point-of-care testing.

B. Management and operations strategy
1. Obtain a strong leadership commitment and seek a consensus regarding the use of diagnostic resources for the entire hospital.
2. Assign tasks to groups strong in process and maintenance abilities and formulate a decision process for space, testing modalities, and workflow.
3. Integrate services within critical care, between care centers, and among all clinical sites.
4. Evaluate the relative performance of quality paths periodically in order to continuously improve the quality of patient care.
5. Use multiskilled clinical and technical partners and hybrid staff to help perform laboratory work and cross-cover patient care functions.
6. Distribute computer resources to each care suite, integrate informatics fully, and incorporate new technologies (e.g., person-side terminals and wireless personal digital assistants).

C. Laboratory medicine principles
1. Assure the accuracy, precision, and interpretability of test results.
2. Guarantee the consistency of biosensor performance (see Kost and Hague[22]), instrument methods, and subject reference intervals.
3. Negotiate the standards to maintain rapid response, accessibility to caregivers (e.g., adequate hours of operation), and efficient communications (e.g., results broadcast, wireless data transmission, and radio voice links).
4. Deploy handheld, portable, and transportable instruments, as well as mobile workstations and automated testing machines when these will improve performance levels and patient outcomes.
5. Develop contingency plans defining two levels of testing for routine tests, additional backup levels for critical tests, and redundant quality paths for disasters.
6. Locate transport systems appropriately, computerize instruments and information, and use remote review[80–80d] to improve efficiency.
7. Fulfill accreditation requirements viewed uniformly for the institution as a whole.
8. Meet federal regulations, state laws, and licensing requirements, but seek waivers or exceptions when the current requirements become outdated or are inappropriate.

Source: Modified from *MLO*[24,106] with permission.

perform the spectrum of these tests needed in patient-focused care settings as well.

28.6. PATIENT-FOCUSED CARE

28.6.1. The Need for Restructuring

The patient-focused care concept[106–108,212–274] originated from 1988 field studies[241–243] that showed hospitals can offer higher levels of care while increasing job satisfaction, streamlining organizational structure, and reducing costs. In these studies, only 16 cents of every dollar spent on hospital personnel actually went toward direct patient care.[107] A patient-focused hospital is based on a decentralized organization where resources are allocated according to patient needs. A narrow set of professional tasks is traded for a set of broader tasks that give the care team ownership of the patient. The key principles are (1) simplify processes, (2) place routine services near the patient, (3) broaden caregiver qualifications, (4) streamline documentation, and (5) reduce demand variability by grouping. These principles establish a hospital value-added profile where the largest component is concentrated in the medical–technical–clinical category.

Patient-focused care presents a unique opportunity for higher-quality and more cost-effective healthcare. Traditional approaches to enhancing hospital performance have focused on incremental departmental improvements rather than improvements in overall hospital quality and efficiency.[241–243] Recent studies show that the primary driver of poor performance is that hospital organizations are structured for high costs.[107] This resulted when fragmented healthcare reimbursements paid for each procedure or test performed. Waste occurs in multiple compartments and management layers and in excess capacity of facilities, equipment, and specialized personnel. Prospective payment by diagnosis, capitation, and managed healthcare are changing the system of funding to reimbursement for complete care. Operational restructuring can relieve cost pressures and initiate step improvement in service levels.

Compartmentalization of functions into small, specialized units served by numerous centralized ancillary and support departments resulted in overly specialized job descriptions, too few employees per classification, limited continuity of care, and operational inefficiency.[107] High "value-added" costs are heavily weighted toward a rigid institutional schedule, nonproductive effort, frictional loses, and underutilized professionals. Caregivers often must compete to deliver patient care. Costs are driven by infrastructure, with little saved by working harder and faster. Unnecessary idle time, communication inefficiencies, redundant information transactions, and administrative burdens are embedded in the current structure of operations, which is incompatible with high-quality, cost-effective service.

In the next decade, successful hospitals and their laboratories will be differentiated by new operating strategies. Sustainable improvement will result primarily from reorganization that simplifies infrastructure, flattens bureaucracy, and eliminates waste associated with process intensity, complexity, and idle time. Rather than being treated merely as objects to be optimized, professionals become empowered problem solvers whose decisions are increasingly relevant to diagnosis and treatment. Care-related components will dominate the value-added cost structure. Several United States hospitals already have implemented patient-focused care centers with favorable results.[213,219,254,256,270] Some are converting entirely to patient-focused care.[213,270] Restructuring and reengineering promote continuity of care, responsiveness, and accountability, while optimizing resources for medical care.

28.6.2. Reengineering

28.6.2.1. CARE PATHS (CLINICAL PATHWAYS). Documentation, most of it clinical, currently consumes about 30% of value-added costs.[107,241–243] With patient focusing, documentation is reduced by charting only exceptions to an established care path (care plan), eliminating redundant narrative entries, and converting to electronic records. Diagnostic–therapeutic processes yield specific care paths developed collaboratively by care teams. The care paths integrate patient data into one document and help track quality drivers, patient outcomes, resource utilization, and length of stay. Efficiency increases through a ≥50% reduction in the number of staff contacts during the hospitalization. Benefits of streamlined documentation include refined patient information, more time for patient care, improved legibility of records, enhanced legal protection, accurate and timely coding, and significant cost reductions.

28.6.2.2. DECENTRALIZATION. Historically, centralized services have introduced prolonged therapeutic turnaround time, wasteful idle time, transportation bottlenecks, and annoying process steps for patient and staff alike. For example, given the traditional remote site of radiology, a routine inpatient x-ray entails a 40-step, 140-minute process[107] that can be replaced by a 5-min procedure when the equipment is readily accessible to the patient in the patient-focused care center. A patient-focused and customer-oriented operation dictates easy access to the majority of high-volume, routine, or predictable services needed by patients (Fig. 28.9). By bringing resources closer to the patient, workflow is simplified. Improved workflow reduces not only the number of ancillary departments competing for patients and the time spent on transportation, scheduling, and coordinating, but also the management, supervision, and staff that previously performed these services elsewhere.

28.6.2.3. HYBRID STAFF. Cross-training of nurses as well as ancillary technicians broadens qualifications, empowers caregivers, and flattens infrastructure. This enables them to make decisions about their patients, to be accountable to each other, and to improve the total quality of care. A multiskilled staff means that the patient interacts with fewer hospital employees. This leads to improved

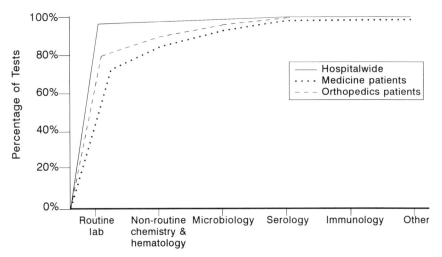

Figure 28.9. Testing trends in patient-focused care. In patient-focused care centers, homogeneous groups of patients have similar diagnostic testing requirements. Most testing is routine, as shown here for orthopedics and medicine patients. Cross-trained staff integrate into the care team when not performing testing and thereby, trim value-added costs. (Redrawn with permission from Ref. 107.)

patient satisfaction, better continuity of care, and decreased documentation. A medical technologist who performs tests in a satellite laboratory on a patient-focused center is a hybrid member of a discrete care team and participates in direct patient care. Other care teams may be composed of registered nurses plus a respiratory care practitioner, licensed vocational nurse, or trained personnel. These teams can cross-cover most services required by the group of patients they serve.

28.6.2.4. OPTIMIZATION.   Reducing   redundancy   and   eliminating   non-productive activities through simplification of process increases the time available for direct patient care. Employees and services are redeployed to multiple patient-focused care centers that act as separate, albeit smaller, "minihospitals". Each care center has the equipment and instrumentation needed to perform high-volume procedures. A satellite laboratory and portable, transportable, mobile, or robotic instruments can provide point-of-care diagnostic testing. Multiskilled managers and clerical workers direct the administrative, hotel, and clinical services provided, for the most part, independently of other hospital functions. Patient-focused care centers require fewer staff, yet provide better coverage of patient needs. With a more homogeneous patient population, the staff is able to respond more efficiently to patient needs, including critical care. Caregiver requirements, use of ancillary services, and support needs tend to be similar within larger care centers operated close to capacity. Rooms are large enough to accept critical care monitoring and bedside computing,[275-283] as well as automated drug dispensaries and on-site care team conferencing. A larger percentage of the staff is deployed at the bedside. Working in this milieu, the patient-focused care team can combine the advantages of responsiveness and knowledge optimization (see below) to produce higher quality, more effective care.

28.6.2.5. IMPACT. Pioneers of the patient-focused hospital approach report a positive and rewarding influence on professional attitudes.[77,83,117,119,133] Care teams are trained to be proficient with a wide spectrum of equipment and medical procedures. Incentive structures reward flexibility, breadth of expertise in several disciplines, and appropriate depth of specialized knowledge. Decentralization of services and simplification of workflow reduce the need for middle managers who are not directly involved in the delivery of patient care. The cross-training of laboratory personnel as care partners obviates idle time in the satellite laboratory within the patient-focused care center and reduces non-value-added activities. Improved instrument designs now allow tests to be performed competently by several levels of qualified and trained operators. Direct involvement of care teams with their patients increases satisfaction and reduces turnover. Each patient has a bedside computer workstation for order entry, the exception-based medical record, and eventually, facilitated analyses of diagnostic–therapeutic processes. Physician productivity and satisfaction improve as a result of faster turn-around times of diagnostic procedures, focused accountability for patient care, strengthened relationships with caregivers, and positive patient feedback. Patients usually interact with as few as 2 or 3 staff per shift, and up to 15 per hospitalization, in contrast to the 60 or more encountered during the course of a traditional hospital stay.[107,241–243] Rather than wasting time scheduling and coordinating phlebotomy, radiology, and respiratory services, care teams provide many of these services themselves, often presenting results to the physicians before they leave the patient-focused care center, the physician capture phenomenon (see below). Test results are produced within one hour for most routine assays. From the physician's vantage point, a patient-focused care center offers an opportunity to interpret test results immediately, change orders quickly, and see actions implemented. This reduces delays and steps in diagnostic–therapeutic processes. Preliminary results from hospitals with patient-focused care show that personnel-related charges are reduced 20–30% hospitalwide and that overall operating expenses are reduced 10%, with a return within 2–3 years.[107,213,219,241–243,254,256,270] Definitive financial data will be needed to validate these early estimates and to establish the economic value of patient-focused care.

28.6.3. The Patient-Focused Care Center

There are several implications of the patient-focused hospital concept for laboratory design. New facility designs should accommodate large patient-focused care centers with decentralized services. The floorplan can include an admissions area, a satellite laboratory, a radiology room, a pharmacy, and the diagnostic and therapeutic facilities required for a preselected patient population. Diagnostic instruments should handle small batches efficiently and economically, and meet the specific needs of particular types of patients. For instance, a cardiac care center might include two or more operating rooms as well as coronary care unit functions embedded in viewable care suites that accommodate point-of-care testing, postoperative critical care devices, and ambulatory cardiac arrhythmia monitors. Existing hospital floors can be successfully remodeled for patient-focused care. This is illustrated with an example. At the Mercy Hospital in San Diego, California, preexisting continuous quality improvement and shared governance programs facilitated restructuring to patient-focused care, known as CARE 2000.[254,256,264] Previously, departmental compartmentalization, patient trips to ancillary services, inefficient infrastructure, and idle time generated expenses that exceeded those for patient care by 2:1. Patient-focusing shifted resources directly to medical care, increased the time caregivers spent with patients, and created an environment that enhanced patient satisfaction, physician effectiveness, and the quality of care. Patient-focused care eliminated unnecessary functions. Caregivers gained both the responsibility and power to improve patient care directly.

Figure 28.10a presents a patient-focused care center from the CARE 2000 program. Clinical and technical partners form "care pairs." A care pair is responsible for the comprehensive health needs of 6–8 patients. A clinical partner is a registered nurse, a medical technologist, or other professional who holds a license. A technical partner works under the supervision of a clinical partner to fulfill patient needs including phlebotomy. Multiskilled care partners, including laboratory personnel, are cross-trained. Each room has a "patient server" housing the medical record, a telephone, medications, supplies, and a computer. Clinical documentation is based on care paths, with charting by exception. Reception, admitting, laboratory, radiology, pharmacy, respiratory therapy, physical therapy, electrocardiography, dietetics, chaplaincy, social services, case management, transportation, housekeeping, and medical records are decentralized. Improved patient satisfaction was documented by a large increase in the Press–Gainey score.

A minilaboratory (Fig. 28.10b) performs 70–80% of the test volume—primarily routine tests needed for the patients in the patient-focused care center. Chemistry, hematology, and hemostasis analyzers, as well as computer and support equipment, are available. Hematology differentials and urinalyses are performed on the bench where microscopes are located. Studies of the first care

---

Figure 28.10. CARE 2000—patient-focused care center. (a) The floorplan shows a CARE 2000 patient-focused care center at Mercy Hospital in San Diego, California. (b) The satellite laboratory, located within the patient-focused care center, provides the majority of tests appropriate for the care center patients. For other tests, specimens travel to the main laboratory via a pneumatic transport system. (Updated by permission from *MLO*.[106])

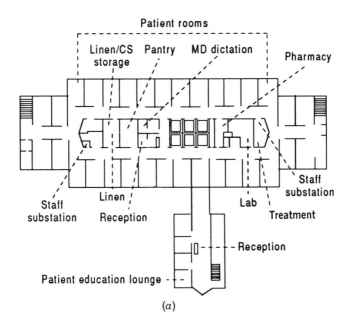

Patient rooms

Linen/CS   Pantry   MD dictation   Pharmacy
storage

Staff
substation

Staff   Linen   Lab
substation   Reception   Treatment

Reception

Patient education lounge

(a)

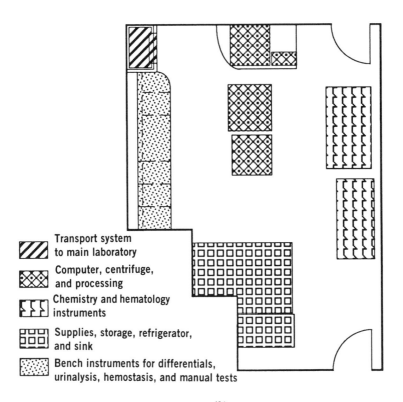

Transport system
to main laboratory

Computer, centrifuge,
and processing

Chemistry and hematology
instruments

Supplies, storage, refrigerator,
and sink

Bench instruments for differentials,
urinalysis, hemostasis, and manual tests

(b)

centers (internal medicine and oncology) showed that on-site testing reduced process steps for a routine chemistry panel from 47 to 23.[256] The frequency of laboratory errors decreased. The turnaround time decreased from 121 to 57 min. The satellite laboratory is staffed two shifts a day, 7 days a week. A transport system connects with the core laboratory and is used for nonroutine tests or at night. The CARE 2000 program now includes several care centers and satellite laboratories. In other hospitals, laboratory professionals working in patient-focused care centers cited several advantages: (1) more efficient communication and interaction, (2) increased patient and physician satisfaction, (3) faster access to testing and results, (4) better diagnostic and monitoring performance, (5) accurate tracking of quality performance, (6) a 10–15% shorter length of stay, and (7) a probable positive impact on morbidity and mortality.

28.6.4. Patient Focusing and Diagnostic Testing

Patient focusing principles are useful and effective in improving the efficiency of diagnostic testing services. Diagnostic instrumentation, which may be duplicated in multiple sites, is one of the most expensive capital expenditures required for the patient-focused care center.[229,236,256] In view of limited test volume, satellite laboratory instrumentation may not be available through leasing for high-volume reagent use. Hence, the integration of diagnostic testing services among care centers will reduce expenses. Management and operations strategies should include ongoing performance improvements that blend point-of-care testing and the workflow within the entire hospital. For example, two adjacent care centers can share one satellite laboratory that is contiguous (vertically or horizontally) or connected by a transport system, in order to achieve more economical test volumes in one site. Alternately, one site can efficiently oversee several other satellite or point-of-care sites by means of computer-facilitated remote review.[80–80d]

In patient-focused care centers with on-site laboratories, physician confidence in ordering tests and then promptly receiving results reduces the consumption of resources by *narrowing the initial spectrum of diagnostic assays*. When test results are available promptly, follow-up tests can be ordered quickly. The conventional hospital operating structure should not limit the ability to improve performance and responsiveness. For instance, any specimen entering the queue of a conventional laboratory that batches its work is unlikely to be expedited. Also, a published turnaround time of, say, 4 h, grossly underestimates the true turnaround time, because tests often must be ordered hours in advance, and published values typically do not reflect actual therapeutic turnaround times. Medical and therapeutic decisions, per se, may not take that long. It is the anticipation and waiting that clinicians find so frustrating. On the other hand, patient-focused satellite laboratories serve client needs directly. Where point-of-care testing is used, response time for highly relevant clusters of whole-blood tests is commonly just 2–5 minutes.[11,95] Fewer delays in treatment and surgery decrease the length of stay,[229,236] a benefit of faster decision cycles.

Patient-focusing policies should be developed for the hospital as a whole and integrated into the hospitalwide quality improvement program. The ease of communication with clinical and technical partners and the proximity and accessibility of testing are pivotal to success. Care teams should have access to hand-held, portable, and transportable instruments, and to mobile workstations for emergencies or special procedures. Backup instrumentation and contingency plans are essential. A transport system is valuable for conveying specimens for nonroutine (or off-shift) tests to another laboratory, or for use when the point-of-care laboratory cannot perform tests. Thus far, patient-focused care centers and their laboratories in several geographic regions have adapted well to accreditation requirements, federal regulations, and state laws. The decentralization of routine testing to care centers and the use of point-of-care testing there allow research and development to focus on technology selection, test development, and advanced strategies (e.g., robotics). Then, restructured resources can be focused to help integrate and optimize diagnostic services for the entire health system.

28.7. TEMPORAL, DIAGNOSTIC–THERAPEUTIC PROCESS, AND OUTCOMES OPTIMIZATION

28.7.1. Linkages

Timely, evidence-based medical decisions are needed to optimize the patient's criticality trajectory (see Fig. 28.7). Efficient *linkages* of time-dependent and process-related events are crucial as the patient progresses through the hospitalization. Linkages also constitute a basic level of connectivity in knowledge optimization. One can not only *identify linkages* inherent in medical illnesses and their critical phases but also *create linkages* that support and optimize patient care. For example, for time-dependent events, we can link the short-term gains from point-of-care testing with the flow of the entire episode of care, or link decreased therapeutic turnaround time with shorter length of stay in critical care. For process-related events, we can link process efficiency with patient outcomes. Two important components of knowledge optimization are temporal optimization and diagnostic–therapeutic process optimization. These two concepts derive their usefulness and validity from fundamentally traceable linkages between pathophysiology and outcome. They are illustrated with examples drawn from clinical research conducted, in part, by means of biosensor-based whole-blood analysis at the point of care during the past decade.[11] Two "man-made" linkages proposed here are hybridization, which emerged early in the point-of-care testing paradigm shift and was discussed above, and a global outcomes optimizer, which is presented below. These also are components of knowledge optimization.

First, we will discuss how timely knowledge of lactate levels can help temporally optimize critical care, and then, how an understanding of the pathophysiology of ionized calcium can help optimize pivotal processes in the diagnosis and treatment of ionized hypocalcemia. The principles of temporal optimization (lactate) and of diagnostic–therapeutic process optimization (ionized calcium) become apparent from these two examples. Temporal optimization and diagnostic–therapeutic process optimization are not mutually exclusive. The principles they identify help link other pivots in the critical care profile to outcome, or help distinguish linkages of individual biochemical to physiological variables. Of course, each variable requires its own fact base (knowledge base).

Following the sections on lactate and ionized calcium, we introduce two outcomes optimization concepts. The first concept is physician capture,[24,25] which emerged historically as a prerequisite for, if not the definition of, point-of-care testing itself. One of the strongest clinical advantages of point-of-care testing is the immediate linkage that it provides between time and process for medical decision making. The second concept is a proposed global outcomes optimizer as a performance team who link temporal optimization and diagnostic–therapeutic process optimization, preferably on-site at the point of patient care, and facilitated by electronic media, software programs, and networking.

28.7.2. Temporal Optimization—Lactate

28.7.2.1. THE CRITICALITY/TIME INDICATOR.   Lactate is a criticality/time indicator[284–389] that the physician and nurse can measure quickly and follow conveniently at the point of care. Lactate levels (1) rapidly identify systemic perfusion deficits, (2) provide an early indication of systemic oxygen debt, (3) help modulate therapy, and (4) predict outcome in critically ill patients. Although there are several potential etiologies for increased lactate in the critically ill patient (e.g., pyruvate dehydrogenase inhibition, drugs, toxins, malignancy, decreased hepatic clearance, and increased glycolysis due to stress or glucose infusion), the primary mechanism is anaerobic metabolism, which supplies the energy substrate, adenosine triphosphate (ATP), when oxygen delivery ($\dot{D}O_2$) is inadequate relative to oxygen consumption ($\dot{V}O_2$). For example, elevated cerebrospinal fluid (CSF) lactate levels (> 3.5 mmol/L) are indicative of hypoxic brain damage and high levels ($> 5.5–5.0$ mmol/L) are ominous.[328] Quantitating lactate levels in CSF can assist in diagnosis, prognosis, treatment, and tracking of therapeutic consequences.[292,301,325,369,373] Therapy aimed at basic metabolic mechanisms may help prevent irreversible cerebral damage.[348,369] Fundamentally, whenever lactate levels are increased, treatment should target the underlying disease.[370]

Lactate levels are important in assessing cardiac status. Sumimoto et al.[371] found that mixed venous oxygen saturation was a better predictor of hyperlactacidemia and survival than cardiac index in critically ill patients with increased $\dot{V}O_2$ and impaired $\dot{D}O_2$ following acute myocardial infarction. In patients with acute myocardial infarction complicated by heart failure or cardiogenic shock, Henning et al.[320] found that patients with lactate levels > 4 mmol/L for ≥ 12 h did not survive regardless of the magnitude of stroke volume, left ventricular filling pressure, or cardiac work. In contrast, patients survived if lactate levels decreased and remained <2 mmol/L. Sustained lactate production may relate to sustained myocardial injury.[345] Elevated peripheral lactate levels correlate with impaired ventricular function.[362] Fluctuations in an individual patient may identify changes in clinical and electrophysiologic status,[362] revascularization,[384] collateralization,[344] or reperfusion.[361,329] Lactate levels also may be useful prognostic markers for risk of recurrent cardiac arrest.[327] Lactate levels help predict survival following successful cardiac resuscitation.[372] In cardiac surgery patients, pre- and postoperative hyperlactatemia is characteristic.[387] In children, postoperative lactate levels correlate with poor outcome following heart surgery.[368]

Lactate levels help triage patients for admission and are quantitative or semiquantitative prognosticators of survival. High lactate levels (> 4.0 mmol/L) can be used to predict the need for hospital admission (with 98.2% specificity) for patients presenting to the emergency department.[285,364–366] In severely injured patients, high lactate levels also can signal the need for invasive monitoring.[284] Lactate levels assist in the evaluation of burn and geriatric patients.[323,343] High lactate levels (> 4.0 mmol/L) predict mortality with 96% specificity in hospitalized nonhypotensive patients.[285,364–366] In hypotensive patients in the emergency department or intensive care unit, high lactate levels (> 4.0 mmol/L) predict mortality with 87.5% specificity.[285] Using 11 definitions of lactic acidosis and sequential cluster analysis, Luft et al.[336a] studied 1467 patients on hospital admission and found that as the definition of lactic acidosis became more restrictive (i.e., higher threshold), the incidence of mortality increased from 30 to 88%, with a 71–88% mortality rate when the level of lactate was ≥ 6 mmol/L. Lactate levels predict survival better than does cardiac index, $\dot{D}O_2$, or $\dot{V}O_2$.[284]. In asphyxiated neonates, the presence of cerebral lactate (by magnetic resonance spectroscopy) indicated a poor outcome.[317] In neonates with severe hypoxemia requiring extracorporeal membrane oxygenation (ECMO), nonsurvivors had persistent and severe hyperlactemia; levels < 25 mmol/L on admission had a 91.3% positive predictive value for survival.[304] Levels > 5 mmol/L support a decision to start ECMO.[378] In some studies,[354] after correction of acidosis[389] persistence or elevation of lactate levels still related to bad prognosis.

Lactic acidosis may represent the best single objective measure of the presence and severity of cardiogenic and other forms of shock.[289,299,303,309,314,331–333,355,383] Figures 28.11 and 28.12 illustrate how temporal trends in lactate levels anticipate and predict survival. In critically ill patients with hepatic dysfunction,[288] lactic acidosis is associated with clinical evidence of shock and increased hospital mortality[334] reaching 100%.[347] Schuster[360] suggested that hyperlactatemia can point to superimposed complications. Lactate levels correlate with results of challenge tests.[380] Lactic acidosis helps identify critical hypoperfusion.[290,291,352] Therapy of critically ill patients with lactic acidosis is designed to improve oxygen delivery (e.g., supranormal O_2[295,298,312a,319,359,366a,367,367a,379a]), increase cardiac index, and maintain hemoglobin levels,[346] in order to reduce microvascular hypoxia.[330–333] Oxygen extraction is crucial.[336] In emergency department patients, Rady et al.[357] found that normalization of hemodynamic variables did not adequately reflect the optimal endpoint of initial therapy in shock. Reduced

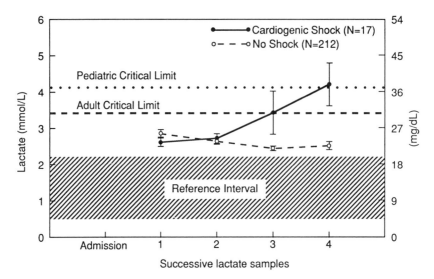

Figure 28.11. Temporal optimization—predicting the development of cardiogenic shock in acute myocardial infarction. Mavric et al.[339] found that lactate levels predicted the development cardiogenic shock. Differences in levels between patient groups were statistically significant at the time of the third successive lactate sample. The next most predictive variable was the peak blood urea nitrogen level. Both lactate and urea can be measured rapidly with a whole blood analyzer at the point of care. The mean critical limits for lactate are from United States surveys of medical centers[204] and children's hospitals,[206] and are 3.4 and 4.1 mmol/L, respectively. The reference interval shown by the horizontal band is 0.5–2.2 mmol/L. (Prepared from data published by Mavric et al.[339])

central venous oxygen saturation and elevated lactate levels suggested persisting global ischemia and cardiac dysfunction. Rady et al.[357] concluded that lactate levels (and central venous oxygen saturation) should be monitored in order to optimize systemic oxygenation and cardiac function during the initial therapy of shock in the emergency department.

Lactate levels increase when oxygen delivery is inadequate to meet demand. The efficient elimination of oxygen debt is crucial to patient outcome.[358,365,366] The rate of clearance of lactate is useful in monitoring a patient's response to therapy.[284,293,312,355,381] The arrest of rising lactate levels is essential to improve patient survival, while the rapid restoration (e.g., > 5% decrease in the first hour of shock reversal[381]) of normal lactate levels indicates good prognosis and is an objective of therapy.[293] Conversely, multiple organ system dysfunction syndrome can slow lactate clearance.[284,356] In trauma patients, Rady[356] advised a target lactate level of < 2 mmol/L for resuscitation of the microcirculation and prevention or attenuation of systemic inflammatory response syndrome. Elevated lactate levels may signal the presence of peripheral shunting of blood, regional hypoperfusion, and inadequate oxygenation.[316,376] In blunt trauma patients, a significant correlation existed between multiple organ failure and lactate lev-

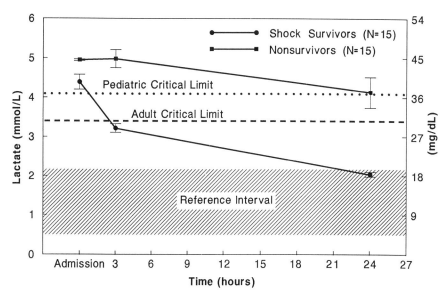

Figure 28.12. Temporal optimization—differentiating clinical progress and outcome in intensive care patients with shock. Cowan et al.[306] found that following admission, serial lactate levels decreased in shock survivors, whereas nonsurvivors showed little change (or in other clinical studies, an increase). A change in the lactate level during the first 3 h of resuscitation was a better predictor of outcome than a single measurement. The decrease in mean lactate level was statistically significant in the group of survivors, most of whom had septic shock. Discriminant function analysis was used to asses predictors in both Figures 28.11 and 28.12. (Reprinted with permission of CRC Press, Boca Raton, FL, from GJ Kost: New whole blood analyzers and their impact on cardiac and critical care. *Crit Rev Clin Lab Sci* 30:153–202, 1993.)

els.[310] For patients with multiple trauma, lactate levels are valuable as prognostic indices.[352] Lactate levels help predict injury severity, fluid requirements, and outcome in trauma victims.[341,342] Resuscitation to restore adequate oxygen supply to ischemic tissues and hepatorenal organ systems is essential for rapid elimination of increased extracellular lactic acid and attenuation of the development of systemic inflammatory response syndrome.[356] In fact, Abramson et al.[284] defined adequate resuscitation as the ability to clear lactate when oxygen delivery is maximized.

A protocol for timed lactate levels is clinically useful. For example, Toffaletti reported[376,378,379] that following pediatric cardiac surgery, serial measurements[374,375] of lactate every 4–12 h help assess recovery and guide cardiotropic, volume, and blood pressure support. Values above 6 mmol/L merit aggressive support, while most should be normal within 24 h.[378] ECMO calls for lactate levels every hour initially, then, every 4–6 h.[378] Rising lactate levels suggest flow, volume, or hematocrit adjustments, or if > 3 mmol/L, a switch from venovenous to venoarterial ECMO.[378] In preterm infants lactic acid helps predict the need for transfusion.[322] Marnitz et al.[338] found that elevated lactate levels during both intraoperative and early postoperative (< 2 h) periods were associated with complications, and if > 4 mmol/L, bad prognosis. Abramson et al.[284] found that for multiple trauma patients, the time required to clear elevated lactate levels predicted survival ($t < 24$ h, 100%; $24 < t < 48$ h, 75%; and $t > 48$ h, 13.6% survival); their results confirmed earlier observations in patients suffering from septic or cardiogenic shock. For critically ill adults, Shirey[364,365] noted that lactate measurement warrants a rapid response. In critical care, lactate results should be available within 30 min or less.[377,381] Diluted blood samples can spuriously lower lactate concentrations.[386] Several lactate methods for whole blood[302,385] are under development.[296,315,337,363] Biosensor-based whole-blood analyzers now provide rapid measurements of lactate with substrate-specific electrodes in 1 or 2 min.[11,285] Direct–undiluted[377] or diluted–hemolyzed[313] lactate measurements[287] appear to be independent of hematocrit. This is important, since hematocrit can vary unexpectedly in critically ill patients, particularly those in shock. Clinically valid lactate results in the first hour of shock can facilitate early diagnosis and treatment and may be pivotal to shock reversal.

28.7.2.2. PRINCIPLES OF TEMPORAL OPTIMIZATION. The clinical evidence presented above demonstrates that lactate is a time-dependent indicator of pathophysiological[324,353] events that are linked fundamentally to patient outcome. While lactate levels correlate with patient criticality, *changes in lactate levels over time* (e.g., appearance, clearance, and trends) and *rates of change* are most important, and help to reveal whether critical care is temporally optimized in the individual patient. The principles of temporal optimization focus on (i) the status of the patient and (ii) survival. The principles related to the clinical status of the patient are (1) elevated absolute levels of lactate indicate the need for the evaluation, admission, invasive monitoring, or supportive intervention of the patient; (2) crossover tiers and their corresponding quantitative decision thresholds are: (a) *normal*—the reference interval of 0.5–2.2 mmol/L,[373a] (b) *critical*—the mean high critical limits of 3.4 (SD 1.3) mmol/L for adults,[204] and 4.1 (SD 1.2) mmol/L for children,[206] and (c) *supercritical*—the zone of approximately 4–8 mmol/L that predicts poor survival and high mortality, especially with levels above 6–8 mmol/L[336a]; (3) rapid biosensor-based whole blood measurements of lactate are essential to continuously differentiate crossover tiers, decision thresholds, and responses to therapy; (4) early and frequent periodic sampling (or continuous measurement) will identify abnormal lactate levels before they become so obvious that the underlying problems are irreversible; and (5) changes and the rates of change in lactate levels are more important than absolute levels (isolated elevations do not necessarily predict impending death[376]), and often are more sensitive than changes in pH.

Temporal optimization principles related to patient survival are (1) knowledge of trends in lactate levels reveal patient status, triage, prognosis, and survival in both hypotensive and nonhypotensive hospitalized patients; (2) trends in lactate levels predict not only the development of cardiogenic or noncardiogenic shock but also its severity; (3) changes in serial lactate levels provide guidance for selection of the type of therapy (including surgical), modulation of its intensity, and detection of unforeseen complications; and (4) additionally, trends in lactate levels provide useful feedback to monitor the efficacy of treatment and the progress of critically ill patients (e.g., trauma victims). The underlying mechanism, or linkage, for these principles is the rapid detection, reversal, and normalization of lactate levels for effective temporal optimization of oxygen delivery and elimination of global or regional oxygen deficiency. In other etiologies of hyperlactatemia (e.g., exercise or seizures), washout typically begins in < 4 min,[288,335] that is, fast enough so as not to be confusing.[308,326] Computer software can assist temporal analysis.[112C–155] Severity of illness scoring and mortality risk prediction[294,311] can help facilitate reasoning and reduce uncertainty.

Clinical evidence indicates that lactate levels can help guide and modulate early and timely interventions that will improve patient outcomes. However, the efficacy of temporal optimization per se will have to be documented. Nevertheless, several of these principles can be generalized. As point-of-care devices incorporate expanded test menus, new diagnostic patterns of temporal change in other biochemical variables will become apparent. Serial data and trend quantitation are more valuable than indirect[321] or isolated observations for identifying the time course of change. As testing evolves from discrete to continuous measurements, lactate[297,300,307,318,340,349–351,382,388] and other biochemical variables will be monitored *ex vivo* or *in vivo* in critically ill patients.[22] Continuous monitoring and telemetry of lactate and of interrelated physiological variables[286,305] will help eliminate unrecognized events associated with rapid or unpredictable[22,189,190] fluctuations, and may reveal adverse changes with sufficient warning and adequate lead time for correction or treatment. Lactate provides a good model of how to apply temporal optimization for biochemical variables coupled or linked, fundamentally, to pathophysiological changes at the cellular level and, ultimately, to patient outcomes. Additionally, temporal optimization focuses on disease evolution, compresses its resolution, and therefore, should help to reveal as yet undiscovered patterns arising in diagnostic-therapeutic processes.

28.7.3. Diagnostic–Therapeutic Process Optimization—Ionized Calcium

28.7.3.1. THE Ca^{2+} CASCADE. A clear understanding of the diagnostic–therapeutic processes associated with ionized hypocalcemia and ionized hypercalcemia is essential to optimize patient outcomes.[11,28] Ionized (free) calcium plays an important role in myocardial contraction and conduction and in the maintenance of vascular smooth muscle tone. There are significant risks associated with calcium treatment if given when not indicated. Additionally, severe ionized hypocalcemia may be associated with cardiac arrest that becomes refractory to resuscitation despite the restoration of ionized calcium levels to normal.[1] Figure 28.13 illustrates the clinical thresholds, pathophysiology, critical limits, and normal reference interval for ionized calcium.[11,28] The solid bars in the cascade represent clinically significant levels of ionized calcium in the studies

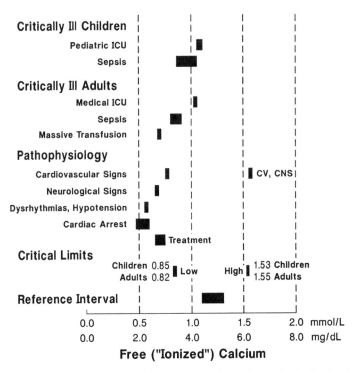

Figure 28.13. Diagnostic—therapeutic process optimization—the ionized calcium cascade. Clinical phenomena and pathophysiology are associated with a cascade of ionized calcium levels—as ionized calcium levels decrease in patients with ionized hypocalcemia, morbidity and mortality worsen. Point-of-care testing is fast enough to enable physicians to optimize diagnostic—therapeutic processes in, for example, the individual critically ill patient or surgical patient receiving massive transfusion, and efficiently correct ionized hypocalcemia. The treatment threshold is 0.70–0.80 mmol/L (see text). Critical limits for ionized calcium were first proposed in 1986[1] and then surveyed in 1992.[28] (Updated from the *Archives of Pathology and Laboratory Medicine,* 1993;117:890–896. Copyright 1993, American Medical Association.)

described next. We start at the top and work down. Sanchez et al.[390] observed that ionized calcium levels of acutely ill children in the pediatric intensive care unit averaged 1.11 mmol/L. Broner et al.[391] found that ionized calcium levels averaged 1.05 mmol/L in nonsurviving critically ill pediatric patients, 46.2% of whom had ionized hypocalcemia. Cardenas-Rivero et al.[392] found that ionized calcium levels ranged from 0.88 to 1.04 mmol/L in septic children, and that mortality was 31% in those with ionized hypocalcemia. Desai et al.[393] observed ionized calcium levels averaging 1.04 mmol/L among critically ill medical intensive care unit adult patients with sepsis, cardiogenic shock, or cardiopulmonary arrest. Ionized calcium levels were significantly lower in hypotensive patients than in normotensive patients.[394] Taylor et al.[395] found that levels of ionized calcium in intensive care unit adult patients with sepsis averaged 0.91 mmol/L. Zaloga and Chernow[396] reported a mortality rate of 50% for adult patients with the combination of sepsis and ionized hypocalcemia, with ionized calcium levels averaging 0.88 mmol/L. Woo et al.[397] observed 100% mortality in adult patients with septic shock and levels of ionized calcium below 0.8 mmol/L. In sepsis, both the total and ionized calcium levels may be depressed, the latter disproportionately and unpredictably. The mortality rate was 71% in massively transfused adult patients with ionized calcium levels less than 0.70 mmol/L.[398]

In critical illness, ionized hypocalcemia results from hypomagnesemia, transient hypoparathyroidism, vitamin D deficiency, and calcium binding, chelation, or cellular redistribution. When levels of ionized calcium decrease below 1.0 mmol/L, neurologic and cardiovascular signs, including dysrhythmias and hypotension appear,[1,399] as shown under the "Pathophysiology" heading in Figure 28.13. Cardiac arrest has been reported when values of 0.47–0.60 mmol/L occur, although the rate of change and clinical circumstances can produce fatal outcomes at other levels.[1,399,400] A low level of ionized calcium is an early predictor of mortality in critically ill surgical patients.[401] Figure 28.13 shows that the adult (0.82 mmol/L) and pediatric (0.85 mmol/L) mean critical limits for ionized hypocalcemia correspond well to the critical clinical phenomena and the acute treatment thresholds. Therefore, the critical limits, which are from a 1992 national survey of United States medical centers and children's hospitals,[27,28] represent sound thresholds for emergency notification of clinicians. An ionized calcium threshold level of 0.70 mmol/L is a reasonable level to initiate calcium repletion in acutely ill patients with symptoms or signs of ionized hypocalcemia, especially low cardiac output and hypotension that are refractory to volume replacement or catecholamines.[402] Calcium treatment typically is not necessary when the ionized calcium level is 0.80 mmol/L or higher,[403] although a more conservative threshold may be necessary for the unconscious patient in whom anesthesia obscures symptoms and signs such as spasms (muscles, airways), tetany, and psychiatric impairment.[1]

28.7.3.2. PRINCIPLES OF DIAGNOSTIC–THERAPEUTIC PROCESS OPTIMIZATION.
The principles of diagnostic–therapeutic process optimization are based on the clinical evidence presented above and the recommendations of several investigators,[1,14,26–28,203–232,378,379,390–419] and focus on (i) diagnostic-therapeutic actions and events and (ii) the use of point-of-care testing. The principles for ionized calcium are (1) the best way to prevent cardiac (and neurologic) catastrophes is to aggressively monitor ionized calcium levels measured directly and anaerobically in whole blood with a 5- to 15-min therapeutic turnaround time; (2) optimal cardiac function depends on appropriate age-specific ionized calcium levels, regardless of whether the patient has heart disease; (3) the safest means of restoring normal cardiac and neurologic function is by patient-specific calcium treatment based on a knowledge of acute trends in the patient's blood levels of ionized calcium; (4) one should interpret ionized calcium levels in light of the pathophysiological interactions of lactate,[286,287,305] pH,[420] citrate, and other metabolites, especially during cardiac arrest, resuscitation,[1,400] transplantation, massive transfusion,[398] and extracorporeal membrane oxygenation[378,379] when endogenous or exogenous (e.g., citrate

in transfused blood) small ligands chelate free calcium and may cause ionized hypocalcemia; and (5) morbidity and mortality should be monitored to effectively deploy ionized calcium testing and maximally improve patient outcomes.

The second set of principles focuses on the diagnostic testing per se.[2,11,28] Laboratory professionals and clinicians not currently performing ionized calcium measurement within their institutions can introduce this test efficiently: (1) by obtaining whole-blood analyzers;[11,14] (2) by designing a uniform strategy for specimen processing;[421–424,424a] (3) by becoming familiar with the National Committee for Clinical Laboratory Standards (NCCLS) and the International Federation of Clinical Chemistry (IFCC) guidelines;[425–427] (4) by targeting important clinical objectives (e.g., pregnancy, prematurity, critical care, surgery, transfusions, parathyroid insufficiency, pancreatitis, renal disease, dialysis, hypotension, hypomagnesemia, seizures, and sepsis[420,428,429]); (5) by cost-effectively integrating and limiting testing (e.g., selective postoperative checks following heart transplantation[378,379]); (6) by measuring ionized calcium simultaneously with several other tests in a critical care profile, which conserves patient blood volume;[111] (7) by prioritizing the use of point-of-care testing and rapid response modalities; and (8) by formatting results to facilitate physician interpretation.[420] A patient diagnostic pattern (Fig. 28.14) pictorially displays ionized calcium and other test results relative to critical limits. Visuals can facilitate fast recognition of critical patient results and alert the clinician to interrelationships of, for example, ionized calcium, lactate, glucose, and acid–base status.[286,303,305]

Ionized calcium provides a good model for diagnostic–therapeutic process optimization. Several of the principles specific to ionized calcium can be generalized to other critical care profile tests. The clinical evidence presented above and summarized in Figure 28.13 suggests that medical sites providing acute patient care also should provide ionized calcium diagnostic testing in house to help optimize critical patient evaluation, intervention, and treatment.[28] Since whole-blood analysis is a practical necessity for ionized calcium,[11] several other rapid response measurements can be performed at the same time (see Section 28.5.3. and Kost and Hague[22]). Measurements of ionized calcium may be needed as frequently as every 5–10 min during transplantation and emergencies requiring significant transfusions.[1] Results should be available within 3–5 min in order to guide calcium replacement after surgery.[378,379] In critically ill intensive care unit patients, measurements may be needed every 1–4 h during calcium repletion[402,403] or more frequently, depending on the initial ionized calcium level,[26–28,399,414,414a] its rate of change,[1] and the severity of cardiovascular insufficiency. Point-of-care testing is the fastest method for the acute surveillance and early detection of ionized hypocalcemia (or hypercalcemia) and its adverse effects. Whole-blood analyzers produce ionized calcium results in 1–2 min.[1,11,14] Point-of-care testing, or other modalities that achieve a therapeutic turnaround time of about 5 min, allow us to link process and temporal optimization by providing ionized calcium results quickly, so that decision thresholds emerge in a nearly continuous manner and are matched with graded and integrated, not empirical, treatment of ionized hypocalcemia.

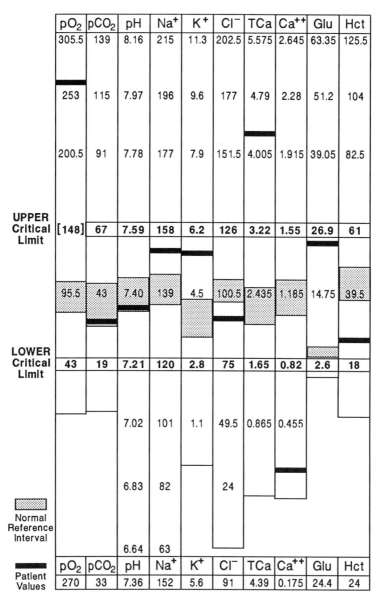

Figure 28.14. The patient diagnostic pattern. The patient diagnostic pattern (PDP) displays critical test results with vertical bands adjusted to align the low and high mean critical limits for individual tests. Normal reference intervals shift according to their relationships to the critical limits. The illustration is from a liver transplant patient[1] who developed severe ionized hypocalcemia, despite increased total calcium, primarily due to an increase in the citrate-bound fraction. The test results are from the period of resuscitation when ionized calcium reached a nadir during the posttransplantation phase, which was complicated by cardiac arrest. High pO_2 was due to mechanical ventilation with high F_{IO_2}. (Reprinted by permission of CRC Press, Boca Raton, FL, from GJ Kost: New whole blood analyzers and their impact on cardiac and critical care. *Crit Rev Clin Lab Sci* 30:153–202, 1993.

28.7.4. Outcomes Optimization

28.7.4.1. PHYSICIAN CAPTURE.   Increasingly, time is an extremely valuable resource to be optimized. Fast, accurate, precise, interpretable, and actionable test results available in pace with rapidly changing diagnostic–therapeutic processes in critical care will *capture the physician's thoughts* before he or she leaves the patient's bedside (Fig. 28.15). This is the definition of *physician capture,* a practical optimizer[11,24,25] that facilitates rapid diagnosis, speeds treatment, and eliminates unnecessary delays and empirical therapies that increase morbidity and prolong intensive care stays.[1,11,175,178,180,194] Physician capture assures that diagnostic testing will not delay critical decisions, interventions, or new clinical objectives. If whole-blood analysis is used, the care team can act almost immediately, treat the patient appropriately, and engage in the next step in the diagnostic–therapeutic process in near real time, without regrouping or refocusing. Cost-effectiveness derives from care team efficiency, shortened length of stay in critical care, and other patient-focusing efficiencies. Physician capture also helps obviate unnecessary tests, blind chases of insignificant abnormalities, costly patient relapses, and "hidden" or "downstream" costs. Continuous quality improvement and information integration are enablers of physician capture. Assuring physician capture helps organize point-of-care testing and partially addresses a related objective, global outcomes optimization.

28.7.4.2. GLOBAL OUTCOMES OPTIMIZER.   Point-of-care testing must be both medically efficacious and economically sound when viewed from the per-

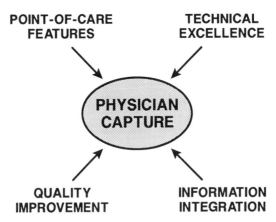

Figure 28.15. Physician capture. Physician capture is a practical optimizer for point-of-care testing. Diagnostic test results must be generated fast enough to capture the physician's thoughts while at the bedside during critical moments. This is not easy, since instruments must be user-friendly, as well as technically excellent on site, and results must be accurate, precise, and interpretable. Information integration is crucial to support the data stream driving the analysis and optimization of diagnostic–therapeutic processes. Quality improvement builds confidence in the new paradigm and encourages collaboration.

spective of the entire health system, the physician network, or the managed care organization. The invention of biosensors and whole-blood analyzers initiated a fundamentally new paradigm in critical care. Then, point-of-care testing spread to fulfill multidimensional needs. Currently, up to 59% of institutions may lack a coordinated point-of-care testing program.[34] In 1992, 43% or more of United States general medical centers did not perform ionized calcium testing in-house for critical care patients.[28] Therefore, many hospitals will be initiating point-of-care testing in critical care and other clinical areas. Although guidelines for the implementation of point-of-care testing now are available,[17,17a] it often is unclear how clinical objectives can be met. The global optimizer concept proposes the formation of an integrated performance team made up of laboratory professionals and physicians who deploy point-of-care testing and manage information to maximize the medical and economic effectiveness of diagnostic testing.

Table 28.7 lists important objectives of a global outcomes optimization performance team. Practical functions include the coordination of testing devices,

---

TABLE 28.7. Global Outcomes Optimization Performance Team

A. Integration
  1. Deploy mobile testing to support emergency resuscitations and monitor utilization.
  2. Coordinate robotic testing workstations in critical care areas, satellite laboratories, and elsewhere—integrated independence.
  3. Organize backup of point-of-care testing to continuously meet priorities and fulfill clinical objectives.
  4. Overview clinical sites, shift staff, and distribute resources efficiently.
  5. Select test clusters, set critical limits, and assure emergency notification.
  6. Design effective performance maps, quality paths, and patient care paths.
  7. Apply patient acuity scoring to adjust point-of-care testing and patient-focused care protocols.
  8. Maintain network or wireless (radio or infrared) access so that clinical teams can use outcomes optimization software programs (and databases) at the point of care.
  9. Merge biochemical and physiological information, trends, and patient diagnoses.
B. Synthesis
  1. Track performance indicators, outcome measures, severity and illness scores, and morbidity and mortality.
  2. Implement clinical information systems (e.g., AcuBase,[430] Project IMPACT,[431] and QuIC[432]) and perform outcome analyses.
  3. Manage predictive algorithms and compare predicted versus actual outcomes.
  4. Provide frequent decision analyses based on prognostic estimates, information databases (knowledge bases), and performance.
  5. Follow patient function after critical care for long-term assessment of outcomes (e.g., frequency of repeated visits or readmission).
  6. Analyze alternatives and their cost-effectiveness for individual critical care areas in comparison to other alternatives and their global impact.
  7. Optimize overall success rates in relation to resource utilization and document performance for review of the quality of care and for accreditation.

(a)

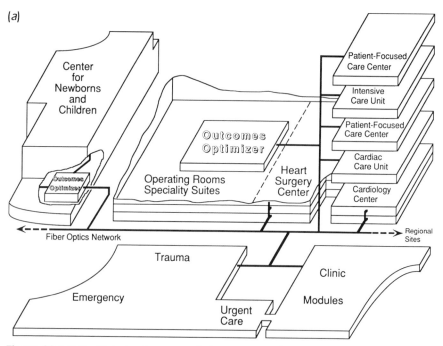

Figure 28.16(a). Global outcomes optimizer concept. One or more performance teams help optimize critical care by using computer-facilitated units (a), distributed universal workstations (b) or a customized hybrid of these two. Fiber optics, other types of networks, or wireless data communications link the sites.

mobile diagnostic carts, robotic workstations, remote review, and satellite laboratories via fiber optics or other types of telecommunication (Figs. 28.16a and 28.16b). For example, one performance team could supervise several geographical sites through the use of remote review,[80–80d] integrate these sites with regional[81–85] laboratories, and manage both instrumentation and information, providing there is adequate computer hardware and software support. Global outcomes optimizer functions can be distributed to, or accessed from, critical care areas via telecommunications systems. It is efficient to consolidate some software and database resources and to access them on a local area or wide area network. Collaboration offers the advantage of globally optimizing quality paths, performance maps, and critical care practice parameters.[430–432] By means of collaborative decision analysis, viewed as an ongoing conversational learning process, the performance team will develop expertise at dynamically fulfilling critical needs and simultaneously optimizing both medical and economic outcomes.

28.8. INTEGRATION ∪ SYNTHESIS ⇒ KNOWLEDGE OPTIMIZATION

Knowledge optimization is intuitive. It systematizes the support of critical care into a paradigm that focuses on patient outcomes. It links temporal optimization

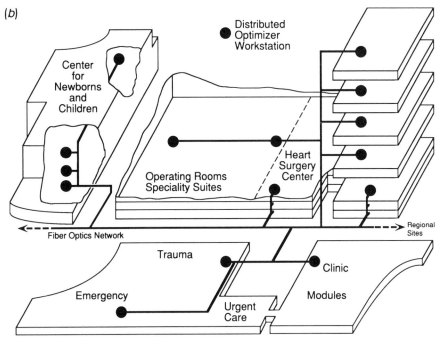

Figure 28.16(b). Network of distributed optimizer workstations. Extension with wireless modalities enhances mobility for efficient integration of point-of-care informatics. Knowledge warehousing facilitates the global integration of outcomes performance.

and diagnostic–therapeutic process optimization through synthesis and draws on the analytic, creative, intuitive, and perceptive skills of the collaborative care team. It integrates point-of-care testing and patient focusing to streamline diagnostic–therapeutic processes. Lactate (temporal optimization) and ionized calcium (process optimization) provide well-documented clinical examples that suggest knowledge optimization can contribute significantly to critical care. These two examples can help us develop performance criteria that are both medical and economic, as well as explicit and quantitative. By establishing sound leadership, satisfying clinical objectives, and preserving quality, hybridization helps link (see 28.7.1) the time-dependent and process-related components of the paradigm. Next, we will outline how the paradigm establishes connectivity among components by blending integration, synthesis, and optimization. Outcomes are integrative. Therefore, integration in anticipation of outcomes improves performance.

• **Integration.**   For clinical effectiveness, integrate the tactical components: (1) point-of-care testing, (2) patient focusing, (3) performance maps and quality paths, and (4) test clusters and critical limits (Fig. 28.17). The objectives of integration are *knowledge continuity* and *knowledge acuity.*

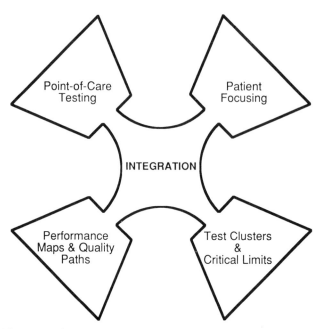

Figure 28.17. Integration. Integration blends point-of-care testing and patient focusing with their operational facets, test clusters and critical limits, and performance maps and quality paths. This produces fast prospective observations linked to patient criticality and appropriate diagnostic–therapeutic strategies, rather than slow retrospective results used for confirmation following empirical treatment.

Clinical integration entails the restructuring and reengineering[433,434] of diagnostic services to support point-of-care testing and patient focusing. Eventually, economic constraints and resource efficiencies will necessitate the automation and robotization of a large proportion of diagnostic testing.[435,436] With few personnel available, the integration of the tactical components (listed above) will be essential for the support of critical care. For example, if a critically ill patient is admitted and progresses from the emergency room to the operating room, and then, to one of several intensive care areas, and if whole-blood analyzers are used in each site, the instruments should yield consistent measurements, so that instrument biases do not mislead physicians into treating "jump" artifacts instead of real changes in medical variables.[17,17a] Bridging space, time, information, and disciplines creates *knowledge continuity.* This is a form of anticipatory problem solving that adds value to the knowledge optimization paradigm by reinforcing the collaborative and multidisciplinary character of modern critical care medicine.

In another example, a critically low potassium result is communicated to a physician, who immediately also receives a point-of-care instrument to perform follow-up electrolyte testing. This quality path creates *knowledge acuity,* another form of future problem solving that enhances the value of knowledge optimization. Because of the potassium critical result, the patient is evaluated urgently, found to have an arrhythmia, treated with potassium and appropriate antiarrhythmics, and placed on a cardiac rhythm monitor until the arrhythmia resolves. A member of the care team performs follow-up potassium testing to monitor the hypokalemia until the potassium level normalizes. On resolution, the instrument is returned to the global outcomes optimizer pool for use with other critical patients. In this application of patient focusing, clinical integration assures that (1) the patient is evaluated urgently, (2) follow-up results are available within the therapeutic turnaround time (near real time) necessary to adjust treatment, (3) dangerous hyperkalemia or other adverse events are avoided, and (4) the crisis is managed cost-effectively. As these examples show, integration merges attention acutely on the patient problem and outcome. Then, point-of-care testing operates mobilely, the way people do in health care, and becomes as much a natural and sensible part of patient evaluation and management as the history, vital signs, and physical exam.

• Synthesis. Focus efforts on synthesis of the information generated from the functional components: (1) temporal optimization and (2) diagnostic–therapeutic process optimization, which are supported by (3) the global outcomes optimizer and (4) hybridization (Fig. 28.18). The objectives of synthesis are *knowledge accessibility, knowledge efficiency,* and *knowledge linkages.*

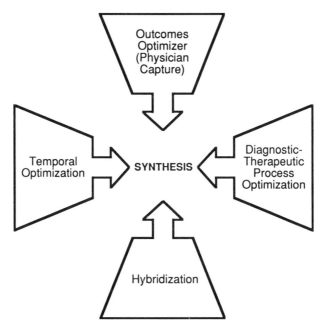

Figure 28.18. Synthesis. Rapid response supported by hybridization captures the physician's thoughts and facilitates patient evaluation and problem solving. Access to timely information is the key to synthesis, which allows the care team to unify temporal optimization and the optimization of diagnostic–therapeutic processes.

Synthesis is the intellectual "engine" of the paradigm. For example, the number of process steps in the patient's criticality trajectory (see Fig. 28.7) generally decreases when physicians quickly perform a synthesis of the clinical observations in order to reveal the pattern of illness and immediately design a strategy for intervention. The resulting *knowledge accessibility* and *knowledge efficiency* are essential to quickly navigate diagnostic-therapeutic processes. This saves time and patient days in critical care. The *knowledge linkages* of synthesis are

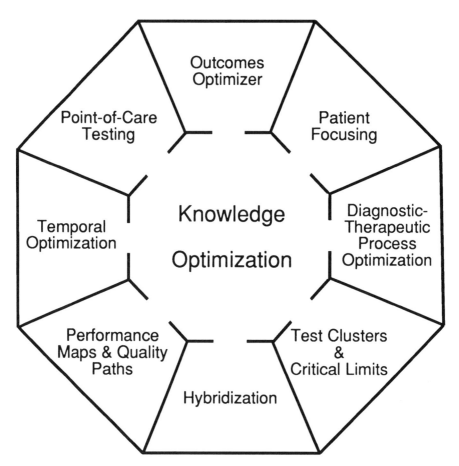

Figure 28.19. Knowledge optimization space. To optimize knowledge, organize components and create new ones that will advance problem solving beyond what was previously possible using fragmented approaches, preexisting technologies, or older patterns of thinking. Two consolidating factors, global outcomes optimization and hybridization, link time-dependent (left) and process-dependent (right) components in critical care. Point-of-care testing and patient focusing insert powerful change agents and are synergistic paradigm shifts. Facing multidimensional components are complementary and tend to balance each other. These components and their connectivity (i.e., linkages, plus integration, synthesis, and optimization) constitute this knowledge structure, which is designed primarily for improving patient outcomes.

temporal optimization and diagnostic–therapeutic process optimization. They relate pathophysiology and treatment fundamentally to outcomes. The global outcomes optimizer (or physician capture) ties the time-dependent and process-related components together, and works in a complementary capacity with hybridization. Hybridization forms the foundation for synthesis by unifying competing disciplines or independent units and by coping with change by creating change.

• Knowledge Optimization.   Optimize the patient's criticality trajectory through the diagnostic-therapeutic processes. Frame actions in terms of overall progress, performance, and success. The objective of knowledge optimization is improved patient outcomes.

The components of the knowledge optimization are interrelated and interdependent (Fig. 28.19). The three primarily time-dependent components are (1) point-of-care testing, (2) temporal optimization, and (3) performance maps and quality paths (left, Fig. 28.19). The three primarily process-related components are (1) patient focusing, (2) diagnostic–therapeutic process optimization, and (3) test clusters and critical limits (right, Fig. 28.19). This paradigm works synergistically with point-of-care testing and patient focusing, which give it sustainable power and momentum. Knowledge optimization helps us create a defensible balance of economic and medical objectives and then, fulfill them effectively and efficiently through the collaborative optimization of outcomes.

28.9. CONCLUSION—THE FUTURE AND THE OPPORTUNITIES

Knowledge Technologies. The currency of the future will be *knowledge.* Perhaps, therefore, point-of-care testing should be considered a *knowledge technology,* since it quickly creates new knowledge that is medically valuable. Point-of-care testing will soon by maturing to a phase where rapid response, consistently high quality results, and economic savings are achieved simultaneously. Therefore, we must look to additional knowledge technologies to help optimize the quality of patient care. Knowledge-based products will be vital. For example, computer-facilitated systems now are available to (1) predict the risk of morbidity and mortality among critically ill patients, (2) link patient outcomes with resource use and expenses, (3) apply patient acuity scoring for management of staffing and treatment protocols, and (4) provide performance reports of quality indicators.[430–432] Importantly, recent objective evidence[437–441] shows that prognostic estimates are helpful in daily clinical decision making and that critical care sites can be compared for severity-adjusted cost-effectiveness—a timely and useful example of knowledge optimization in action. The judicious use of these new knowledge technologies will differentiate the future problem solvers ("pioneers") in this paradigm and will enhance patient survival, as well as physician success, in the highly competitive era ahead. Knowledge technologies add substantially to the notion of knowledge optimization, which here focused primarily on diagnostic testing, biosensor-based whole-blood analysis, and how to implement these effectively.

Knowledge Performance. Integrated healthcare systems, managed care, and capitation are imposing limitations on critical care resources. Economic incentives are becoming strong enough to motivate many, if not all, medical professionals and their organizations to design performance teams made up of multidisciplinary individuals who focus on *integration* and *synthesis* in order to *optimize* outcomes and the use of resources. There is a parallel national effort to improve performance. The Joint Commission on Accreditation of Healthcare Organizations (JCAHO) increasingly stresses satisfactory patient outcomes as a criterion for hospital accreditation. The Society of Critical Care Medicine recently launched Project IMPACT, a performance-tracking national database for critical care.[431] Project IMPACT allows both local tracking of outcomes and, by means of a national registry, peer comparisons with other critical care services, health systems, and geographic areas. Peer comparisons provide incentives to improve morbidity rates, mortality rates, and other measures of the quality of medical care in order to compete better at the local and national levels. Knowledge optimization will be fundamental to the successful attainment of enhanced performance and the fulfillment of these national objectives.

Knowledge Creation. Knowledge optimization blends current technological and medical trends in a fundamental paradigm that helps identify several valuable opportunities for laboratory professionals. First, it encourages careful analysis of clinical observations. Thus, the laboratory consultant or clinical pathologist can contribute substantially to our understanding of temporal optimization and the role of diagnostic testing in optimizing diagnostic–therapeutic processes. This also will facilitate wise selection of alternative testing modalities, test clusters, and instrument formats. Second, the knowledge optimization paradigm encourages collaboration. The laboratory professional is a natural member of the performance team (or teams) overseeing outcomes optimization and is well prepared to continuously improve the quality of point-of-care testing in critical care and other disciplines. Explicit specialty-specific performance criteria for accuracy, precision, response time, test clusters, and other factors are essential and can only be established and accomplished jointly with clinicians. Third, knowledge optimization calls for clinical integration in the form of practice guidelines, care paths, and treatment algorithms. These can help determine how, when, and where whole-blood analysis and point-of-care testing should be implemented. They also improve cost-effectiveness. It is essential to incorporate leadership from laboratory professionals who are familiar with the economics of diagnostic testing and the advantages and disadvantages of new diagnostic technologies. Fourth, knowledge optimization merges this clinical integration with synthesis. The clinical pathologist can facilitate synthesis by helping the care team learn how to best use immediate test results to accelerate critical decision cycles and treatment. Fifth, the paradigm focuses on outcomes optimization from a global perspective. This perspective is appropriate for the laboratory professional, who provides services to the entire healthcare system and thereby, can help remove inconsistency and variance. Finally, knowledge optimization will help improve the efficiency with which laboratory professionals fulfill shared goals—creating new knowledge and maximizing patient welfare.

ACKNOWLEDGMENT

I am indebted to Kathryn Marr and Kate Maney for several of the illustrations. Judith Welsh and Julia Barry provided valuable library assistance. I thank the staff of the Health Sciences Library and the Interlibrary Loan Department. Over the years many colleagues have contributed to these concepts. I thank them all.

REFERENCES

1. Kost GJ, Jammal MA, Ward RE, Safwat: Monitoring of ionized calcium during human hepatic transplantation: critical values and their relevance to cardiac and hemo-dynamic management. *Am J Clin Pathol* 86:61–70, 1986.

2. Kost GJ: Point-of-care testing for ionized calcium in cardiac and critical care. *Lab-Medica Internatl* 12:18–21, 1995.

3. Forrest ARW, Shenkin A: Dangerous pseudohyponatremia. *Lancet* 2:1256, 1980.

4. Frier BM, Steer CR, Baird JD, Bloomfield S: Misleading plasma electrolytes in diabet-ic children with severe hyperlipidemia. *Arch Dis Child* 55:771–775, 1980.

5. Weisberg LS: Pseudohyponatremia: A reappraisal. *Am J Med* 86:315–318, 1989.

6. Kost GJ: Accurate and efficient diagnosis of hyperosmolar coma. *Audio-Digest Intern Med* 38(10), May 22, 1991.

7. Grateau G, Bachmeyer C, Taulera O, Sarfati G, Cremer G, Sereni D: Pseu-dohyponatremia and pseudohyperphosphatemia in a patient with human immu-nodeficiency virus infection. *Nephron* 46:640, 1993.

8. Vaswani SK, Sprague R: Pseudohyponatremia in multiple myeloma. *South Med J* 86:251–252, 1993.

9. Sachs C, Levillain P: The real cause of discrepancy between plasma sodium results obtained by ISE and "dilution" techniques: an error in the dilution factor. *AACC Electrolyte/Blood Gas Division Newslett* 9:2–4, 1994.

10. Kost GJ: Role of new whole blood analytical techniques in critical care. *Clin Chem* 35:1232–1233, 1989.

11. Kost GJ: New whole blood analyzers and their impact on cardiac and critical care. *Crit Rev Clin Lab Sci* 30:153–202, 1993.

12. Kost GJ: Point-of-care testing: patient focusing for the future. In Howanitz PJ, McBride JH, eds: *Professional Practice in Clinical Chemistry: A Review.* Washington, DC: Amer-ican Association for Clinical Chemistry Press, 1994, pp. 443–454.

13. Hall JR, Shapiro BA: Acute care/blood gas laboratories: Profile of current operations. *Crit Care Med* 12:530–533, 1984.

14. Kost GJ, Shirey TL: New whole-blood testing for laboratory support of critical care at cardiac transplant centers and US hospitals. *Arch Pathol Lab Med* 114:865–868, 1990.

15. Kost GJ: New stat laboratory instrumentation: We can and should satisfy clinicians' demands for rapid response. *Am J Clin Pathol* 94:522–523, 1990.

16. Kost GJ: The impact of whole-blood testing on response time: a challenge for the new College of American Pathologists Q-Probes program. *Arch Pathol Lab Med* 114:921–922, 1990.

17. Kost GJ: Guidelines for point-of-care testing. *Proc Society Critical Care Medicine*

Educational and Scientific Symp 24:8, 1995; audio recording. Palm Desert, CA: Convention Cassettes Unlimited.

17a. Kost GJ: Guidelines for point-of-care testing: Improving patient outcomes. *Pathol Patterns, Am J Clin Pathol* 104:S111–S127, 1995.

18. Shirey TL: Critical care profiling for informed treatment of severely ill patients. *Pathol Patterns, Am J Clin Pathol* 104:S79–S87, 1995.

19. Kost GJ, Trent JKT, Saaed D: Indications for measurement of total carbon dioxide in arterial blood. *Clin Chem* 34:1650–1652, 1988.

20. Zaloga GP: The ideal critical care profile. *Proc Society Critical Care Medicine Educational and Scientific Symp* 24:8, 1995; audio recording. Palm Desert, CA: Convention Cassettes Unlimited.

20a. Castro HJ, Oropello JM, Halpern N: Point-of-care testing in the intensive care unit: the intensive care physician's perspective. *Pathology Patterns, Am J Clin Pathol* 104:S95–S99, 1995.

21. Arnold MA: New developments and clinical impact of noninvasive monitoring. In: Kost GJ, ed. *Handbook of Clinical Automation, Robotics, and Optimization.* New York: John Wiley and Sons, Inc.; 1996: Chapter 26.

22. Kost GJ, Hague C: *In vitro, ex vivo,* and *in vivo* biosensor systems. In: Kost GJ, ed. *Handbook of Clinical Automation, Robotics, and Optimization.* New York: John Wiley and Sons, Inc.; 1996: Chapter 27.

22a. Kost GJ, Hague C: The current and future status of critical care testing and patient monitoring. *Pathol Patterns, Am J Clin Pathol* 104:S2–S17, 1995.

23. Vogt W, Nagel D, Sator H: *Cluster Analysis in Clinical Chemistry: A Model.* New York: Wiley, 1987.

24. Kost GJ: The hybrid laboratory: Shifting the focus to the point of care. *MLO (Medical Laboratory Observer)* 24(9S):17–28, 1992.

25. Kost GJ: The hybrid laboratory: The clinical laboratory of the 1990's is a synthesis of the old and the new. *Arch Pathol Lab Med* 116:1002–1003, 1992.

25a. Thiebe L, Vinci K, Gardner J: Point-of-care testing: improving day-stay services. *Nurs Management* 24(12):54,56, 1993.

26. Kost GJ: The challenges of ionized calcium: cardiovascular management and critical limits. *Arch Pathol Lab Med* 111:932–934, 1987.

27. Kost GJ: Ionized calcium: Cardiac significance, critical limits and clinical challenges. *Clin Chem* 38:926–927, 1992.

28. Kost GJ: The significance of ionized calcium in cardiac and critical care: availability and critical limits at US medical centers and children's hospitals. *Arch Pathol Lab Med* 177:890–896, 1993.

29. Bachner P, Howanitz PJ: A response to challenge for the College of American Pathologists new Q-Probes program: The impact of whole-blood testing on response time. *Arch Pathol Lab Med* 114:1195–1197, 1990.

30. Cembrowski GS, Steindel S: *Emergency Department Turnaround Time: Preliminary Report of Results.* Q-Probes 90-13A. Northfield, IL: College of American Pathologists, 1990.

31. Howanitz PJ, Steindel SJ, Cembrowski GS, Long TA: Emergency department stat test turnaround times: A College of American Pathologists' Q-Probes study for potassium and hemoglobin. *Arch Pathol Lab Med* 116:122–128, 1992.

32. Howanitz PJ, Cembrowski GS, Steindel SJ, Long TA: Physician goals and laboratory test turnaround times: A College of American Pathologists Q-Probes study of 2763 clinicians in 722 institutions. *Arch Pathol Lab Med* 117:22–28, 1993.

33. Jahn M: Turnaround time down sharply, yet clients want results faster. *MLO* 25(9):24–29, 1993.

34. Jahn M: CLIA after year 1: No help to patients, and a hindrance to labs. *MLO* 26(5):20–26, 1994.

35. *Blood Gas Monitoring: Economic Assessment and Market Strategies.* Washington, DC: The Lash Group, 1992.

36. McAllister E: *Point of Care (POC) Testing Report.* Plymouth Meeting, PN: IMS America, Health Care Division, 1994.

37. *Operational Laboratory Benchmarking Project.* Oak Brook, IL: University Hospital Consortium. Sept 1994.

37a. Cummings JP: *Technology Report, Point-of-Care Testing: Whole-blood Clinical Analyzers.* Oak Brook, IL: University Hospital Consortium; 1995.

38. Tsai WW, Nash D, Last JV: Point-of-care testing: Barriers and facilitators to implementation. *American Clinical Laboratory. Perspectives in Laboratory Management,* 1994.

39. Bickford GR: Decentralized testing in the 1990s. A survey of United States hospitals. *Clin Lab Management Rev* 8(4):327–338, 1994; *Clinics Lab Med* 14:623–645, 1994.

40. Weetall HH: The biosensor technology program at the National Institute of Standards and Technology (NIST). *Biosens Bioelectron* 8:xii–xiii, 1993.

41. Kricka LJ, Wilding P: Micromechanics and nanotechnology. In: Kost GJ, ed. *Handbook of Clinical Automation, Robotics, and Optimization.* New York: John Wiley and Sons, Inc.; 1996: Chapter 3.

42. Ansell J, Tiarks C, Hirsch J, et al: Measurement of the activated partial thromboplastin time from a capillary (fingerstick) sample of whole blood: A new method for monitoring heparin therapy. *Am J Clin Pathol* 95:222–227, 1991.

43. Nardella A, Unser S, Cyr J, et al: Implementing near-patient coagulation monitoring. *MLO* 24:1–4, 1992.

44. Oberhardt BJ: Advancing blood coagulation testing to the point of care in response to molecular biology-driven development of pharmaceuticals. *Clin Chem* 39:1982–1984, 1993.

45. Reich DL, Yanakakis MJ, Vela-Cantos FP, DePerio M, Jacobs E: Comparison of bedside coagulation monitoring tests with standard laboratory tests in patients after cardiac surgery. *Anesth Analg* 77:673–679, 1993.

46. Rose VI, Dermott SC, Murray BF, McIver MM, High KA, Oberhardt BJ: Decentralized testing for prothrombin time and activated partial thromboplastin time using a dry chemistry portable analyzer. *Arch Pathol Lab Med* 117:611–617, 1993.

47. Arkin CF: Coagulation screening tests. *Am J Clin Pathol* 102:150–151, 1994.

48. Despotis GJ, Santoro SA, Spitznagel E, et al: Prospective evaluation and clinical utility of on-site monitoring of coagulation in patients undergoing cardiac operation. *J Thor Cardiovasc Surg* 107:271–279, 1994.

49. Werner M, Gallagher JV, Ballo MS, Karcher DS: Effect of analytic uncertainty of conventional and point-of-care assays of activated partial thromboplastin time on clinical decisions in heparin therapy. *Am J Clin Pathol* 102:237–241, 1994.

50. Oberhardt BJ: Thrombosis and hemostasis testing at the point of care. *Pathol Patterns, Am J Clin Pathol* 104:S72–S78, 1995.

51. Gong AK: Near-patient measurements of methemoglobin, oxygen saturation, and total hemoglobin: Evaluation of a new instrument for adult and neonatal intensive care. *Crit Care Med* 23:193–201, 1995.

52. Handorf CR: Background—Setting the stage for alternate-site laboratory testing. *Clin Lab Med* 14:451–465, 1994.

53. *Alternate Site Testing Conference: Venturing Beyond the Boundaries of the Clinical Laboratory.* Arlington, VA: College of American Pathologists, Jan, 1995. (Reprinted in *Arch Pathol Lab Med* 119:867–983, 1995.)

54. Herring K, McLellan W, Plaut D: QC and new technology: Do the old rules still apply? *MLO* 25(9S):7–15, 1993.

55. Jacobs E: Total quality management and point-of-care testing. *MLO* 25(9S):2–6, 1993.

56. Handorf CR: Quality control and quality management of alternate-site testing. *Clin Lab Med* 14:539–558, 1994.

57. Jones BA: Testing at the patient's bedside. *Clinics Lab Med* 14:473–492, 1994.

58. Pikul FJ: CLIA and point-of-care testing. *MLO* 25(9S):42–47, 1993.

59. Hamlin WB: Regulatory and accreditation implications of alternate-site laboratory testing. *Clin Lab Med* 14:605–622, 1994.

60. Ehrmeyer SS, Laessig RH: Regulatory requirements (CLIA'88, JCAHO, CAP) for decentralized testing. *Pathol Patterns, Am J Clin Pathol* 104:S40–S49, 1995.

61. Clarke WL, Cox D, Gonder-Frederick LA, Carter W, Pohl SL: Evaluating clinical accuracy of systems for self-monitoring of blood glucose. *Diabetes Care* 10:622–628, 1987.

62. Koschinsky T, Dannehl, Gries FA: New approaches to technical and clinical evaluation of devices for self-monitoring of blood glucose. *Diabetes Care* 11:619–629, 1988.

63. Ting C, Nanji AA: Evaluation of the quality of bedside monitoring of the blood glucose level in a teaching hospital. *Can Med Assoc J* 138:23–26, 1988.

64. Chu S, Edney-Parker H: Evaluation of the reliability of bedside glucose testing. *Lab Med* 20:93–96, 1989.

65. Colagiuri R, Colagiuri S, Jones S, Moses RG: The quality of self-monitoring of blood glucose. *Diabetes Med* 7:800–804, 1990.

66. Fogh-Anderson N, Wimberley PD, Thode J, Siggaard-Anderson O: Direct reading glucose electrodes detect the molality of glucose in plasma and whole blood. *Clin Chim Acta* 189:33–38, 1990.

67. Phillipou G, Farrant RK, Phillips PJ: Computer based quality assessment of hospital capillary blood glucose monitoring. *Diabetes Med* 7:234–237, 1990.

67a. Atkin SH, Dasmahapatra A, Jaker MA, Chorost MI, Reddy S: Fingerstick glucose determination in shock. *Ann Int Med* 114:1020–1024, 1991.

68. Havlin CE, Parvin CA, Cryer PE: The accuracy of blood glucose monitoring devices. *Clin Diabetes* 9:92–93, 1991.

69. Kost GJ, Wiese DA, Bowen TP: New whole blood methods and instruments: glucose measurement and test menus for critical care. *J Internatl Fed Clin Chem* 3:160–172, 1991.

70. Vallera DA, Bissell MG, Barron W: Accuracy of portable blood glucose monitoring: Effect of glucose level and prandial state. *Am J Clin Pathol* 95:247–252, 1991.

71. Lewandrowski K, Cheek R, Nathan DM, et al: Implementation of capillary blood glucose monitoring in a teaching hospital and determination of program requirements to maintain quality testing. *Am J Med* 93:419–426, 1992.

72. Tate PF, Clements CA, Walters JE: Accuracy of home blood glucose meters. *Diabetes Care* 15:536–538, 1992.

73. Jones BA, Bachner P, Howanitz PJ: Bedside glucose monitoring: A College of American Pathologists Q-Probes study of the program characteristics and performance in 605 institutions. *Arch Pathol Lab Med* 117:1080–1087, 1993.

74. Watts NB: Bedside monitoring of blood glucose in hospitals: Speed vs precision and accuracy. *Arch Pathol Lab Med* 117:1078–1079, 1993.

75. American Diabetes Association: Self-monitoring of blood glucose. *Diabetes Care* 17:81–86, 1994.

76. Bernbaum M, Albert SG, McGinnis J, et al: Laboratory assessment of glucose meters does not predict reliability of clinical performance. *Lab Med* 25:32–34, 1994.

77. Genter PM, Ipp E: Accuracy of plasma glucose measurements in the hypoglycemic range. *Diabetes Care* 17:595–598, 1994.

77a. Maser RE, Butler MA, DeCherney GS: Use of arterial blood with bedside glucose reflectance meters in an intensive care unit: Are they accurate? *Crit Care Med* 22:595–599, 1994.

77b. Sylvain HF, Pokorny ME, English SM et al: Accuracy of fingerstick glucose values in shock. *Am J Crit Care* 4:44–48, 1995.

78. Chmielewski SA: Advances and strategies for glucose monitoring. *Pathol Patterns, Am J Clin Pathol* 104:S59–S71, 1995.

79. Nichols JH, Howard C, Loman K, Miller C, Nyberg D, Chan DW: Laboratory and bedside evaluation of portable glucose meters. *Am J Clin Pathol* 103:244–254, 1995.

79a. Stott RAW, Hortin GL, Wilhite TR, Miller SB, Smith CH, Landt M: Analytical artifacts in hematocrit measurements by whole-blood chemistry analyzers. *Clin Chem* 41:306–311, 1995.

79b. Wilding P: Point-of-care testing: Reality or dream. *Clin Lab News.* 21:4, 1995.

80. Felder RA: Robotic automation of near-patient testing. In: Kost GJ, ed. *Handbook of Clinical Automation, Robotics, and Optimization.* New York: John Wiley and Sons, Inc.; 1996: Chapter 24.

80a. Felder RA: Robotics and automated workstations for rapid response testing. *Pathol Patterns, Am J Clin Pathol* 104:S26–S32, 1995.

80b. Boyd JC, Felder RA, Margrey KS, Holman W, Savory J: Use of fully-automated laboratories to provide cost-effective testing at the point of care. Charlottesville, NC: Medical Automation Systems, Inc., 1995. (International Federation of Clinical Chemistry Meeting, Melbourne, Australia.)

80c. Kisner HJ: Medical automation systems' RALS. *Clin Management Lab Rev* 9(2):130–133, 1995.

80d. *UVA Study Confirms RALS System Responsible for Significant Reductions in Turnaround Times for Blood Gas Analysis and Ventilator Weaning Protocols.* Charlottesville, VA: Medical Automation Systems; 1995.

81. Steiner JW: *A Conceptual Framework for a Province-Wide Laboratory Services Delivery System.* Toronto: Chi Laboratory Systems, Inc. and GSA Consulting; 1994.

82. *Laboratory Services Review. Report to the Ministry of Health.* Toronto: Queen's Printer for Ontario (Catalog No. 2227248); 1994.

83. Steiner JW, Root JM, Buck E: The regionalization of laboratory services. *MLO* 26(6):22–29, 1994.

84. Steiner JW, Root JM, Buck E: Lab regionalization: Structural options for the age of managed competition. *MLO* 26(7):48–51, 1994.

85. Steiner JW, Root JM, Buck E: Lab networks: models of regional cooperation. *MLO* 26(8):38–42, 1994.

86. Craig TM: The economics of near-patient testing. In Marks V, Alberti SMM, eds: *Clinical Biochemistry Nearer the Patient.* New York: Churchill-Livingstone, 1985, Chap 15, pp. 162–167.

87. Goldschmidt HMJ, Vuysters FAM, Leijten JF: Cost of laboratory monitoring tests evaluated with regard to the medical information present. In Salamon R, Blum B, Jorgensen M, eds: *Proc 5th Conf Medical Informatics.* New York: North-Holland, 1986, pp. 266–270.

88. Statland B, Brzys K: Evaluating stat testing alternatives by calculating annual laboratory costs. *Chest* 97:198S–203S, 1990.

88a. Winkelman JW, Woo J, Tirabassi CP, O'Connell M: Centralization and decentralization of the hospital clinical laboratory. In Vonderschmitt DJ, ed: *Laboratory Organization-Automation.* New York: Walter deGruyter, 1991, pp. 81–98.

89. Greendyke RM: Cost analysis: bedside glucose testing. *Am J. Clin Pathol* 97:106–107, 1992.

89a. Greendyke RM: Cost analysis of bedside glucose testing. *Am J Clin Pathol* 98:384, 1992.

89b. May ME: Cost analysis of bedside glucose testing. *Am J Clin Pathol* 98:383, 1992.

90. McIntire T: Cost analysis of bedside glucose testing. *Am J Clin Pathol* 98:383–384, 1992.

91. Popper C: Using cost-effectiveness analysis to weigh testing decisions. *MLO* 24(9S):29–35, 1992.

91a. Rabbitts DG: Point-of-care testing: Needs and cost-benefit analysis. *Clin Lab Sci* 6:228–230, 1993.

92. Roizen MF, Schreider B, Austin W, Carter C, Polk S: Pulse oximetry, capnography, and blood gas measurements: reducing cost and improving quality of care with technology. *J Clin Monit* 9:237–240, 1993.

93. Coalition for Critical Care Excellence: *ICU Cost Reduction: Practical Suggestions and Future Considerations.* Anaheim, CA: Society of Critical Care Medicine, 1994.

94. *Cost Benefit Analysis of the GEM Premier Blood Gas and Electrolyte Analyzer.* Salt Lake City, UT: The International Healthcare Consulting Group, 1994.

95. Frankel HL, Rozycki GS, Ochsner MG, et al: Minimizing admission laboratory testing in trauma patients: use of a microanalyzer. *J Trauma* 37:728–736, 1994.

96. Gipe BT, Harris S: Accurate cost accounting for critical care medicine. *Crit Care Med* 22:A40, 1994.

97. Keffer JH: *Economic Aspects of Decentralized Testing.* Washington, DC: American Association for Clinical Chemistry Teleconference, Nov 15, 1994.

97a. Lee-Lewandrowski E, Laposata M, Eschenbach K, et al: Utilization and cost analysis of bedside capillary glucose testing in a large teaching hospital: implications for managing point of care testing. *Am J Med* 97:222–230, 1994.

98. Shapiro BA: Blood gas monitors: Justifiable enthusiasm with a note of caution. *Am J Resp Crit Care Med* 149:850–851, 1994.

99. Shapiro BA: Evaluation of blood gas monitors: Performance criteria, clinical impact, and cost/benefit. *Crit Care Med* 22:546–548, 1994.

100. Simpson KN, LaVallee RL, Halpern MT, et al: *The Economic and Clinical Efficiency of Point-of-Care Testing for Critically Ill Patients: GEM Premier versus Usual Laboratory Testing Procedures* (Executive Summary). Ann Arbor, MI: Mallinckrodt Sensor Systems, 1994.

100a. Tsai WW, Nash DB, Seamonds B, Weir GJ: Point-of-care versus central laboratory testing: an economic analysis in an academic medical center. *Clin Ther* 16:899–910, 1994.

101. Winkelman JW, Wybenga DR, Tanasijevic MJ: The fiscal consequences of central vs distributed testing of glucose. *Clin Chem* 40:1628–1630, 1994.

101a. *Control Destiny: Control Cost.* Society of Critical Care Medicine 24th Educational and Scientific Symposium, 1995. Video produced by Abbott Critical Care Systems, Chesterfield, MI.

101b. Fleisher M, Schwartz MK: Automated approaches to rapid response testing: a comparative evaluation of point-of-care and centralized laboratory testing. *Pathol Patterns, Am J Clin Pathol* 104:S18–S25, 1995.

102. Keffer JH: The economic aspects of new delivery options for diagnostic testing. In: Kost GJ, ed. *Handbook of Clinical Automation, Robotics, and Optimization.* New York: John Wiley and Sons, Inc.; 1996: Chapter 23.

102a. Keffer JH: Economic considerations of point-of-care testing. *Pathol Patterns, Am J Clin Pathol* 104:S107–S110, 1995.

103. Nosanchuk JS, Keefner R: Cost analysis of point-of-care laboratory testing in a community hospital. *Am J Clin Pathol* 103:240–243, 1995.

104. Shapiro BA: Clinical and economic performance criteria for intraarterial and extraarterial blood gas monitors, with comparison with *in vitro* testing. *Pathol Patterns, Am J Clin Pathol* 104:S100–S106, 1995.

105. Smith I: The economics of pulse oximetry. *J. Resp Care Pract* 73–79, Jan 1995.

106. Kost GJ, Lathrop JP: Designing hybrid laboratories, performance maps, and quality paths for patient-focused care. *MLO* 25(9S):16–26, 1993.

107. Lathrop JP: *Restructuring Health Care: The Patient-Focused Paradigm.* San Francisco: Jossey-Bass, 1993.

108. Bishop MS, Husain I, Aldred M, Kost GJ: Multisite point-of-care potassium testing for patient-focused care. *Arch Pathol Lab Med* 118:797–800, 1994.

109. Kuhn TS: *The Structure of Scientific Revolutions.* Chicago: University of Chicago Press, 1970.

110. Barker JA: *Future Edge: Discovering the New Paradigms of Success.* New York: William Morrow, 1992.

111. Salem M, Chernow B, Burke R, et al. Bedside diagnostic testing: Its accuracy, rapidity, and utility in blood conservation. *JAMA* 266:382–389, 1991.

112. Herr DM, Newton NC, Santrach PJ, Hankins DG, Burritt MF: Airborne and rescue point-of-care testing. *Pathol Patterns, Am J Clin Pathol* 104:S54–S58, 1995.

112a. Burritt MF, Santrach PJ, Hankins DG, Herr D, Newton NC: Evaluation of the i-STAT portable clinical analyzer for use in a helicopter. *Scand J Clin Lab Invest,* in press.

112b. Kost GJ: Artificial intelligence and new knowledge structures. In: Kost GJ, ed.

Handbook of Clinical Automation, Robotics, and Optimization. New York: John Wiley and Sons, Inc.; 1996: Chapter 8.

112c. Albert A, Chapelle JP, Bourguignat A: Dynamic outcome prediction from repeated laboratory measurements made on intensive care unit patients. I. Statistical aspects and logistic models. *Scan J Clin Lab Invest* 44 (Suppl 171):259–268, 1984.

113. Ash D, Gold G, Seiver A, Hayes-Roth B: Guaranteeing real-time response with limited resources. *Artif Intell Med* 5:49–66, 1993.

114. Autio K, Kari A, Tikka H: Integration of knowledge-based system and database for identification of disturbances in fluid and electrolyte balance. *Comput Method Programs Biomed* 34:201–209, 1991.

115. Beyer J, Schulz G, Strack T, Kustner E, Schrezenmeir J: Computer-assisted diabetes therapy—a challenge for modern medicine. *Z Gesamte Inn Med* 45:673–677, 1990.

116. Blum RL: Induction of causal relationships from a time-oriented clinical database: an overview of the RX project. *Proc 2nd Natl Conf Artificial Intelligence* (Pittsburgh, PA), 1982, pp. 355–357.

116a. Bourguignat A, Albert A, Chapelle JP: Dynamic outcome prediction from repeated laboratory measurements made on intensive care unit patients. III. Application to severe head injury. *Scand J Clin Lab Invest* 44 (Suppl 171):279–287, 1984.

116b. Chapelle JP, Albert A, Bourguignat A: Dynamic outcome prediction from repeated laboratory measurements made on intensive care unit patients. II. Application to acute myocardial infarction. *Scan J Clin Lab Invest* 44 (Suppl 171):269–278, 1984.

117. Coiera E: Intelligent monitoring and control of dynamic physiological systems. *Artif Intell Med* 5:1–8, 1993.

117a. Connelly DP, Rhodes JB: Decision making in clinical monitoring: Experts, expert systems and statistics. In Kerkhof PLM, van Dieijen-Visser MP, eds: *Laboratory Data and Patient Care.* New York: Plenum Press, 1988; pp. 171–176.

118. Das AK, Musen MA: A temporal query system for protocol-directed decision support. *Meth Info Med* 33:358–370, 1994.

119. Deutsch T, Boroujerdi MA, Carson ER, et al: The principles and prototyping of a knowledge-based diabetes management system. *Comput Meth Programs Biomed* 29:75–88, 1989.

120. Deutsch T, Lehmann ED, Carson ER, Roudsari AV, Hopkins KD, Sonksen PH: Time series analysis and control of blood glucose levels in diabetic patients. *Comput Meth Programs Biomed* 41:167–182, 1994.

120a. East T, Morris A, Wallace J, et al: Computerized decision support systems are an effective tool for the standardization of critical care. *Crit Care Med* 23:A25, 1994.

120b. Eddy DM: Timing of repeated monitoring tests. *Scand J Clin Lab Invest* 44 (Suppl 171):131–152, 1984.

121. Friesdorf W, Konichezky S, Gross-Alltag F, Fattroth A, Schwilk B: Data quality of bedside monitoring in an intensive care unit. *Internatl J Clin Monit Comput* 11:123–128, 1994.

122. Furukawa T: Revolution of paradigm in clinical diagnosis—from the mechanization to the intelligent being. *Rinsho Byori* 39:1044–1048, 1991.

123. Gardner RM: Computerized management of intensive care patients. *MD Comput* 3:36–51, 1986.

124. Groth T, Moden H: A knowledge-based system for real-time quality control and fault diagnosis of multitest analyzers. *Comput Meth Programs Biomed* 34:175–190, 1991.

125. Groth T, Collison PO: Strategies for decision support for fluid and electrolyte therapy in the intensive care unit-approaches and problems. *Internatl J Clin Monit Comput* 10:3–15, 1993.

126. Hayes-Roth B, Washington D, Ash R, et al: Guardian: a prototype intelligent agent for intensive-care monitoring. *Artif Intell Med* 4:165–185, 1992.

127. Hayes-Roth B, Uckun S, Larsson JE, et al: Guardian: an experimental system for intelligent intensive care unit monitoring. *Proc Annu Symp Comput Appl Med Care,* 1994, p 1004.

128. Hazen GB: Factored stochastic trees: a tool for solving complex temporal medical decision models. *Med Decision Making* 13:227–236, 1993.

129. Hovorka R, Svacina S, Carson ER, Williams CD, Sonksen PH: A consultation system for insulin therapy. *Comput Meth Programs Biomed* 32:303–310, 1990.

130. Howorka K, Thoma H, Grillmayr H, Kitzler E: Phases of functional, near-normoglycaemic insulin substitution: What are computers good for in the rehabilitation process in type I (insulin-dependent) diabetes mellitus? *Comput Methods Programs Biomed* 32:319–323, 1990.

130a. Imami ER, Komer K, Martin M: Computer assisted ICU patient management: physician progress notes, summaries, quality improvement and billing. *Crit Care Med* 22:A26, 1994.

131. Kohane IS: Temporal reasoning in medical expert systems. In Salamon R, Blum B, Jorgensen M, eds: *Proc 5th Conf Medical Informatics.* New York: North-Holland, 1986.

132. Koski EM, Sukuvaara T, Makivirta A, Kari A: A knowledge-based alarm system for monitoring cardiac operated patients—assessment of clinical performance. *Internatl J Clin Monit Comput* 11:79–83, 1994.

133. Lau F: A clinical decision support system prototype for cardiovascular intensive care. *Internatl J Clin Monit Comput* 11:157–169, 1994.

134. Lehmann ED, Deutsch T, Carson ER, Sonksen PH: Combining rule-based reasoning and mathematical modeling in diabetes care. *Artif Intell Med.* 6:137–160, 1994.

135. Martin JC, Maguire LC: Fuzzy logic expert systems. In: Kost GJ, ed. *Handbook of Clinical Automation, Robotics, and Optimization.* New York: John Wiley and Sons, Inc.; 1996: Chapter 7.

136. Moret-Bonillo V, Alonso-Betanzos A: Uncertainty based approach for symbolic classification of numeric variables in intensive care units. *J Clin Eng* 15:361–369, 1990.

136a. Mutimer D, McCauley B, Nightingale P, Ryan M, Peters M, Neugerger J: Computerized protocols for laboratory investigation and their effect on use of medical time and resources. *J Clin Pathol* 45:572–574, 1992.

137. Nykanen P, Boran G, Pince H, et al: Interpretative reporting and alarming based on laboratory data. *Clin Chim Acta* 222:37–48, 1993.

138. Patil RS, Szollovits P, Schwartz WB: Modeling knowledge of the patient in acid-base and electrolyte disorders. In Szolovits P, ed: *Artificial Intelligence.* Boulder, CO: Westview Press, 1982, pp 191–226.

138a. Rollo JL, Fauser BA: Computers in total quality management. Statistical process control to expedite stats. *Arch Pathol Lab Med* 117:900–905, 1993.

139. Russ TA: A system for using time-dependent data in patient management. In Salamon R, Blum B, Jorgensen M, eds: *Proc 5th Conf Medical Informatics.* New York: North-Holland, 1986, pp. 165–169.

140. Shahar Y, Musen MA: A temporal-abstraction system for patient monitoring. *Proc Ann Symp Comp Appl Med Care,* 1992, pp 121–127.

141. Shahar Y, Das AK, Tu SW, Kraemer FB, Musen MA: Knowledge-based temporal abstraction for diabetic monitoring. *Proc Ann Symp Comput Appl Med Care,* 1994, pp 697–701.

142. Sittig DF, Gardner RM, Pace NL, Morris AH, Beck E: Computerized patient care in a complex, controlled clinical trial in the intensive care unit. *Comput Meth Programs Biomed* 30:77–84, 1989.

143. Sittig DF, Pace NL, Gardner RM, Beck E, Morris AH: Implementation of a computerized patient advice system using the HELP clinical information system. *Comput Biomed Res* 22:474–487, 1989.

144. Sukuvaara T, Koski EM, Makivirta A, Kari A: A knowledge-based alarm system for monitoring cardiac operated patients-technical construction and evaluation. *Internatl J Clin Monit Comput* 10:117–126, 1993.

145. Tate KE, Gardner RM, Weaver LK: A computerized laboratory alerting system. *MD Comput* 7:296–301, 1990.

146. Timcenko A, Reich DL: Real-time expert system for advising anesthesiologists in the cardiac operating room. *Proc Ann Symp Comput Appl Med Care,* 1994, p 1005.

147. Uckun S, Dawant BM: Qualitative modeling as a paradigm for diagnosis and prediction in critical care environments. *Artif Intell Med* 4:127–144, 1992.

148. Uckun S, Dawant BM, Lindstrom DP: Model-based diagnosis in intensive care monitoring: the YAQ approach. *Artif Intell Med* 5:31–48, 1993.

149. Uckun S: Instantiating and monitoring treatment protocols. *Proc. Ann Symp Comput Appl Med Care,* 1994, pp 689–693.

150. Uckun S: Model-based reasoning. In: Kost GJ, ed. *Handbook of Clinical Automation, Robotics, and Optimization.* New York: John Wiley and Sons, Inc.; 1996: Chapter 6.

151. Ursino M, Artioli E, Avanzolini G, Potuto V: Integration of quantitative and qualitative reasoning: an expert system for cardiosurgical patients. *Artif Intell Med* 61 (Suppl 1):229–247, 1994.

152. Vertosick FT: Neural networks. In: Kost GJ, ed. *Handbook of Clinical Automation, Robotics, and Optimization.* New York: John Wiley and Sons, Inc.; 1996: Chapter 4.

152a. Vitek PJ, Lennard-Jones P: Disciplining time-related clinical and laboratory data. In Kerkhof PLM, van Dieijen-Visser MP, eds: *Laboratory Data and Patient Care.* New York: Plenum Press, 1988; pp 165–170.

153. Wade TD, Byrns PJ, Steiner JF, Bondy J: Finding temporal patterns—a set-based approach. *Artif Intell Med.* 6:263–271, 1994.

154. Winkel P: A programming language and a system for automated time- and laboratory test level dependent decision-making during patient monitoring. *Comput Biomed Res* 23:426–446, 1990.

155. Zarkadakis G, Carson ER, Cramp DG, Finkelstein L: ANABEL: intelligent blood-gas analysis in the intensive care unit. *Internatl J Clin Monitor Comput.* 6:167–171, 1989.

156. Friedman BA, Mitchell W: Integrating information from decentralized laboratory testing sites: the creation of a value-added network. *Am J Clin Pathol* 99:637–642, 1993.

157. Roberts DE, Bell DD, Ostryznuik T, et al: Eliminating needless testing in intensive care—an information-based team management approach. *Crit Care Med* 21:1452–1458, 1993.

158. Bauer S: A blood gas network: Using blood gas and electrolyte analyzers at the point of care. *MLO* 26(9S):2–9, 1994.

159. Elevitch FR: Multimedia communications networks: Patient care through interactive point-of-care testing. *Clinics Lab Med* 14:559–568, 1994.

160. Hortin GL, Utz C, Gibson C: Managing information from bedside testing. *MLO* 27:28–32, 1995.

161. Jacobs E: Information integration for point-of-care and satellite testing. In: Kost GJ, ed. *Handbook of Clinical Automation, Robotics, and Optimization.* New York: John Wiley and Sons, Inc.; 1996: Chapter 25.

161a. Jacobs E, Laudin A: The satellite laboratory and point-of-care testing—Integration of information. *Pathol Patterns, Am J Clin Pathol* 104:S33–S39, 1995.

162. Liscouski J: *Laboratory and Scientific Computing: A Strategic Approach.* New York: Wiley, 1995, Chapter 25.

163. Holtzman S: *Intelligent Decision Systems.* Reading, MA:Addison-Wesley, 1989.

164. Seiver A, Holtzman S: Decision analysis: A framework for critical care decision assistance. *Internatl J Clin Monit Comput* 6:137–156, 1989.

165. Howard RA: From influence to relevance to knowledge. In Oliver RM, Smith JQ, eds: *Influence Diagrams, Belief Nets, and Decision Analysis.* New York: Wiley, 1990, Chap 1, pp 3–23.

165a. Shachter RD, Hendrickson MR: A decision theoretic perspective on clinicopathologic diagnosis. *Proc Internatl Workshop on Principles of Diagnosis,* 1990.

166. Seiver A: A decision class analysis of critical life-support decision-making. *Internatl J Clin Monit Comput* 10:31–66, 1993.

167. Belkora JK, Fehling MR, Esserman LJ: Assuring medical decision quality through decision analysis for patient and physicians. In: Kost GJ, ed. *Handbook of Clinical Automation, Robotics, and Optimization.* New York: John Wiley and Sons, Inc.; 1996: Chapter 29.

168. Kroll MH: Medical decision analysis. In: Kost GJ, ed. *Handbook of Clinical Automation, Robotics, and Optimization.* New York: John Wiley and Sons, Inc.; 1996: Chapter 30.

169. Kroll MH. Automated-facilitated causal reasoning in diagnosis and management. In: Kost GJ, ed. *Handbook of Clinical Automation, Robotics, and Optimization.* New York: John Wiley and Sons, Inc.; 1996: Chapter 31.

170. Yang JM, Lewandrowski KB, Laposata M: Algorithmic diagnosis. In: Kost GJ, ed. *Handbook of Clinical Automation, Robotics, and Optimization.* New York: John Wiley and Sons, Inc.; 1996: Chapter 32.

170a. Cordell JL: A guide to developing clinical pathways. *MLO* 27:35–39, 1995.

171. Hillborne LH, Oye RK, McArdle JE, et al: Evaluation of stat and routine turnaround times as a component of laboratory quality. *Am J Clin Pathol* 91:331–335, 1989.

172. Hillborne LH, Oye RK, McArdle JE, et al: Use of specimen turnaround time as a

component of laboratory quality: a comparison of clinician expectations with laboratory performance. *Am J Clin Pathol* 92:613–618, 1989.

173. Steindel S: *Analytical Turnaround Time (TAT) Data Analysis and Critique (CSF)*. Q-Probes 89-03A. Northfield, IL: College of American Pathologists, 1989.

174. Valenstein PN, Emancipator KA: Sensitivity, specificity, and reproducibility of four measures of laboratory turnaround time. *Am J Clin Pathol* 91:452–457, 1989.

175. Zaloga GP, Hill TR, Strickland RA, et al: Bedside blood gas, electrolyte monitoring in critically ill patients. *Crit Care Med* 17:920–925, 1989.

176. Fleisher M, Schwartz MK: Strategies of organization and service for the critical-care laboratory. *Clin Chem* 36:1557–1561, 1990.

177. Fletcher AB: The essential role of the laboratory in the optimal care of the sick neonate. *J Internatl Fed Clin Chem* 2:166–172, 1990.

178. Zaloga GP: Evaluation of bedside testing options for the critical care unit. *Chest* 97:185S–190S, 1990.

179. Jacobs E, Sarkozi L, Colman N: A centralized critical care (stat) laboratory. *Crit Care Rep* 2:397–405, 1991.

180. Zaloga GP: Monitoring versus testing technologies: present and future. *MLO* 23:20–31, 1991.

181. Bluth EI, Lambert DJ, Lohmann TP, et al: Improvement in "Stat" laboratory turnaround time: a model continuous quality improvement project. *Arch Intern Med* 152:837–840, 1992.

182. Jahn M: Stats too high, yet labs cope. *MLO* 25:33–38, 1993.

183. Zaloga GP, Dudas L, Roberts P, Bortenschlager L, Black K, Prielipp R: Near-patient blood gas and electrolyte analyses are accurate when performed by non-laboratory individuals. *J Clin Monitor* 9:341–346, 1993.

184. Trotto NE: Stats: tolerable for some, a major headache for others. *MLO* 26:20–24, 1994.

185. Trotto N: Stat testing triumphs and disappointments. *MLO* 26:26–31, 1994.

186. Cooney MM: Managed healthcare: Managing the risks of laboratory testing in an integrated delivery system. *Pathol Patterns, Am J Clin Pathol* 104:S50–S53, 1995.

187. Kost GJ: Theory of network planning for laboratory research and development. *Am J Clin Pathol* 79:353–359, 1983.

188. Kost GJ: Application of Program Evaluation and Review Technic (PERT) to laboratory research and development planning. *Am J Clin Pathol* 86:186–192, 1986.

189. Thorson SH, Marini JJ, Pierson DJ, Hudson LD: Variability of arterial blood gas values in stable patients in the intensive care unit. *Chest* 84:14–18, 1983.

190. Sasse SA, Chen PA, Mahutte CK: Variability of arterial blood gas values over time in stable medical intensive care unit patients. *Chest* 106:187–193, 1994.

191. Kost GJ, Evans BD, Biltz JH, et al: Pattern recognition ("fingerprinting") for continuous quality improvement of point-of-care whole blood testing. *Proc Oak Ridge Conf Advanced Analytical Concepts for the Clinical Laboratory,* 1992, p. 20.

192. Evans BD, Blitz J, Becker R, MacDonald P, Coleman R, Kost GJ: Pattern recognition ("fingerprinting") for continuous quality improvement of point-of-care testing. *Clin Chem* 38:1029–1030, 1992.

193. Speicher CE: Practice parameters. An opportunity for pathologists to take a leadership role in patient care. *Arch Pathol Lab Med* 114:823–824, 1990.

194. Strickland RA, Hill TR, Zaloga GP: Bedside analysis of arterial blood gases and electrolytes during and after cardiac surgery. *J Clin Anesth* 1:248–252, 1989.

195. Kost GJ: The future is now! Patient-centered testing result of automation, robotics. *ADVANCE Med Lab Prof* 10–11,18, April 1994.

195a. Bailey TM: Implementing point-of-care testing at Methodist Hospital. *Proc Amer Soc Clin Pathol* (New Orleans), 1995, A158.

196. Hammond JE, Simmons RC, McLendon WW: Critical care laboratory services in a central laboratory: use of dedicated pneumatic tube and instrument-microcomputer-laboratory information system interface. *Info Pathol* 2:15–22, 1987.

197. Keshgegian AA, Bull GE: Evaluation of a soft-handling computerized pneumatic tube specimen delivery system. *Am J Clin Pathol* 97:535–540, 1992.

198. Eschenbach K, Missiano D: Implementing a pneumatic tube system: maintenance. *Adv Admin Lab* 3:45–48, 1994.

199. Winkelman JW, Wybenga DR: Quantification of medical and operational factors determining central versus satellite laboratory testing of blood gases. *Am J Clin Pathol* 102:7–10, 1994.

200. Weber D: Logistics and transport. In: Kost GJ, ed. *Handbook of Clinical Automation, Robotics, and Optimization.* New York: John Wiley and Sons, Inc.; 1996: Chapter 9.

201. Travers EM, Wolke JC, Johnson R, et al: Changing the way lab medicine is practiced at the point of care. *MLO* 26:33–40, 1994.

202. Bedell SE, Deitz DC, Leeman D, et al: Incidence and characteristics of preventable iatrogenic cardiac arrests. *JAMA* 265:2815–2820, 1991.

203. *Near Patient Testing: A Partnership for Quality Care.* Video. Washington, DC: American Association for Clinical Chemistry, 1992.

204. Kost GJ: Critical limits for urgent clinician notification at US medical centers. *JAMA* 263:704–707, 1990.

205. Critical limits studied. *Clin Chem News* 16:6, 1990.

206. Kost GJ: Critical limits for emergency clinician notification at United States children's hospitals. *Pediatrics* 88:597–603, 1991.

207. Kost GJ: Strategies to reduce hyperkalemia-induced cardiac arrhythmias in premature infants and newborns. *Pediatrics* 89:1130–1131, 1992.

208. Table of critical limits. In Wallach JB: *Interpretation of Diagnostic Tests: A Handbook Synopsis of Laboratory Medicine.* Boston: Little, Brown, 1992, Chap 2, pp 28–29.

209. Kost GJ: Using critical limits to improve patient outcome. *MLO* 25(3):22–27, 1993.

210. Table of critical limits. *MLO* (Clinical Laboratory Reference) 1994–1995, p 5.

211. Critical Limits. *Adv Admin Lab* 3:18, 1994.

211a. Nanji AA, Poon R, Hinberg I: Decentralized clinical chemistry testing: quality of results obtained by residents and interns in an acute care setting. *J Intensive Care Med* 3:272–277, 1988.

212. *Managing Patient-Focused Laboratory Services.* Video. Chicago: American Society of Clinical Pathologists, 1993.

213. Operational restructuring: 19 pioneering models. *Healthcare Forum J* July/Aug 1992.

214. Patient-focused care—a comparison study. *Hosp Food Nutr Focus* 11:6–7, 1994.

215. Patient focused care. Health management guide. *Health Serv J* 104:1–12, 1994.

216. Roles of health information managers and coders in patient-focused care. *J AHIMA* 64(Suppl 2), 1993.

217. Bernd DL: Patient-focused care pays hospital-wide dividends. *Health Care Strategic Management* 10:9–12, 1992.

218. Bickler B: Putting patient-focused care into practice. *AORN J* 60:242–245, 1994.

219. Borzo G: Patient-focused hospitals begin reporting good results. *Health Care Strategic Management* 10:1, 17–22, 1992.

220. Boyer ST: Patient-focused work design: hospital and pharmacy department restructuring. *Top Hosp Pharm Management* 14:20–27, 1994.

221. Brider P: The move to patient-focused care. *Am J Nurs* 92:26–33, 1992.

222. Cousar JB, Peters TH: Laboratories in patient-centered units.*Clin Lab Med* 14:525–538, 1994.

223. Esler R, Bentz P, Sorensen M, Van Orsow T: Patient-centered pneumonia care: a case management success story. *Am J Nurs* 94:34–38, 1994.

224. Farris BJ: Converting a unit to patient-focused care. *Health Prog* 74:22–25, 1993.

225. Galloway M, Moffitt GK: Integrating TQM and patient focused care. *Rev Patient Focused Care Assoc* Fall:14–16, 1992.

226. Galloway M, Tinstman TC: Helping hospitals spread the word about their patient focused care programs. Communicating effectively with physicians. *Rev Patient Focused Care Assoc* Fall:18–20, 1992.

227. Galloway MG: Designing patient focused reward systems. *Rev Patient Focused Care Assoc* Spring:2–5, 1993.

228. Galloway M, Leander WJ: The state of innovation: the outlook for patient focused restructuring. *Rev Patient Focus Care Assoc* Winter:12–13, 1993.

229. Gomberg F, Miller K: Focused care centers, decentralization, cross-training, and care paths define "World Class Healthcare" at Florida's Lee Memorial. *Strategies Healthcare Excellence* 5(3):1–7, 1992.

230. Goodemote E: The evolutionary development of patient focused managers. *Rev Patient Focused Care Assoc* Summer:17–20, 1993.

231. Harrell A: Building a patient record system. New information technologies will support development of patient-focused care. *Health Prog* 75:51–54, 1994.

232. Jacobsen TJ: Integrating patient-focused information systems in a open-architecture environment. *Comput Healthcare* 12:38–42, 1991.

233. Janower ML: Patient-focused care: radiology department beware. *Radiology* 187:313–314, 1993.

234. Jirsch D: Patient-focused care: the systemic implications of change. *Health Management Forum* 6:27–32, 1993.

235. Johnson PE, Rearson MB: Pharmacy's role within a multidisciplinary, patient-focused model for health care. *Top Hosp Pharm Management* 10:67–74, 1991.

236. Johnson W, Miller K: Lee Memorial Hospital records positive early results for first of several "Focused Care Centers," foundation of hospitalwide conversion. *Strategies Healthcare Excellence* 5(10):1–8, 1992.

237. Jones WJ, Bullard M: *New Century Hospital: Patient-Focused Planning and Design.* San Francisco: New Century Healthcare Press, 1992.

238. Kerfoot K: Risk management and the nurse manager: the role of patient-focused care. *Nurs Econ* 11:173–175, 1993.

239. Koska MT: Patient-centered care: Can your hospital afford not to have it? *Hospitals* 64:48–54, 1990.

240. Lansky D: A patient-focused approach to measuring the quality of cardiac care. *Qual Lett Healthcare Lead* 5:18–23, 1993.

241. Lathrop JP: The patient-focused hospital. *Healthcare Forum J* 34:17–21, July/Aug 1991.

242. Lathrop JP, Seufert GE, MacDonald RJ, Martin SB: The patient-focused hospital: a patient care concept. *J Soc Health Syst* 3:33–50, 1991.

243. Lathrop JP: The patient-focused hospital. *Healthcare Forum J* 35:76–78, May/June 1992.

244. Leander WJ: Helping hospitals spread the word about their patient focused care programs. *Rev Patient Focused Care Assoc* Summer:21–23, 1992.

245. Leander WJ, Rees RT: Effective education for patient focused staff. *Rev Patient Focused Care Assoc* Fall:2–6, 1992.

246. Leander WJ: Exploring the economic aspects of patient focused restructuring. *Rev Patient Focused Care Assoc* Winter:14–19, 1993.

247. Leander WJ: Patient focused care team design. Critical aspects of a cost-effective design strategy. *Rev Patient Focused Care Assoc* Summer:10–15, 1993.

248. Lee JG, Clarke RW, Glassford GH: Physicians can benefit from a patient-focused hospital. *Physician Exec* 19:36–38, 1993.

249. Matsch G: Patient-focused care and pharmaceutical care: How do they organizationally work together? *Top Hosp Pharm Management* 14:28–35, 1994.

250. McQueen J: Overcoming the barriers to implementing patient-focused care. *Health Info Management* 7:17–21, 1993.

251. Moffitt GK, Galloway M: Patient focused care and total quality management. *Rev Patient Focused Care Assoc* Summer:2–6, 1992.

252. Moffitt GK, Daly PB, Tracey L, Galloway M, Tinstman TC: Patient-focused care: key principles to restructuring. *Hosp Health Serv Admin* 38:509–522, 1993.

253. Morgan G: The implications of patient focused care. *Nurs Stand* 7:37–39, 1993.

254. Ollier C: Ambitious "Care 2000" initiative decentralizes work process at San Diego's Mercy Hospital & Medical Center. *Strategies Healthcare Excellence* 5:1–7, 1992.

255. Pack DA: Patient-focused care and the future of radiology. *Radiol Technol* 65:375–379, 1994.

256. Parker L: *CARE 2000*. Patient Focused Planning Forum No. 6, December 1992; video available from Ratcliff Architects, Emeryville, CA.

257. Saksen L: EDI (electronic data interchange) and patient-focused care. *Healthcare Exec* 8:40, 1993.

258. Snyder GM: Patient-focused hospitals: an opportunity for respiratory care practitioners. *Resp Care* 37:448–454, 1992.

259. Suh YS: Integrated delivery networks. *Health Prog* 74:51–60, 1993.

260. Talley CR: Patient-focused care and pharmacy. *Am J Hosp Pharm* 50:2317, 1993.

261. Thielke TS: Automation support of patient-focused care. *Top Hosp Pharm Management* 14:53–59, 1994.

262. Thompson CA: Conference explores patient-focused computing. *Am J Hosp Pharm* 51:274–276, 1994.

263. Tidikis F, Strasen L: Patient-focused units improve service and financial outcomes. *Healthcare Finan Management* 48:38–44, 1994.

264. Tornabeni J: Care 2000—a patient-focused care model. *Calif Hosp* 8:12–13, 1994.

265. Townsend MB: Patient-focused care: is it for your hospital? *Nurs Management* 24:74–80, 1993.

266. Troup N: Patient-focused care. A macro approach to productivity and quality improvement. *Healthcare Exec* 7:24–25, 1992.

267. Troup N: Working smarter with patient-focused care. *South Hosp* 58:13–27, 1992.

268. Troup NC: World Class Healthcare—revolutionizing the way hospitals do business. *J Healthcare Inform Management Syst Soc* 1992.

269. Vogel DP: Patient-focused care. *Am J Hosp Pharm* 50:2321–2329, 1993.

270. Weber DO: Six models of patient-focused care. *Healthcare Forum J* 34:23–32, July/Aug 1991.

271. Weber DO: Palomar Pomerado Health System employs second generation knowhow to achieve patient-focused care. *Strategies Healthcare Excellence* 7:1–9, 1994.

272. Weber DO, Weber AL: Reshaping the American hospital—a compendium on patient-focused care. *Healthcare Forum J* 37:49–57, Sep/Oct 1994.

273. Weisman E, Hagland M: Built-in care. One hospital sees the future in patient-centered design. *Hosp Health Network* 68:54–58, 1994.

274. Wimpsett J: Nursing case management: outcomes in a rural environment. *Nurs Management* 25:41–43, 1994.

275. Arnold WP: Perioperative biochemical monitors. In Lake CL, ed: *Clinical Monitoring for Anesthesia and Critical Care.* Philadelphia: Saunders, 1994, pp 539–560.

276. Bria WF, Rydell RL: *The Physician-Computer Connection.* Chicago: American Hospital Association, 1992.

277. Bria W: Person-side terminals: The missing link in patient care information systems. *Healthcare Info,* May 1993.

278. Dennis KE, Sweeney PM, Macdonald LP, Morse NA: Point of care technology: Impact on people and paperwork. *Nurs Econ* 11:229–237, 1993.

279. Eddleman DW, Tucker DM, McEachern M: A patient monitoring system designed as a platform for application development. *Internatl J Clin Monit Comput* 7:233–240, 1990.

280. Gardner E: Bedside ICU computers aid direct care. *Mod Healthcare* 21:26, 1991.

281. Griffin JZ, Woolery LK: Point of care documentation: A viable alternative. *Missouri Med* 91:76–77, 1994.

282. Jacobsen TJ: Workstations as enabling technologies for the computer-based patient record (CPR): point of care approaches across the patient care continuum—nursing's perspective. *Internatl J Bio-Med Comput* 34:123–129, 1994.

283. Stefanchik MF: Point-of-care revolution. *Comput Healthcare* 12:19–24, 1991.

284. Abramson D, Scalea TM, Hitchcock R, Trooskin SZ, Henry SM, Greenspan J: Lactate clearance and survival following injury. *J Trauma* 35:584–589, 1993.

285. Aduen J, Bernstein WK, Khastgir T, et al: The use and clinical importance of a substrate-specific electrode for rapid determination of blood lactate concentrations. *JAMA* 272:1678–1685, 1994.

286. Aduen J, Berstein WK, Miller JA, et al: Relationship between blood lactate concentrations and ionized calcium, glucose, and acid-base status in critically ill and noncritically ill patients. *Crit Care Med* 23:246–252, 1995.

287. Aduen J, Wiese J, Kerzner R, Aktman M, Chernow B: Discordance between increased circulating lactate concentrations and lactic acidosis: Results from a large clinical data base (n = 1,424). *Crit Care Med* 23(1S):A103, 1995.

288. Almenoff PL, Leavy J, Weil MH, Goldberg NB, Vega D, Rackow EC: Prolongation of the half-life of lactate after maximal exercise in patients with hepatic dysfunction. *Crit Care Med* 17:870–873, 1989.

289. Afifi AA, Chang PC, Vinnie YL, da Luz PL, Weil MH, Shubin H: Prognostic indexes in acute myocardial infarction complicated by shock. *Am J Cardiol* 33:826–832, 1974.

290. Astiz ME, Rackow EC: Assessing perfusion failure during circulatory shock. *Crit Care Clin* 9:299–312, 1993.

291. Astiz MA, Rackow EC, Kaufman B, Falk JL, Weil MH: Relationship of oxygen delivery and mixed venous oxygenation to lactic acidosis in patients with sepsis and acute myocardial infarction. *Crit Care Med* 16:655–658, 1988.

292. Bailey EM, Domenico P, Cunha BA: Bacterial of viral meningitis? Measuring lactate in CSF can help you know quickly. *Postgrad Med* 88:217–223, 1990.

293. Bakker J, Coffernils M, Leon M, Gris P, Vincent J-L: Blood lactate levels are superior to oxygen-derived variables in predicting outcome in human septic shock. *Chest* 99:956–962, 1991.

294. Barriere SL, Lowry SF: An overview of mortality risk prediction in sepsis. *Crit Care Med* 23:376–393, 1995.

295. Bishop MH, Shoemaker WC, Appel PL, et al: Relationship between supranormal circulatory values, time delays, and outcome in severely traumatized patients. *Crit Care Med* 21:56–63, 1993.

296. Bonora R, Panteghini M: An enzymatic method for lactate in whole blood adapted to the Cobas Bio. *Clin Chem* 35:324–325, 1989.

297. Boycks E, Michaels S, Weil MH, Shubin H, Marbach EP: Continuous-flow measurement of lacatate in blood: A technique adapted for use in the emergency room. *Clin Chem* 21:113–118, 1975.

298. Boyd O, Grounds RM, Bennett ED: A randomized clinical trial of the effect of deliberate perioperative increase of oxygen delivery on mortality in high risk surgical patients. *JAMA* 270:2699–2707, 1993.

299. Broder G, Weil MH: Excess lactate: An index of reversibility of shock in human patients. *Science* 143:1457–1459, 1994.

300. Campanella L, Tomassetti M, Mazzei F: Biosensor for direct determination of glucose and lactate in undiluted biological fluids. *Biosens Bioelectron* 8:307–314, 1993.

301. Chang WH: Cerebrospinal fluid lactate, acid-base and gases unbalance in severe head injury. *Chung Hua Wai Ko Tsa Chih* 31:759–762, 1993.

302. Chariot P, Ratiney R, Ammi-Said M, Herigault R, Adnot S, Gherardi R: Optimal handling of blood samples for routine measurement of lactate and pyruvate. *Arch Pathol Lab Med* 118:695–697, 1994.

303. Chernow B: Lactate: The ultimate blood test in critical care? *Crit Care State of the Art* 15:253–268, 1995.

304. Cheung P-Y, Finer NN: Plasma lactate concentration as a predictor of death in neonates with severe hypoxemia requiring extracorporeal membrane oxygenation. *J Ped* 125:763–768, 1994.

305. Cooper DJ, Walley KR, Dodek PM, et al: Plasma ionized calcium and blood lactate concentrations are inversely associated in human lactic acidosis. *Intern Care Med* 18:286–289, 1992.

306. Cowan BN, Burns HJG, Boyle P, et al: The relative prognostic value of lactate and hemodynamic measurements in early shock. *Anesthesia* 39:750–755, 1984.

307. DeBoer J, Korf J, Plijter-Groendijk H: In vivo monitoring of lactate and glucose with microdialysis and enzyme reactors in intensive care medicine. *Internatl J Artif Organs* 17:163–170, 1994.

308. Druml W, Grimm G, Laggner AN, Lenz K, Schneeweiss B: Lactic acid kinetics in respiratory alkalosis. *Crit Care Med* 19:1120–1124, 1991.

309. Drummond AJ, Bernard GR, Russell JA: Decreasing lactate is associated with lower mortality of patients who have sepsis syndrome. *Chest* 104:57S, 1993.

310. Dunham CM, Frankenfield D, Belzberg H, Wiles CE, Cushing B, Grant Z: Inflammatory markers: superior predictors of adverse outcome in blunt trauma patients? *Crit Care Med* 22:667–672, 1994.

311. Dunn DL: Predicting mortality in septic patients. *Crit Care Med* 23:228–229, 1995.

312. Falk JL, Rackow EC, Leavy J, et al: Delayed lactate clearance in patients surviving circulatory shock. *Acute Care* 11:212–215, 1985.

312a. Fleming A, Bishop M, Shoemaker W, et al: Prospective trial of supranormal values as goals of resuscitation in severe trauma. *Arch Surg* 127:1175–1179, 1992.

313. Foxdal P, Bergqvist Y, Eckerbom S, Sandhagen B: Improving lactate analysis with the YSI 2300 GL: Hemolyzing blood samples makes results comparable with those for deproteinized whole blood. *Clin Chem* 38:2110–2114, 1992.

314. Friedman G, Berlot G, Kahn RJ, Vincent J-L: Combination of blood lactate levels and pHi in severe sepsis. *Crit Care Med* 22:A112, 1994.

315. Gerlo E, Gorus F, De Meirleir K: Automated micro-method for determining L-(+)-lactate in arterialized whole blood. *Clin Chem* 33:188–189, 1987.

316. Goeneveld ABJ, Kester ADM, Nauta JJP, Thijs LG: Relation of arterial blood lactate to oxygen delivery and hemodynamic variables in human shock states. *Circ Shock* 22:35–53, 1987.

317. Groenendaal F, Veenhoven RH, van der Ground J, Jansen GH, Witkamp TD, de Vries LS: Cerebral lactate and *N*-acetyl-aspartate/choline ratios in asphyxiated full-term neonates demonstrated *in vivo* using proton magnetic resonance spectroscopy. *Ped Res* 35:148–151, 1994.

318. Hakanson H, Kyrolainen M, Mattiasson B: Portable system for continuous *ex vivo* measurements of lactate. *Biosens Bioelectron* 8:213–217, 1993.

319. Hayes MA, Timmins AC, Yau EHS, Palazzo M, Hinds CJ, Watson D: Elevation of systemic oxygen delivery in the treatment of critically ill patients. *N Engl J Med* 330:1717–1722, 1994.

320. Henning RJ, Weil MH, Weiner F: Blood lactate as a prognostic indicator of survival in patients with acute myocardial infarction. *Circ Shock* 9:307–315, 1982.

321. Iberti TJ, Leibowitz AB, Papadakos PJ, Fischer EP: Low sensitivity of the anion gap as a screen to detect hyperlactatemia in critically ill patients. *Crit Care Med* 18:275–277, 1990.

322. Izraeli S, Ben-Sira, L, Harell D, Naor N, Ballin A, Davidson S: Lactic acid as a predictor for erythrocyte transfusion in healthy preterm infants with anemia of prematurity. *J Ped* 122:629–631, 1993.

323. Jeng JC, Lee K, Frankel H, Silva CA, Jablonski K, Jordan MH: Hemoconcentration suggests inadequate resuscitation of burn patients: application of a point of care laboratory instrument. *Crit Care Med* 23:A88, 1995.

324. Jensen JC, Buresh C, Norton JA: Lactic acidosis increases tumor necrosis factor secretion and transcription *in vitro. J Surg Res* 49:350–353, 1990.

325. Karkela J, Pasanen M, Kaukinen S, Morsky P, Harmoinen A: Evaluation of hypoxic brain injury with spinal fluid enzymes, lactate, and pyruvate. *Crit Care Med* 20:378–386, 1992.

326. Katz J, Wolfe RR: On the measurement of lactate turnover in humans. *Metabolism* 37:1078–1080, 1988.

327. Kessler KM, Kozlovskis P, Trohman RG, Myerburg RJ: Serum lactate: prognostic marker for recurrent cardiac arrest? *Am Hear J* 113:1540–1544, 1987.

328. Khodas MI, Leonova SF, Vysotskii MV, Dement'eva II, Tverskoi AL: Prognostic significance of lactate concentration and indicators of acid-base balance in air embolism of cerebral vessels. *Anesteziol Reanimatol* 1:34–37, 1993.

329. Kodama K, Komamura K, Naka M: Serial myocardial lactate metabolic changes after intracoronary thrombolysis in evolving myocardial infarction. *Jpn Circ J* 52:695–701, 1988.

330. Koike A, Wasserman K, Taniguchi K, Hiroe M, Marumo F: Critical capillary oxygen partial pressure and lactate threshold in patients with cardiovascular disease. *J Am Col Cardiol* 23:1644–1650, 1994.

331. Kost GJ: *Hypothesis Relating Skeletal Muscle Fiber Types to the Mechanism of Irreversibility in Hemorrhagic Shock.* Berkeley, CA, 1977.

332. Kost GJ: Utilization of surface pH electrodes to establish a new relationship for muscle surface pH, venous pH, and arterial pH. *Proc San Diego Biomedical Symp* 16:25–33, 1977; *IEEE Trans Biomed Eng* 25:110, 1977.

333. Kost GJ: Surface pH of the medial gastrocnemius and soleus muscles during hemorrhagic shock and ischemia. *Surgery* 95:183–190, 1984.

334. Kruse JA, Zaidi SAJ, Carlson RW: Significance of blood lactate levels in patients with liver disease. *Am J Med* 83:77–82, 1987.

335. Leavy JA, Weil MH, Rackow EC: "Lactate washout" following circulatory arrest. *JAMA* 260:662–664, 1988.

336. Logan A, Edwards JD: Oxygen extraction ratio vs blood lactate as a predictor of survival in shock. *Crit Care Med* 23(1S):A134, 1995.

336a. Luft D, Deichsel G, Schmulling RM, Stein W, Eggstein M: Definition of clinically relevant lactic acidosis in patients with internal diseases. *Am J Clin Pathol* 80:484–489, 1983.

337. Luzi L, Ripamonti M, Marconi C, et al: Whole blood L-lactate assay by a new differential pH method: application to metabolic investigations. *Acta Diabet Latina* 27:129–138, 1990.

338. Marnitz U, Dauberschmidt R, Mrochen H: The value of blood lactate determination in the postoperative phase. *Anesthesiol Reanim* 19:103–109, 1994.

339. Mavric Z, Zaputovic L, Zagar D, Matana A, Smokvina D: Usefulness of blood lactate as a predictor of shock development in acute myocardial infarction. *Am J Cardiol* 67:565–568, 1991.

340. Meyerhoff C, Bischof F, Mennel FJ, et al: On-line continuous monitoring of blood lactate in men by a wearable device based upon an enzymatic amperometric lactate sensor. *Biosens Bioelectron* 8:409–414, 1993.

341. Milzman D, Boulanger B, Wiles C, Hinson D: Admission lactate predicts injury severity and outcome in trauma patients. *Crit Care Med* 20:S94, 1992.

342. Milzman D, Boulanger B, Wiles CE, Mitchell K: Admission lactate predicts fluid requirements for trauma victims during the initial 24 hours. *Crit Care Med* 22:A73, 1994.

343. Milzman D, Manning D, Presman D, Lill D, Howell J, Shirey T: Rapid lactate can impact outcome prediction for geriatric patients in the emergency department. *Crit Care Med* 23:A32, 1995.

344. Mizuno K, Horiuchi K, Matui H, et al: Role of coronary collateral vessels during transient coronary occlusion during angioplasty assessed by hemodynamic, electrocardiographic and metabolic changes. *J Am College Cardiol* 12:624–628, 1988.

345. Mishima M, Kodama K, Nanto S, Hirayama A, Asada S: Serial transcardiac lactate metabolism in post-reperfused stunned myocardium in evolving myocardial infarction. *Jpn Circ J* 55:930–935, 1991.

346. Mizock BA, Falk JL: Lactic acidosis in critical illness. *Crit Care Med* 20:80–93, 1992.

347. Moreau R, Hadengue A, Soupison T, et al: Septic shock in patients with cirrhosis: hemodynamic and metabolic characteristics and intensive care unit outcome. *Crit Care Med* 20:746–750, 1992.

348. Nakada T: Compounds and method for protection of cells and tissues from irreversible injury due to lactic acidosis. US Patent 5,312,839, May 17, 1994.

349. Nguyen AL, Luong JHT: Development of mediated amperometric biosensors for hypoxanthine, glucose and lactate: a new format. *Biosens Bioelectron* 8:421–432, 1993.

350. Palmisano F, Centonze D, Zambonin PG: An in situ electrosynthesized amperometric biosensor based on lactate oxidase immobilized in a poly-o-phenylenediamine film: determination of lactate in serum by flow injection analysis. *Biosens Bioelectron* 9:471–479, 1994.

351. Pandey PC, Pandey V, Mehta S: An amperometric enzyme electrode for lactate based on graphite paste modified with tetracyanoquinodimethane. *Biosens Bioelectron* 9:365–372, 1994.

352. Pasch T, Mahlstedt J, Pichl J, Buheitel G, Pscheidl E: Can the outcome after trauma or sepsis be predicted from biochemical or hormonal parameters? *Prog Clin Biol Res* 236B:85–95, 1987.

353. Paty PB, Banda MJ, Hunt TK: Activation of macrophages by L-lactic acid. *Surg Forum* 39:27–28, 1988.

354. Peretz DI, Scott HM, Duff J, Dossetor JB, MacLean LD, McGregor M: The significance of lacticacidemia in the shock syndrome. *Ann NY Acad Sci* 1133–1141, 119.

355. Rackow EC, Weil MH: Physiology of blood flow and oxygen utilization by peripheral tissue in circulatory shock. *Clin Chem* 36:1544–1546, 1990.

356. Rady MY: Patterns of oxygen transport in trauma and their relationship to outcome. *Am J Emerg Med* 12:107–112, 1994.

357. Rady MY, Rivers EP, Martin GB, Smithline H, Appelton T, Nowak RM: Continuous central venous oximetry and shock index in the emergency department: use in the evaluation of clinical shock. *Am J Emerg Med* 10:538–541, 1992.

358. Raskin MC, Bosken C, Baughman RP: Oxygen delivery in critically ill patients: relationship to blood lactate and survival. *Chest* 87:580–584, 1985.

359. Ronco JJ, Fenwick JC, Tweeddale MG, et al: Identification of the critical oxygen delivery for anaerobic metabolism in critically ill septic and nonseptic humans. *JAMA* 270:1724–1730, 1993.

360. Schuster HP: Prognostic value of blood lactate in critically ill patients. *Resuscitation* 11:141–146, 1984.

361. Serruys PW, Suryapranata H, Piscione F, et al: Myocardial release of hypoxanthine and lactate during percutaneous transluminal coronary angioplasty. *Am J Cardiol* 63:45E–51E, 1989.

362. Sheps DS, Conde C, Cameron B, et al: Resting peripheral blood lactate elevation in survivors of prehospital cardiac arrest: correlation with hemodynamic, electrophysiologic and oxyhemoglobin dissociation indexes. *Am J Cardiol* 44:1276–1282, 1979.

363. Shimojo N, Naka K, Nakajima C, et al: Test-strip method for measuring lactate in whole blood. *Clin Chem* 35:1992–1994, 1989.

364. Shirey TS: *Meeting the New Demands for Stat Critical Care Testing.* Waltham, MA: NOVA Biomedical, 1991.

365. Shirey TS: *Stat Lactate: The Earliest Indicator of Oxygen Deficiency and Circulatory Shock.* Waltham, MA: NOVA Biomedical, 1991.

366. Shirey TS: *Stat Lactate: The Best Indicator of O_2 Deficiency and Circulatory Shock is Now Available as Part of The Blood Gas Panel.* Waltham, MA: NOVA Biomedical, 1994.

366a. Shoemaker WC, Appel PL, Kram HB, Waxman K, Lee TS: Prospective trial of supranormal values of survivors as therapeutic goals in high-risk surgical patients. *Chest* 94:1176–1186, 1988.

367. Shoemaker WC, Appel PL, Kram HB: Hemodynamic and oxygen transport in survivors and nonsurvivors of high-risk surgery. *Crit Care Med* 21:977–990, 1993.

367a. Shoemaker WC, Appel PL, Kram HB, Bishop M, Abraham E: Hemodynamic and oxygen transport monitoring to titrate therapy in septic shock. *New Horizons* 1:145–159, 1993.

368. Siegel LB, Hauser GJ, Hertzog JH, Hopkins RA, Hannan RL, Dalton HJ: Initial postoperative serum lactate predicts outcome in children after open heart surgery. *Crit Care Med* 23(1S):A205, 1995.

369. Siesjo BK: Mechanisms of ischemic brain damage. *Crit Care Med* 16:954–963, 1988.

370. Stacpoole PW, Wright EC, Baumgartner TG, et al: A controlled clinical trial of dichloroacetate for treatment of lactic acidosis in adults. *New Engl J Med.* 327:1564–1569, 1992.

371. Sumimoto T, Takayama Y, Iwasaka T, et al: Mixed venous oxygen saturation as a guide to tissue oxygenation and prognosis in patients with acute myocardial infarction. *Am Heart J* 122:27–33, 1991.

372. Sun S, Weil MH, Tang W, Lindermann R, Yang L: Arterial blood lactate predicts survival following successful cardiac resuscitation. *Crit Care Med* 22:A134, 1994.

373. Tang LM: Serial lactate determinations in tuberculous meningitis. *Scand J Infect Dis* 20:81–83, 1988.

373a. Tietz NW: *Clinical Guide to Laboratory Tests.* Philadelphia: Saunders.

374. Toffaletti J, Christenson RH, Mullins S, Harris RE: Relationship between serum lactate and ionized calcium in open heart surgery. *Clin Chem* 32:1849–1853, 1986.

375. Toffaletti J, Abrams B: Effects of in vivo and in vitro production of lactic acid on ionized, protein-bound, and complex-bound calcium in blood. *Clin Chem* 35:935–938, 1989.

376. Toffaletti JG: Blood lactate: biochemistry, laboratory methods, and clinical interpretation. *Crit Rev Clin Lab Sci* 28:253–268, 1991.

377. Toffaletti J, Hammes ME, Gray R, Lineberry B, Abrams B: Lactate measured in diluted and undiluted whole blood and plasma: comparison methods and effect of hematocrit. *Clin Chem* 38:2430–2434, 1992.

378. Toffaletti J: Physiology and regulation: ionized calcium, magnesium and lactate measurements in critical care settings. *Pathol Patterns, Am J Clin Pathol* 104:S88–S94, 1995.

379. Toffaletti J, Hansell D: Interpretation of blood lactate measurements in pediatric open-heart surgery and in extracorporeal membrane oxygenation. *Scand J Clin Lab Invest* 55:301–307, 1995.

379a. Tuchschmidt JA, Mecher CE: Predictors of outcome from critical illness. Shock and cardiopulmonary resuscitation. *Crit Care Clin* 10:179–185, 1994.

379b. Tuchschmidt J, Fried J, Astiz M, Rackow E: Elevation of cardiac output and oxygen delivery improves outcome in septic shock. *Chest* 102:216–220, 1992.

380. Vallet B, Chopin C, Curtis SE, et al: Prognostic value of the dobutamine test in patients with sepsis syndrome and normal lactate values: a prospective, multicenter study. *Crit Care Med* 21:1868–1875, 1993.

381. Vincent J-L, Dufaye P, Berre J, Leeman M, Degaute J-P, Kahn RJ: Serial lactate determinations during circulatory shock. *Crit Care Med* 11:449–451, 1983.

382. Waite RI, Waite LR, Lim SP, et al: A catheter-based enzyme-coupled electrode for measurement of lactate. *Biomed Instrum Technol* 25:461–464, 1991.

383. Weil MH, Afifi AA: Experimental and clinical studies on lactate and pyruvate as indicators of the severity of acute circulatory failure (shock). *Circulation* 51:989–1001, 1970.

383a. Wiener K: Blood sample tubes for blood lactate assay. *Clin Chem* 41:483, 1995.

384. Wiener L, Walinsky P, Kasparian H, et al: Therapeutic implications of myocardial lactate metabolism in patients considered candidates for emergency myocardial revascularization. *J Thor Cardiovasc Surg* 75:612–620, 1978.

385. Wiese J, Kerzner R, Chernow B: The use of different anti-coagulants in storing blood samples to be used for lactate analysis. *Crit Care Med* 23(1S):A44, 1995.

386. Wiese J, Miller J, Bhatiani A, et al: Proper handling of blood samples for lactate determinations: a prospective, controlled trial. *Crit Care Med* 23(1S):A32, 1995.

387. Wiese J, Sigal B, Davison L, Bernstein W, Aduen J, Chernow B: Increased blood lactate concentrations in cardiac surgery patients: Results of a prospective, longitudinal study. *Crit Care Med* 23(1S):A45, 1995.

388. Xie B, Harborn U, Mecklenburg M, Danielsson B: Urea and lactate determined in 1-microL whole-blood samples with a miniaturized thermal biosensor. *Clin Chem* 40:2282–2287, 1994.

389. Zilva JF: The origin of the acidosis in hyperlactataemia. *Ann Clin Biochem* 15:40–43, 1978.

390. Sanchez GJ, Venkataraman PS, Pryor RW, Parker MK, Fry HD, Blick KE: Hypercalcitonemia and hypocalcemia in acutely ill children: Studies in serum calcium, blood ionized calcium, and calcium-regulating hormones. *J Ped* 114:952–956, 1989.

391. Broner CW, Stidham GL, Westenkirchner DF, Tolley EA: Hypermagnesemia and hypocalcemia as predictors of high mortality in critically ill pediatric patients. *Crit Care Med* 18:921–928, 1990.

392. Cardenas-Rivero N, Chernow B, Stoiko MA, Nussbaum SR, Todres ID: Hypocalcemia in critically ill children. *J Ped* 114:946–951, 1989.

393. Desai TK, Carlson RW, Geheb MA: Prevalence and clinical implications of hypocalcemia in acutely ill patients in a medical intensive care setting. *Am J Med* 84:209–214, 1988.

394. Desai TK, Carlson RW, Thill-Baharozian M, Geheb MA: A direct relationship between ionized calcium and arterial pressure among patients in an intensive care unit. *Crit Care Med* 16:578–582, 1988.

395. Taylor B, Sibbald WJ, Edmonds MW, Holliday RL, Williams C: Ionized hypocalcemia in critically ill patients with sepsis. *Can J Surg* 21:429–433, 1978.

396. Zaloga GP, Chernow B: The multifactorial basis for hypocalcemia during sepsis: studies of the parathyroid hormone-vitamin D axis. *Ann Intern Med* 107:36–41, 1987.

397. Woo P, Carpenter MA, Trunkey D: Ionized calcium: The effect of septic shock in the human. *J Surg Res* 26:605–610, 1979.

398. Wilson RF, Binkley LE, Sabo FM, et al: Electrolyte and acid-base changes with massive blood transfusions. *Am Surg* 58:535–545, 1992.

399. Drop LJ: Ionized calcium, the heart, and hemodynamic function. *Anesth Analg* 64:432–451, 1985.

400. Urban P, Scheidegger D, Buchmann B, Barth D: Cardiac arrest and blood ionized calcium levels. *Ann Intern Med* 109:110–113, 1988.

401. Burchard KW, Gann DS, Colliton J, Forester J: Ionized calcium, parathormone, and mortality in critically ill surgical patients. *Ann Surg* 212:543–550, 1990.

402. Zaloga GP: Hypocalcemic crisis. *Crit Care Clin* 7:191–200, 1991.

403. Zaloga GP: Hypocalcemia in critically ill patients. *Crit Care Med* 20:251–262, 1992.

404. Drop LJ, Laver MB: Low plasma ionized calcium and response to calcium therapy in critically ill man. *Anesthesiology* 43:300–306, 1975.

405. Gray TA, Paterson CR: The clinical value of ionised calcium assays. *Ann Clin Biochem* 25:210–219, 1988.

406. Lynch RE: Ionized calcium: Pediatric perspective. *Ped Clin N Am* 37:373–389, 1990.

407. Forman DT, Lorenzo L: Ionized calcium: Its significance and clinical usefulness. *Ann Clin Lab Sci* 21:297–304, 1991.

408. Meliones JN, Moler FW, Custer JR, et al: Hemodynamic instability after the initiation of extracorporeal membrane oxygenation: Role of ionized calcium. *Crit Care Med* 19:1247–1251, 1991.

409. Boink ABTJ, Buckley BM, Christiansen TF, et al: Recommendations on blood sampling, transport and storage for the determination of the substance concentration of ionized calcium. In Mass AHJ et al, eds: *Methodology and Clinical Applications of Ion-Selective Electrodes.* Vol 8, *Proc IFCC Workshop.* Gaz: Radiometer (Private Press), 1987, pp 81–87.

410. Boink ABTJ, Buckley BM, Christiansen TF, et al: IFCC recommendation on sampling, transport and storage for the determination of the concentration of ionized calcium in whole blood, plasma, and serum. *Ann Biol Clin* 49:434–438, 1991; *Clin Chim Acta* 202:S13–S22, 1991; *Eur J Clin Chem Clin Biochem* 29:767–772, 1991; *J Internatl Fed Clin Chem* 4:147–152, 1992.

411. Lang RM, Fellner SK, Neumann A, Bushinsky DA, Borow KM: Left ventricular contractility varies directly with blood ionized calcium. *Ann Intern Med* 108:524–529, 1988.

412. Hughes WG, Ruedy JR: Should calcium be used in cardiac arrest? *Am J Med* 81:285–296, 1986.

413. Paraskos JA: Cardiovascular pharmacology. III. Atropine, calcium, calcium blockers, and beta-blockers. *Circulation* 74(Suppl 4):IV86–IV89, 1986.

414. Merchant MR, Hutchinson AJ, Butler SJ, Boulton H, Hintchliffe R, Gokal R: Calcium, magnesium mass transfer and lactate balance study in CAPD patients with reduced calcium/magnesium and high lactate dialysis fluid. *Adv Peritoneal Dialysis* 8:365–368, 1992.

414a. Zaloga GP: Critical electrolyte disturbances. *Proc Soc Crit Care Med Educ Sci Symp* 23:134–143, 1994.

415. Casandy M, Forster T, Julesz J: Reversible impairment of myocardial function in hypoparathyroidism causing hypocalcemia. *Br Heart J* 63:58–60, 1990.

416. Connor TB, Rosen BL, Blaustein MP, Applefield MM, Doyle LA: Hypocalcemia precipitating congestive heart failure. *N Engl J Med* 307:869–872, 1982.

417. Ginsburg R, Esserman LJ, Bristow MR: Myocardial performance and extracellular ionized calcium in a severely failing human heart. *Ann Intern Med.* 98(Part 1):603–606, 1983.

418. Carlon GC, Howland WS, Goldiner PL, Kahn RC, Bertoni G, Turnbull AD: Adverse effects of calcium administration. *Arch Surg* 113:882–885, 1978.

419. Katz AM: Is calcium beneficial or deleterious in patients with cardiac arrest? *Ann Intern Med* 109:91–92, 1988.

420. Muller-Plathe O: Improving the acceptance of "ionized calcium" for routine clinical practice. *Scand J Clin Lab Invest* 53(Suppl 214):95–98, 1993.

421. Masters PW, Payne RB: Comparison of hypertonic and isotonic reference electrode junctions for measuring ionized calcium in whole blood: a clinical study. *Clin Chem* 39:1082–1085, 1993.

422. Swanson JR, Heeter C, Limbocker M, Sullivan M: Bias of ionized calcium results from blood gas syringes. *Clin Chem* 40:669–670, 1994.

423. Landt M, Hortin GL, Smith CH, McClellan A, Scott MG: Interference in ionized calcium measurements by heparin salts. *Clin Chem* 40:565–570, 1994.

423a. Toffaletti J, Ernst P, Hunt P, Abrams B: Dry electrolyte-balanced heparinized syringes evaluated for determining ionized calcium and other electrolytes in whole blood. *Clin Chem* 37:1730–1733, 1991.

424. Toffaletti J: Use of novel preparations of heparin to eliminate interference in ionized calcium measurements: have all the problems been solved? *Clin Chem* 40:508–509, 1994.

424a. Toffaletti J, Thompson T: Effects of blended lithium-zinc heparin on ionized calcium and general clinical chemistry tests. *Clin Chem* 41:328–329, 1995.

425. Graham GA, Bergkuist C, Cormier AD, et al: *Ionized Calcium Determinations: Precollection Variables, Specimen Choice, Collection, and Handling*. Villanova, PA: National Committee for Clinical Laboratory Standards, Document C31, 1993.

426. Moran RF, Bergkuist C, Graham GA, Misiano DR, O'Connell KO, Sena SF: *Considerations in the Simultaneous Measurement of Blood Gases, Electrolytes, and Related Analytes in Whole Blood*. Villanova, PA: National Committee for Clinical Laboratory Standards, Document C32, 1993.

427. Burnett RW, Covington AK, Fogh-Andersen N, et al: Recommendations on whole blood sampling, transport, and storage for simultaneous determination of pH, blood gases, and electrolytes. International Federation of Clinical Chemistry Scientific Division. *J Internatl Fed Clin Chem* 6:115–120, 1994.

428. Burritt MF: Electrolytes and blood gases (ionized calcium). *Anal Chem* 65:409R–411R, 1993.

429. Dahlman T, Sjobert HE, Bucht E: Calcium homeostasis in normal pregnancy and puerperium. A longitudinal study. *Acta Obstet Gynecol Scand* 73:393–398, 1994.

430. *AcuBase*. Seattle, WA: Clinical Information Systems, Inc.

431. *Project IMPACT. A National Critical Care Database Developed by the Society of Critical Care Medicine (SCCM) and Tri-Analytics, Inc.* Anaheim, CA: SCCM, 1995.

432. *Quality Intensive Care (QuIC) System*. Redmond, WA: SpaceLabs Medical.

433. Hammer M, Champy J: *Reengineering the Corporation: A Manifesto for Business Revolution*. New York: HarperCollins, 1993.

434. Farnsworth RE, Maguire LC: Re-engineering clinical laboratory processes. In: Kost GJ, ed. *Handbook of Clinical Automation, Robotics, and Optimization*. New York: John Wiley and Sons, Inc.; 1996: Chapter 21.

435. Felder RA: Overview and challenges. In: Kost GJ, ed. *Handbook of Clinical Automation, Robotics, and Optimization*. New York: John Wiley and Sons, Inc.; 1996: Chapter 1.

436. Markin RS: Historical perspectives and critical issues. In: Kost GJ, ed. *Handbook of Clinical Automation, Robotics, and Optimization*. New York: John Wiley and Sons, Inc.; 1996: Chapter 2.

437. Lemeshow S, Klar J, Teres D, et al: Mortality probability models for patients in the intensive care unit for 48 or 72 hours: a prospective, multicenter study. *Crit Care Med* 22:1351–1358, 1994.

438. Rapoport J, Teres D, Lemeshow S, Gehlbach S: A method for assessing the clinical performance and cost-effectiveness of intensive care units: a multicenter inception cohort study. *Crit Care Med* 22:1385–1391, 1994.

439. Wagner DP, Knaus WA, Harrell FE, Zimmerman JE, Watts C: Daily prognostic estimates for critically ill adults in intensive care units: results from a prospective, multicenter, inception cohort analysis. *Crit Care Med* 22:1359–1372, 1994.

440. Zimmerman JE, Shortell SM, Rousseau DM, et al: Improving intensive care: observations based on organizational case studies in nine intensive care units. A prospective, multicenter study. *Crit Care Med* 21:1443–1451, 1993.

441. Zimmerman JE, Wagner DP, Draper EA, Knaus WA: Improving intensive care unit discharge decisions: supplementing physician judgment with predictions of next day risk for life support. *Crit Care Med* 22:1373–1384, 1994.

CHAPTER

29

Assuring Medical Decision Quality through Decision Analysis for Patients and Physicians

JEFFREY K. BELKORA, MICHAEL R. FEHLING, AND
LAURA J. ESSERMAN

ACKNOWLEDGMENT

This work was supported by a grant from the Charitable Lead Trust of Boston, MA.

CONTENTS

Handbook of Clinical Automation, Robotics, and Optimization, Edited by Gerald J. Kost with the collaboration of Judith Welsh.
ISBN 0-471-03179-8 © 1996 John Wiley & Sons, Inc.

29.1. INTRODUCTION

The healthcare industry is beginning to realize that it is not so different from other industries in that it seeks to meet consumer demand for high-quality goods and services.[1] The services that medical professionals provide include decision support. The evolution of decision analysis practice has led to an understanding of six dimensions of decision quality. Decision analysis tools (Section 29.2) can be used by patients to achieve the necessary conditions for optimal decision quality. In order to achieve the sufficient conditions for optimal decision quality, patients may require more competent decision support from physicians.

We present a comprehensive framework (Section 29.3) for evaluating the quality of certain classes of medical decisions, and explaining what features of a medical practice promote high-quality decisions. In this framework, decision analysis establishes the standard for decision quality for simple dichotomy and test/treat decisions. Medical practitioners' decisions, when presented with fully specified simple dichotomy and test/treat cases, are compared to the optimal decision analytic solutions to those cases. In this way, the variation from optimality and differences in decision quality among practitioners can be studied.

This use of decision analysis should complement patients' use of decision quality tools to help patients achieve both necessary and sufficient conditions for optimal decision quality. We suggest that the evaluative framework for medical decisions be deployed by means of a survey. The survey is designed to include predictor variables whose association with responses is to be investigated. The survey sample design allows researchers to incorporate variables associated with different medical practice contexts so that their effect on decision making can be examined. We illustrate these concepts with a survey for breast cancer decision making.

29.2. DECISION QUALITY THROUGH DECISION ANALYSIS
FOR PATIENTS

A discussion of decision quality will require some precise decision language. A decision can be defined using terms from the field of decision analysis.[2] A distinction is the specification of conditions for classification of any phenomenon into one of many mutually exclusive and collectively exhaustive states. At any given time, various distinctions constitute a person's state of information. From time to time, that state of information changes due to events. A decision maker is a person who designs action to influence future events.

The decision maker uses a frame, or description of the decision, to design action. The first feature of a frame is the interval of time, or epoch, over which the decision maker wishes to think prospectively. This is sometimes called the "horizon."

A frame can feature one decision or a series of related decisions, or choices among alternatives, by one particular decision maker. All the other events in the frame are "uncertainties." The possibilities are all the possible states of information at the end of the epoch. Prospects are the decision maker's descriptions of what each possibility means.

The "rules of actional thought," or axioms of decision analysis, require a decision maker to reduce every alternative under consideration to mutually exclusive and collectively exhaustive prospects, associate with each prospect a probability, order the prospects according to preference, establish reference prospects that are equivalent to those at hand, use the equivalent prospects as a basis for evaluating the alternatives, and choose the most preferred alternative.[3] Subscription to these norms buys a decision maker a body of derived knowledge that allows the application of engineering mathematics for simple, powerful, representation and modeling of the preferences, information, and alternatives that form the basis for the decision at hand.

Many authors have thoroughly exposed the fundamental norms and derivations of decision analysis.[2,4,5] In this chapter, our first aim is to illustrate how patients can use decision analysis to achieve decision quality. Next we suggest a framework for the quality improvement of specific classes of medical decisions, to be employed by physicians learning to improve their decision competence.

29.2.1. Understanding Optimal Decision Quality

One of the first lessons that decision analysts learn is to separate the quality of a decision from the quality of the events that succeed it. Popular wisdom invariably confounds the two. For example, a decision to postpone an outdoor party is usually judged on the basis of whether rain falls, not on the quality of the decision at the time it was made.

A basis on which to judge decisions at the time they are made includes the alternatives, information, and preferences that a decision maker finds it prudent to analyze at the time that a decision is declared. In the early days of decision analysis, practitioners focused on perfecting their methodology, which consisted of a decision analysis cycle of basis formulation, analysis, and appraisal.[6]

After decades of practice, leading practitioners of decision analysis have converged on an understanding of six dimensions of decision quality.[7] The first dimension is the decision frame, that is, what is to be included and excluded from the decision analysis. The decision basis contributes three more dimensions: preferences, alternatives, and information. The execution of the analysis cycle is another. Finally, the decision maker's commitment to action determines whether the quality of the previous dimensions is realized.

Decision quality can be measured along the six dimensions represented in Figure 29.1, which shows a decision quality "spider diagram." The practitioners who defined decision quality provide the best explanation of the spider diagram:

> The six spokes radiating from the center represent each of the six elements [of decision quality]. The outer rim represents 100% quality (the point where additional efforts at improvement would not be worth their cost). The hub represents zero percent. The goal is to get as close to 100% in each of the requirements as possible; acceptable decision quality is achieved when the cost of improvement exceeds the marginal benefit of the improvement.[7]

Note that Creswell and McNamee, the authors quoted above, implicitly propose necessary and sufficient conditions for achieving optimal decision quality. Optimal decision quality is attained when the marginal benefit of further effort equals marginal cost, on all the dimensions. The dimensions of decision quality are briefly described in Table 29.1, with references given for the tools necessary to achieve optimality.

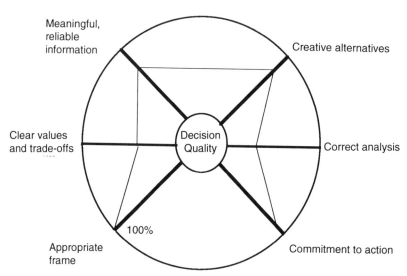

Figure 29.1. The decision quality spider diagram. (Copyright—Strategic Decisions Group. Reprinted by permission.)

TABLE 29.1. The Decision Quality Toolkit

Decision Quality Dimension	To Achieve Quality in This Dimension Is to	Tools to Achieve Quality in this Dimension Include	References
Frame	Examine the right problem in a timely manner	The decision hierarchy	7
Preferences	Use decision maker's preferences, tradeoffs, and risk attitude	Value hierarchy, value functions, utility functions, discounting	5
Information	Scrutinize information for value, relevance	Value of information calculations	8, 9
Alternatives	Consider diverse feasible alternatives	Strategy tables	2
Analysis	Employ validated tools of analysis correctly	Decision diagrams, decision trees, computer software	6, 10
Commitment to action	Implement the resulting recommendation	Organizational learning	11

29.2.2. Achieving Optimal Decision Quality

For the purposes of understanding how the tools of decision quality may be applied, consider the hypothetical case of Lucy, a woman who discovers a suspicious lump in her breast while taking a shower one day. Using the tools in the decision quality toolkit, a decision maker like Lucy can confidently achieve the necessary conditions for optimal decision quality. Lucy's is a fictitious case that patients or experts may find lacking for reasons unrelated to decision-making considerations.

Suppose that, on detecting her suspicious lump, Lucy suspends her showering activity to gather her thoughts. Aware of the need to screen for breast cancer through self-examinations, Lucy frames the lump problem as a potential indication of cancer. Beyond her cursory reading of a breast self-examination pamphlet, which she has misplaced, Lucy has no further information.

One of Lucy's first thoughts is to see her gynecologist. Another alternative that occurs to her is to wait and watch the lump herself over the next few days and weeks. Her preference is to see a doctor as quickly as possible, regardless of the cost or inconvenience. Lucy does no further analysis, gets out of the shower and calls her gynecologist to make an appointment through the assistant who answers the phone.

Lucy was lucky enough, or well-educated enough, to know that breast cancer is a highly prevalent disease that can manifest itself through detectable breast

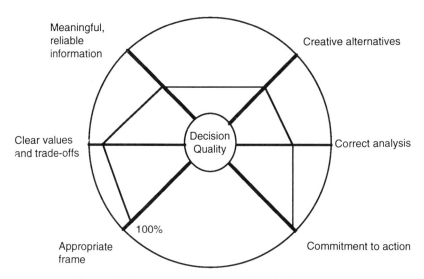

Figure 29.2. Appraisal of Lucy's initial decision quality.

lumps. Her frame was optimal; a broad range of experts would agree that no amount of additional effort would have led her to a better frame. Lucy's preferences featured aversion to undertaking much risk of missing a possible cancer, and not much aversion to generating a false alarm. Again, further exploration of her preferences at this stage would apparently not have led to any material insights. Lucy demonstrated clear commitment to action by implementing her decision without procrastination. So from a decision analytic point of view, Lucy's frame, values, and commitment to action were very close to optimal, represented by scores close to 100% on the spider diagram shown in Figure 29.2.

Along three dimensions, however, Lucy might agree that she could have achieved much higher decision quality at extremely low cost. With a little more analysis, Lucy could have reasoned that she could spend half an hour deliberating before taking further action. This would have allowed her to employ other tools of decision analysis, and notably to generate some creative alternatives. For example, Lucy thought to call her gynecologist out of familiarity and habit. When she did call, she made the appointment through an assistant. Another alternative would have been to speak with the gynecologist, assessing her expertise in palpating lumps, before either going ahead with the appointment or asking for a referral to a breast cancer specialist.

Lucy could also have hunted for her self-examination pamphlet, or found public sources that could provide more information by telephone. This deliberation would have cost almost nothing and had the potential to send Lucy along a much better path to diagnosis and treatment than an appointment with a nonspecialist who might be qualified, but then again might unduly reassure or alarm

Lucy. So on the dimensions of alternatives, information, and analysis, Lucy's decision quality might justifiably be deemed suboptimal.

29.2.3. Implications of Lucy's Initial Decision Quality

Lucy's initial decision about whether to seek assistance resulted in an action that most breast cancer experts would applaud. The event that succeeded this decision was that Lucy got an appointment with her gynecologist. However, if consulted, a decision analyst would want to help evaluate the quality of Lucy's decision regardless of what resulted, so as to identify opportunities for improvement.

Indeed, Lucy might have stumbled into a relatively favorable situation. This is hardly the last important decision she will have to make. If Lucy does not have a high-quality decision-making process, she could be vulnerable in her next decision.

In our example above, Lucy may have been satisfied both with her decision making, and with the result. That does not preclude the assessment that she could have used tools to achieve better, or even optimal, decision quality. Therefore, we revisit Lucy's decision to explore how she might have proceeded using tools of decision quality.

29.2.4. The Decision Hierarchy Framing Tool

The decision hierarchy is a tool used to identify the decision to be analyzed among the many decisions presented by a problem or opportunity (see Fig. 29.3). One way to distinguish the strategic frame from the tactical, and the tactical from the operational, is to consider the question of what is the appropriate time horizon.

A strategic frame looks broadly and deeply at the elements of a situation and

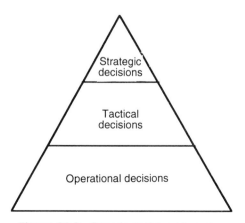

Figure 29.3. Generic decision hierarchy.

challenges all assumptions and decisions. It considers very long-term goals, and the uncertainties that can intervene. A tactical frame accepts certain elements as fixed by previous strategic decisions, and strives to focus on the most important ways that decisions in a particular situation can serve the long-term strategy. An operational frame accepts strategic and tactical decisions as fixed, and seeks to optimize actions with respect to the given strategy and tactics.

Lucy, discovering her suspicious lump during a self-examination, might want to structure her frame using the decision hierarchy. Her longest-term concern about the breast lump might ultimately be her survival, as opposed to, say, her appearance or her career.

Working back from that strategic frame, Lucy might conclude that with regard to her survival, and given her breast lump, seeking medical assistance is the real issue. A competing tactical frame might be to think about what decisions she faces concerning her spiritual care, given her concerns about survival and her breast lump.

At the operational level, Lucy recognizes that, whatever her tactical frame, she will have to make some decisions about whom to call or what to do first. For example, if she resolves the issue of whether to seek medical assistance by determining to call a physician, she must then figure out which one to call. Lucy's decision hierarchy is illustrated in Figure 29.4.

Let's assume Lucy settles on "seek medical assistance" as the appropriate frame for her decision, and analyzes her alternatives, information, preferences, and commitment to action within the bounds of that frame. Lucy's decision quality should be improved by her understanding of different frames, and her willingness to reframe her decision if it becomes necessary.

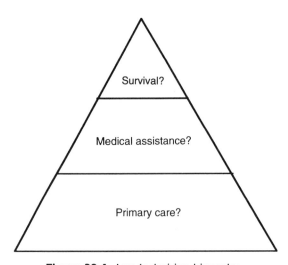

Figure 29.4. Lucy's decision hierarchy.

29.2.5. The Strategy Table for Creating Alternatives

Several recent best-selling books discuss how to foster creativity and come up with creative ideas. Practitioners of decision analysis have incorporated some of the lessons from the creativity field into a tool known as the *strategy table*.[2]

The strategy table features columns, each of which (except the first) represents one dimension of the decision at hand, that is, one area with respect to which various actions can be taken. The columns should be headed with a description of the action dimension (except for the first, to be named later). Underneath, the decision maker adds actions theoretically possible along that dimension without worrying about their feasibility. When this has been done for each column, or action dimension, it will be observed that a particular action from any one column would be coherent with particular actions from other columns. These can be joined with a line indicating a strategy trajectory, labeled in the first column. Three or four feasible trajectories constitute a good set of alternatives to evaluate when analyzing the decision (see Fig. 29.5).

Lucy, having initially framed the decision as whether to seek medical assistance, could have used a strategy table to investigate her options. By dividing and conquering the space of possible actions, she could well identify piecemeal some alternatives she never would have thought of holistically.

The strategy table shown in Figure 29.6 illustrates how Lucy might have identified four general areas in which she could act. First, she could engage her family in different ways. She could communicate with medical professionals. That communication could be done at various times, and in various ways.

In each area, Lucy then thinks of as many actions as she can, putting aside for a moment any judgment of them. Later, a couple of coherent alternatives emerge, which she names. Lucy's decision quality has been improved by the clarification of the alternatives that she wishes to analyze.

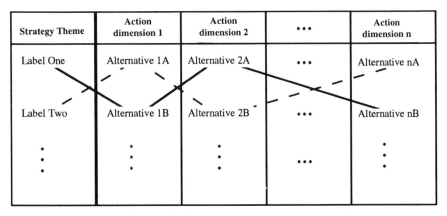

Figure 29.5. A generic strategy table.

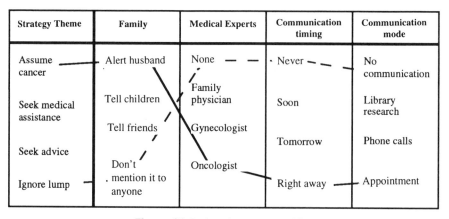

Figure 29.6. Lucy's strategy table.

29.2.6. Decision Diagrams for Communication and Computation of the Basis

The dimension of analysis in decision quality was for a long time handled by decision trees that spawned probability distributions on prospects for decisions, from which a variety of sensitivity analyses could be conducted. Trees, however useful for computations, are difficult to "build" and do not fit on a page if they are at all complicated.

The development of decision diagrams represented a major breakthrough for decision analysis, as they embody formal mathematical models but also communication-friendly representations. A few rules must be followed to enhance the interpretability of the diagram as a representation, and allow it to drive automatic computations of the model.

First, each dimension of the decision basis is represented by a different figure. Decisions or possible actions are represented by squares. Uncertainties are represented by circles, and values are represented in diamond or octagonal or hexagonal nodes. The value node represents an uncertain quantity, because it consists of a set of rules for assigning values based on the resolution of uncertainties and decisions (see Fig. 29.7).

Arrows are differentiated according to whether they link two uncertainties, two decisions, an uncertainty to a decision, a decision to an uncertainty, a decision to a value or an uncertainty to a value. Decision diagram rules state that an arrow must be drawn between two uncertainties when knowing how one resolves changes the decision maker's beliefs (or probability distribution) on the other. This kind of arrow is a relevance arrow. When a decision maker or expert indicates that an arrow should be drawn between two uncertainties, the uncertainties are said to be "mutually relevant."

An arrow must be drawn from a decision node to an uncertainty when the probability distribution over the uncertainty will differ depending on the course of action chosen. Such an arrow is known as an "influence."

Finally, an arrow must be drawn between two decisions when the decision at the foot of the arrow will be made before the decision at the head of the arrow. This is known as an "informational" arrow. An arrow with its foot in an uncertainty and its head at a decision is also known as an informational arrow, since it indicates that the uncertainty will be resolved before the decision in question gets made.

The very experience of building a decision diagram often adds tremendous value to the decision client. What was a complex, uncertain mess benefits from order, completeness, and transparency. Every element of the decision can be pointed to and accounted for.

In particular, all the uncertainties in the model must pass the clarity test. The idea behind the clarity test is that an event should be defined and specified so clearly and unambiguously that a hypothetical clairvoyant could answer "yes" or "no" when asked if the event was going to occur, without needing any further clarification and without using judgment. Thus, by most standards, the uncertainty "rain tomorrow" fails the clarity test, while the uncertainty "at least one inch of precipitation recorded between 3 and 4 a.m. Pacific Standard Time on Saturday the 11th of December 1993 by the meteorologist on duty at San Francisco International Airport" passes the clarity test. Many failures of decision analyses are ultimately traced to confusion over to what an uncertainty in the model actually referred.

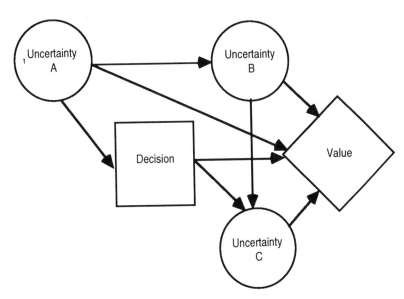

Figure 29.7. Generic decision diagram.

At this point, most decision diagrams feature many uncertain nodes, and to encode probability distributions on all of them would require many resources. Fortunately, the value node contains a formula expressing value as a function of all the decisions and uncertainties in the decision model. The presence of a value node distinguishes a decision diagram from a relevance or inference diagram because deterministic sensitivity analysis allows the decision analyst to focus the decision client's attention on the most impactful uncertainties, for which probability distributions are duly encoded from the client or experts.

Deterministic sensitivity analysis involves swinging each uncertain value in the model from its lowest possible value to its highest and noting the impact on value. Most decisions, no matter how complex or uncertain, derive most of their uncertainty from three to seven uncertainties. All other uncertainties in the model can be set to "medium" levels since in any event their impact is practically negligible.

Finally, from all the individual probability distributions on uncertainties assessed piecemeal, an overall probability distribution on value for each alternative being considered can be calculated, and the decision made according to the risk attitude of the decision client. Further sensitivity analyses can be conducted for insight.

Lucy, deciding whether to seek medical assistance concerning her newly discovered breast lump, could have used a decision diagram to structure her decision. A software package might facilitate this task. First, she would have to identify uncertainties that she thinks are relevant to her decision situation. Suppose she is uncertain as to whether the lump is suspicious, as to whether she has breast cancer, and as to the stage of her cancer if and when it is detected. Next, Lucy's decision is whether to seek medical assistance. If she decides to seek medical assistance, she will determine what kind in a later decision analysis.

Lucy wants all her distinctions to pass the clarity test, so she specifies that a lump is suspicious if, in the course of three successive trials with her eyes closed, she can draw rings around it that overlap to a specified extent. Otherwise the lump is not suspicious, because it doesn't feel different enough from the rest of her breast for her to be able to isolate it.

Next she resolves that she would consider herself to have breast cancer if a pathologist reported that she did after conducting tests, now or later. Otherwise she would consider herself free of cancer. Similarly, which of four stages the cancer had reached would be determined by a pathologist's report, with all variables duly specified.

Lucy can now identify and rank the prospects she faces, from best (no suspicious lump, no cancer of any stage) to worst (no suspicious lump, stage IV cancer when eventually detected). She can express each prospect in terms of a reference prospect so that they may be compared meaningfully. For example, an intermediate prospect of suspicious lump, seek medical assistance, breast cancer, stage I when detected, could be expressed as equivalent to some probability of the best versus a complementary probability of the worst prospect.

Lucy knows that she will observe the result of her "suspicious lump" diagnostic before she has to make her decision and draws an information arrow from that uncertainty to her decision. Her belief about having breast cancer changes according to the result of her diagnostic, so she insists on a relevance between those two uncertainties. Also, Lucy's beliefs about the stage of her breast cancer when it is detected change according to whether she seeks medical assistance now and whether she in fact has breast cancer, so an influence and relevance, respectively, are required. Finally, all the uncertainties as well as the decision are relevant to her value judgment of any particular prospect, so arrows are needed from those nodes to the value node (see Fig. 29.8).

At the level of this frame, Lucy faces a simple yet uncertain decision, and so foregoes deterministic sensitivity analysis. Lucy can now encode her probability assessments for uncertainties, if she wishes to pursue the analysis.

For example, given a suspicious lump, Lucy might believe there is a 20% chance it is cancer, whereas if she cannot isolate a lump she feels she has a 1% chance of having cancer. Given that she has cancer and seeks medical assistance, the chance that it is stage I she assesses to be 50%, whereas if she does not have cancer and seeks medical assistance, she feels that if she ever is detected with cancer it will be stage I with a probability of 90%, as this scare will induce her to begin regular screening.

These are just illustrative assessments. Lucy will have to make 32 assessments if she completes this analysis before observing whether her lump is suspicious.

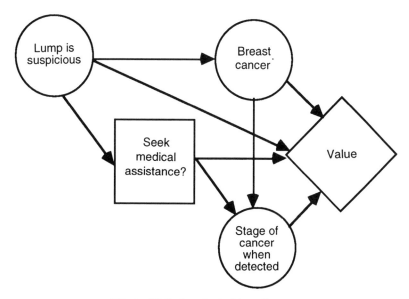

Figure 29.8. Lucy's decision diagram.

Lucy will probably want to consult an expert in the domain of breast cancer while making these assessments.

If Lucy were willing to express her values as "preference probabilities," her decision analysis software could generate overall probability distributions based on Lucy's "marginal" assessments to show Lucy's beliefs about achieving particular levels of value for particular actions. From this Lucy could choose the course of action whose combination of possibilities she valued the most. However, Lucy could stop short of using the decision diagram in this way, as a computational model and simply use it to represent the decision precisely.

The decision diagram thus provides a locus around which a decision maker's reflections about the quality of an analysis can revolve. Using a decision diagram to structure an analysis almost always makes sense, assuming the decision maker knows how to draw one; the extent to which probability and preference assessments will add value varies widely. In short, decision diagrams can add tremendous value to the quality of analysis, and thus to the quality of a decision.

29.2.7. Achieving Commitment to Action

Decision consultants agree that the decision maker should be happy to follow the recommendation that results from a high-quality decision analysis. After all, the decision model is just a "divide and conquer" approach to ensuring that a decision maker makes a decision consistent with preferences expressed to the analysts. In particular, the decision maker must agree at the outset to use probabilities to express belief or information, express all prospects relative to reference prospects, order the prospects according to preference, and choose the action that has associated with it the highest equivalent probability of the best prospect.

If the decision maker balks at a recommendation, then because the decision model is transparent, the cause for the concern can usually be traced to a mistaken or out-of-date probability assignment, or value judgment in need of revision.

29.2.8. Conclusion

The hypothetical case of Lucy, a breast cancer patient, illustrates how some of the tools of decision analysis can be used to satisfy the necessary conditions for optimal decision quality. Achieving the sufficient conditions for optimal decision quality is another matter. To do so, Lucy may want to delegate some aspects of her decisions to medical professionals.

Medical professionals, in turn, can use decision analysis to support decision quality. For classes of decisions known as "simple dichotomous" and "test/treat" decisions, standard decision analysis can lead to organizational learning to assure decision quality through decision analysis for physicians.

29.3. DECISION QUALITY THROUGH DECISION ANALYSIS FOR PHYSICIANS

29.3.1. Simple Dichotomy Medical Decisions

A large class of medical decisions is "simple dichotomous," and can be addressed through efficient, quantitative analyses. Such analyses lead to tools for learning how to access and improve the quality of decision support for simple dichotomous decisions. A medical decision is "simple dichotomous" if it satisfies the following:

1. The first condition for a medical decision to be simple dichotomous is that it must be explicitly described or framed. A decision frame is best understood using terms from the field of decision analysis.[2] (See Section 29.2.) The possibilities are all the possible states of information at the end of the epoch. They are shown at the ends of the branches of the decision tree depicted in Figure 29.9. The prospects are the decision maker's description of what the possibilities mean.

2. One decision A is considered in a simple dichotomous medical decision frame. It features two alternatives; treat ($A = a$) and not treat ($A = \neg a$). Another decision T may become available, whether to perform a test ($T = t$) or not ($T = \neg t$). This test/treat situation will be analyzed later. There is one uncertainty of interest, S, in the frame, and it has two degrees. Assume the uncertainty of interest is disease state, and that the disease can be present or absent, denoted

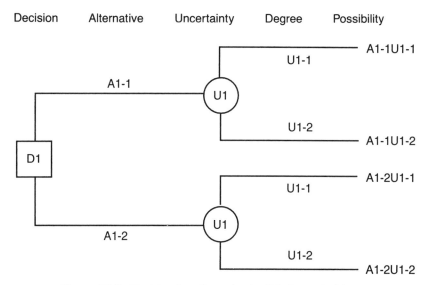

Figure 29.9. Decision tree for a simple dichotomy decision.

@ and Ø respectively (see Fig. 29.10). The possibilities in the decision frame are that the patient gets treated and has the disease (a, @); gets treated and does not have the disease (a, Ø); gets no treatment and has the disease (¬a, @); or gets no treatment and does not have the disease (¬a, Ø). The prospects are the patient's interpretation of what the possibilities mean. Treatment a could be toxic and interfere with the patient's activities of daily life; disease state @ could mean that the patient faces a high risk of death. A prospect can be "expressed" in terms of other prospects. For example, as we shall see, prospect (a, Ø) might be comprehensible to the decision maker as being equivalent to an uncertain event featuring prospect (¬a, Ø) with probability x and prospect (¬a, @) with probability $1 - x$.

3. The patient has sole and recognized authority for decision making, and may delegate part or all of the decision making to medical professionals. The patient understands the decision prospects and can communicate preferences about them. Whoever assists with the decision agrees to serve the patient's preferences.

4. The decision maker has beliefs about the uncertain events in the decision frame. These beliefs can be represented by probability distributions. A probability distribution assigns a probability between zero and one to each of the collectively exhaustive and mutually exclusive degrees of an uncertain event. The probabilities assigned to such degrees must sum to one (1), and must be proportional to the decision maker's belief in the likelihood that the uncertain event will transpire in that degree. For most uncertain events in medical deci-

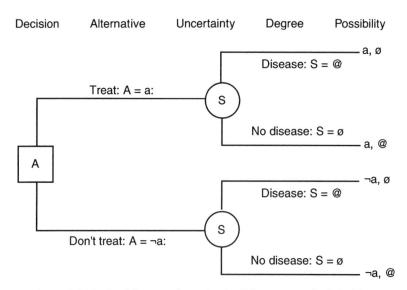

Figure 29.10. Decision tree for a simple dichotomy medical decision.

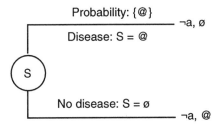

Figure 29.11. Probability assessments depicted in a tree.

sions, a decision maker will want to consult experts who can provide better probability assessments. Experts tend to concentrate their probability assessments on fewer degrees of an uncertain event than do nonexperts. For a tractable simple dichotomous medical decision, a decision maker will have to assess the probability of being in the disease state, denoted $\{@\}$, and the probability of being disease-free, denoted $\{\varnothing\}$ (see Fig. 29.11). The decision maker may want to consult medical specialists, who in turn may want to consult journal articles reporting on experiments.

5. The patient is amenable to communicating preferences using preference probabilities, which are derived from von Neumann–Morgenstern expected utility theory.[3] Specifically, the decision maker must be able to rank the prospects in order of preference; and designate a best and a worst prospect. Then the decision maker must consider an artificial uncertain event featuring as degrees the best and worst prospects. For every intermediate prospect, the decision maker's preference probability is the probability of best prospect that would leave the decision maker indifferent between facing the intermediate prospect and the artificial uncertain event. (see Fig. 29.12). Essentially what this procedure does is allow the decision maker to describe all prospects in "units" of best versus worst prospect. That is, the decision maker can state that intermediate prospect $(a, \varnothing)$ "corresponds" to the prospect of an uncertain event featuring a 0.6 chance of the best prospect $(\neg a, \varnothing)$ and a 0.4 chance of the worst prospect $(\neg a, @)$. The statement of correspondence is denoted by $\sim$.

6. The decision maker can express each alternative as being equivalent to an uncertain event featuring as degrees the best and worst prospects, and compute for each alternative the equivalent probability of the best prospect. The aggregation of preference probabilities and probabilities to give an uncertainty equivalent to an alternative is done using the e-value operation. We use the term "e-value" rather than "expectation" to describe the aggregating operation to emphasize that it is a mathematical abstraction and does not yield anything "expected." Indeed, the e-value operation takes as an argument any set of decision prospects described by numerical measures and returns the average of the numerical measures weighted by their probabilities. Once preference probabilities have been assigned to each prospect, they can be treated as numerical

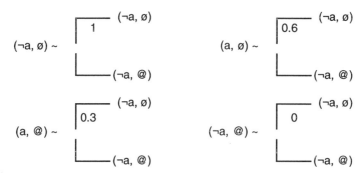

Figure 29.12. Preferences in a tractable simple dichotomous medical decision. The most preferred prospect is (¬a, ∅), the least preferred prospect is (¬a, @), and the second and third best preferred prospects are (a, ∅) and (¬a, @). Equivalence is denoted ~.

measures and averaged. The average measure that results can still be interpreted as representing the decision maker's preference probability for the reduced prospect in terms of the best and worst prospects. The probability of a prospect is the joint probability of all the event degrees constituting that prospect. Figures 29.13 and 29.14 show the decision tree for a simple dichotomous medical decision with a full set of prospects, and the reduced tree resulting from *e*-value aggregation.

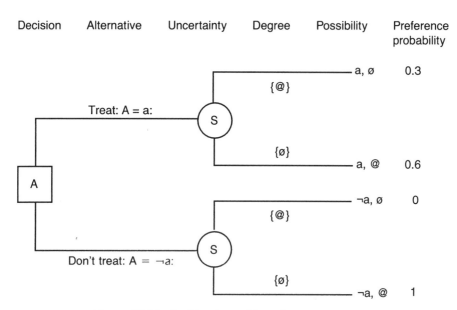

Figure 29.13. Decision tree with preference measures.

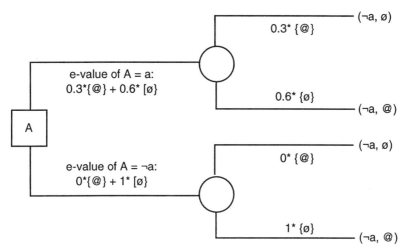

Figure 29.14. Decision tree with alternatives reduced.

7. The final condition for a medical decision to qualify as tractable simple dichotomous is that the patient be someone who would accept decision analysis as the best available choice process. The implication of this is that the patient, after satisfactorily assigning preference probabilities and probabilities and executing computations, would always choose the alternative with the highest *e*-value of preference probabilities. A decision maker who would do so is said to subscribe to the decision analysis rules of actional thought.[3] Such a decision maker must describe the uncertainty associated with possibilities using probabilities; must be able to rank order the decision prospects; must be willing to assign probabilities to deals so as to express indifference between receiving a prospect for certain and a lottery between any better and any worse prospect; must be willing to substitute equivalent deals for prospects; and, when offered two deals featuring only two prospects, must choose the deal with the highest probability of the best prospect.

Even a decision maker who found onerous the tasks required by the rules of actional thought could use decision analysis as a benchmark for quality in decision making, for decision analysis provides an optimal solution to simple dichotomous medical decisions. This optimal solution is a standard against which existing simple dichotomy medical decision support can be evaluated.

29.3.2. Evaluative Framework for Simple Dichotomy Medical Decisions

In general, decision quality is thought to have six dimensions[7] (see Fig. 29.1). A decision is declared optimal when the cost of further improvement along any of the dimensions outweighs the benefits. An optimal decision features a decision maker who gets the optimal frame, expresses preferences optimally, obtains all the affordable, valuable information, generates an optimal set of alternatives, performs optimal analysis, and acts on the recommended decision.

A medical decision that satisfies the simple dichotomy conditions is fixed in three of the six dimensions of decision quality. Specifically, a simple dichotomous medical decision is by assumption correctly framed, the patient preferences accurately represented, and the alternatives proscribed by the state of the art in medicine. Therefore, improving the quality of simple dichotomous medical decisions is a question of improving the ability of physicians and patients to integrate *information* into their analysis to generate *action* recommendations.

This ability to analyze information and generate action recommendations can be summarized analytically, for simple dichotomy decisions, by the decision maker's *policy threshold,* or probability of disease at which the preferred action switches from a to $\neg a$. The policy threshold is derived from decision analysis calculations.

Assume that a patient has ranked the prospects, assigned preference probabilities to each, described uncertain events with a probability distribution, computed the e-value or expected value of the preference probabilities for each alternative, and chosen the alternative with the highest aggregate preference probability. Then the variation of the preference probability associated with each alternative can be plotted as a function of the probability assigned to one of the degrees of an uncertainty. The function will be linear in any single probability, as the e-value function is a linear operation.

The convex epigraph of the sensitivity functions reveals the optimal policy for a decision maker whose state of information on a particular uncertainty may vary. In other words, for any given state of information, a decision maker can use the results of this type of sensitivity analysis to determine the best alternative. In particular, for simple dichotomy decisions, a decision maker can calculate the probability threshold at which the preferred action switches from alternative a to alternative $\neg a$.

Consider Figure 29.15 depicting sensitivity analysis for a simple dichotomous medical decision. For $\{\varnothing\}$ between 0 and X, the best alternative is $\neg a$, while for $\{\varnothing\}$ between X and 1 the best alternative is a. This analysis yields recommended actions as a function of state of information on S, with X being the decision maker's policy threshold.[12–14]

Before using policy thresholds as a measure of a decision maker's competence, we must examine how to evaluate the quality of the information being used to determine action recommendations and policy thresholds. In most medical practices, the provision of information is agreed to be central to the role of a physician.[15] Therefore, improving the information component of simple dichotomous decision quality is a matter of improving the ability of doctors to provide valuable information.

For a simple dichotomy medical decision, the state of information about the uncertainty of interest can be summarized by the patient's (or physician's) prob-

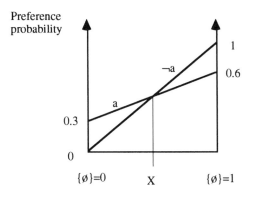

Figure 29.15. Sensitivity of preference probability to probability of ∅.

ability distribution over the degrees of the distinction of interest. This will be two numbers, the probability of being disease positive, denoted {@} and the probability of being disease negative, denoted {∅}.

Physicians should be well calibrated and well resolved in their probability estimates with respect to the best probability assessments available from research. "Well calibrated" means that the average of the estimates should be near the average of the assessments. "Well resolved" means that no single probability estimate is too far away from its corresponding probability assessment. Thus one way to measure the decision quality associated with a physician's practice is to determine the doctor's calibration and resolution with respect to a set of "gold standard" probability assessments.

Calibration can be measured by comparing the average of a set of probability estimates P to the average of the corresponding correct probability assessments P'. Resolutions can be compared by computing the average squared deviation of estimates P from assessments P'.

The calibration and resolution of each physician's probability estimates can be calculated through a comparison with the assessed probabilities. Given probability estimates P and probability assessments P', two simple statistics, C and R, respectively describe calibration and resolution:

Calibration

$$C = \sum_{i=1}^{n} (P_i - P'_i)$$

Resolution

$$R = \frac{1}{n} \sum_{i=1}^{n} (P_i - P'_i)^2$$

A method for comparing resolution and calibration is to compute the difference of the averages of a set of estimates and corresponding assessments and compare it to the average of the absolute differences between each estimate and its corresponding assessment. Thus

$$C' = \frac{1}{n} \sum_{i=1}^{n} (P_i - P_i')$$

$$R' = \frac{1}{n} \sum_{i=1}^{n} |P_i - P_i'|$$

$$C' - R' \begin{cases} \text{positive indicates better calibration than resolution} \\ \text{negative indicates better resolution than calibration} \end{cases}$$

For a set of simple dichotomy cases solved using decision analysis, the optimal actions (derived from decision analysis) can be compared with the actions recommended by a set of physicians. A simple measure for quality of action recommendations might be the sensitivity and specificity of classification for the physicians, or their positive and negative predictive value, as described in Table 29.2.

As for policy thresholds, the quality of current decision practices could also be evaluated by comparing the recommended policies of the decision maker to the optimal policies yielded by decision analysis. Since policies are summarized by probability thresholds at which optimal actions switch, the quality of the recommended policies can be judged from their calibration and resolution as probability estimates.

The calibration and resolution of a respondent's action thresholds can be computed to determine an absolute measure of variation from decision analysis optimality. As with information quality, two simple statistics summarize calibration and resolution. Denoting the set of threshold assignments X, and the set of decision analytic optimal threshold assessments X', we obtain

Calibration

$$C^X = \sum_{i=1}^{n} (X_i - X_i')$$

Resolution

$$R^X = \frac{1}{n} \sum_{i=1}^{n} (X_i - X_i')^2$$

For thresholds, too, calibration and resolution can be compared using the following measures:

TABLE 29.2. Summary Statistics for Quality of Action Recommendations

Recommended	Optimal		
	a	$\neg a$	
"a"	Correct action	Incorrect action	*Positive predictive value*
	(CA)	(IA)	$= CA/(CA + IA)$
"$\neg a$"	Incorrect inaction	Correct Inaction	*Negative predictive value*
	(II)	(CI)	$= II/(II + CI)$
	Sensitivity =	*Specificity* =	
	$CA/(CA + II)$	$IA/(IA + CI)$	

$$C^{X'} = \frac{1}{n} \sum_{i=1}^{n} (X_i - X_i')$$

$$R^{X'} = \frac{1}{n} \sum_{i=1}^{n} |X_i - X_i'|$$

$$C^{X'} - R^{X'} \begin{cases} \text{positive indicates better calibration than resolution} \\ \text{negative indicates better resolution than calibration} \end{cases}$$

In general, decision analysis is complex and costly, and the required assessments and computations may not be feasible. However, decision analysis always provides a transparent, normative basis for decision making. In the case of simple dichotomous medical decisions, it provides powerful analytical results with relatively few assessments, and relatively simple computations.

A clear measure of decision quality associated with a practice could be obtained by performing a decision analysis for a set of simple dichotomy cases subsequently presented to physicians and comparing the decision analysis optimal actions with the physicians' recommendations. The information or probabilities of disease used in the decision analysis case studies could be culled from the relevant literature, and compared to physicians' probability assessments for the same cases.

Finally, the decision analytic policy thresholds could be computed and compared to the physicians' policy thresholds. For simple dichotomy decisions, the probabilities, action recommendations, and policy thresholds constitute a robust framework for evaluating the quality of simple dichotomy decision support.

29.3.3. Survey to Describe Existing Simple Dichotomy Decision Quality

The evaluative framework for simple dichotomy medical decisions can be deployed through the administration and analysis of a survey. The survey presented in this section will later be amended to cover test/treat decisions.

The survey is analogous to an academic examination in that it asks respondents to solve a problem and then compares their solution to a "correct" answer derived from decision analysis. Operationally, the way this works is to include in each survey several case descriptions featuring different demographic and physiologic profiles, and different preferences. Then for each case, each respondent is invited to estimate the probability of disease and indicate the recommended action and action threshold.

For each case, each respondent's estimate and recommendations are compared to the decision analytic solution. The decision analytic solution combines the best available probability estimates for risk of disease with the patient preferences to determine the optimal action and policy. The elements of the survey design and analysis are described below for a generic survey of simple dichotomy medical decisions. The general approach is later illustrated with a specific example for breast cancer simple dichotomy decisions.

29.3.3.1. SURVEY DESIGN.   In current medical practice, formal decision analysis is rarely performed. Medical professionals know from anecdotal evidence that, given a particular case, any two practitioners may differ in their recommendation for that patient. Which decision-making practice best serves the patient's interests? How can practitioners learn from each other to improve their decision making? These questions can be explored by inviting practitioners from very different practice styles to solve hypothetical but realistic cases for which the decision analytic solutions have also been computed. Decision analysis provides a basis for characterizing the respondents' solutions.

Indeed, responses can be analyzed to understand which practice styles lead to the greatest deviation from the decision analysis standard. For by varying the case descriptions, it is possible to study how practitioners incorporate into their decision recommendations information about tests and patient preferences, physiology, and demographics.

The survey sample can be designed to include medical professionals from practices with known differences in (for example) number of patients seen, degree of compensation for procedures, and likelihood of malpractice suits. Sending the same case descriptions to such a survey sample makes it possible to examine the effects of experience, compensation, and regulatory environment on how respondents incorporate into their decision recommendations information about patients and tests.

The analysis of such a survey should enable practitioners to see specific opportunities for improvement in their decision making. The survey will reveal which predictor variables (for example, experience, compensation, and regulatory environment) explain variation in decision making, and which combinations allow practitioners best to serve patient interests.

29.3.3.2. GENERIC SURVEY OF SIMPLE DICHOTOMY DECISION QUALITY.
Consider the case of a patient with enclosed medical examination results. Suppose this patient faces a simple dichotomous medical decision featuring two alternatives, treat ($A = a$) and not treat ($A = \neg a$). There is one uncertainty S, and it has

two degrees. Assume the uncertainty of interest is disease state, and that the disease can be present ($@$) or absent ($\varnothing$).

The patient feels that the best prospect is ($\neg a$, $\varnothing$), while the worst prospect is ($\neg a$, $@$). The patient is indifferent between the prospect (a, $\varnothing$) and an uncertainty featuring an x chance of ($\neg a$, $\varnothing$) and a [$1 - x$] chance of ($\neg$a, $@$). The patient is indifferent between the prospect (a, $@$) and an uncertainty featuring a y chance of ($\neg a$, $\varnothing$) and a [$1 - y$] chance of ($\neg$a, $@$) (x and y are variables in the survey design).

1. Given the case description, what is your estimate of the probability that the patient is in disease state $@$?
2. Given the case description, which of the actions a and $\neg a$ would you recommend to the patient?
3. Given the case description, at what probability of disease state $@$ would your action change from a to $\neg a$ or from $\neg a$ to a?

29.3.4. Evaluating Decision Quality Survey Responses

The *solutions* for each case in the survey will include an assessment of disease risk from the relevant literature; a decision analytic recommended action; and a policy threshold or statement of how the recommended action should vary with probability of disease state. The survey *responses* will include a probability estimate of disease risk; an action recommendation; and a policy threshold which is the probability of disease at which the respondent's recommended action switches from a to $\neg a$.

The survey responses can be compared to each other and to the corresponding optimal solutions (see Fig. 29.16). Note that for the moment the issue is to evaluate and compare the decisions of each respondent. The investigation of hypotheses about the effects of predictor variables on decision recommendations will follow.

Analyses of the information dimension of decision quality can provide an indication of the differences in practice styles surveyed, as well as a measure of the variation from the decision analysis "gold standard." The survey returns will reveal the probability estimates for each case made by the various respondents. For each case, the probabilities will also have been assessed by a panel of experts, or established through research. The calibration and resolution of the respondents will provide measure of information quality. In addition, probability estimates can be graphed in a scatterplot against the assessed probabilities to reveal variation from optimality (see Fig. 29.17). Later investigation of hypotheses may include looking for patterns in probability estimates among respondents with a common predictor variable value.

Respondents can be characterized by the ROC (receiver operating characteristic) curve plotting sensitivity against their specificity (see Fig. 29.18). Alternatively, their positive and negative predictive values could be averaged or otherwise summarized.

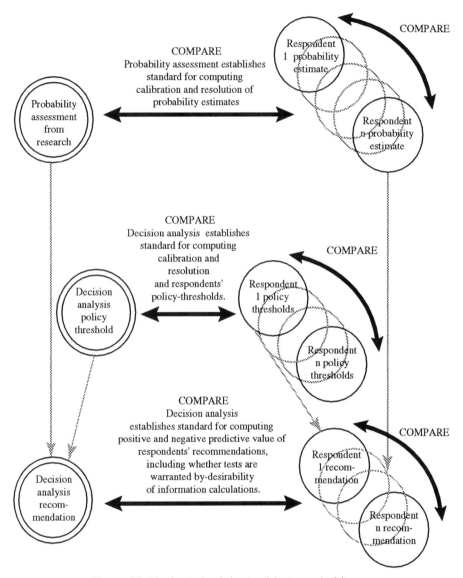

Figure 29.16. Analysis of simple dichotomy decisions.

The quality of performance reflected by an ROC curve can be summarized by the area under the curve, or C-statistic.[16,17] For relative measures of performance, note that one curve may be dominated by another, that is, reflect a higher sensitivity for any given level of specificity. Also, investigations of hypotheses can aggregate respondents according to common predictor variable values, and compare the ROC curves for one type of respondent versus another.

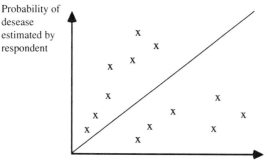

Probability of desease estimated by respondent

Probability of desease assessed from experiments or research

Figure 29.17. Information quality for various medical practices. Responses can be shown with an x. Estimates matching assessments would fall on the line shown.

For each case and physician, the probability threshold for switching actions or "action threshold" can also be compared with the optimal threshold, again in a scatterplot (see Fig. 29.19). Such a graph can reveal patterns during the investigation of hypotheses.

The simple dichotomy evaluative framework provides a rich characterization of decision quality. Survey respondents can be judged both in terms of their variation from optimal decision quality and their differences in decision quality. Survey respondents can learn from the differences and variation how to serve decision quality by subscribing to the methodology of decision analysis.

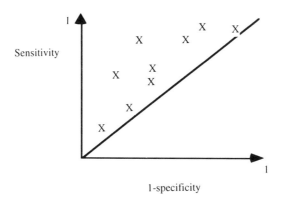

Sensitivity

1-specificity

Figure 29.18. Receiver operating characteristic (ROC) curve. This graph can be used to show the performance of one respondent's recommendations for different types of cases, or the performances of many respondents with similar predictor variable values evaluating the same cases. The line shows the performance of a recommender choosing between *a* and ¬*a* by coin toss.

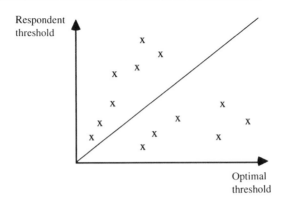

Figure 29.19. Differences and variation in policy quality. Responses can be shown with an x, while the line indicates practice that matches decision analytic optimality.

29.3.5. Evaluative Framework for Test/Treat Decisions

To obtain an evaluative framework for test/treat decisions, the only required addition to the tractable simple dichotomy medical decision framework is the introduction of another decision T with alternatives test ($T = t$) and no test ($T = \neg t$). The test can yield results R with known likelihoods $\{R|S\}$. The introduction of these new alternatives leads to a two-threshold optimal policy.

The two-policy thresholds can be denoted X_1 and X_2, and are defined such that for $\{\varnothing\}$ between 0 and X_1, ($A = \neg a, T = \neg t$) is optimal; for $\{\varnothing\}$ between X_1 and X_2, ($A = \neg a, T = t$) is optimal; and for $\{\varnothing\}$ greater than X_2, ($A = a, T = \neg t$) is optimal (see Fig. 29.20). The test must satisfy "tractability conditions" ensuring that its administration changes only the decision maker's state of information on

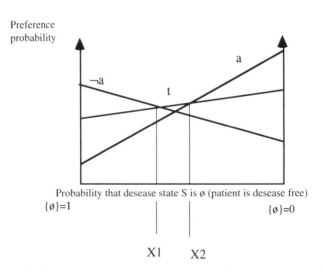

Figure 29.20. Sensitivity of preference probability to probability of $\varnothing$.

the single uncertainty of interest to the decision maker.[18] The test is assumed to have no monetary cost.

29.3.6. Desirability of Information

Associated with any test/treat medical decision is the notion of desirability of information (DOI).[18] Indeed, the desirability of a "tractable" test in a test/treat decision is the chance that it will cause a decision maker to change from an initial default to a new action, times the benefit of the change in action, summed over the possible changes in action.

Thus, if the initial default action is (no treatment, no test), the desirability of a test in the test/treat decision is the preposterior probability of any test result times the difference in preference probabilities for the corresponding optimal versus the initial action, summed over all possible results R.

DOI is a measure of the desirability of information associated with a diagnostic test because it provides a criterion by which a decision maker can tell whether the test is at all worthwhile (DOI > 0) and which of several tests under consideration is most worthwhile (the one with the highest DOI). Thus, to the extent that a decision maker finds it valuable to prioritize or rank-order various tests under consideration with respect to a particular decision, the decision maker may want to use DOI as a measure of the desirability of the information associated with a test.

It is worth noting that DOI provides no guidance to a decision maker interested in how much better one test is than another, or what the magnitude of DOI means. This is because the decision maker's preference probabilities or u-values express the prospects in terms (or units) of the best and worst prospects. Differences in preference probabilities do not correspond to prospects that can be expressed in units of best/worst prospect. The implication is that DOI is not a measure or approximation of monetary value of information. Specifically, no conclusion should be drawn as to what a decision maker should pay for a test on the basis of its DOI. DOI should not be confused with a measure of the value of information.

As an example, consider a simple dichotomy medical decision in which the decision maker's state of information prior to testing $\{\emptyset|\&\}$ leads to an optimal action $A = \neg a$ as in the Figure 29.21 where & denotes the conditioning state of information. The decision maker's preference probabilities are denoted by $u°$ for the default action and u^* for the action under the optimal policy.

Suppose also that the test under consideration leads to one of two results, R_1 and R_2, and that these results update the decision maker's state of information to posteriors $\{\emptyset|R_1, \&\}$ or $\{\emptyset|R_2, \&\}$. The former posterior leads to no change in action from the default, whereas the latter causes the decision maker optimally to take action a. Then the desirability of information DOI associated with the test given the decision maker's preferences and initial state of information, is

$$\text{DOI} = \{R_2\} \times [u^*(T = t, \{\phi|R_2\}, C_t) - u°(T = \neg t, \{\phi|R_2\}, C_t)]$$
$$+ (\{R_1\} \times [u°(T = t, \{\phi|R_1\}, C_t) - u°(T = \neg t, \{\phi|R_1\}, C_t)])$$

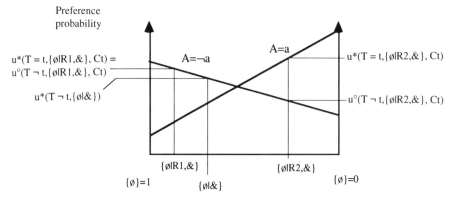

Probability that disease state S is ø (patient is disease free)

Figure 29.21. Sensitivity of preference probability to state of information on ∅.

In general, for a test with any number of possible test results R, and whose likelihood characteristics $\{R|S\}$ are known, the desirability of information associated with ordering a test when at some default action can be written as a function of the optimal policy derived through decision analysis.

$$\text{DOI} = \sum_{i=1}^{n} \{R_i\} \times [u^*(T = t, \{S|R_i\}, C_t) - u^\circ(T = \neg t, \{S|R_i\}, C_t)]$$

Note that for the simple dichotomous medical decision:

$$\{R_i\} = \{R_i|\varnothing\}\{\varnothing\} + \{R_i|@\}\{@\}$$

where i can take on the values 1 or 2.

The decision maker's preference probabilities at various states of information can be interpolated from the original preference probability assessments. If a decision maker has preference probabilities $u(A = a, S = \varnothing)$ and $u'(A = a, S = @)$, then the preference probability at state of information $\{\varnothing\}$ for action a is

$$u(A = a, \{\varnothing\}) = \min(u, u') + (|u - u'|)^*\{\varnothing\}$$

These results give us the means to easily compute the desirability of information associated with a test being considered in the simple dichotomy medical decision frame.

29.3.6.1. SURVEY IMPLEMENTATION   The only modification required to convert a survey of simple dichotomy decisions into a survey of test/treat decision making is the inclusion of a question asking the respondent whether, for a given case including a description of an available test, the test should be performed or not. The test must change nothing about the decision except the decision maker's state of information. How it does so must be specified:

> The test T has the characteristics that if the disease is present, the test will yield result R_1 with likelihood [insert variable p], and if the disease is absent, the test will yield result R_2 with likelihood [insert variable q].

The test is assumed to be available at no monetary cost.

29.3.7. The Quality of Test/Treat Decisions

The entire analysis evaluating and comparing simple dichotomy medical decisions can be repeated for a frame featuring two decisions, where the second decision is whether to administer some test whose characteristics are well known. Now decision analysis provides a rich normative framework against which to evaluate test ordering practice.

29.3.7.1. SURVEY ANALYSIS.   The full panoply of measures to evaluate and compare simple dichotomy decisions applies to test/treat decisions. For example, the positive and negative predictive value of respondents' test recommendations can be established by comparing the responses with the appropriate decision analysis conclusions. As for action recommendations in the simple dichotomy situation, ROC curves can be generated to summarize respondents' performances.

In addition, test ordering practice can be evaluated through a computation of the association between respondents' test recommendations and the decision analytic desirability of information DOI. This association can be illustrated graphically as in Figure 29.22. Statistical measures are available to quantify the

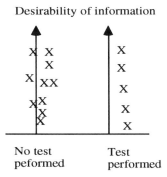

Figure 29.22. Association between test ordering and desirability of information can be displayed for various responses.

association. As usual, hypotheses can be investigated by aggregating respondents with similar predictor variable values.

29.3.8. Exploring and Explaining the Quality of Breast Cancer Decisions

Several important classes of decisions in breast cancer diagnosis and treatment can be classified as test/treat decisions. For example, for a patient with an abnormal mammogram, the decision of whether to biopsy, order a fine-needle aspiration, or follow up in 6 months can be structured in the test/treat framework.

Although test/treat decisions are relatively easily solved by decision analysis, few physicians know it, and even if they did, obtaining meaningful preference probabilities from patients has proved in other settings to be a formidable, if surmountable, challenge. Therefore, as an alternative to teaching everyone involved in test/treat decisions the technology of decision analysis, it is worth exploring how far physicians stray from serving patient preferences. It may be possible to pinpoint what leads them astray. And understanding what causes them to stray from serving patient preferences will presumably help them to serve better.

Figure 29.23 shows a model for explaining why respondent probability estimates, action thresholds, and action recommendations vary from optimality and differ from one another. The association between any two of the observable nodes in the model can be explored and hypotheses tested.

For example, the model in Figure 29.23 proposes that a respondent's estimate of risk of breast cancer in a patient is estimated from patient demographics, mammographic findings, patient physiology, and number of breast cancer patients seen. These predictor variables can be controlled in a survey sample so that the source of variation from best research assessments of risk (frequencies or consensus risk assessments) can be isolated.

Now consider Figure 29.24. It shows a plot of hypothetical data to illustrate the association of risk estimates or action thresholds with some predictor variable like age. Mammographic finding or number of patients seen could also have been used as the predictor variable. Statistical measures of association are available, in addition to graphical exploratory data analysis of the type shown here.

One hypothesis is that respondents' experience, as measured by number of patients seen, has a bearing on the accuracy of their risk estimates. Another plausible hypothesis is that respondents' risk estimates are significantly more accurate for older than for younger patients.

A plausible hypothesis for the association depicted in Figure 29.25 might be that respondents adhere to patient preferences more closely for young patients than for old.

A plausible hypothesis for the association depicted in Figure 29.26 might be

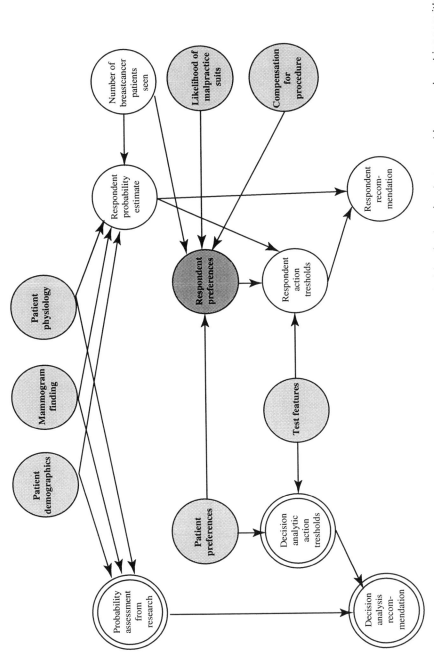

Figure 29.23. Explaining breast cancer decision making. The test/treat decision is choosing between biopsy and no biopsy, with possibility to conduct a fine-needle aspiration. Circles represent variables. An arrow between two circles indicates probabilistic relevance. The dotted circles show survey predictor variables, controlled as part of the survey design. The shaded circles show unobserved variables. Double-rimmed circles show variables computed using decision analysis based on inputs. Other circles show survey response variables.

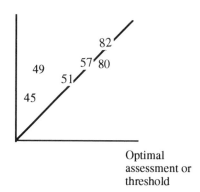

Figure 29.24. Are respondent errors in risk of cancer estimates or in action thresholds associated with age of patient? Estimates can be plotted against optimal assessments using age of the patients to mark each response. Optimal responses would fall along the 45° line depicted.

that respondents adhere more closely to patient preferences for patients with low levels of cancer risk than for those with high levels of risk.

A plausible hypothesis for Figure 29.27 would be that respondents understand patient preferences better for older patients than for the young.

A plausible hypothesis for Figure 29.28 is that, for the particular respondent depicted, there was a possible inconsistency between what the respondent's action threshold was stated to be, and what it in fact was in practice.

A plausible hypothesis for Figure 29.29 might be that respondents in practices with low incidence of malpractice suits order and do not order tests appropriately, whereas respondents facing a high risk of malpractice suits order tests without regard to their desirability of information.

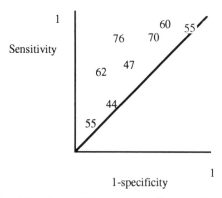

Figure 29.25. Is action driven by age? Average age of respondents' cases can be used to mark each respondent's performance in choosing recommendations that correspond to decision analytic optimality. Performance of doctors choosing between *a* and ¬*a* by coin flip would fall along the 45° line depicted.

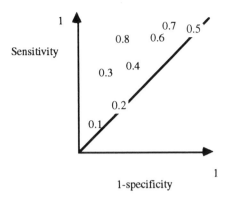

Figure 29.26. Is action associated with information? Average estimate of cancer risk for respondents' cases can be used to mark each respondent's performance in choosing recommendations that correspond to decision analytic optimality. Performance of recommendations to choose between ¬a and ¬a by coin flip would fall along the 45° line.

29.3.9. Hypotheses Generated by Pilot Survey of Breast Cancer Physicians

The following hypotheses were generated after piloting these tools on two breast cancer physicians. They are reproduced here to illustrate how exploration of associations between dimensions of decision quality can be used to generate hypotheses for further testing.

29.3.9.1. CANCER CANCER ESTIMATES

1. Respondents' estimates of risk of cancer agree with research assessments more often and more closely as number of patients seen increases.

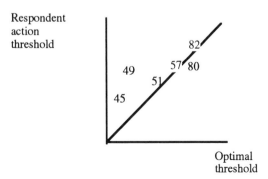

Figure 29.27. Are assignments and policies driven by age? Patient age can be used to mark responses vis-à-vis decision analytic optimality.

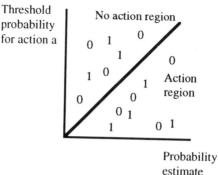

Figure 29.28. Consistency of actions with policies. The line separates the regions of probability of disease for which the respondent's espoused policy is to recommend *a* from that for which the policy is to recommend ¬*a*. Each 1 indicates when the respondent in fact recommended *a*, while each 0 indicates a threshold/probability estimate pair for which the respondent in fact recommended ¬*a*.

2. Respondents' estimates of risk of cancer agree with research assessments more closely as degree of compensation for procedures decreases.
3. Respondents' estimates of risk of cancer agree with research assessments less often and less closely as regulatory environment becomes more punitive.

29.3.9.2. BIOPSY RECOMMENDATIONS

1. Respondents' propensity to biopsy agrees with patient preferences less often as the regulatory environment becomes more punitive.

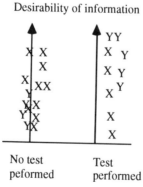

Figure 29.29. Association between test ordering and desirability of information for two different types of respondents. *X* could depict performance of respondents in practices with high incidence of malpractice suits, with *Y* depicting performance of "low malpractice"-type respondents.

2. Respondents' aversion to biopsy agrees with patient preferences more often as the regulatory environment becomes more punitive.

3. Respondents' biopsy recommendations agree with patient preferences more often as degree of compensation for procedures decreases.

4. Respondents' biopsy recommendations agree with patient preferences more often as number of patients seen increases.

29.3.9.3. POLICY THRESHOLDS

1. Respondents' policy thresholds agree with patient preferences less often and less closely as regulatory environment becomes more punitive.

2. Respondents' policy thresholds agree with patient preferences more often and more closely as degree of compensation for procedures decreases.

3. Respondents' policy thresholds agree with patient preferences more often and more closely as number of patients seen increases.

29.3.9.4. TEST RECOMMENDATIONS

1. Respondents' propensity to order tests agrees with patient preferences more often as degree of compensation for procedures decreases.

2. Respondents' aversion to ordering tests agrees with patient preferences more often as degree of compensation for procedures decreases.

3. Respondents' test ordering recommendations agree with patient preferences less often as regulatory environment becomes more punitive.

4. Respondents' test ordering recommendations agree with patient preferences more often as number of patients seen increases.

29.4. CONCLUSIONS

Decision analysis can be used to help patients arrive at optimal decision quality for simple dichotomous and test/treat decisions. Used as an evaluative framework, decision analysis can help organizations explore the quality of decisions, and assess the variation from optimality and difference in decision support competence among physicians. The analytical tools suggested in this chapter, including simple graphics and statistics, should allow physicians to generate hypotheses concerning the quality of their decision support, and therefore lead to well-founded efforts toward quality improvement.

REFERENCES

1. Ellig DH: *Patient's Handbook.* Mesa: Med. Ed., 1988.
2. Howard RA: Decision analysis: practice and promise. *Management Sci* 34:679–695, 1988.

3. Howard RA: In praise of the old-time religion. Edwards W, ed: *Utility Theories: Measurements and Applications*. Boston: Kluwer Academic Publishers, 1992.

4. Clemen RT: *Making Hard Decisions: An Introduction to Decision Analysis*. Boston: PWS-KENT, 1991.

5. Keeney RL. *Value-Focused Thinking: A Path to Creative Decisionmaking*. Cambridge, MA: Harvard University Press, 1992.

6. Howard RA: Decision analysis: applied decision theory. In Hertz DB, Melese J, eds: *International Conference on Operational Research*. New York: Wiley-Interscience, 1966, pp 55–71.

7. Creswell D, McNamee P: Decision quality and decision tools: making the right choices. *PC AI* 40–43, 1991.

8. Howard RA: Information value theory. *IEEE Trans Sys Sci Cybernetics* SSC-2:22–26, 1966.

9. Howard RA: Value of information lotteries. *IEEE Trans Syst Sci Cybernetics* SSC-3:54–60, 1967.

10. Howard RA: From influence to relevance to knowledge. *Conf Influence Diagrams for Decision Analysis, Inference, and Prediction*. Berkeley, CA, 1988.

11. Argyris C, Schon D: *Organization Learning: A Theory of Action Perspective*. Reading, MA: Addison-Wesley, 1978.

12. Pauker SG, Kassirer JP: The threshold approach to clinical decision making. *N Engl J Med* 302:1109–1117, 1980.

13. Sackett DL, Haynes RB, Trigwell, P: *Clinical Epidemiology: A Basic Science for Clinical Medicine*. Boston: Little, Brown, 1985.

14. Eisenberg JM, Hershey JC: Derived thresholds. Determining the diagnostic probabilities at which clinicians initiate testing and treatment. *Med Decision Making* 3:155–168, 1983.

15. Smith C: Legal review: informed consent—a shift from paternalism to self-determination? *Top Health Rec Management* 11:71–75, 1990.

16. Fink DJ, Galen RS: Probabilistic Approaches to clinical decision support. In Williams BT, ed: *Computer Aids to Clinical Decisions*. Boca Raton, FL: CRC Press, 1980, pp 1–65.

17. Poses R, Bekes C, Winkler R, Scott W, Copare F: Are two (inexperienced) heads better than one (experienced) head? Averaging house officers' prognostic judgments for critically ill patients. *Archives of Intern Med* 150:1874–1878, 1990.

18. Belkora JK: *Calculating Value of Information: Analysis and Derivations*. Stanford, CA: Department of Engineering-Economic Systems, Stanford University, 1994.

30

Medical Decision Analysis

MARTIN H. KROLL

CONTENTS

30.1. CLASSIC DECISION ANALYSIS

"The only certainty is that nothing is certain."[1] This quotation comes from the ancient world, but is still true today and perhaps better appreciated. Humans, for their survival and prosperity, have always had to make good and proper deci-

Handbook of Clinical Automation, Robotics, and Optimization, Edited by Gerald J. Kost with the collaboration of Judith Welsh.
ISBN 0-471-03179-8 © 1996 John Wiley & Sons, Inc.

sions. Medicine, like many other areas of human endeavor demands decisions in the face of uncertainty, that is, not knowing all the facts. Also, wise clinicians must make their decisions with an overabundance of facts, although not all the facts, and in a complex web of relationships. Making decisions with all of these complications requires sound judgment. The deans of medicine have always pursued and honored sound judgment. The current trend has been to raise the overall level of medical judgment by incorporating the judgment of the best clinicians into a uniform body of language that can supplement all physician practices. Academic physicians have driven this unification of judgment, in their quest to improve the education of physicians. Federal and local governments have driven this unification in their pursuit of improved quality of care. And health maintenance organizations, insurers, and consumer-action groups have drive this unification in their pursuit of controlling healthcare costs and minimizing mistakes. All these groups have made use of an important statistical tool known as *decision analysis*. Classic decision analysis portrays results simple enough to allow most physicians to use them with ease. Modern decision analysis, is either a result of automation or makes use of automated means. Whether classic or modern, decision analysis originates in the manipulation the unknown facts in terms of probability to give the user the best "chance" of arising at the appropriate decision.

The concept of probability incorporates the unknown from two sorts of random processes. One random process is the random variable. A random variable is a function where each numerical value of the function takes different probabilities.[2] These differing probabilities can be thought of as individual samplings. Each sampling is separate and independent of the prior and subsequent samplings.

The second source of random error is the random sampling. Every time a blood sample is taken from a patient to measure an analyte, the sampling is random in both time and volume. One assumes the sample is a decent representation of the average concentration or activity of the analyte.

Both of these sources of randomness—the random variables and random sampling—are uncontrollable sources of error. Probability allows one to deal with these errors by obtaining descriptive statistics for a large number of samples. Even though the error is uncontrollable for any individual case, one can make predictions by applying the probabilities.

Physicians order laboratory tests to decrease their uncertainty about their patients diagnosis or condition. Physicians monitor patients so they can alter treatment to maintain effectiveness of their therapies and avoid complications of the disease process.

With laboratory tests, uncertainty as to their interpretation arises in part from the random error dealing with sampling and analysis. More important, though, in the interpretation of laboratory tests is the uncertainty of the state of nature. The use of laboratory tests often invokes a relationship between a set of results and the condition of the patients. Typically, when a patient presents with an illness, several states are possible. The states consist of one state of health and anywhere from one to many states of disease. The physician is ignorant in which state of nature the patient belongs, whether in a state of health or one of disease, and if disease, which among the many. A laboratory test is much easier to interpret when one knows the state of nature the patient is in. Such interpretation of laboratory tests is a form of retrospective thinking. Physicians can often deal with their ignorance of the state of nature by applying the available information in the form of probabilities. As an hypothetical example, consider a case of a young woman presenting with lower abdominal pain and having missed her last menstrual period. The physician is uncertain whether the patient has a self-limited disease, such as a gastroenteritis that does not require therapy, has disorder requiring immediate therapy such as appendicitis, is pregnant, or has an ectopic pregnancy. Physicians can have prior information about the prevalence of disease in the population they see; for instance, the probability of self-limited disease is high, as in pregnancy in young women who have missed one menstrual period. The physician may know that the incidence of ectopic pregnancy in the population of pregnant women is as high as 2%. When a pregnancy test is positive, the probability of pregnancy goes up to 100%. The physician observes the patient. Because in early pregnancy the βHCG should double every 2 days, a decreased rate of rise of βHCG provides information indicating that an ectopic pregnancy is more likely, while a normal rate of rise provides information that an ectopic pregnancy is less likely. The physician will choose other tests such as ultrasound or leukocyte counts to further delineate the type of disease process the patient has. By rearranging the appropriate probabilities, which represent the available information, the physician can arrive at probabilities of disease and weigh the cost of different actions. Such reasoning is the basis for applying decision theory.[3]

One can envision that treating medical patients is akin to staking claims at a betting table. It takes resources to treat patients. Each forward progress in the patient's condition is like each betting event, in that the event must occur and one must place a bet; in other words, the evolution of the patient is inevitable, but one does have some control over the course of that evolution. Consider the game of roulette. One can pick a number, high-priced bet, a range of numbers, a lower-priced bet, or a color, for the lowest-priced bet. One plays against the odds. If one wins a high-priced bet, one also is greatly rewarded. If one wins a low-priced bet, one is modestly rewarded. Before the placing of bets, one has no knowledge beyond the initial odds what the probable outcomes are. When playing roulette, the probabilities of winning and losing are obvious. When caring for patients, the probabilities for making the necessary decision—that is, to win or lose in taking care of patient—is not obvious. Part of the purpose of decision analysis is to make these probabilities more apparent. We discuss the exact definitions of these probabilities in Section 30.1.1. We want to play medicine to our greatest advantage, and utilize any information available to improve our odds. In the roulette game, if half the black positions are removed, the odds of being on red go up from 1:1 to 2:1. One does a lot better betting on red than black, but one needs to have knowledge beforehand. Decisions analysis puts the knowledge about the odds into a formal context so that the physician can take advantage of knowledge about prior relationships.

30.1.1. Probability and Bayes Theorem

The essential problem in interpreting a laboratory test is deciding if the patient has or does not have the disease given the result. Ideally, there is a clear separation of results for the population between those with and without disease. The phrase "without disease" is used because one cannot assume that their group is healthy, for they may have other diseases or conditions such that one would want to separate from the specific disease of interest. When there is a clear separation between the test results, then a positive test indicates that the patient has the disease and a negative result indicates that the patient does not. In reality, the test results for the sets for with disease and without disease overlap. As an example, a certain segment of the population is at high risk for developing coronary heart disease while the rest of the population is not. There are many causes for the development of coronary heart disease, some known such as smoking, hypertension, and altered lipid metabolism. There are some causes of coronary heart disease that are not known and for which we have no marker. The Cholesterol Education Program strongly suggests using cholesterol as a marker for altered lipid metabolism. For cholesterol to be an ideal marker, all patients who are not at risk for developing coronary heart disease would have cholesterol concentrations within a certain reference range, <200 mg/dL, and those patients who are at risk due to coronary heart disease from altered lipid metabolism would have an elevated cholesterol, >240 mg/dL (Fig. 30.1). Of course, such a clear separation is not the case and there is significant overlap between the two groups (Fig. 30.1). When presumed distributions of the at-risk and not-at-risk groups are plotted separately, it appears that adequate discrimination between the diseased and nondiseased groups could be performed (Fig. 30.1). When the two distributions are combined, as shown in the third part of Figure 30.1, there is not even a hint of a separation and a significant borderline high region must be considered.[4] The diseased and nondiseased sets overlap for most diseases and most laboratory tests, so it is important to have ways to separate the information.

Because the diseased and nondiseased sets for any laboratory test overlap and we are ignorant of the true state of nature as it relates to health and disease for the patient, we need a rational method to convert the data we obtain to information about the patient. Bayes theorem deals with the way to convert data from a sample of the population to individual probabilities[5] (Table 30.1). The percentage of true positives for all with disease is the sensitivity, the percentage of true negatives for all without disease is the specificity, and the number or percentage of people with disease is the prevalence[6,7] (Fig. 30.1, Table 30.2). The type of questions to answer when interpreting a laboratory test is what is the predictive value of a positive test and what is the predictive value of a negative test results (Table 30.2). The answers to these questions are using in decision making and the construction of diagnostic trees or algorithms.

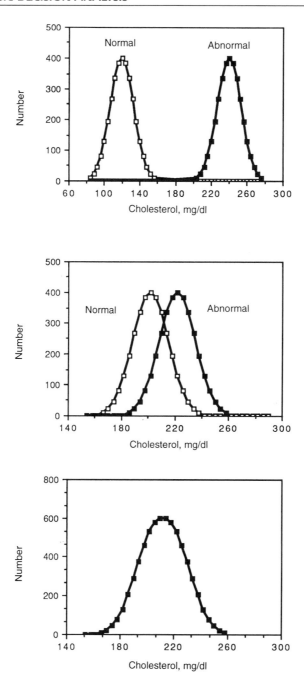

Figure 30.1. Population distributions for cholesterol. *Upper panel:* When the distributions are far apart, it is easy to differentiate between normal and abnormal. *Middle panel:* In reality the distributions are closer together, resulting in overlap. *Lower panel:* When the two distributions are merged, there is not apparent separation between normal and abnormal.

TABLE 30.1. Basic Nomenclature in Terms of Probability

$P\{D\}$	= probability of disease, the prevalence
$P\{R\}$	= probability of a positive test result
$P\{ND\}$	= probability of not having the disease
$P\{NR\}$	= probability of a negative test result
$P\{D/R\}$	= probability of having the disease given that the test result is positive = predictive value of a positive test.
$P\{ND/NR\}$	= probability of not having the disease given that the test result is negative = predictive value of a negative test

The calculation of the predictive values of positive or negative tests depends on the prevalence and the sensitivity and specificity of the test, respectively (Table 30.3). Bayes theorem informs one that the prevalence of the disease must always be taken into consideration. The predictive values can be calculated from the prevalence, sensitivity, and specificity of a test or from the number of true positives (*TP*), true negatives (*TN*), false positives (*FP*), and false negatives (*FN*) (see also Fig. 30.2).

30.1.2. Errors and Diagnosis

There are two major sources of error or variation in laboratory tests. The analytical performance of the test gives rise to analytical errors, which can either be random errors or errors of bias. The analytical errors can be quantitated and communicated to the clinician.

The true concentration or activity of analytes, whether from well or diseased patients, varies over time. Such variation is known as the *biological variation,* and it has been expressed as a standard deviation with mean or coefficient of

TABLE 30.2. Derived Entities in Terms of Probability

$P\{R/D\}$	= probability of a positive test result given the patients sampled have the disease = sensitivity = $TP/(TP + FN)$
$P\{NR/ND\}$	= probability of a negative test result given the patients sampled do not have the disease = specificity = $TN/(TN + TP)$
$1 - P\{R/D\}$	= 1 − sensitivity = false-negative rate
$1 - P\{NR/ND\}$	= 1 − specificity = false-positive rate

True positives (*TP*) = prevalence × sensitivity
False positives (*FP*) = (1 − prevalence) × (1 − specificity)
False negatives (*FN*) = prevalence × (1 − sensitivity)
True negatives (*TN*) = (1 − prevalence) × specificity

TABLE 30.3. Predictive Value of Positive and Negative Test Results[5]

	Sensitivity
$P\{D \text{ and } R\}$	$= P\{D\} \cdot P\{R/D\}$
$P\{D/R\}$	$= P\{D \text{ and } R\}/P\{R\}$
	$= P\{D\} \cdot P\{R/D\}/P\{R\}$
	$= \text{prevalence} \times \text{sensitivity/total positives}$
	$= TP/(TP + FP)$
	Specificity
$P\{ND \text{ and } NR\}$	$= P\{ND\} \times P\{NR/ND\}$
$P\{ND/NR\}$	$= P\{ND \text{ and } NR\}/P\{NR\}$
	$= P\{ND\} \cdot P\{NR/ND\}/P\{NR\}$
	$= TN/(TN + FN)$

variation.[8] Physicians typically do not know the biological variation of the patients they treat, and unfortunately, the degree of biological variation varies among patients.[9]

Physicians must juggle these two sources of error along with their ignorance of the true state of nature of the patient every time they diagnose or treat a patient. The physician's judgment depends on the relative ability to juggle the uncertainties. One of the goals of medical decision analysis is to bring all physicians up to a minimal standard of decision making, forcing them to consider all probabilities.[10]

Decision analysis provides physicians with uniform information concerning

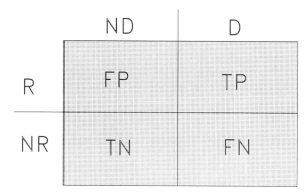

Figure 30.2. *Results table:* There are four ways a result can be interpreted. They depend on the absence (*ND*) or presence of disease (*D*) and whether the result is positive (*R*) or negative (*NR*). The results can be a true positive (*TP*), true negative (*TN*), false positive (*FP*), or false negative (*FN*).

the assessment of the prior and posterior likelihood. The prior likelihood is the probability that the patient has the disease prior or before the result of the test is known, $P\{D\}$, the prevalence of disease for the population in question. Most physicians know the prevalence in rough, general terms, and the prevalence is usually obtained from limited studies. By observing and tabulating the patient's outcome with a computerized data management system, one could determine the prevalence for each appropriate subpopulation and physicians could retrieve the information through the computer system. After the test results are known, the probability of disease is altered and is known as the *posterior likelihood*. Here, too, a computer system could assess the posterior likelihood using sensitive and specificities appropriate for the patient's subpopulation.

30.1.3. Decision Trees

Decision theory uses the Bayes theorem as a basis. The key elements require knowledge of the possible outcomes; the cost measured in dollars, pain and suffering, benefits or other resources; the employable strategies; and the posterior likelihood.[11] Knowledge of the strategies is critical and can be arranged into the tree. Because of the influence of computer programs, most of these trees follow an algorithmic structure with yes/no answers. For example, a decision tree for the evaluation of chest pain could include duration of pain, site of pain, previous history, electrocardiogram changes, and creatine kinase results. The trees can become complicated, and so it sometimes is better to concentrate on the consequences of one decision at a time. In the decision tree for creatine kinase, MB fraction, and assessment for chest pain, myocardial infarction is assumed as the disease entity, but all four possibilities—true positive, false positive, true negative, and false negative—must be considered (Fig. 30.3). The patient who has the myocardial infarct may die or recover spontaneously. For care, one must consider both death and survival as potential outcomes. One then uses Bayes theorem to estimate the probabilities of each outcome (not shown in Fig. 30.3). The next factor is cost. In Figure 30.3, the costs are given in relative terms. One can consider costs as a relative weight but can factor in the true costs if they are known. To assess the effect of each decision in the decision tree, one multiplies the probability of that decision by the cost and weight of the outcome. If the outcome appears to tip the balance away from a favorable appearance, the strategy should be reexamined, or cutoff for the test criteria should be altered. ROC curves are helpful in reassigning cutoff values.

Automation has affected laboratory tests in many ways; it has decreased analytical variation by improved precision and accuracy and extension of reportable ranges for tests, low thyroid stimulating hormone (TSH) results for example. Automation has decreased the costs for tests, which means that more tests are equal in price than before, and thereby, it may be more difficult to decide which tests to use. In addition, it is less expensive to repeat tests and test repetition must be included in the decision process. The equalization of many different laboratory tests, many of which test for similar disease conditions, mean that

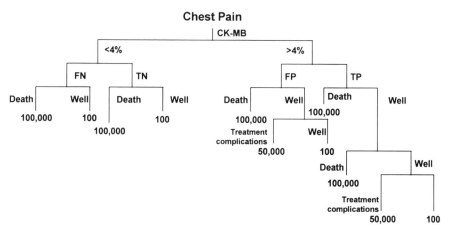

Figure 30.3. Decision tree for chest pain. The decision tree considers the two types of error—false positive or false negative—and the two types of correct answers—true positive or true negative—and displays the relative cost for each decision.

there are more test strategies for a physician to choose from. By analyzing the problem through the decision tree format, the strategies can be optimized and improved. Over a decade ago, cholesterol was the main analyte used to assess for coronary heart disease risk, because determination of HDL (high-density lipoprotein)–cholesterol was difficult and expensive. Improvements in automation made cholesterol measurements better, and thereby, improved the measurement of HDL–cholesterol. Even though some of the steps in the measurement of HDL–cholesterol are still manual (but probably not for long), the cost of performing the test has decreased, and it is recommended that it be included as part of the screen for coronary heart disease.[12]

30.1.4. ROC Curves

Receiver operator characteristic (ROC) curves are formed by plotting the sensitivity against (1 − specificity) and varying the cutoff used for positive for a given data set.[13] Both sensitivity and (1 − specificity) are functions of the prevalence even though specificity is (1 − prevalence) in the denominator. The slope for the ROC curve is the likelihood ratio. A likelihood ratio of greater than one (>1) increases the probability of disease.[6] Figure 30.4 shows a theoretical ROC curve and the effect of changing the cutoff or criteria for positive. ROC curves minimize the error in terms of the predictive value of a test.[13] Because the slope of the ROC curve represents the likelihood ratio and a test with a likelihood ratio of >1 increases the probability of disease, one test is better than another if it moves the curve further to the left from the line of identity (the 45° line, which has a slope of 1). ROC curves are a convenient means of comparing methods, especially, as mentioned above, since automation has improved the turnaround times, decreased the costs, and facilitated the operations of many tests in differ-

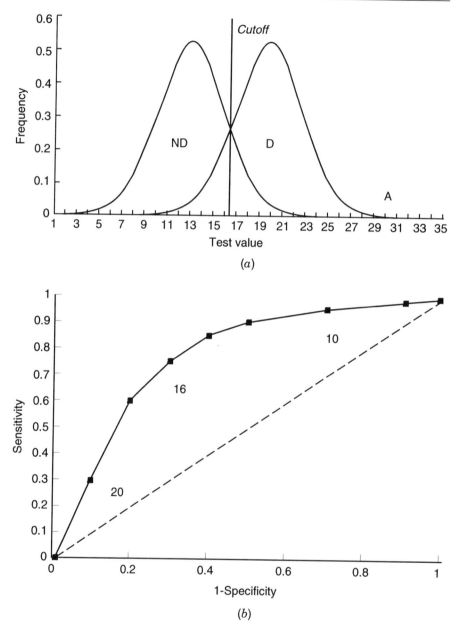

Figure 30.4. Receiver operation characteristic (ROC) curve. (A) In the presence of overlap between the diseased and nondiseased group, one has control over the sensitivity or specificity for the test because one can manipulate the cutoff line—the line that separates positive and negative for the test. (B) ROC curve. The closer the curve is to the upper left-hand corner, the better the test is in discriminating between diseased and nondiseased groups. The number along the curves represents the location of the cutoff along the x axis of panel A.

ent locations (point-of-care testing and satellite laboratories, for example, can be sites of operations).

30.2. MODERN DECISION ANALYSIS

30.2.1. Standardization of Medical Care

There is a strong driving force to standardize medical care. This drive has arisen from the overwhelming demand for medical services, the need to control costs, and inconsistencies in judgment among physicians. Physicians often perceive different observations about patients, but even more disturbing is that, given a certain set of symptoms, including abdominal pain, a physician who has recently seen a patient with porphyria is more likely to overestimate the prevalence of porphyria in the general population.[6] Studies have shown that physicians overestimate the probability of diseases, especially diseases they have been familiar with.[14] We can likewise believe that physicians are likely to miss a diagnosis if they do not have practical experience with the disease. Further, many physicians fail to make appropriate adjustments to their patient management as new information is provided.[15]

30.2.2. The Effect of Laboratory Automation

Automation has brought about a standardization of results in the laboratory. Most tests are performed with similar or with comparable methods. Even when methods differ, the outcome or results of those methods are typically similar. Automation has improved precision, reduced the cost and increased the ease of obtaining laboratory results. The number of pieces of data that a physician has the potential of obtaining has increased dramatically. So have medical costs. Unfortunately, the ways of arranging that data in presentation format for the physician has not improved that much. In an effort to maintain the same level of quality in the management of patients, more use of computer programs is necessary, either as a rational-based thinking adjunct or as a way of massaging the data into more recognizable information.

30.2.3. Implementation of Decision Analysis in Standardization

Decision analysis can be a great adjunct in the standardization of medical care. Beyond the thought processes involved, implementation of decision analysis can be greatly assisted by computer-based methods.[16] A simple type of program available for mainframe or personal computers is an expert system, which acquire and store data and information in a format designated by an expert in the field. Expert systems have been developed for internal-medicine use.[17,18] To program an expert system, one must write the algorithm in the common language, and once written, these algorithms are fixed.

A neural network consists of a group of nodes, each node representing a factor or condition in a model of the problem. For example, a neural network for the evaluation of chest pain might include electrocardiogram results, creatinine kinase activity, and shortness of breath. A bank of input nodes (20–30 of them), one for each test result or piece of information, is connected to a second bank of nodes (half as many as before), which connect to one node. This last node outputs the probability. Each inner-bank node receives multiple inputs and sends an output through a transfer function. A trainer of the neural network assigns a value to each connection. The trainer uses a data set of patients with known outcomes, and runs them through the neural network, changing the value of the connections each time until the best set of values is attained. The neural network is then able to diagnose the taught disease state within certain error limits. Neural networks have been developed for the diagnosis of chest pain and dementia.[19,20] Neither expert systems nor neural networks are a replacement for physicians, for they have difficulties dealing with the subtleties and aberrant bits of information that are so typical of true medical situations, but they may serve as an adjunct in the diagnostic process.

Software is available for developing decision trees that can automatically construct decision trees based on information provided the program.[21] The author of this program suggests that one list all possible results for diagnostic test with branches at each possibility.[21]

Any program for developing decision trees or algorithms must be based on outcome data. The designer of such systems should base the structure of the program on the results of carefully tailored clinical trials of laboratory tests. One must prove the efficacy of laboratory tests in a fashion similar to the clinical trials for medications. Bayes theorem and decision analysis provide a structured way to incorporate the positive and negative outcomes. Decision analysis is invaluable in the development of standardization schemes.

Standardization in medicine is a growing trend because of the changing trend toward managed care, the implication of healthcare reform, and the move toward controlling healthcare costs.[22] It has been assumed that standardization will minimize costs while maximizing favorable outcomes. Such an occurrence will be true only if the standardization group makes the correct selection of strategies and correct assumption about the probabilities.

When a proper standardization is adopted, its success will depend less on the quality of the protocol and more on the ease with which the protocol can be put to use. An automated system through a user-friendly computer offers a good solution to the problem of making management accessible. Such a system should provide the physician with the ability to input patient information and laboratory requests. The laboratory test results should go to the computer, where posttest probabilities are calculated (Fig. 30.5). The information bank of the computer should provide the prevalence of the subpopulation, as well as the sensitivity and specificity. The computer organizes the information into presentable form for the physician. The physician inputs into the computer manage-

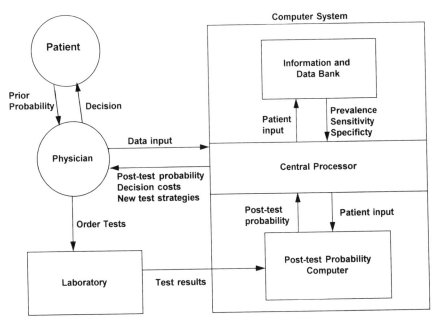

Figure 30.5. Interaction flow diagram for interaction between the physician and a computer system that facilitates medical decision making. The physician collects data and information from the patients and passes it to the computer. In addition, the physician orders laboratory tests. The computer combines the laboratory test results with population information and provides the physician with the posttest probabilities, new test strategies, and cost of decision.

ment strategies, and the computer responds with projected probabilities based on the proposed decisions. The physician can decide whether the projected probabilities are acceptable and modify the management plan if they are not. In addition, the information bank would provide the physician with descriptive statistics of national and local diagnoses as well as the physician's individual record. Such a system would provide feedback to the physician (Fig. 30.5).

30.2.4. Optimization Theory for Laboratory Tests

Decision analysis appears to be an excellent approach to achieving standardization in patient analysis and laboratory test utilization. Surely, the process of examining all possible outcomes and assigning weights for a given decision is an important exercise; however, the process is not perfect. Practice parameters, to be effective, must be comprehensive and specific.[10] A proper decision tree should have four possible results for each test result (*TP, FP, TN, FN*). Each generation in the tree increases the number of possibilities by 4. The second generation has 16, the third 64 (Fig. 30.6), with a general formula of $N = 4^G$,

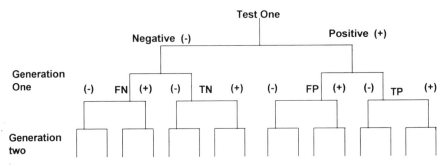

Figure 30.6. Decision tree growth. The first generation yields four possibilities and the second generation, 16 possibilities. Decision tree possibilities grow with $N = 4^G$, with N the number of possibilities and G is the generation number of each decision.

where N is the number of branches and G is the generation number. Typically, in the development of a practice protocol, the protocol becomes too complex to be manageable or so simple that it is trivial.[10]

In spite of the problems associated with decision analysis, it still provides a logical scheme for the establishment of management protocols. When using decision analysis and decision trees, one must keep in mind these techniques are a subset of optimization theory.

Optimization theory is the study of the general minimum–maximum problem (min–max problem), specifically, finding all the local minima and maxima on the surface generated by the information. Assume that the local maxima represent the maximum efficiency of the test utilization process. Then, the goal is to find the maximum efficiency for the surface; however, this is impossible because the methods used are able to find only local maxima. If two or more maxima are present on the surface, the current optimization methods zero in on one local maximum, ignoring the others.

In most complex problems, there are many competing local maxima. Thus, ultimately, we must improve the theory in decision analysis to make it a better tool. The existence of more than one laboratory test for the same disease category is one source of the multiple maxima, as is different possible treatments.

The result is that standardization of medical practice requires many decision trees. A multiplicity of laboratory tests implies that broad coverage is necessary and, further, that there is no pure linear independence among laboratory tests or treatments.

To be used wisely, medical decision analysis should generate many decision trees because of the realization that multiple local maxima exist. The existence of multiple local maxima implies that there are many ways to efficiently utilize laboratory tests in patient management, that many ways may be correct, and that it is a mistake to choose one sole way to manage a clinical problem. The use of multiple decision trees has advantages, for it retains physician individuality while applying efficient methods and retains the individuality of patient management. Automation—as a computer thinking process—will be necessary to wisely generate and use the complex array of medical decision trees.

REFERENCES

1. *Pliny the Elder.* Historia Naturalis, Book 2, Chap 7.
2. Bielmer, MG: *Principles of Statistics.* New York: Dover, 1979, pp 29–44.
3. Chernoff H, Moses LE: *Elementary Decision Theory.* New York: Dover, 1959, pp 119–196.
4. The Expert Panel. Report of the National Cholesterol Education Program Expert Panel on Detection, Evaluation, and Treatment of High Blood Cholesterol in adults. *Arch Intern Med* 148:36–69, 1988.
5. Feller W: *An Introduction to Probability Theory and Its Applications,* 3rd ed, Vol 1. New York: Wiley. 1968, pp 114–145.
6. Sox HC: Probability theory in the use of diagnostic tests. *Ann Intern Med* 104:60–66, 1986.
7. Hillner BE: Medical decision making: a Bayesian approach to laboratory testing. *Proc Annu Meet Meds Sect, Am Council Life Insurance,* 1987, pp 27–37.
8. Fraser CG: Biological variation in clinical chemistry. An update: collated data, 1988–1991. *Arch Pathol Lab Med* 116:916–923, 1992.
9. Wasenius A, Stugaard M, Otterstad JE, Froyshov D: Diurnal and monthly intraindividual variability of the concentration of lipids, lipoproteins and apoproteins. *Scand J Clin Lab Invest* 50:635–642, 1990.
10. Werner M: Can medical decision be standardized? Should they be? *Clin Chem* 39:1361–1368, 1993.
11. Fisher LD, van Belle G: *Biostatistics: A Methodology for the Health Sciences.* New York: Wiley, 1993, pp 665–673.
12. The Expert Panel. Summary of the second report of the National Cholesterol Education Program (NCEP) Expert Panel on Detection, Evaluation, and Treatment of High Blood Cholesterol in Adults (Adult Treatment Panel II). *JAMA* 269:3015–3023, 1993.
13. Zweig MH, Campbell G: Receiver-operating characteristic (ROC) plots: a fundamental evaluation tool in clinical medicine. *Clin Chem* 39:561–577, 1993.
14. Desmet AA, Fryback DG, Thornbury JR: A second look at the utility of radiographic skull examination for trauma. *Am J Radiol* 132:95–99, 1979.
15. Tversky A, Kahnman D: Judgement under uncertainty: heuristics and biases. *Science* 1985:1124–1131, 1974.
16. Marquardt VC, Jr: Artificial intelligence and decision-support technology in the clinical laboratory. *Lab Med* 24:777–782, 1993.
17. Waxman HS, Worley WE: Computer-assisted adult medical diagnosis: subject review and evaluation of a new microcomputer-based system. *Medicine* 69:125–136, 1990.
18. Barnett GO, Amino JJ, Hupp JA, et al: DX plain: an evolving diagnostic decision-support system. *JAMA* 258:67–74, 1987.

19. Furlong JW, Dupuy ME, Heinsimer JA: Neural network analysis of serial cardiac enzyme data: a clinical application of artificial machine intelligence. *Am J Clin Pathol* 96:134–141, 1991.

20. Mulsant BH: A neural network as an approach to clinical diagnosis. *MD Comput* 7:25–36, 1990.

21. Sonnenberg FA, Hagerty G, Kulikowski CA: An architecture for knowledge-based construction of decision models. *Med Decision Making* 14:27–39, 1994.

22. Altschuler CH: Data utilization, not data acquisition, is the main problem. *Clin Chem* 40:1616–1620, 1994.

CHAPTER
31

Automated–Facilitated Causal Reasoning in Diagnosis and Management

MARTIN H. KROLL

CONTENTS

31.1. CAUSAL REASONING

Causal reasoning in medicine is a thought process that invokes the knowledge and understanding of physiology in the solution of clinical problems.[1] Essen-

Handbook of Clinical Automation, Robotics, and Optimization, Edited by Gerald J. Kost with the collaboration of Judith Welsh.
ISBN 0-471-03179-8 © 1996 John Wiley & Sons, Inc.

tially, the knowledge and understanding of physiology means physicians can use first principles.[1] Some even surmise that this causal reasoning is the major way we solve problems.[1] To understand and facilitate the power of causal reasoning and how it relates the physiologic changes in the patient to subsequent changes in laboratory values, one must review the mental process.

In thinking about the causes of disease, physicians must have a clear idea of the normal physiology to expect in their patients. In addition, physicians possess an extensive knowledge of the diseased physiologic states. In evaluating the patient, the physician compares the patient's physiology with the normal physiology and appropriate pathophysiologic states.

There are many causes of edema, some of which are listed in Table 31.1.[2] Each cause represents a different mechanism. The physician compares the normal physiology, such as no edema, to the different pathological states. If the patient has no evidence of heart disease, the physician can rule out congestive heart failure; if the liver appears normal, the physician can rule out cirrhosis; if there are no signs of hypothyroidism (e.g., normal free T_4 and TSH), the physician rules out hypothyroidism; and so on.

The general process in causal reasoning is the collection of information (see Table 31.2), such as the chief complaint of the patient. After hearing the chief complaint, the physician begins to narrow down the possibilities. The physician takes a careful history, delineating the time relationships among all the events of the disease progress. The physician begins to form a differential diagnosis and asks particular questions to ferret out more information pertinent to the pathological possibilities. The physician performs a physical, paying particular attention to signs that would support the possible diagnosis.

After performing the history and physical, the physician has usually formed a fairly narrow number of diseases in the differential diagnosis. The physician will try to determine the degree of sickness of the patient. The degree of illness is important because if the patient is very ill, the physician will want to admit the patient to the hospital for immediate treatment. If the patient's life is not in danger, then the physician will want to treat the patient as an outpatient. If the patient feels ill, but is not suffering from a disease, the physician will want to improve the mental health of the patient. The physician will do additional information gathering consisting of other tests—those from the laboratory, radiology, and functional, such as electrocardiogram (EKG). The purpose of these additional tests is twofold: (1) if the physician is fairly certain of the diagnosis, it is to

TABLE 31.1. A Brief Differential Diagnosis of Edema

Congestive heart failure
Cirrhosis
Renal disease
Hypothyroidism
Diabetes mellitus
Capillary leak syndrome (septicemia or interleukin-2 therapy)

TABLE 31.2. Physician Fact Gathering

Patient's chief complaint(s)
History
Physical exam
Tests—further diagnosis and documentation
Laboratory
Radiology
Functional

document the disease; and (2) if the diagnosis is not certain, it is to rule in or rule out appropriate diseases. In interpreting the laboratory tests, the physician is looking for results that would be either incompatible with the course of the disease or expected with only one or several diseases. In terms of number, if the physician is thinking of two possible diseases and knows two laboratory tests where the values would be abnormal for one test with one disease and for the other test with the other disease, it should be fairly easy to discriminate between the two.

31.2. PATIENT CASE

31.2.1. Chief Complaint

A 27-year-old man previously in good health reported to the emergency room complaining of nausea, vomiting, and muscular aches and pains. (These symptoms are so general that they could represent many different diseases.)

31.2.2. Additional History

The patient did not suffer from a runny nose nor headache, nor did he have a cough (something one would expect with an infection). He had felt well enough the previous night to have been out drinking with his "buddies." (Such information excludes a chronic illness as a cause.) Review of symptoms revealed that the patient's urine was reddish-brown and was another reason why the patient sought medical attention. (The discolored urine represents an important factor because many diagnoses can be excluded because of it.) On urinalysis, the urine tested positive for hemoglobin. (Considering the patient's complaints and the positive finding of hemoglobin in the urine, the physician assumes that the patient is very ill until proven otherwise. The physician decides to further work up the patient's disease in the emergency room.) Results of laboratory tests were elevated potassium, alanine aminotransferase (ALT), aspartate aminotransferase (AST) and lactate dehydrogenase (LDH), creatinine of 2.5 mg/dL, creatine kinase $> 30,000$ IU/L, and positive toxicology screen for ethanol. (The elevated potassium is disturbing and indicates the seriousness of the illness. Together the elevated potassium and lactate dehydrogenase frequently constitute a harbinger of hemolysis because both are present at high concentrations in erythrocytes. Frequently, the hemolysis is the result of damage when collecting the sample and represents in vitro hemolysis. *In vitro* hemolysis is a false cause of elevated potassium, and LDH and makes the sample unreliable. Less commonly, the hemolysis is from an *in vivo* process, as one might find in a patient with an artificial aortic valve or autoimmune disorder. Hemolysis is high on the list because of the hemoglobin found in the urine. Hemolysis, whether *in vitro* or *in vivo*, however, would not give rise to such significantly elevated ALT and AST as seen with this patient. The elevation of both ALT and AST is frequently seen with hepatic diseases, because hepatocytes have high concentrations of both enzymes. The sky-high creatine kinase provides most of the information, though, because it is found in significant concentrations only in muscle. One usually thinks of elevated creatine kinase as being associated with myocardial infarction; however, when the creatine kinase is so greatly elevated, one thinks of skeletal muscle because skeletal muscle makes up 90% of the muscle mass. In myocardial infarction, the activity of creatine kinase goes as high as 1000 IU/L, but rarely up to 2000 IU/L. One could try to differentiate cardiac from skeletal muscle injury by determining creatine kinase isoenzyme activity or concentration, except when the activity of creatine kinase is so elevated the results of isoenzyme studies is often misleading. The elevated potassium, lactate dehydrogenase, ALT, AST, and creatine kinase are all consistent with an acute necrotizing polymyopathy (otherwise known as *acute rhabdomyolysis*). The positivity of the urine for hemoglobin is consistent with the peroxidase activity of hemoglobin. Skeletal muscle, in addition to creatine kinase, contains large amounts of myoglobin. Myoglobin, which is biochemically similar to hemoglobin, has peroxidase activity and will appear positive on the chemical strip used for detecting hemoglobin in urine. The ultimate cause of the acute rhabdomyolysis was probably binge drinking the night before, as evidenced by the positive toxicology screen for alcohol. Rhabdomyolysis is also seen after crushing trauma and freezing in subzero weather.)

31.2.3. Hospital Course

The creatinine, which was mildly elevated at the start, continued to rise until it reached a maximum of 6.0 mg/dL. (The myoglobin is excreted in the kidneys but often is nephrotoxic, being a cause of acute tubular necrosis.)

The thought processes in this case went from one compatible and likely diagnosis to another (Fig. 31.1). A large part of the thinking was what pathologies would be consistent with the entire picture. The laboratory tests are not infallible because the elevated potassium, lactate dehydrogenase, ALT, AST, hemoglobin on urine chemistry stick, and creatine kinase can all have different interpretations, depending on the disease entity one considers. The physician typically tries to fit the information to clinical and pathophysiological scenarios. Another important element is the timeframe. The physician is searching for evidence of cause and effect, expecting to see a cause followed in time by some

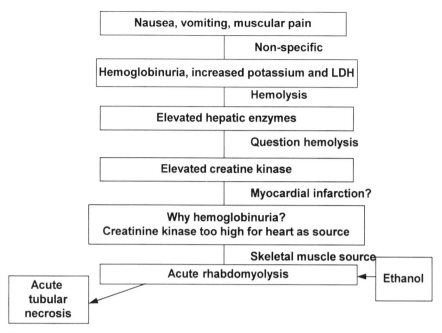

Figure 31.1. Reasoning process for patient case. The process uses information from physiology to reach a conclusion.

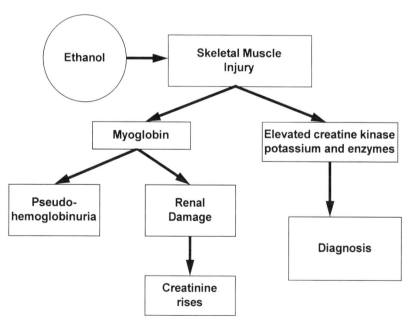

Figure 31.2. Cause–effect relationship in a patient. Time progresses downward in the figure.

effect. As in this case, the drinking binge caused an acute muscular injury; the muscular injury caused muscular pain and the release of creatine kinase, myoglobin, potassium, and other enzymes; the elevated creatine kinase served as a marker for the pathological process; the myoglobin colored the urine and caused renal damage; and the renal damage caused the creatinine to rise (Fig. 31.2).

Physicians use causal thinking all the time, and it is important to study the thinking processes if one is interested in simulating them.[3] Part of the appeal of the causal thinking of the physician is that the experienced physician can efficiently use the available information, considering only the facts that would make or break the case for the diagnosis.[3]

31.3. AUTOMATED FACILITATION OF DATA PRESENTATION

Physicians need to utilize their time and energy wisely. Today, there is more pressure than ever for physicians to spend less time in the evaluation process (cognitive thinking) about their patients because of growing restraints on resources. This philosophy makes sense because physicians should spend most of their time treating and communicating with their patients, rather than doing work that a computer could. In the previous section, we showed how a physician could convert data into information; information, into understanding the disease process; and understanding of the disease process, into decisions (Fig. 31.3).

Automation currently provides the facilitation of converting data into informa-

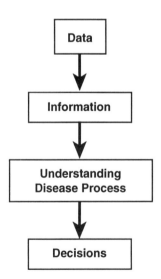

Figure 31.3. Goals of cognitive thinking are to convert data to decisions through understanding the disease process.

TABLE 31.3. Calculated Data

Urea/creatinine
> 20 prerenal azotemia
< 20 renal or postrenal pathology
Anion gap = (sodium + potassium) − (chloride + total bicarbonate)
< 16 meq/L normal
> 16 meq/L metabolic acidosis
Magnesium deficiency, certain drugs, etc.
LDL–cholesterol = total cholesterol − (HDL–cholesterol + TG/5),
where TG is the triglyceride concentration

tion when the cognitive processes are relatively simple. One of the simplest types of automation is reporting calculations with the laboratory results: the urea:creatinine ratio indicates the presence or absence of prerenal azotemia, the anion gap, the presence of certain acids, and the Friedenwald equation, the concentration of low-density lipoprotein or LDL–cholesterol (Table 31.3). In addition to these calculated results, many laboratory or hospital computer systems are capable of automatically graphing laboratory data, usually through values versus time. All of these methods facilitate the decision-making process by making the data easier to perceive.

The production of graphs for serial data is especially important. Many physicians use a glucose tolerance test to make decisions about the ability of their patients to handle glucose. In the glucose tolerance test, a fasting blood sample is drawn for glucose determination, the patient ingests 75 g of glucose, and another blood sample is drawn 2 h later. If the glucose concentration in the fasting sample is > 120 mg/dL, the patient has diabetes mellitus. If the fasting sample glucose is < 120 mg/dL but the 2-h postdose blood glucose is between 140 and 200 mg/dL, the patient has impaired glucose tolerance; however, if the patient 2-h postdose blood glucose is > 200 mg/dL, the patient has diabetes mellitus. Such data can be neatly and automatically presented.

The serial pattern of estradiol data is important in assessing ovulation status for women undergoing *in vitro* fertilization. The prognosis for pregnancy is improved when the estradiol follows one of four patterns after stimulation with gonadotropin-releasing hormone agonists (GnRHa).[4] Women whose estradiol rose and then fell between days 2 and 5 poststimulation had more than threefold greater live birth rate (38%) than did those women whose estradiol rose continuously (11%) or did not rise at all (6%).[4] The increased live birth rate occurs in the former group because the fall in estradiol is a marker of the down-regulation of the pituitary gonadotropin-releasing hormone receptors after the FSH and LH surge.[5]

Other temporal changes are important in the interpretation of laboratory tests. After a myocardial infarction, one expects to see the creatine kinase rise and fall during the first 24 h after the event. In dehydration, one often sees the urea concentration rise. Patients who have had an internal crush injury as from an automobile accident (e.g., a ruptured spleen) frequently have internal hemorrhaging. The internal hemorrhaging is often not apparent but can be suspected or followed by watching a falling hemoglobin or hematocrit. In the diagnosis of prostatic cancer, the value of the prostate-specific antigen (PSA) is > 4 ng/mL, but recurrence after prostatic resection is indicated by the velocity of increase of the PSA.[6] It is important to diagnose ectopic pregnancy before it ruptures. The change in value of β-HCG over time in ectopic is less than that in a normal pregnancy and can be used to diagnose the condition.[7] In all these cases, the technology to graphically display this data in an automatic fashion is currently available. Further, the laboratory could make interpretations about the results.

31.4. AUTOMATED FACILITATION OF CAUSAL REASONING

Automation in the laboratory has had profound effects on test usage. It has greatly decreased the necessary turnaround time for tests, with some analyzers able to determine many of the analytes in < 5 min.

Automation has greatly decreased the costs and expertise needed to perform many laboratory tests. The decreased cost and expertise for these laboratory tests makes the tests more available at many sites and increases utilization of these tests. Finally, laboratory automation has decreased the required sample volumes, which is especially important in pediatrics.

The progress in informatics has been just as dramatic. Computers have replaced paper reports, and data storage and retrieval is a distinct possibility when utilized.

The attempts at the facilitation of causal reasoning have progressed slower than that of data storage and retrieval because of the essential difference between the automation of data organization, such as a graph or computerized report and the conversion of data into information. The conversion of data into information (Fig. 31.3) requires appropriate models of the underlying physiology. Groth developed a model that relates the synthesis, release and elimination of analytes (8,9) (Fig. 31.4). One can write a set of equations that relate the concentration or activity of the analyte to its synthesis, release into the blood, and elimination from the blood (Table 31.4). When the analyte is released into the blood, the concentration depends on the balance between the rate of release and the rate of elimination. The release is a linear function of the enzyme concentration in the cell. Thus, if the cellular enzyme concentration is high (e.g., creatine kinase in skeletal muscle), the release—especially the release under injury—assumes a high value. If the cellular enzyme concentration is low, the release assumes a low value, but never less than zero. The blood concentration is a balance between release and elimination. When the elimination is given as a linear dependency on the enzyme concentration, the elimination rate will be higher at higher concentrations of enzyme, although never less than zero.

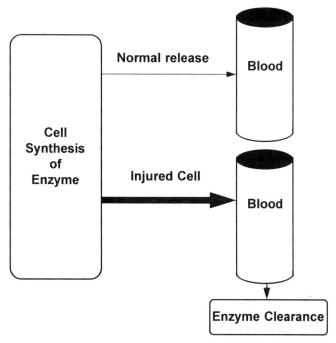

Figure 31.4. Biodynamics model of an enzyme marker for cell injury.

The equations in Table 31.4 represent differential equations for the concentrations of enzymes in cell and blood. As such, at the steady state, i.e., where there is no change in enzyme concentration in the blood, $(r_n + r_i)$ [enzyme]$_{cell}$ = $e \cdot$[enzyme]$_{blood}$, where the rate constants are r_n for normal release, r_i for injury release and e for enzyme elimination. When the value of the right-hand side of the equation exceeds that of the left-hand side, enzymes will accumulate in the blood. This model represents a basic linear synthesis and elimination differential equation and has been used with some success by many investigators (Table 31.5). Cramp et al. have emphasized physicians should use these models as an auxiliary to their thinking process—in a sense a human–machine interaction.[18] He also described these models as control models.[18]

TABLE 31.4. Biodynamics of Analyte Equation

Cell concentration rate = synthesis − normal release − injury release
Blood concentration rate = normal release + injury release − elimination
    Assume elimination = $e \cdot$ [enzyme]$_{blood}$
    release = $(r_n + r_i)$ [enzyme]$_{cell}$
At steady state
    $(r_n + r_i)$ [enzyme]$_{cell}$ = $e \cdot$ [enzyme]$_{blood}$

TABLE 31.5. Synthesis and Elimination Linear Model

Interpretation	Reference
Complement in inflammatory conditions	10
Fluid resuscitation in trauma	11
Internal hemorrhage from urea	12
Thyroid disease	13
Amylase turnover	14
Allopurinol kinetics	15
Pharmacokinetics	16, 17

It is important to consider control models, for these models were the first type to be utilized in the simulation of biological systems. The subject begins with an analysis of biologic or intraindividual variation. Cotlove and coworkers observed that the value for many analytes varied over time for the same subject.[19,20] For any given population, such as would make up a reference range, there are three sources of variation: analytical (from the determination of the specimen), interindividual (among individuals), and intraindividual (for the same subject) (19) (Fig. 31.5). The intraindividual variation is larger than one

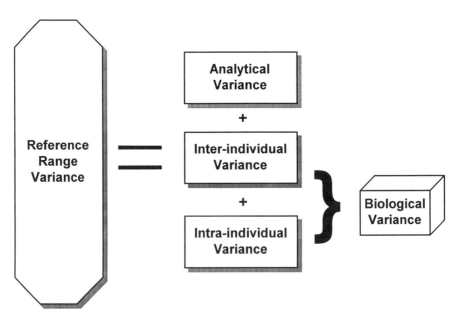

Figure 31.5. Components of variation: Var = variance; Var (analytic) + Var (intrain-dividual) + Var (interindividual) = total variance.

would usually expect, with the average intraindividual variation/average interindividual ratio ranging between 0.4 and 1.2 for most analytes.[19] They interpreted the intraindividual variation in light of the homeostatic control model.[20] In their interpretation, the average value one obtains for an analyte in an individual is the controlled value determined by the set-point of the control system.[20] Their homeostatic model is essentially the model of a control system (Fig. 31.6). The set-point (S_1) represents the fixed input into the system; S_2 represents the feedback of the control loop. The error signal is equal to $S_1 - S_2$. If $S_2 = S_1$, the error signal is zero and no change is effected on the homeostatic system. When $S_2 > S_1$, that is, when the value of the analyte is greater than that of the set-point, a negative error signal is sent to the effector and the effector changes the system in such a manner as to let the value of the analyte fall. The controlled signal is then the new value of the analyte and represents the output signal and is fed back as S_2. When S_2 is less than S_1, the error signal ($S_1 - S_2 > 0$) is positive and the effector acts on the system to raise the value of the controlled signal. Control systems like this one (or in one's home thermostat) can keep the output signal almost identical to the set-point, except for two elements. All control systems are typified by a time delay, so these systems can oscillate. Also, the disturbance, as indicated in Fig. 31.6, can perturb the system away from the set-point.[21] In the original designation of the control systems, the disturbances were believed to be large perturbations from the outside environment that pushed the output signal away from the set-point and the controls system slowly stepped closer and closer to the set-point, until it was finally reached. Mathematically speaking, it follows an oscillating decay pattern (Fig. 31.7). Cotlove's group interpreted the disturbance differently. Rather than being large and outside, they believed the disturbances to be small and internal to the organism but outside the control mechanism and the result of random processes.[20]

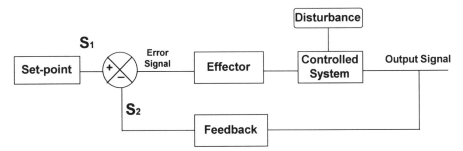

Figure 31.6. Homeostatic control model. The average analyte concentration or activity is determined by the set-point. The effector modifies the system to produce more or less of the analyte, and the controlled signal is the result. The environment can disturb the controlled system, thus altering the output signal. The output signal is fed back to the input. The error signal = $S_1 - S_2$.

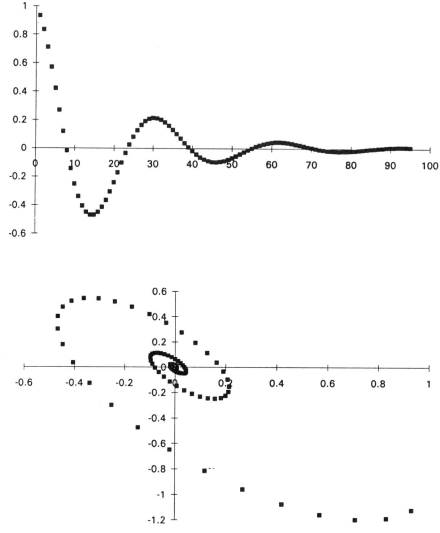

Figure 31.7. Decaying oscillations for a disturbed homeostatic control system for an analyte: (*A*) output signal plotted against time—the disturbed signal decays down to the set-point; (*B*) the velocity of the output signal plotted against the output signal results in a phase plot. The disturbed signal spirals down to zero.

31.5. INNOVATIVE FACILITATED CAUSAL REASONING

One might accept the homeostatic model of intraindividual variation, except not all observed intraindividual variation is random. Instead, many analytes demonstrate circadian rhythms, which, by definition, are not random.[22] Thus, there is empirical evidence the homeostatic-control model is inadequate to explain intraindividual variation. Moreover, this model does not adequately explain the shifts seen in disease. The disturbance could increase in size, but that would not change the mean value, but only the standard deviation. The set-point could change, but we do not know why, nor do we even know where the original value of the set-point originated. Finally, the control system itself could break, but then again, we would expect to see wildly different values in disease, although we do not see them in actuality.

West proposed that current theory in biodynamics should be based on nonlinear models because they are closer representations of biological systems.[23] We modify the original biodynamic model to include nonlinear modifiers at both the synthesis and elimination step; these modifiers represent receptors for the analyte (Table 31.6). F_1 represents the negative feedback one usually sees in negative feedback control for synthesis; F_2 represents the receptor for the analyte in the elimination system. When the receptor for the analyte is overloaded or destroyed, the analyte can no longer be removed at the same rate and the analyte accumulates.

As an example, consider lactate in circulatory shock (see Fig. 31.8). Mortality is higher for those patients with lactate concentration greater than 4.4 mmol/L.[24] But there is considerable overlap in the initial values of lactate between those who survive and those who die.[25] Serial measurements of lactate are better predictors of outcome than initial values because the serial values of survivors fall while those of nonsurvivors fail to decrease.[25] Further, only survivors of septic shock show a decrease in blood lactate in the final stages of septic shock.[26] Lactate synthesis increases in shock, but the real culprit is lactate elimination decreases in hepatic dysfunction.[27] The hepatic dysfunction can follow many insults, including trauma, circulatory shock, surgery, or infection.[27] The primary hepatic dysfunction is due to the initial injury, while the second phase, occurring several days after the initial insult, is due to a systemic inflammatory response with multiple organ failure.[27] Lactate increases in nonsurvivors of shock because the liver enters into progressive failure with decreased clearance.[27] The lactate fails to fall during the systemic inflammatory response because even though hepatic clearance of lactate increases, the patient is in hypermetabolic state and may have increased synthesis of lactate.[26] The systemic inflammatory phase is typified by a circular feedback mechanism, while the transition from systemic inflammatory response to progressive organ failure is a major change in state, with mortality of the former being 40–60%; and the latter, 90–100%.[27]

TABLE 31.6. Nonlinear Biodynamic Model for an Analyte

Cell concentration rate = k_1 synthesis $\cdot F_1 - k_2$ [analyte]$_{cell}$
Blood concentration rate = k_2 [analyte]cell $- k_3$[analyte] $\cdot F_2$
  where k_1, k_2, k_3 = constants
        F_1, F_2 = nonlinear factors related to receptors for the analyte

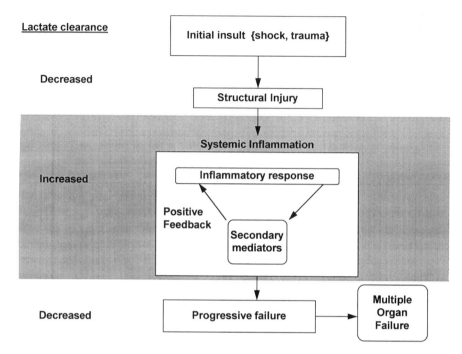

Figure 31.8. Effects of shock and hepatic failure on hepatic lactate clearance. Shock leads to systemic inflammation and multiple organ failure. Lactate clearance varies depending on the stage of the disease.

The processes involved in hepatic dysfunction after shock are complex and difficult to model, but recently investigators have modeled complex systems that show the circulatory feedback as seen in the systemic inflammatory response and the transition from one physiologic state to another.

In circulatory feedback, the values appear to oscillate over time. One can get a view of the character of the oscillations by observing the position and shape of the structure formed in the phase space. The phase space is constructed by plotting the rate of change of the values vs. the values. The phase space analysis can also be performed by plotting X_{t+1} versus X_t where X_t is a value at time t of the analyte.[28,29] The second panel in Figure 31.7 shows the phase space analysis for a linear control system. As an example of nonlinear dynamics, Figure 31.9 shows the phase plots from three different cases of chronic granulocytic leukemias.[30–32]

Harnes and coworkers created phase plots of PTH with different types of

Figure 31.9. Phase plots of WBC counts for three different patients[30–32] with chronic myelogenous leukemia. The scale for the first plot is 10^4, the second is a log scale, and the third is 10^2 WBC/mm^3. The shapes for the first- and third-phase plots are similar.

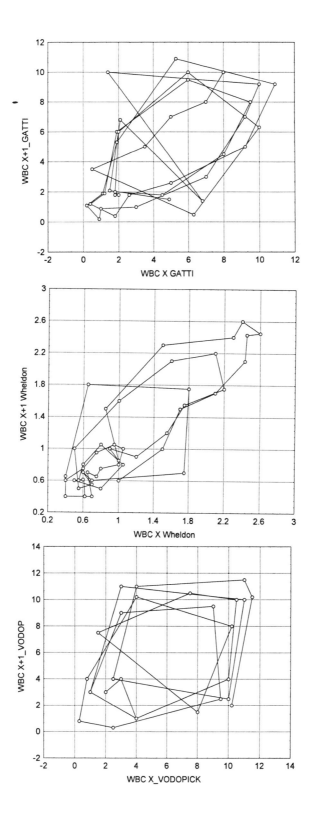

patients. They found a clear separation in the phase space between the normal and osteoporotic subjects.[33] The patient's PTH values had been in the normal range, and the clear separation of the two groups was achieved by reduction of the time-dependent date to the phase space.[33] The osteoporotic group demonstrated a lower dynamic structure than the normal group.[33]

Seif studied euthyroid, hypothyroid, hyperthyroid, and treated hyperthyroid patients in response to TRH stimulation.[34] The first three groups all showed unimodal distributions, while the treated hyperthyroid distribution was clearly bimodal.[34] He noted that hyperthyroid patients, although treated until their T_4, T_3, and TSH levels were within the reference range, showed a significantly decreased response to TRH stimulation, identical to that of the hyperthyroid state.[34] The patients, although successfully treated biochemically, were not functionally cured. The bimodal states for the treated group implies, with one peak showing TRH responsiveness characteristic of euthyroid patients and the other, of hyperthyroid patients, that there exist two different, distinct, discontinuous and stable states.[34] Seif suggested that the treated hyperthyroid patients could be brought back to the TRH responsive euthyroid state by making them temporarily hypothyroid.[34] This example demonstrates that two discontinuous stable states may exist in the phase space, and one must take the proper pathway to go from one state to the other.

The innovative methods of causal reasoning elicit new information, information about the physiologic state of the patient by computer manipulation of the data. Computer-facilitated manipulation of data offers the potential to study the functional states of individual patients. At present, methods such as phase space analysis are experimental, but they offer the potential of investigating patients' individual dynamics and improving healthcare.

REFERENCES

1. Kassirer JP, Kopleman RI: The case for causal reasoning. *Hosp Pract* 22:25–36, 1987.

2. Epstein M, Perez GO: Pathophysiology of the edema-forming states. In Narins NG, ed: *Maxwell's and Kleeman's Clinical Disorder of Fluid and Electrolyte Metabolism,* 5th ed. New York: McGraw-Hill, 1994.

3. Kuipers B, Kassirer JP: Causal reasoning in medicine: Analysis of a protocol. *Cogn Sci* 8:363–385, 1984.

4. Padilla SL, Bayati J, Garcia J: Prognostic value of the early serum estradiol response to leukopoietin acetate in invito fertilization. *Fertil Steril* 53:288–294, 1990.

5. Lemay A, Metha AE, Tobis G, Favre N, Labrie F, Fazekas AJ: Gonadotropins and estradiol responses to a single intramuscular or subcutaneous administration of a luteinizing hormones-releasing hormone agonist in the early follicular phase. *Fertil Steril* 39:668, 1983.

6. Carter HB, Pearson JD, Metter EJ, et al: Longitudinal evaluation of prostate specific antigen levels in men with and without prostate disease. *JAMA* 267:2515–2520, 1992.

7. Gronlund B, Marushak A: Serial human chorionic gonadotropic determination in the diagnosis of ectopic pregnancy. *Austral NZ Ob Gynaecol* 33:312–314, 1993.

8. Groth T: The probe of formal biodynamic models in laboratory medicine. *Scand J Clin Invest* 44:175–192, 1984.

9. Groth T, deVerdier CH: Biodynamic models as pre-processors of clinical laboratory data. In Heusghem C, Albert A, Benson ES, eds: *Advanced Interpretation of Clinical Laboratory Data.* New York: Marcel Dekker, 1982, pp 151–170.

10. Wiener F, Groth T, Nilsson V: A knowledge-based system for automatic interpretation of an analytical profile of complement factors. *J Clin Lab Anal* 3:287–295, 1989.

11. Hedlund A, Zaar B, Groth T, Arturson G: Computer simulation of resuscitation in trauma. I. Description of an extensive pathophysiological model and its first validation. *Comput Meth Programs Biomed* 27:7–21, 1988.

12. Groth T, deVerdier CH: Quantitative assessment of internal hemorrhage or necrosis from serial observations of urea and some relevant auxiliary components. In Heusghem C, Albert A, Benson ES, eds: *Advanced Interpretation of Clinical Laboratory Data.* New York: Marcel Dekker, 1982, pp 223–246.

13. Carson ER, Edwards PR, Finkelstein L: A model-based approach to the interpretation of clinical measures of thyroid disease. In Heusghem C, Albert A, Benson ES, eds: *Advanced Interpretations of Clinical Laboratory Data.* New York: Marcel Dekker, 1982, pp 193–221.

14. Jacobson G, Groth T, Wahlberg J: Amylase turnover in pancreatitis. A study by computer simulation. *Scand J Clin Lab Invest* 44:398, 1984.

15. van Waeg G, Groth T, Niklasson F, deVerdier CH: Allopurinol kinetics in humans as a means to assess liver function: comparison of different models. *Am J Physiol* 253:R352–R360, 253.

16. Koup JR: Disease states and drug pharmacokinetics. *J Clin Pharmacol* 29:674–679, 1989.

17. Leeman TD, Blaschke TF: Semi-quantitative simulation for reasoning about physiological models of drug kinetics and effects. *Schweiz med Wschr* 120:1849–1852, 1990.

18. Cramp DG, Nicolosi E, Leaning MS, Carson ER: Design requirements for a user-friendly computer aided decision support system in laboratory medicine. In Salamon R, Blum B, Jorgensen M, eds: *MedInfo 86. Proc 5th Conf Medical Informatics.* Amsterdam: North-Holland, 1986, pp 204–208.

19. Harris EK, Kanofsky P, Shakarji G, Cotlove E: Biological and analytical components of variation in long-term studies of serum constituents in normal subjects. II. Estimating biological components of variation. *Clin Chem* 16:1022–1027, 1970.

20. Cotlove E, Harris EK, Williams GZ: Biological and analytical components of variation in long-term studies of serum constituents in normal subjects. III. Physiological and medical implications. *Clin Chem* 16:1028–1032, 1970.

21. Stolwijk JAJ, Hardy JD: Regulation and control in physiology. In Mountcastle VB, ed: *Medical Physiology,* Vol 2, 13th ed. St Louis: Mosby, 1974, pp 1343–1358.

22. Kanabrocki GL, Scheving LE, Halberg F, Brewer RL, Bird TJ: Circadian variations in presumably health men under conditions of peace-time army reserve unit training. *Space Life Sci* 4:258–270, 1973.

23. West BJ: *An Essay on the Importance of Being Nonlinear.* Berlin: Springer-Verlag, 1985, pp 9–12.

24. Peretz DI, Scott HM, Duff J, et al: The significance of lactic acidemia in the shock syndrome. *Ann NY Acad Sci* 119:1133, 1965.

25. Vincent JL, Dufaye P, Berre J, Leeman M, Degaute JP, Kahn RJ: Serial lactate determinations during circulatory shock. *Crit Care Med* 11:449–451, 1983.

26. Bakker J, Coffernils M, Leon M, Gris P, Vincent JL: Blood lactate levels are superior to oxygen-derived variables in predicting outcome in human septic shock. *Chest* 99:956–962, 1991.

27. Bankay PE, Cerra FB: Hepatic dysfunction in shock and organ failure. In Schlag G, Redl H, eds: *Pathophysiology of Shock, Septic, and Organ Failure.* Berlin: Springer-Verlag, 1993, pp 948–960.

28. Roux JC, Simoyi RH, Swinney HL: Observation of a strange attractor. *Physica* 3D:257–266, 1983.

29. Packard NH, Crutchfield JP, Farmer JD, Shaw RS: Geometry from a time series. *Phys Rev Lett* 45:712–716, 1980.

30. Vodopick H, Rupp EM, Edwards L, Goswitz FA, Beauchamp JJ: Spontaneous cyclic leukocytosis and thrombocytosis in chronic granulocytic leukemia. *N Engl J Med* 286:284–290, 1972.

31. Wheldon TE: Mathematical models of oscillatory blood cell production. *Math Biosci* 24:289–305, 1975.

32. Gatti RA, Robinson AS, Deinare AS, Nesbit JJ, McCullough JJ, Ballow M: Cyclic leukocytosis in chronic myelogenous leukemia. *Blood* 41:771–782, 1973.

33. Harms HM, Prank K, Brora V, Schlinke E, Neubauer O, Brabant G, Hesch RD: Classification of dynamical diseases by new mathematical tools: application of multidimensional phase space analysis to the pulsatile secretion of parathyroid hormone. *Eur J Clin Invest* 22:371–377, 1992.

34. Seif FJ: Cusp bifurcation in pituitary thyrotropin secretion. In Guttinger W, Eikemeier H, eds: *Structural Stability in Physics.* Berlin: Springer-Verlag, 1979, pp 275–289.

CHAPTER

32

Algorithmic Diagnosis

JANE M. YANG, MICHAEL LAPOSATA, AND
KENT B. LEWANDROWSKI

CONTENTS

It has been estimated that up to 30% of laboratory tests are unnecessary or are performed in such a way as to render their result of no clinical value. Studies have shown that as little as 5% of laboratory data are actually utilized by physicians in patient management.[1-3] Healthcare reform and pressures for cost containment require optimal approaches for utilizing laboratory services. The use of diagnostic algorithms has been advocated as a method to control overutilization of selected laboratory tests and to assist in the differential diagnosis of clinical problems. A number of books and pocket manuals are available providing algorithmic approaches for various clinical situations.[4-6]

Handbook of Clinical Automation, Robotics, and Optimization, Edited by Gerald J. Kost with the collaboration of Judith Welsh.
ISBN 0-471-03179-8 © 1996 John Wiley & Sons, Inc.

32.1. TYPES OF DIAGNOSTIC ALGORITHMS

Algorithms may be designed with either of two purposes in mind. First, an algorithm can be constructed to provide a recommended approach for the diagnosis of a specific clinical problem. This type of algorithm is usually employed by the physician (is physician-based) and requires little from the laboratory except the performance of the desired tests. Typically, these strategies employ a systematic integration of clinical, radiologic, and laboratory data, culminating in a definitive diagnosis. An example of a physician-based algorithm for the differential diagnosis of cough is shown in Figure 32.1.[6] The only input from the laboratory is the result of the sputum in one arm of the decision tree. There is little opportunity to automate this type of algorithm in the laboratory since the strategy involves input from clinical findings, radiological data, and laboratory data. Physician-based algorithms may reduce utilization by eliminating unnecessary tests or by streamlining the diagnostic workup, but their usual purpose is to assist in differential diagnosis. Presumably, the quality of care is also enhanced since the efficiency of the workup is increased with more rapid institution of appropriate treatment.

The second type of algorithm is laboratory-based. In this case, the physician does not specifically order the tests but rather requests that the laboratory perform a diagnostic workup such as a thyroid screen or a hypercoagulopathy evaluation. Laboratory algorithms assist in clinical decision making and reduce

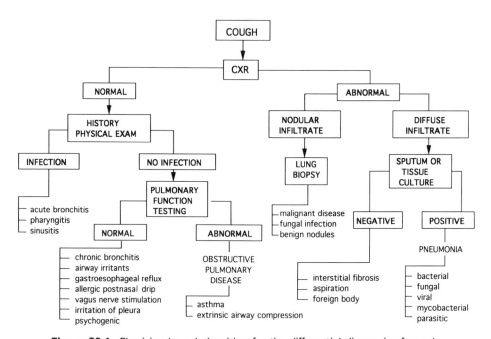

Figure 32.1. Physician-based algorithm for the differential diagnosis of cough.

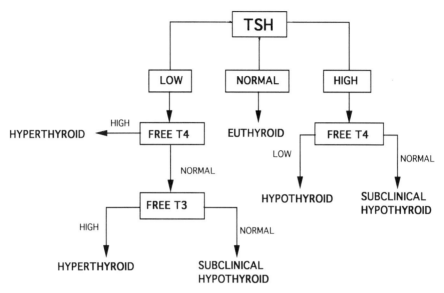

Figure 32.2. Algorithm for thyroid function screening.

laboratory test utilization. Unlike the physician-based algorithm, the laboratory determines the appropriate tests, in what order they will be performed, and may provide an interpretation of the findings. An example of a laboratory-based screening algorithm for thyroid disease is shown in Figure 32.2.[7] The algorithm employs thyroid stimulating hormone (TSH) as a screening test followed by free thyroxine (FT_4) and free T_3 (FT_3) depending on the results of the initial TSH. Although different institutions may substitute other tests for FT_4 and FT_3, the overall approach is widely used. The thyroid screening algorithm involves a sequential decision-making process by the laboratory. The physician orders the thyroid screen but thereafter does not directly select the tests. Thus, the role of the laboratory may be passive with a physician-based algorithm, or it may play a central role in the selection and triage of the tests and in the interpretation of the results. Some algorithms represent a hybrid between the two types. Either type of algorithm may eliminate unnecessary laboratory tests, but the laboratory-based algorithm presents far greater opportunities to reduce utilization and control costs through automation and standardization of the diagnostic process.

Although diagnostic algorithms have intuitive appeal, in practice these strategies are subject to a number of potential problems that may prevent their acceptance by the clinical community or produce a less-than-expected impact on the utilization of laboratory services (Table 32.1). This chapter will review some of the factors that influence the selection and effectiveness of diagnostic algorithms in the clinical laboratory. To illustrate these concepts, we will present our experience with the thyroid screening algorithm shown in Figure 32.2. The discussion will include our observations concerning the selection of the algo-

**TABLE 32.1. Factors that May Limit the Utility and Impact
of a Diagnostic Algorithm**

1. Physician acceptance of the algorithm
2. Questionable medical principles within the algorithm
3. Inadequate consideration of the patient mix of the population
4. The use of an algorithm on inappropriate patients
5. Selection of an algorithm that does not fit with the laboratory operation
6. Selection of algorithms that target low-cost or low-volume tests
7. Selection of an algorithm that substitutes an expensive test for an inexpensive test
8. Failure to develop mechanisms to accommodate complex or rare cases
9. Inadequate analysis of laboratory unit costs and revenues when predicting the impact
   of the algorithm
10. Failure to analyze test ordering patterns by physicians
11. Applying algorithms to problems better addressed by other methods
12. Failure to consider the impact of an algorithm on nonlaboratory aspects of patient
    care

rithm, and the impact on costs, revenues, and utilization. We will also present our perspective on the role of computers and laboratory automation in supporting implementation of diagnostic algorithms.

32.2. SELECTING AN ALGORITHM

The first step in selecting an algorithm is the recognition of a goal or problem that requires a solution. This may include diagnostic questions or issues concerning misuse or overuse of laboratory services. On several occasions we have been asked to develop algorithms to reduce test utilization. However, in some cases it was not initially clear that utilization was either excessive or inappropriate. The decision to implement an algorithm should therefore come after, not before, an analysis of test utilization patterns. Not all problems are best addressed with algorithms, and consequently, alternative approaches should be considered. Constructing an algorithm requires a thorough understanding of laboratory operations and knowledge of the medical issues relevant to the clinical problem. Algorithms that are medically inappropriate or that are constructed in a manner that is inconsistent with the functioning of the laboratory are destined to failure and may be detrimental to the patient. In many cases, algorithms for a given problem have been previously developed and published in the medical literature. In cases where an algorithm has not been previously published, we recommend forming a working group of clinicians and clinical pathologists to develop a strategy to address the specific problem.

Algorithms are especially suited to problems involving multiple tests, particularly when the need for some tests is dependent on the results of other tests in the group. Thus, one or more tests may be eliminated by the results of another, provided that the tests can be performed in an appropriate sequence. For example, thyroid testing may include a combination of TSH, T_4, T_3, T_3-resin uptake (T_3RU), FT_4, FT_3, and FT_4-index. Only three of these tests (TSH, FT_4, FT_3) are necessary for the routine evaluation of thyroid disease, and in most cases only TSH is required.[7] The other tests may have clinical utility in more specialized situations.

Algorithms are also useful when there are many different types of tests available to address a clinical problem, especially when there is confusion over which tests are most appropriate. In this situation, an algorithm may assist the clinician in selecting the best test for a given problem. For example, some tests are best used as screening tests (those with high sensitivity), whereas others are better suited for confirming a diagnosis (those with high specificity) despite the fact that they may be less sensitive. A typical algorithm could start with a more sensitive screening test to exclude patients without disease, and follow with the more specific confirmatory tests on a smaller number of patients to confirm or rule out the diagnosis suggested by the screening test. The clinician may be unaware of the relative sensitivity and specificity of the various tests and, as a result, might order both tests on all patients. Not only is this wasteful of laboratory resources, but in some cases, false-positive screening tests could confuse the physician, prompting further testing.

In our institution, we observed that some physicians were routinely ordering four or five thyroid function tests and, in some cases, the most useful test (TSH) was not requested. A different situation was observed at McLean Hospital, an affiliated psychiatric institution. At McLean Hospital, all inpatient admissions were screened for thyroid disease with a combination of TSH, T_4, and T_3RU. Since the vast majority of these patients had normal thyroid function, institution of the screening algorithm dramatically reduced overall thyroid test utilization. Substituting free hormone measurements for the less useful T_4 and T_3RU provided for more optimal testing for those patients with abnormal TSH values. The two hospital situations described above were ideal for the application of the thyroid screening algorithm because there was both overutilization and misutilization of the thyroid function tests.

Selection of an algorithm requires a careful consideration of the types of patients that may be tested. The thyroid screening algorithm shown in Figure 32.2 is not appropriate for all patients, especially those with hypothalamic and pituitary disorders who require more extensive evaluation. Thus, the algorithm should be used only for screening patients for common thyroid disorders and is inappropriate for evaluating complex or unusual cases. Similar types of exceptions occur with most published algorithms, especially those intended for screening large populations.

Most algorithms have difficulty classifying unusual cases. This is because algorithms assume as a starting point a limited set of well-defined hypotheses, and cannot deal with more ill-structured diagnostic problems.[1] However, rare or complex cases will inevitably present for evaluation. The physician and the laboratory should be aware of the limitations of diagnostic algorithms to prevent algorithm misuse on inappropriate patients. It must also be noted that some patients will present with ambiguous or seemingly contradictory findings that do not flow with the algorithm. For example, a patient with a pituitary TSH-secreting adenoma will present with an elevated TSH, suggesting hypothyroidism in the thyroid screen, but the follow-up FT_4 would be elevated. The algorithm shown in Figure 32.2 provides no mechanism to resolve this discrepancy.

The implementation of diagnostic algorithms requires the active involvement of the clinical laboratory. In many cases, physicians are aware of the existence of an algorithm, but the laboratory may not be prepared to perform the tests as indicated. For example, if the thyroid algorithm is not followed in response to the TSH value, the physician must either call the laboratory to request follow-up tests, or worse, call the patient back to provide an additional specimen. Likewise, if the physicians are not aware that the laboratory performs the algorithm, or are unaware of its appropriate use, then they will continue to order tests according to old habits. Therefore the selection and implementation of an algorithm requires close communication between the physician and the laboratory.

Some algorithms may reduce test numbers, but in the case of highly automated tests may produce little cost savings, or may substitute an expensive test in the place of a less expensive test(s). Furthermore, the cost-effective use of medical services includes many factors other than the laboratory. Little is accomplished if an increase in the efficiency of one service is offset by a decrease in the efficiency of another. When considering the selection of an algorithm, the laboratory must be viewed as only one part of a much larger system. The decision as to whether an algorithm is appropriate in any given setting may be relatively straightforward or may require a careful consideration of many factors that operate in a complex manner unique to the institution.

32.2.1. Physician Factors

The underlying assumption of diagnostic algorithms is that there exists an optimal system for evaluating a given clinical problem and that most parties can agree on the strategy. However, there is often more than one valid approach to a clinical problem. The literature is replete with proposed algorithms, yet in only a few cases do different physicians employ the same approach to a problem. In most cases, there is no consensus at either the national, local, or institutional level. These differences in practice patterns make implementation of algorithms difficult or produce poor compliance with the recommendations in the algorithm, thus reducing its effectiveness. Only rarely has a proposed algorithm gained widespread national acceptance. An example is the thyroid screening algorithm shown in Figure 32.2. Thus, the initial problem in implementing a diagnostic algorithm is gaining consensus on its clinical acceptability and identifying the clinical situation in which it will apply. Since physicians are responsible for ordering tests, physician acceptance is essential. Gaining consensus may be relatively easy or may be extremely difficult depending on a number of factors (listed in Table 32.2). Large academic medical centers are notorious for their decentralized decision making apparatus. At the Massachusetts General Hospital (MGH), we have more than 2000 residents and staff physicians representing multiple departments and clinical divisions. The diffusion of authority within the institution makes consensus building extremely challenging. In contrast, in smaller practice groups or managed care organizations, the decision-making apparatus is likely to be more streamlined. In some of these organizations, the physicians are employees of an institution or health plan and are subject to an executive decision-making structure. In community hospitals, on the other hand, physicians may be entirely autonomous with no centralized decision-making apparatus. The growth of managed care with capitated risk sharing contracts involving physicians will assist in consensus building as cost containment pressures increase. Recently we have been approached by several physician practice groups to develop algorithms for common outpatient diagnostic problems. These requests were brought about by a perceived need on the part of the physicians to reduce utilization in response to capitation.

One final caveat concerning the ordering of tests in an algorithm. Ordinarily, physicians are responsible for ordering laboratory tests. When an algorithm is employed, the physician delegates authority for test ordering to the laboratory. In some cases, this may affect the ability of the laboratory to bill for the tests since reflexed tests are not directly ordered by the physician. The simple solution to this problem is to institute a standing order by the hospital or laboratory medical director authorizing the performance of the appropriate testing as directed by the clinical laboratory.

TABLE 32.2. Questions to Address When Assessing Consensus for a Proposed Diagnostic Algorithm

1. Has the algorithm been endorsed by a national physician organization representing the subspecialty of interest?
2. Is there a wide body of literature to support the use of the algorithm?
3. Do local experts and opinion leaders in the specialty field endorse the algorithm?
4. Is there a central decision-making authority in the institution such as a Clinical Practice Council or Chief of Service to support the use of the algorithm?
5. Is partial compliance from some physicians acceptable, or is universal compliance required?
6. Can physicians with practice patterns contrary to the algorithm be accommodated?
7. To which physicians does the algorithm apply (house staff, staff, subspecialists, private practicioners, etc)? In general, the smaller the physician group, the easier it will be to gain consensus.
8. Do physicians have a direct financial stake in reducing utilization?
9. Does the algorithm assist in clinical decision making by organizing the approach to a complex or confusing clinical problem?

32.3. EFFECTS OF ALGORITHMIC DIAGNOSIS ON UTILIZATION

32.3.1. Effects on Utilization

Algorithms may produce different effects on test utilization in different institutions. Predicting the effect of an algorithm on the number of laboratory tests requires a careful analysis of test ordering patterns and an understanding of the reasons why physicians order certain tests. The thyroid screening algorithm shown in Figure 32.3 was recently implemented at McLean Hospital. Prior to establishing the algorithm, all admissions to the hospital were screened for thyroid disease with a panel of tests including TSH, T_4, and T_3RU. Of these, approximately 10% of TSH values were abnormal (mostly elevated, suggesting hypothyroidism). A much larger percentage of T_4 and T_3RU values were abnormal because many patients had poor nutritional status or exhibited euthyroid sick syndrome. The high incidence of abnormal T_4 and T_3RU values resulted in considerable confusion and in many cases, prompted repeat testing and requests for internal-medicine consultations. In theory, the algorithm would be expected to reduce thyroid function tests by approximately 63% since in most cases, three tests would be replaced by one plus an occasional follow-up free hormone assay (Table 32.3). The Chief of Medicine actively promoted the use of the algorithm to the clinical staff, and the predicted reduction in tests was realized within one month. In addition, the quality of care was also enhanced because the algorithm eliminated two frequently abnormal but often misleading tests (T_4 and T_3RU). At MGH, a similar algorithm was introduced. Owing to a combination of factors at the MGH, notably the large number of complex endocrine cases, and the difficulties of ensuring compliance with the algorithm in a large multidisciplinary institution, the impact of the algorithm on test volume in the first few months after its introduction was more modest (15% reduction in tests). It required 2 years to fully implement. At both MGH and McLean, utilization was reduced, but the percent of tests eliminated and the speeds with which this reduction occurred were dramatically different. Thus the actual impact of an algorithm on test utilization may vary from the predicted effect as a result of a variety of factors. As a second example, we instituted an anemia screening algorithm shown in Figure 32.3 at McLean Hospital. Prior to implementation of the algorithm, all inpatient admissions were evaluated with a complete blood count, a serum B_{12} (vitamin B_{12}), and a folate assay. The latter two tests were being ordered largely because of old practice patterns for admission protocols and were clearly grossly overutilized. Most patients were not anemic and only rarely

TABLE 32.3. Effect of a Thyroid Screening Algorithm on Test Utilization in a Psychiatric Institution

	TSH	T_4	T_3RU	FT_4	FT_3	Total
Before algorithm	3400	3400	3400	0	0	10,200
After algorithm	3400	0	0	340	34	3,774

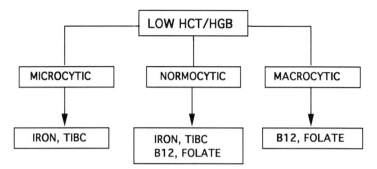

Figure 32.3. Algorithm for anemia screening.

were they either B_{12}- or folate-deficient. The purpose of the new screening algorithm was to reduce the use of two expensive sendout tests for the majority of admissions while adding two less expensive but clinically appropriate tests for patients with evidence of iron-deficiency anemia. From a preliminary analysis of abnormal values, we estimated an approximately 50% reduction in test volume related to the diagnosis of anemia and a much larger reduction in laboratory costs. Compliance with the algorithm was initially disappointing, and it ultimately required a mandate from the Chief of Internal Medicine to produce the expected reductions. A similar anemia screening algorithm is being considered for use in the outpatient setting at MGH. In this case, our primary intention is not to reduce test utilization but to provide physicians with enough initial information for the differential diagnosis of common anemias. By having the laboratory automatically perform the appropriate series of tests on the initial specimen, we hope to reduce delays in diagnosis, decrease return visits by the patients, and reduce the need to obtain additional specimens for follow-up studies. Presumably the increased efficiency of patient care will offset any increase in test volumes. In the final analysis, we expect to do more tests but on fewer samples. To be effective, this algorithm will need to be restricted to a limited subset of patients and will require close cooperation between the clinicians and the laboratory.

The thyroid and anemia screening algorithms illustrate several important points concerning the impact of diagnostic algorithms on laboratory utilization. First, the impact of an algorithm may be difficult to predict and may vary from one institution to another or between patient populations within an institution. Second, a careful analysis of test ordering patterns is necessary to predict the impact of the algorithm on test volumes. Third, algorithms may effect costs and utilization patterns both inside and outside the clinical laboratory. In some cases test volumes may actually increase, but this may result in an improvement in the quality or efficiency of care. The ultimate goal of managing laboratory test utilization is not exclusively to reduce the volume of tests performed, but rather to ensure that the most optimal cost-effective utilization of laboratory services is provided.

32.3.2. Effects on Laboratory Costs

Reducing the number of clinical laboratory tests performed may in some cases have relatively little impact on costs. Winkleman[8] estimated that a 50% reduction in automated tests would produce only a 10% reduction in costs. For example, eliminating magnesium from a 12-test chemistry panel would reduce test volume by 8.3%, but the impact on costs would be trivial since the specimen would still require phlebotomy, transport, processing, accessioning, analysis, and reporting for 11 other analytes. Furthermore, since the magnesium test is performed as part of a panel on a single analyzer, the savings incurred as a result of eliminating the test is limited to the small cost of the reagents for the magnesium assay. On the other hand, if magnesium tests were being frequently ordered as a single test, rather than as part of a chemistry panel, the specimen could be eliminated including the costs of phlebotomy, transport, accessioning, analysis, and reporting. Therefore, algorithms should be designed either to eliminate whole panels of tests, and thus specimens, or should target overutilized expensive tests to ensure that only the appropriate tests are performed for the clinical condition. Reducing a high-volume test that is part of a panel that is inexpensive to perform will have little effect on costs other than to raise the apparent unit cost of the remainder of the laboratory operation. Although this point may seem obvious to laboratory directors, we have frequently observed physicians and managed care organizations target a presumably overutilized test that is part of a chemistry panel for utilization reduction initiatives.

In order to estimate the impact of a diagnostic algorithm on laboratory costs, it is necessary to understand the unit cost of the individual tests performed and not to simply target reductions in test volume. Unfortunately, few hospital laboratories have even a basic understanding of unit costs. In some cases, estimating the unit cost of a test may be relatively straightforward, particularly for tests sent out to reference laboratories and performed for a fixed fee. For tests performed in house, the calculations are more difficult and require an analysis of both the fixed and variable costs of the test and application of an appropriate overhead value. An example of a cost analysis for a serum glucose test is shown in Table 32.4. Note that this cost analysis includes the costs of phlebotomy and transport and indirect costs. Also note that the cost is the average unit cost for the test and not the marginal cost. It is critical to distinguish between the average unit cost of a test (obtained by simply dividing the total cost by the volume of tests) and the marginal unit cost (the cost of adding or subtracting one additional test to a preexisting operation). For example, a laboratory performing 1000 tests for a total cost of $10,000 would have an average unit cost of $10. If the laboratory were to perform 1001 tests the cost of the added test would most likely be less than $10 since additional employees and instruments would not be required. Thus the marginal cost of an additional test is less than the average cost. The same principle applies when reducing test volume at the margin. Eliminating 10 tests from the laboratory would not save $100 because many costs such as technologists and instruments would not be eliminated. Although these calcula-

**TABLE 32.4. Cost Analysis (in U.S. Dollars)
of Serum Glucose Testing in a Clinical Laboratory**

Labor cost	
Collection and transport	0.85
Test performance	0.79
Supply cost	0.15
Instrumentation	<u>0.43</u>
Total direct costs	2.22
Indirect costs	
Nonoverhead	1.14
Overhead	<u>0.48</u>
Total indirect costs	1.62
Total cost	3.84

Source: Adapted from E Lewandrowski, et al, reprinted with permission from *American Journal of Medicine* 97:222–230, 1994.

tions may be difficult to perform, an analysis of the effect of an algorithm on laboratory costs without an understanding of the marginal unit cost is likely to be highly inaccurate. The usual approach to this dilemma is to perform a simplified calculation based on a rough estimate of the costs of reagents, consumables, labor, and other direct costs. The estimate does not need to be absolutely precise to permit an estimation of its approximate impact on laboratory costs. One pitfall when estimating savings based on reducing labor requirements is that typically the laboratory may be either unable or unwilling to eliminate personnel to realize the savings related to labor.

A cost analysis for the thyroid screening algorithm used at McLean Hospital is shown in Table 32.5. Test costs were determined using an institutional rate charged by a commercial vendor since all of these tests were sent out to a reference laboratory. Overall, the algorithm produced a 10% reduction in reference laboratory charges, a 4% reduction in direct laboratory costs, and a $28,000 savings for the institution per year. The cost for testing related to thyroid disease was reduced by 39%. This example shows the potentially large impact on labora-

**TABLE 32.5. Effect of a Thyroid Screening Algorithm on Laboratory Costs
in a Psychiatric Institution**

Before Algorithm			After Algorithm		
Test	Volume	Cost ($)	Test	Volume	Cost ($)
TSH	3400	10.65	TSH	3400	10.65
T_4	3400	7.00	FT_4	340	20.00
T_3RU	3400	4.00	FT_3	34	50.00
Total	10,200	73,610	Total	3774	44,710

tory costs that may be obtained with a well-selected algorithm that targets testing that is significantly overutilized.

Not all algorithms save money by reducing laboratory costs. In many cases an algorithm is designed to assist in clinical decision making by providing guidelines for evaluating a clinical problem and indicating which tests are most helpful in achieving an accurate diagnosis quickly. Laboratory testing may not be reduced in these situations, but the overall efficiency of care is improved. This may translate into savings related to a decrease in the length of stay or fewer outpatient follow-up visits. In some cases, laboratory costs may actually increase, but the overall cost of care in the institution is reduced.

The increasing role of capitated managed care contracts necessitates a reassessment of laboratory costs in a manner different from the traditional approach of viewing the laboratory as an isolated cost center. The clinical laboratory must be viewed as a provider of information that facilitates the overall process of patient care. Algorithms are best used to promote the most cost-effective care and should not be viewed as impacting only the clinical laboratory.

32.3.3. Effects on Revenues

The effect of diagnostic algorithms on laboratory revenues is complex. Factors to be considered include the type of institution, the difference between inpatient versus outpatient test volumes, and the payer mix of the institution. In the simplest case, a reduction in test volume will result in a corresponding decrease in revenues. However, this is not invariably the case. For example, capitated contracts pay a fixed rate per insured member regardless of the number of tests ordered. Thus, in these situations there is a significant incentive to perform as few tests as possible. The optimum net revenue is obtained when no inappropriate laboratory tests are ordered. The laboratory will lose money when the cost of services exceeds the capitated rate. As an example, we recently agreed to a capitated rate of $3.50 per member per month for outpatient testing services provided to a local managed care plan. A diagnostic algorithm that reduces utilization for this patient population will have a positive effect on revenue.

The type of institution influences the impact of algorithms on laboratory revenues. Most hospitals are subject to diagnosis-related groups (DRGs) covering medicare inpatient admissions. The hospital receives a fixed reimbursement that varies with the DRG code. Each admission is, in effect, capitated, and as a result, net revenues increase as utilization is reduced. Some hospitals are not subject to DRGs and are permitted to bill for all laboratory services. In this situation, a diagnostic algorithm will have a negative effect on laboratory revenues. Table 32.6 shows the impact of a thyroid screening algorithm on McLean Hospital revenues. At the time that the algorithm was instituted, the institution could bill for all inpatient laboratory services because it is a long-term inpatient psychiatric facility. The effect on revenues shown in Table 32.6 assumes 100% payment of billed services. In practice, this is seldom the case because certain tests are reimbursed by third-party payers at a rate less than the standard institu-

TABLE 32.6. Effect of a Thyroid Screening Algorithm on Laboratory Revenues in a Psychiatric Institution

Before Algorithm			After Algorithm		
Test	Volume	Charge ($)	Test	Volume	Charge ($)
TSH	3400	63.00	TSH	3400	63.00
T_4	3400	31.00	FT_4	340	29.00
T_3RU	3400	19.00	FT_3	34	64.00
Total	10,200	384,200	Total	3774	226,236

tional charge and because patients without insurance do not always pay their bills. Assuming 100% reimbursement, overall revenue decreased by $157,964, which was roughly 7% of the total laboratory revenue. Thus, the thyroid screening algorithm appears to have decreased revenues at McLean by a much larger amount than it decreased costs ($28,000). However, recently the institution has shifted its payer mix to include a much larger percentage of managed care and capitated plans. Now this shift alters the cost–revenue relationship in favor of reducing costs.

The effect of DRGs on inpatient revenue does not apply to outpatient laboratory testing. In the case of outpatients, all laboratory tests can be billed, creating an incentive toward excessive test ordering. Algorithms applied to this population will have a negative impact on revenue. For this reason, physician office laboratories (POLs), many of which were established to generate revenue for a clinical practice, have little incentive to adopt algorithms unless they have a significant number of patients covered under capitated contracts. Likewise, commercial reference laboratories that service outpatients or hospital-based accounts have little incentive to control utilization unless they or their clients are capitated.

Most hospitals currently accept both inpatients and outpatients from a variety of third-party payers. This creates a complex mix of payers and reimbursement systems including DRGs, capitated contracts, self-paying patients, and multiple private insurance contracts. The revenue that the laboratory receives from each of these sources for the same laboratory test may be different. For this reason, it is extremely difficult to predict the impact of algorithms on laboratory revenues without a careful analysis of the payer mix within the institution and a knowledge of the utilization patterns of the physician practices.

32.4. ROLE OF THE LABORATORY COMPUTER

Algorithms require decisions based on data. For this reason, it is possible to automate laboratory-based algorithms. This is best accomplished with computer technology to direct instruments concerning which tests to perform and to make decisions based on the results of the tests. Laboratory information systems (LISs) are becoming increasingly sophisticated, and in the future, computers will play an integral role in the implementation of laboratory-based algorithms. On the other hand, physician-based algorithms are difficult to automate unless the laboratory computer is interfaced with a hospital information system (HIS) to make nonlaboratory data available to the clinician and to allow the laboratory to inquire about clinical information.

Although most laboratory algorithms can be managed manually by knowledgeable laboratory personnel, the computer permits the entire process to be automated. Automation is best suited for situations involving repetitive tasks that generate large amounts of information (see examples listed in Table 32.7) and require decisions that are relatively straightforward. Algorithms that target tests of low volume benefit little from computer technology. Likewise, test selection decisions that are highly complex or subjective in nature are very difficult to automate even with sophisticated artificial intelligence technologies. The basic components of a computer-assisted laboratory-based algorithm for thyroid screening are shown in Figure 32.4. The LIS must be bidirectionally interfaced to an automated immunoassay system capable of performing all the tests in the algorithm. If tests are performed on more than one instrument or in more than one laboratory, then a more sophisticated arrangement is required to achieve full automation. The process begins with the physician who requests a thyroid screen. In hospitals utilizing an order entry system, the request is entered into the HIS along with patient demographic information, and the information is passed to the LIS. A bar-code label is then generated that contains all the necessary data to permit the laboratory to process the specimen. Once the specimen is received in the laboratory, it is processed and routed to the immunoassay analyzer. The LIS directs the instrument to perform a TSH; receives the result; orders dilutions or repeat analyses if necessary; determines whether the TSH is elevated, normal, or low; orders appropriate follow-up tests as needed; receives these results; and reports the values with or without an interpretation to the HIS to make the data available to the physician. This level of automation is currently

TABLE 32.7. Operational Aspects of Diagnostic Algorithms that May Be Improved by Automated Instrumentation and Computerization

1. Specimen transport, accessioning, and processing
2. Specimen identification (bar coding)
3. Routing of specimens to instruments (conveyor systems)
4. Specimen handling at the instrument (robotics)
5. Performance of tests and reporting of results to the host computer through a bidirectional interface
6. Interpreting tests by the computer
7. Ordering of follow-up tests by the computer
8. Reporting of results to the physician
9. Maintaining records of test data

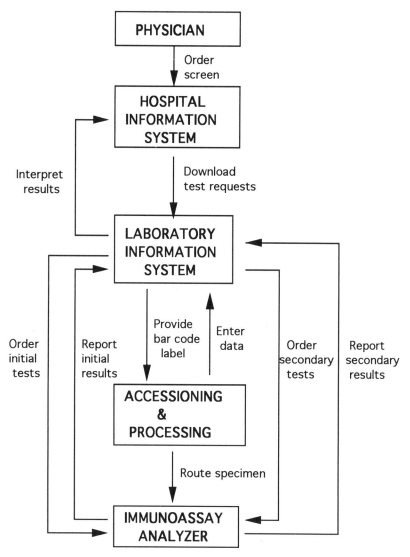

Figure 32.4. Components of a computer-assisted laboratory-based algorithm.

within the capability of most laboratory and hospital computers. In the near future, even greater degrees of automation will become possible through the use of automated specimen processing technologies and conveyor-belt systems to route specimens directly to robots that load the specimens on to instruments. The anemia algorithm shown in Figure 32.3 could theoretically be set up in a similar manner. However, additional enhancements to the LIS would dramatically improve the effectiveness of this algorithm. For example, many patients are evaluated with multiple CBCs either as inpatients or during the course of a prolonged outpatient management. Once the diagnosis of anemia has been established and classified, further evaluations on subsequent specimens are most likely to be unnecessary. In this case, the computer could query the LIS archival database to determine whether the patient had a prior anemia evaluation or could query the HIS to limit anemia evaluations to selected types of patients. For example, the LIS could query the HIS to exclude patients not in the operating room or immediately postoperative. Thus, the computer would be used to screen candidates for suitability to avoid unnecessarily triggering the algorithm. This degree of computer sophistication is within the capabilities of current technology but most hospitals have not developed this type of capability. In the case of the anemia algorithm, there are no instruments currently available that can perform all the tests required for the algorithm. Thus, the anemia algorithm is limited more by instruments than by computer technology. This problem can be circumvented by employing a computer-directed conveyor-belt system utilizing robotic technology as described earlier. Robotic technology is not yet available in most laboratories, but a number of systems are under rapid development to bring this capability into the laboratory.

32.5. EXPERT SYSTEMS AND ALGORITHMIC DIAGNOSIS

Algorithms represent one method of formalizing medical knowledge and providing a systematic structure for the efficient utilization of laboratory services. Most laboratory information systems are adequate for the implementation of simple algorithms. For more complex problems, especially those requiring integration of clinical data with laboratory findings, a higher level of computer sophistication is needed. The development of systems utilizing artificial intelligence offers promise as a method to integrate clinical and laboratory information to support complex diagnostic algorithms.

Artificial intelligence provides a method to develop computer systems to simulate the complex analytic and decision-making processes of humans. Artificial intelligence permits the development of computers to do the things that make people seem intelligent. Artificial-intelligence programs may be classified according to the method of knowledge representation. These include expert systems and neural networks, both of which have potential applications to computer-aided medical diagnosis.

Algorithms are commonly criticized for their inability to resolve diagnostic problems in patients with unusual presentations or rare disorders, or those with more than one disease. Computer programs utilizing artificial intelligence may permit the development of more sophisticated algorithms capable of evaluating nonroutine cases. Simple laboratory algorithms are based on a set of rules designed to produce a specific output (diagnosis) from a specific input (test results). Some types of expert systems that represent knowledge as a set of ordered rules emulate this form of diagnostic reasoning and therefore may be viewed as complex algorithms managed by artificial-intelligence techniques. In contrast, models of artificial intelligence based on neural networks are less suited for the type of knowledge inherent in clinical algorithms because these represent, store, and use knowledge to recognize complex patterns.

Simply defined, expert systems are artificial-intelligence programs that represent and apply the knowledge of experts to solve problems in a particular domain. A domain is a field of human expertise that may be broad-based (e.g., internal medicine) or more focused (e.g., acid–base disorders). Expert systems assist in medical decision making by relating specific patient data (input) to a knowledge base in order to generate output in the form of probable diagnoses, explanations, or recommended actions. Probability-based reasoning may be incorporated to assist in making predictions or to report potential diagnoses in conjunction with a certainty factor.

The success of programs utilizing expert systems depends, in part, on the knowledge base. Ideally, knowledge bases contain large amounts of different information such as knowledge derived from textbooks (factual knowledge), the ability to recognize patterns, and heuristic knowledge. Heuristic knowledge represents experimental knowledge or that gained from trial-and-error methods. As such, it encompasses knowledge reflecting good medical judgment that is gained from training and empirical observation.

The database in expert systems is input by the user. Depending on the user and the domain, data may include the patient history, physical findings, procedure results and laboratory data. The input of data may also be a part of the ongoing decision-making process. For example, the internal medicine expert system, INTERNIST-1, may generate a tentative diagnosis based on initial data. It then queries the user for other pertinent findings in order to evaluate the pending hypothesis. As another example, an expert system for rheumatology and endocrinology (EXPERT) requires the entry of an initial set of findings and formulates a preliminary hypothesis about the diagnosis. This system may be used to initiate a laboratory testing algorithm.[10]

Examples of expert systems that emphasize the use of laboratory data are shown in Table 32.8. Some expert systems operate by displaying comments

TABLE 32.8. Examples of Expert Systems that Utilize Laboratory Data

System	Domain
ABEL	Acid–base/ electrolytes
ANEMIA	Anemia
PHEO-ATTENDING	Pheochromocytoma
EXPERT	Serum proteins
PRO.M.D.	Lipoprotein metabolism
EXPERT	Outpatient testing

Source: Adapted from Reference 1.

describing the use of proposed tests and diagnostic procedures (reactive systems). In PHEO-ATTENDING, the user requests decision support, and the output may be in the form of a critique of the users evaluation and planned course of action. Either proactive or reactive systems may offer consultative support to inform and educate users and to improve the efficient utilization of laboratory services. To the extent that expert systems guide physicians through a patient evaluation in an orderly stepwise fashion, compliance with clinical algorithms is facilitated. However, the performance of currently available expert systems has been disappointing.[11]

Clinical pathologists have training in computer technology and clinical diagnostics, and have an understanding of laboratory operations. Because of this unique knowledge base, clinical pathologists should play an important role in developing and implementing computer-assisted diagnostic strategies.

REFERENCES

1. Winkel P: Application of expert systems in the clinical laboratory. *Clin Chem* 8:1595–1601, 1989.
2. Dixon R, Lazlo J: Utilization of clinical chemistry services by medical house staff. *Arch Intern Med* 134:1064–1067, 1974.
3. Durbridge T, Edwards F, Edwards R, Atkinson M: Evaluation of benefits of screening tests done immediately on admission to hospital. *Clin Chem* 22:968–971, 1976.
4. Laposata M, Connor A, Hicks D, Phillips D: *The Clinical Hemostasis Handbook*. Chicago: Year Book Medical Publishers, 1989.
5. Liu P: *Blue Book of Diagnostic Tests*. Philadelphia: Saunders, 1986.
6. Healey P, Jacobson E: *Common Medical Diagnoses: An Algorithmic Approach*. Philadelphia: Saunders, 1990.
7. Toft A: Use of sensitive immunoradiometric assay for thyrotropin in clinical practice. *Mayo Clin Proc* 63:1035–1042, 1988.
8. Winkelman J: Less utilization of the clinical laboratory produces disproportionately small true cost reductions. *Human Pathol* 15:499–501, 1984.
9. Schechtman J, Paulson L: The cosy effectiveness of three thyroid function testing strategies for suspicion of hypothyroidism in a primary care setting. *J Gen Intern Med* 5:9–15, 1990.
10. van Lente F, Castellani W, Chou D, Matzen R, Galen R: Application of the EXPERT consultation system to accelerated laboratory testing and interpretation. *Clin Chem* 32:1719–1725, 1986.
11. Berner E, Webster G, Shugerman A, Jackson J, et al: Performance of four computer-based diagnostic systems. *New Engl J Med* 330:1792–1797, 1994.